3D Virtual Treatment Planning of Orthognathic Surgery

Gwen R.J. Swennen
Editor

3D Virtual Treatment Planning of Orthognathic Surgery

A Step-by-Step Approach for Orthodontists and Surgeons

With Contributions by Martin Gaboury

Springer

Editor
Gwen R.J. Swennen
Division of Maxillofacial Surgery and Facial Plastic Surgery
Department of Surgery, General Hospital St-Jan Bruges-Ostend, Belgium

Bruges Cleft and Craniofacial Centre, Bruges, Belgium

Private Practice in Facial Cosmetic Surgery, Clinic Tilleghem, Bruges, Belgium

Associate Professor, Department of Oral and Maxillofacial Surgery
Hannover Medical School, Hannover, Germany

Affiliate Professor, Department of Oral and Maxillofacial Surgery
University of Catalunya, Barcelona, Spain

ISBN 978-3-662-47388-7 ISBN 978-3-662-47389-4 (eBook)
DOI 10.1007/978-3-662-47389-4

Library of Congress Control Number: 2016957321

Printed on acid-free paper

This Springer imprint is published by Springer Nature
The registered company is Springer-Verlag GmbH Berlin Heidelberg

First of all, I want to dedicate this book to my lovely wife Valérie and my sons Joaquin and Cédrique.

I also want to dedicate this colour atlas and manual to my former chairman, colleague and above all personal good friend, Professor Calix De Clercq.

Gwen R. J. Swennen

Foreword I

In the first half of the previous century, radiographic cephalometry moved the focus of orthodontists from malocclusions towards underlying skeletal disharmonies. Linear and angular measurements were not only used to study the dento-alveolar structures in relation to the jaws but also the jaws in relation to the rest of the cranio-facial complex. Data collected from longitudinal growth studies were used to better understand complex facial changes and establish reference values for "normality". For many decades, these cephalometric values and proportions were the bases for a better diagnosis of cranio-facial malformations, the planning of orthognathic surgery and the long-term evaluation of treatment outcome. However, cephalometric analyses are limited to 2 dimensions.

With the introduction of the cone-beam CT, reduction of the costs for the hardware and reduction of the radiation dose, 3D imaging became available for a growing group of clinicians and a standard tool for diagnosis and treatment planning in several disciplines. Colour maps generated after registration of 2 consecutive CBCTs on stable structures in the anterior cranial base give us new tools to assess in detail hard and soft tissue changes over time. This is a revolution for future research to study growth modifications induced by dento-facial orthopaedic appliances, treatment outcome and long-term stability after orthognathic surgery. The correction of cranio-facial malformations and asymmetries by surgical repositioning of both jaws, and complex rotations in 3 planes, can now virtually be simulated with high accuracy. Intermediate wafers made by CAD/CAM or 3D printing are the link between the virtual simulation and the surgeon in the operating room.

Gwen Swennen has written a masterpiece helping us to better explore all new potentials of 3D imaging for the planning of orthognathic surgery. With splendid illustrations and step-by-step procedures, this is the perfect guide for all clinicians, young and old, to improve their skills in extracting and implementing all these data for further improvement of the quality of patient care. This atlas and manual is the result of many years of enthusiastic research by the author. His input for the development of adapted software makes this technology available to all of us. We are grateful to the author willing to share his expertise with us.

Professor Hugo De Clerck, DDS, PhD
Orthodontic Private Practice,
Brussels, Belgium
Adjunct Professor, Department of Orthodontics,
Chapel Hill NC, USA
August 2016

Foreword II

I first met Gwen Swennen in May 2009, at the Spanish Association of Oral and Maxillofacial Surgery meeting in Bilbao. At that moment, I was still conventionally planning my surgeries with good results and was deeply convinced that computers would just unnecessarily complicate my routine work, besides being eventually time consuming. It was in that precise occasion that I had the opportunity to attend Gwen's lecture on 3D virtual planning which was utterly enlightening. The speaker's clear and rigorous demonstration of the concept's sequence, the high quality of the images proposed, and the compelling logic of the processes forced me to a critical revision of my own everyday activities. That young and clever surgeon had literally enchanted me, thanks to his technical knowledge and his passionate application of 3D virtual planning of orthognathic surgery.

We became good friends and, since then, we have been taking advantage of congresses and meetings around the world to meet, to reinforce our mutual consideration and respect, while sharing professional and private experiences with a touch of irony and *joie de vivre*. All occasions were perfect to spend some spare time with Gwen and Valérie, his precious wife, in Bruges or in Knokke.

It was in 2011 that, after passionately devouring all Gwen Swennen's articles and publications, I finally decided to convert to 3D virtual planning. I attended one of his courses in Bruges which definitely convinced me, and from that moment I dived into 3D virtual planning. I was helped by two valid surgeons and friends in this quest: Prof. Dr. Federico Hernandez Alfaro and, above all, Dr. Simonas Gribauskas. Moreover, I witnessed Dr. Bill Arnett, to whom I have tremendous respect, also making the same change. My personal shift to 3D virtual planning happened, and today, after 3 years of its routine clinical application, I have become absolutely convinced.

Anyway, after this personal digression, let us focus on Gwen Swennen's book. It was in Melbourne, last October, during the ICOMS 2015 congress that I assisted to the first presentation of his "integrated" work. Once more, Gwen surprised me with the lucidity and clarity with which he systematized his pioneering work.

First, it is an atlas, a manual notwithstanding its impressive dimension. The author's experience is so deep that the manuscript focuses on all aspects of 3D virtual planning of orthognathic surgery. The division in thematic chapters is prone to a rapid consultation on specific topics. All subjects are exemplified with illustrations and easily understandable to a general public. Diagnosis, transition from clinical practice to digital representation, orthodontical and surgical planning, and risk evaluation are clearly analyzed. Moreover, tricks but also potential pitfalls, risks, mistakes, and their prevention are included in the treatise. Finally, a great variety of cases are shown as examples in Chap. 6.

In short, all clinical relevant topics are critically analyzed by the author, who has been rationally applying his knowledge to his everyday clinical routine practice, going from first intuitions to actual simplification and moreover evaluation of potential future applications. Prof. Gwen Swennen with his well-known and recognized generosity is offering the reader his fatigue, his knowledge, and his vast clinical experience toward this subject. I am definitely suggesting his book to anyone who approaches 3D virtual planning in orthognathic surgery, ensuring that he will find in this work a theological "summa" on the subject.

Moreover, even those surgeons who still rely on conventional planning technique are advised to read Gwen Swennen's book since they may find in these pages, that sort of flash of inspiration which leads to a substantial change, besides benefiting from practical information to improve their own clinical practice in maxillofacial deformity surgery.

Professor Mirco Raffaini, MD
Maxillofacial Surgery, University of Florence, Florence, Italy
Founder and Director, Face Surgery Center, Parma, Italy
August 2016

Preface

> … Existing paradigms are held by a scientific community. They explain observations, are the basis for communication and guide future research …
> … Observations that don't fit the paradigm are ignored, or are explained in ways that fit the paradigm …
> … A crisis occurs when the existing paradigms no longer explains the observations and new theories arise. A revolution occurs and new paradigms are accepted …
> … Once a paradigm shift has occurred, a veritable explosion of new ideas and information leads to rapid advances in the field …

Thomas S. Kuhn:
The Structure of Scientific Revolutions.
The University of Chicago Press. 1996

When I reflect on this new project, I realise that I was already playing with the idea and preliminary outline of this book in my mind since 2009. This would definitely have been too early, and the book would most probably have been outdated already. The idea of our "Colour Atlas and Manual on Three-Dimensional Cephalometry (2005)" was an attempt to bridge conventional cephalometry with the 3D virtual approach and 3D cephalometry. It is amazing that after more than 10 years the concept of this latter atlas is currently more than actual for both orthodontists and surgeons.

With this new book, I hope to offer a comprehensive, systematic, standardised and above all individualised approach towards 3D virtual planning of orthognathic surgery in the daily clinical routine. This book is based on my personal experience having being involved in more than 2700 clinical cases on virtual planning since almost 20 years. Moreover, I was fortunate to be continuously triggered over all these years by my colleagues, residents, fellows, surgeons and orthodontists all over the world during scientific meetings, courses and workshops.

The concept towards "step-by-step" individualised and integrated 3D virtual treatment planning of orthognathic surgery outlined in this book aims to make once again the bridge between conventional and 3D virtual treatment planning:

1. ($3D\text{-}VPS_1$) "3D Cephalometry of the Patient's Hard Tissues and Teeth (Sect. 2.2.2)" can be compared to conventional cephalometric tracing.
2. ($3D\text{-}VPS_2$) "3D Cephalometry of the Patient's Soft Tissues (Sect. 2.2.3)"can be compared with direct or indirect anthropometric assessment of the patient.
3. ($3D\text{-}VPS_3$) "3D Virtual Osteotomies (Sect. 3.2)" can be compared to some extent with conventional "orthognathic model surgery".
4. ($3D\text{-}VPS_4$) "3D Virtual Occlusal Definition (Sect. 3.3)" can be compared with conventional occlusal definition on plaster dental models.
5. ($3D\text{-}VPS_5$) "10 Step-by-Step Individualised 3D Virtual Treatment Planning (Sect. 3.5)" finally attempts to provide the clinician a manner to integrate 3D virtual planning in daily clinical routine based on the concepts of conventional treatment planning.

The underlying philosophy of this colour atlas and manual is not to dogmatise but to push forward "the paradigm shift" that truly occurred in treatment planning of orthognathic surgery and especially stimulate further development and innovation in "3D Virtual Treatment Planning of Orthognathic and Orthofacial Surgery" to further improve patient care.

Professor Gwen R.J. Swennen, MD, DMD, PhD, MSc, FEBOMFS
Bruges, Belgium
August 2016

Acknowledgements

I especially wish to thank my teachers and mentors Professor Jarg-Erich Hausamen (former chair, Department of OMF and Plastic Surgery, Hannover Medical University, Hannover), Professor Henning Schliephake (Department of OMF and Plastic Surgery, Georg-August University, Göttingen), Professor Albert De Mey (former chair, Deparment of Plastic Surgery, University Hospital Brugmann and Queen Fabiola Children's University Hospital, Brussels) and Professor Chantal Malevez (former chair, Department of OMF Surgery, Queen Fabiola Children's University Hospital, Brussels) who taught me the importance of working hard to try to become not only an excellent surgeon and clinician but also a good researcher. I am also very grateful to Peter Brachvogel (former staff member, Department of OMF and Plastic Surgery, Hannover Medical University, Hannover) and Hannes Berten (former staff member, Department of Orthodontics, Hannover Medical University, Hannover) for teaching and sharing their clinical and scientific knowledge on orthognathic surgery with me during my training.

I want to thank my associate colleagues Professor Calix De Clercq, Johan Abeloos, Philippe Lamoral, Nathalie Neyt, Krisztian Nagy, Joke De Ceulaer, all our residents, international fellows and Professor Jan Casselman (chair, Department of Radiology and Medical Imaging, GH Hospital St-Jan Bruges) and his team for their continuous support. I am also very grateful to Bill Arnett (Santa Barbara, USA) and Mirco Raffaini (Florence, Italy) for sharing with me their knowledge and for all the stimulating discussions that we had together all over the world.

From all the fellows who have visited our department over the last 10 years since I have been in Bruges, I particularly want to thank Raquel Guijarro Martinez (Barcelona, Spain) and Martin Gaboury (Quebec, Canada). I am very proud that I had the opportunity to be together with my personal friend, Professor Federico-Hernandez Alfaro (Barcelona, Spain), director of the first Spanish OMF European PhD thesis conducted by Raquel on "Cone-beam computerized tomography evaluation of the upper airway in the context of orthognathic surgery". Moreover I am very grateful to Martin Gaboury for his critical reviewing of this project; his contribution to Chaps. 1, 2 and 4; and his collaboration in the videos, which are of major importance to the clinical reader of this book and would otherwise have never been realised without his help and efforts. I wish to thank all my referring orthodontists and colleagues for having been working together so nicely for the last 10 years in Bruges, and I look forward to close collaboration in the future.

I want to thank in particular S.O.R.G. (Strasbourg Osteosynthesis Research Group) and especially Professor Paul Stoelinga (former chair, Department of OMF Surgery, Radboud University, Nijmegen, and former chair, S.O.R.G. Orthognathic Section), Oliver Scheunemann and all my co-members of both the orthognathic and cranio-facial section of S.O.R.G for the excellent and stimulating collaboration over the years. I would also like to express my special thanks to Filip Schutyser, Wouter Mollemans and their engineering team for their invaluable support over almost 20 years. Finally, I wish to thank Christian Leibinger for his belief in me and the opportunity as a clinician to develop IPS CaseDesigner, which I truly believe is the next level of 3D virtual planning software.

Last but not least, I need to thank Springer for their trust, boundless patience and collaboration in publishing this new project.

Professor Gwen R.J. Swennen, MD, DMD, PhD, MSc, FEBOMFS
Bruges, Belgium
August 2016

Introduction

"3D Virtual Treatment Planning of Orthognathic Surgery" offers a "step-by-step" guide towards three-dimensional (3D) diagnosis, treatment planning and evaluation of maxillofacial deformity to orthodontists and orthognathic and orthofacial surgeons. Vertical cone-beam CT imaging has definitely revolutionised the treatment planning of orthognathic surgery. Moreover, it allows unprecedented evaluation of treatment outcome in patients with maxillofacial deformity. This colour atlas and manual attempts to provide clinicians a comprehensive, systematic, standardised and above all individualised "step-by-step" approach towards 3D virtual diagnosis, treatment planning and outcome assessment of orthognathic surgery. In Chap. 1, the 3D imaging workflow is explained along with how it can be integrated in the daily clinical routine. Systematic CBCT virtual diagnosis of the patient's deformity, anatomy and pathology (including 3D airway and TMJ) is described in a comprehensive way in Chap. 2. Moreover, 3D cephalometric analysis of the patient's soft and hard tissues and teeth and the potential of 3D mirroring and colour distance maps for enhanced patient diagnostics are elaborated. Chapter 3 focuses on the "Virtual Natural Head Position (ν-NHP) and Planning Head Position (PHP)"; "3D Virtual Osteotomies and 3D Virtual Occlusal Definition"; "the Principles of 'Roll', 'Yaw' and 'Pitch' in the 3D Virtual Scene"; and finally "10-Step-by-Step Individualised 3D Virtual Treatment Planning". In Chap. 4, the transfer of the 3D virtual treatment plan towards the patient in the operation theatre is explained. Chapter 5 shows the unprecedented potential towards 3D virtual evaluation of treatment outcome of orthognathic surgery. Finally, after having provided this essential background information to the reader, Chap. 6 illustrates the application of the 3D virtual approach in different types of maxillofacial deformity. Based on almost 20 years of personal experience, the author discusses and shares with the reader the clinical relevant potential but also the current limits and actual pitfalls of 3D virtual diagnosis, treatment planning and evaluation of treatment outcome of orthognathic surgery throughout this book.

List of Videos

Video N° 1: 3D-VPS$_{1-2}$: Chapter 2
Video N° 2: NHP-PHP: Chapter 3
Video N° 3: 3D-VPS$_3$: Chapter 3
Video N° 4: 3D-VPS$_4$: Chapter 3
Video N° 5: 3D-VPS$_5$: Chapter 3

Videos can be found in the electronic supplementary material in the online version of the book.

On http://springerlink.com enter the DOI number given on the bottom of the chapter opening page. Scroll down to the Supplementary material tab and click on the respective videos link.

In addition, all videos to this book can be downloaded from http://extras.springer.com. Enter the ISBN number and download all videos.

Contents

Abbreviations

AM	Additive manufacturing
AUM	Augmented model
CAD/CAM	Computer-aided design/computer-aided manufacturing
CBCT	Cone-beam computed tomography
CCW	Counterclockwise
CR	Centric relation
CW	Clockwise
DICOM	Digital imaging and communications in medicine
FOV	Field of view
ICP	Iterative closest point
IO-CBCT	Intra-operative cone-beam computed tomography
IO-MSCT	Intra-operative multi-slice computed tomography
MSCT	Multi-slice computed tomography
NHP	Natural head position
c-NHP	Clinical natural head position
v-NHP	Virtual natural head position
PACS	Picture archiving and communication system
PHP	Planning head position
PSI	Patient-specific implant
RPT	Rapid prototyping technology
STI	Surface to image
STL	Standard tessellation language
VOI	Volume of interest
VOXEL	Volumetric pixel
VPS	Virtual planning step

Contributor

Martin Gaboury, DMD, MSc, FRCDc
Private Practice in Maxillofacial and Facial Cosmetic Surgery, OroSphère, Quebec, Canada

Division of Oral and Maxillofacial Surgery, Department of Surgery, Hôtel-Dieu de Lévis, Lévis, Canada

Clinical Fellow, Division of Maxillofacial and Facial Plastic Surgery, Department of Surgery, General Hospital St-Jan Bruges-Ostend, Belgium

Imaging Workflow for 3D Virtual Treatment Planning of Orthognathic Surgery

Gwen R.J. Swennen and Martin Gaboury

G.R.J. Swennen (ed.), *3D Virtual Treatment Planning of Orthognathic Surgery*,
DOI 10.1007/978-3-662-47389-4_1

1.1 Image Acquisition for 3D Virtual Treatment Planning of Orthognathic Surgery

1.1.1 Image Acquisition and Virtual Rendering of the Patient's Head

For proper orthognathic and orthofacial surgery planning, the patient's head needs to be scanned without deformation of the facial soft tissue mask, with the mandible in "centric relation (CR)" and ideally in its individual "natural head position (NHP)":

1. "Without deformation of the facial soft tissue mask" implements that the patient is scanned in a vertical seated or standing position, without distortion of the facial mask especially lip morphology and posture. With the advent of "cone-beam CT imaging (CBCT)" in a seated or standing position, this has become feasible. Multi-slice CT (MSCT) scanning, which is performed in a horizontal position and also CBCT apparatus that scan the patient in a supine position, inherently falsify the 3D facial soft tissue mask of the patient due to the effects of gravity. On the other hand, careful attention should be paid that wax-bite wafers or registration devices do not disturb lip position neither lip morphology (◘ Figs. 1.1 and 1.2).
2. To ensure that the patient is scanned with the mandible "in CR", the patient needs to be scanned with a wax-bite wafer. This wax-bite wafer is not different than the one used in conventional orthognathic surgery planning. It is, however, important that this wax-bite wafer is meticulously trimmed in order to avoid deformation of the facial soft tissue mask by interference with the cheeks or lips (◘ Fig. 1.3). A CBCT scout view is made prior to scanning of the patient to assure that the wax-bite wafer is adequately in place and that the patient's mandible is in CR (◘ Fig. 1.4).
3. Based on the author's personal experience, the patient's head position during image acquisition never corresponds to its true clinical "NHP". Therefore, a "step-by-step" approach is described to virtually modify the patient's head position towards its individual clinical NHP (► see also Sect. 3.1), prior to start 3D virtual treatment planning.

Accurate "3D virtual treatment planning of orthognathic surgery" starts with proper image acquisition.

Image Acquisition and Virtual Rendering of the Patient's Head

To illustrate the workflow towards (1) image acquisition of the patient's head, (2) additional image acquisition of the patient's dentition and occlusion and finally (3) additional image acquisition of the texture of the patient's head, volunteer M.G. will be used throughout this chapter.

On the other hand, the routine clinical imaging workflow for 3D virtual treatment planning of orthognathic surgery will be demonstrated on *Case 1* (Patient V.E.W.) which will be used throughout this book (► Chaps. 2, 3, 4, 5 and 6).

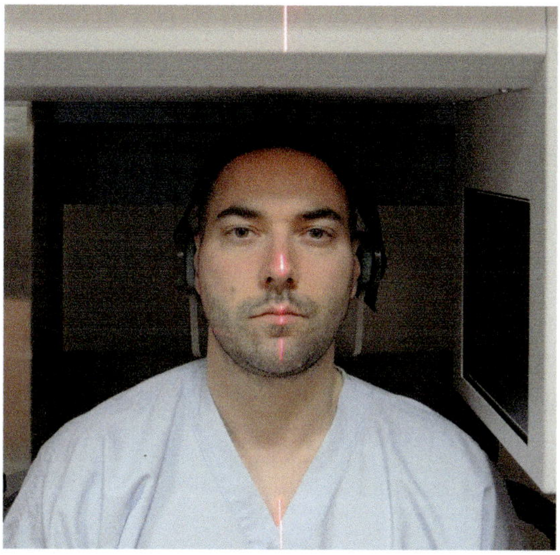

Fig. 1.1 Full face CBCT scanning of the patient, with a wax-bite wafer in CR, needs to be performed in a vertical position (seated or standing) without distortion of the facial soft tissue mask. To avoid movement artefacts, it is crucial that the patient is stabilised by a headrest in the back and a frontal headband. Note that although attempted to scan volunteer M.G. is its individual NHP, in a seated position with the use of laser lines, the shoulders were still distorted which caused a small "Yaw" rotation (► see also Sect. 3.4) to the left (i-CAT, Imaging Sciences International Inc., volunteer M.G.)

> Stabilisation of the patient's head is crucial during CBCT scanning.
> Do not use chin supports neither frontal bands that cover the forehead.

Image Acquisition and Virtual Rendering of the Patient's Head

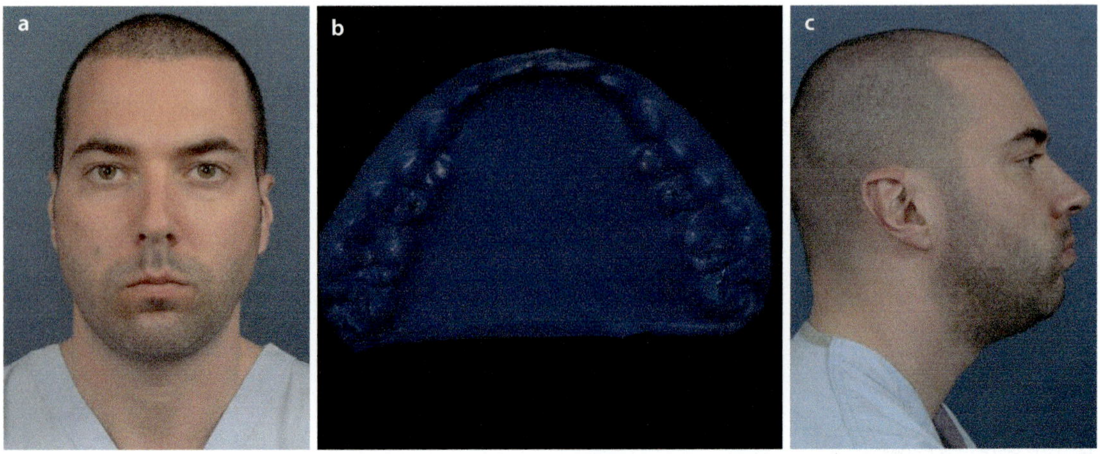

Fig. 1.2 A wax-bite wafer (Delar Corp., Lake Oswego, USA) was taken in CR as in conventional treatment planning to ensure adequate CR during CBCT scanning (**b**). Note the significant distortion of the lips and the cheeks when the wax-bite wafer is not trimmed (**a**, **c**) (volunteer M.G.)

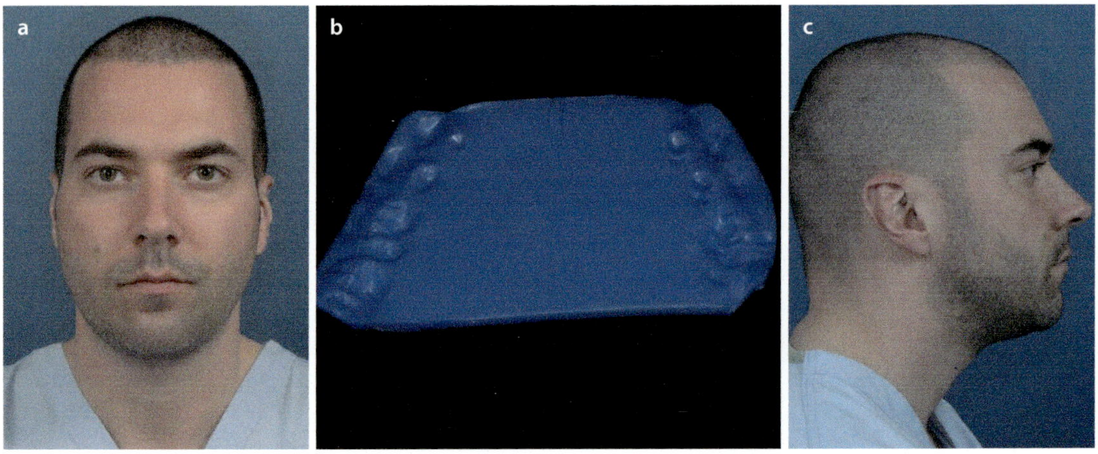

Fig. 1.3 A wax-bite wafer (Delar Corp., Lake Oswego, USA) was taken in CR as in conventional treatment planning to ensure adequate CR during CBCT scanning. The wax-bite wafer was meticulously trimmed to remove all parts that could interfere with the lips and cheeks during CBCT scanning (**b**). Note that there is no distortion of the lips neither of the cheeks (**a**, **c**) (► see also Sect. 1.1.3) (volunteer M.G.)

Image Acquisition and Virtual Rendering of the Patient's Head

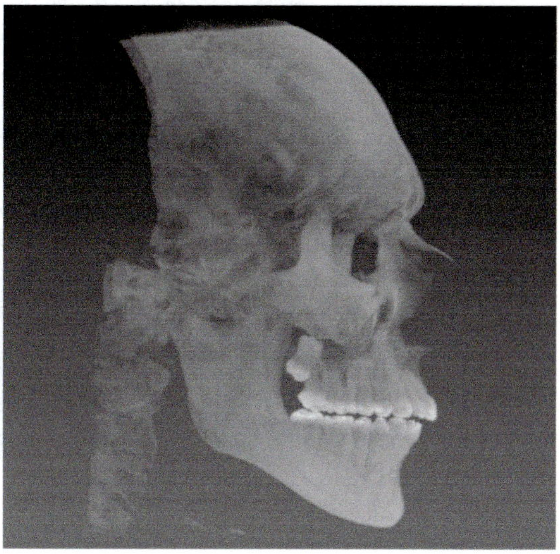

Fig. 1.4 CBCT profile scout view, to ensure that the wax-bite wafer is adequately in place and that the patient's mandible is in CR prior to CBCT scanning (i-CAT, Imaging Sciences International Inc., volunteer M.G.)

Always
Take a scout view prior to CBCT scanning of the patient to verify:
1. Adequate CR
2. Adequate positioning of the wax-bite wafer

Virtual Rendering of the Patient's Head in a "3D Virtual Scene Approach"

An appropriate "3D virtual visualisation paradigm" (Swennen and Schutyser 2007) is needed to visualise the DICOM CBCT data, but also additional image data (▶ see also Sects. 1.1.2. and 1.1.3) that can be acquired from other 3D imaging sources.

A "3D Virtual Scene Approach" is therefore adopted in which the "3D virtual space" is considered as a "3D virtual scene" with "medical image data" as "actors" (Schutyser 2005). This "3D virtual scene" is viewed with a virtual camera and the resulting views are shown on the computer screen. The virtual camera can be moved around in the "3D virtual scene" to image and inspect the structures of interest from various angles and positions.

Besides visualising the patient's image data with the virtual camera, the "3D virtual visualisation paradigm" and the "3D Virtual Scene Approach" allow other actions and interactions in the "3D virtual scene" such as indicating 3D cephalometric landmarks of the patient's hard tissues and teeth (3D-VPS$_1$) (▶ see also Sect. 2.2.2), indicating 3D cephalometric landmarks of the patient's soft tissues (3D-VPS$_2$) (▶ see also Sect. 2.2.3), performing 3D virtual osteotomies (3D-VPS$_3$) (▶ see also Sect. 3.2), indicating 3D virtual occlusal definition (3D-VPS$_4$) (▶ see also Sect. 3.3) and moving bone fragments with additional soft tissue simulation, towards the "step-by-step" individualised 3D virtual treatment planning (3D-VPS$_5$) of orthognathic surgery (▶ see also Sect. 3.5).

After proper image acquisition of the patient's head, CBCT imaging results in a 3D volume of DICOM (Digital Imaging and Communications in Medicine) data, consisting of a collection of "cube-like blocks" called "voxels". Each voxel has a certain height, width and depth. A typical voxel size of a CBCT scan of the patient's head is $[v_x, v_y, v_z] = [0.4\ \text{mm}, 0.4\ \text{mm}, 0.4\ \text{mm}]$.

Virtual Rendering of the Patient's Head

The CBCT DICOM data can be "rendered" to generate a 3D virtual image of the patient's head by (1) "surface rendering" or (2) "volume rendering".

1. **"Surface rendering"** is an indirect way for reconstruction of 3D structures by segmentation (◘ Figs. 1.5 and 1.6) based on the grayscales of the image data towards surfaces that are drawn on the computer screen given a viewing direction of the virtual camera (◘ Fig. 1.7). "Surface rendering" has the advantage that it allows additional actions and interactions in the "3D virtual scene" such as indicating 3D cephalometric landmarks, performing 3D virtual osteotomies, 3D virtual occlusal definition, moving bone fragments with additional soft tissue simulation and 3D superimposition of datasets. Moreover, axial, coronal, sagittal and multiplanar reslices can be calculated and added to the "3D virtual scene". Finally, "surface rendering" allows to integrate the results from surface scanning hardware for additional image acquisition of the patient's dentition and occlusion (▶ see also Sect. 1.1.2) or texture of the patient's head (▶ see also Sect. 1.1.3) in a straightforward way.
2. **"Volume rendering"** is a more direct way for reconstruction of 3D structures by rendering a volume of voxels. Towards each voxel, a colour and opacity is assigned based on shading algorithms. According to the viewing direction of the virtual camera in the "3D virtual scene", a projection image is computed and presented on the computer screen. Compared to "surface rendering", "volume rendering" has the advantage that the transitions between several tissues (e.g. teeth and bone) are smooth which results in more detailed anatomy of the teeth and interdental spaces (◘ Figs. 1.8 and 1.9). It however does not allow actions and interactions such as indicating 3D cephalometric landmarks, performing 3D virtual osteotomies, 3D virtual occlusal definition, moving bone fragments with additional soft tissue simulation and 3D superimposition of datasets.

For optimal 3D virtual treatment planning of orthognathic surgery, both "surface rendering" and "volume rendering" are combined.

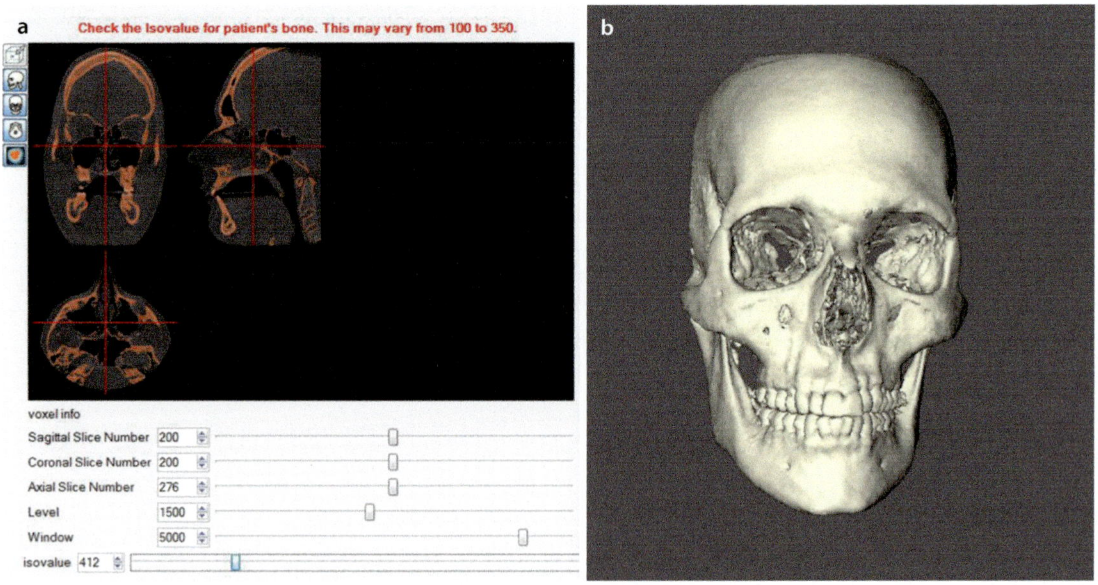

◘ **Fig. 1.5** "Surface rendering" (Maxilim v. 2.3.0.3) of the hard (**a**, **b**) and soft (**c**, **d**) tissues of the head of volunteer M.G. after CBCT image acquisition. For the hard tissue rendering, the isovalue was set at 412, while for soft tissue rendering, it was set at -560 (i-CAT^{TM}, Imaging Sciences International, Inc., Hatfield, USA, "extended field" modus; FOV, 17 cm diameter – 22 cm height; scan time 2 × 20 s; voxel size 0.4 mm at 120 kV according to DICOM field, 0018,0060 KVP, and 48 mA according to DICOM field, 0018,1151 XRayTubeCurrent) (volunteer M.G.)

Virtual Rendering of the Patient's Head

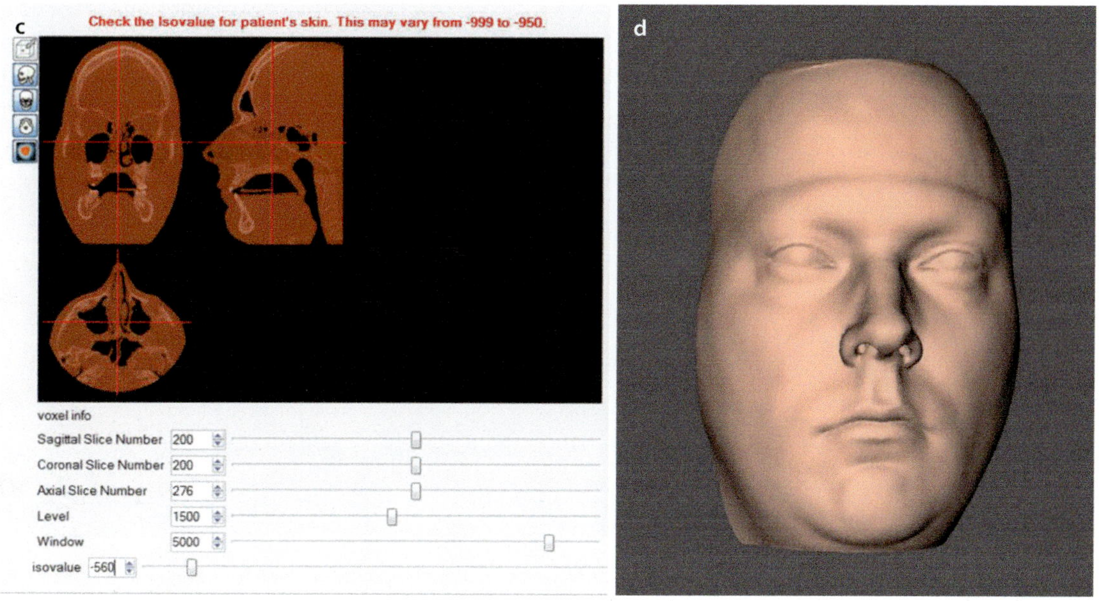

Fig. 1.5 (continued)

During the "surface rendering" process, the "threshold" is adjusted to optimise the visualisation of the 3D hard (Fig. 1.5a and 1.6) and soft tissue (Fig. 1.5c) surface representations of the patient's head.

"Thresholding" is the process of creating a "black-and-white image" out of a "grayscale image" consisting of setting exactly those pixels to white whose value is above a given threshold while setting the other pixels to black. Finally, a colour can be assigned to the reconstructed 3D hard (Figs. 1.5b, 1.6 and 1.7) and soft tissue (Figs. 1.5d and 1.7) surface representations.

Virtual Rendering of the Patient's Head

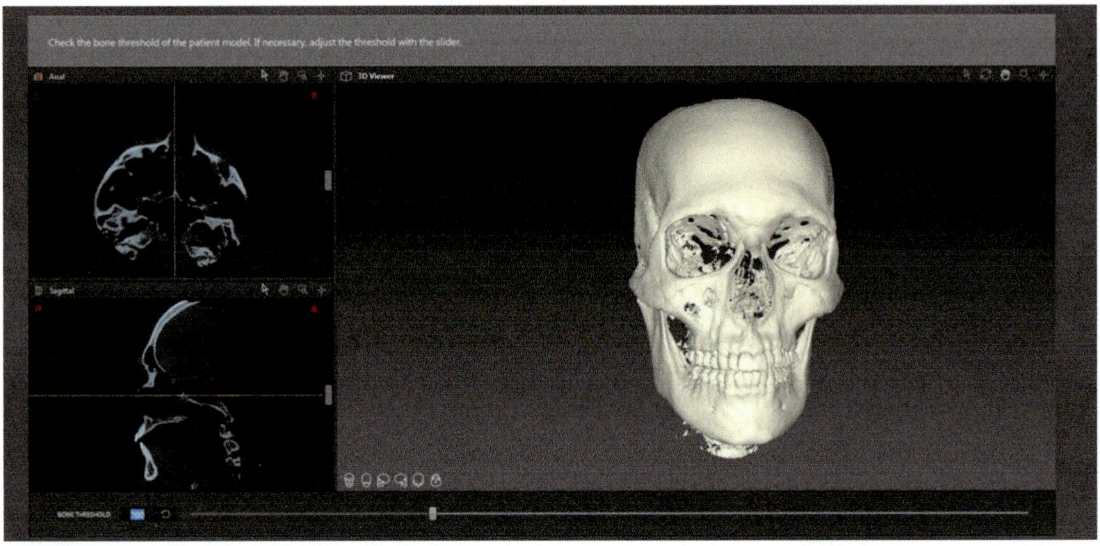

Fig. 1.6 "Surface rendering" (IPS CaseDesigner ALPHA version) of the hard tissues of the head of volunteer M.G. after CBCT image acquisition. The threshold is adjusted to optimise the visualisation of the hard tissues (i-CAT™, Imaging Sciences International, Inc., Hatfield, USA, "extended field" modus; FOV, 17 cm diameter – 22 cm height; scan time 2 × 20 s; voxel size 0.4 mm at 120 kV according to DICOM field, 0018,0060 KVP, and 48 mA according to DICOM field, 0018,1151 XRayTubeCurrent) (volunteer M.G.)

Virtual Rendering of the Patient's Head

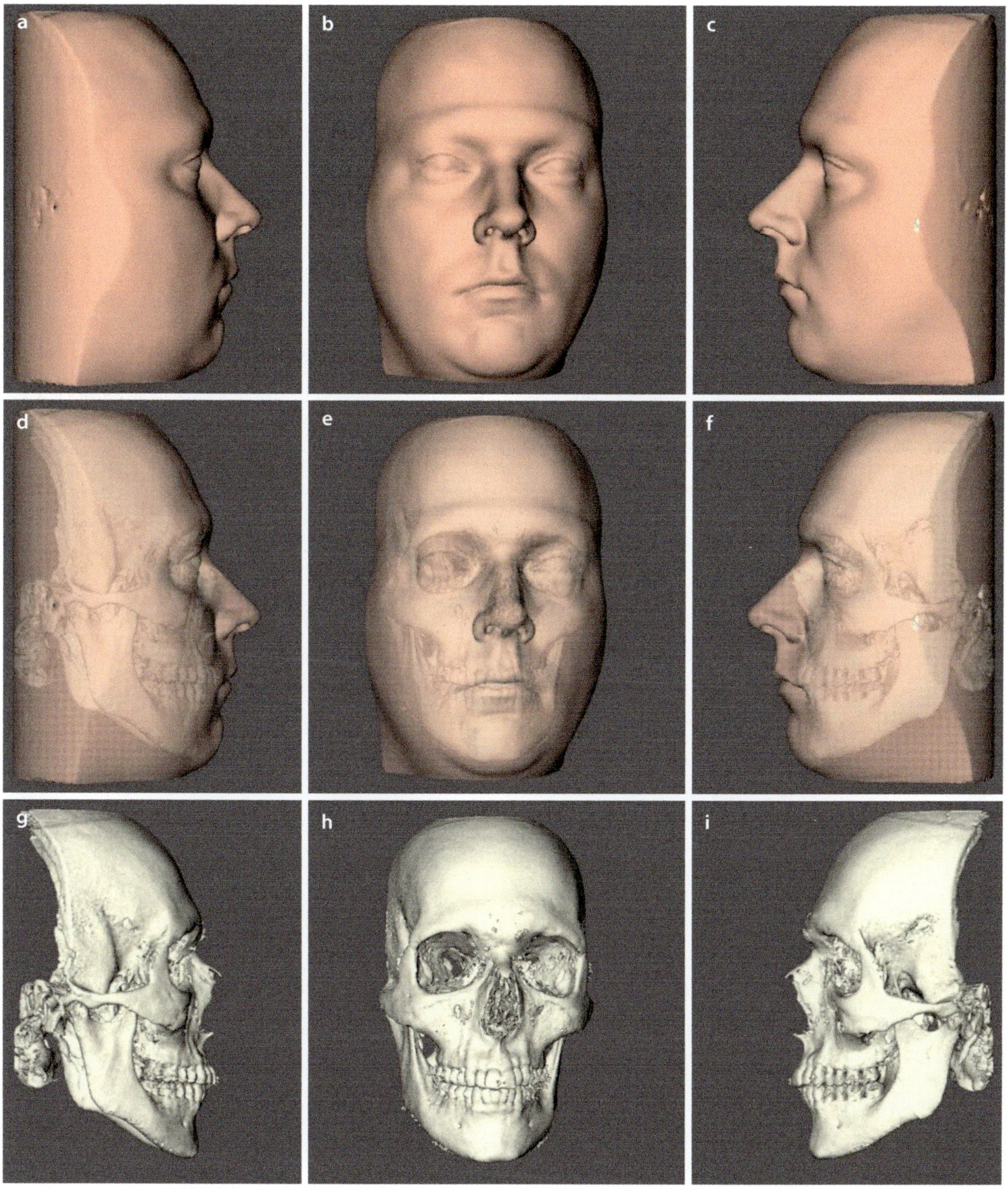

Fig. 1.7 3D "surface-rendered" (Maxilim v. 2.3.0.3) soft and hard tissues representations of the head of volunteer M.G., as acquired during CBCT image acquisition (i-CAT^{TM}, Imaging Sciences International, Inc., Hatfield, USA). Volunteer M.G. was vertically scanned with a wax-bite wafer in place in a natural seated position using a standardised CBCT scanning protocol ("extended field" modus; FOV, 17 cm diameter – 22 cm height; scan time 2 × 20 s; voxel size 0.4 mm at 120 kV according to DICOM field, 0018,0060 KVP, and 48 mA according to DICOM field, 0018,1151 XRayTubeCurrent) (volunteer M.G.). Right profile (**a**, **d**, **g**), frontal (**b**, **e**, **h**) and left profile (**c**, **f**, **i**) views. Note the incorrect position and orientation of the head ("Yaw" rotation to the left, ► see also Sects. 3.1 and 3.4) although it was attempted to scan volunteer M.G. in his correct NHP. Also note the presence of artefacts at the dentition level although volunteer M.G. does not have orthodontic brackets neither dental reconstitution materials

Virtual Rendering of the Patient's Head

During the "volume rendering" process, a colour and opacity are assigned towards each voxel (◘ Figs. 1.8 and 1.9) based on shading algorithms.

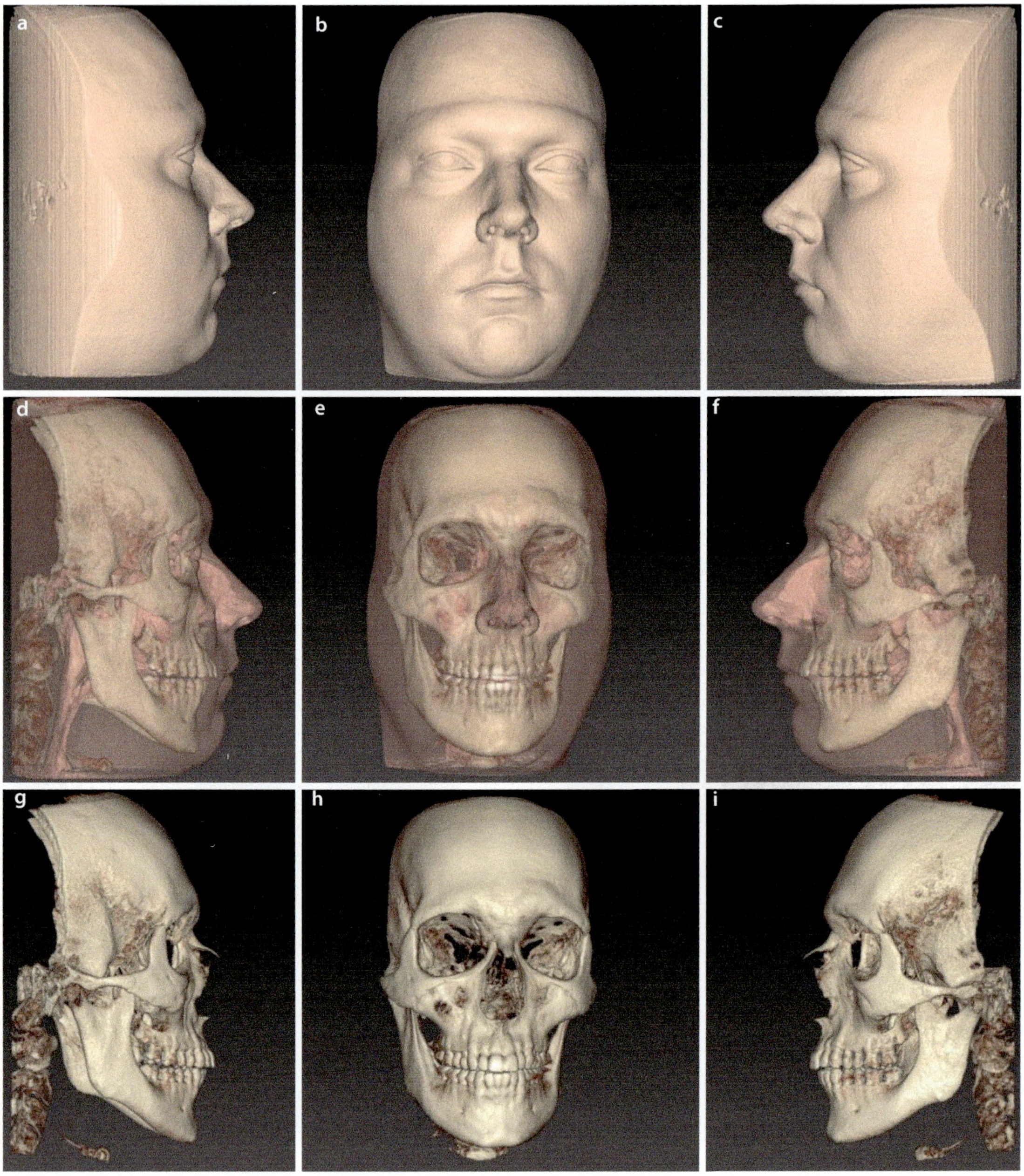

◘ **Fig. 1.8** 3D "volume-rendered" (IPS CaseDesigner ALPHA version) soft and hard tissues representations of the head of volunteer M.G., as acquired during CBCT image acquisition (i-CAT™, Imaging Sciences International, Inc., Hatfield, USA). Volunteer M.G. was vertically scanned with a wax-bite wafer in place in a natural seated position using a standardised CBCT scanning protocol ("extended field" modus; FOV, 17 cm diameter – 22 cm height; scan time 2 × 20 s; voxel size 0.4 mm at 120 kV according to DICOM field, 0018,0060 KVP, and 48 mA according to DICOM field, 0018,1151 XRayTubeCurrent) (volunteer M.G.). Right profile (**a**, **d**, **g**), frontal (**b**, **e**, **h**) and left profile (**c**, **f**, **i**) views. Note that "volume rendering" produces less artefacts at the dentition level

Virtual Rendering of the Patient's Head

Attention
Towards 3D virtual diagnosis, 3D virtual treatment planning and 3D outcome evaluation, both "surface rendering" and "volume rendering" are necessary and need to be combined.

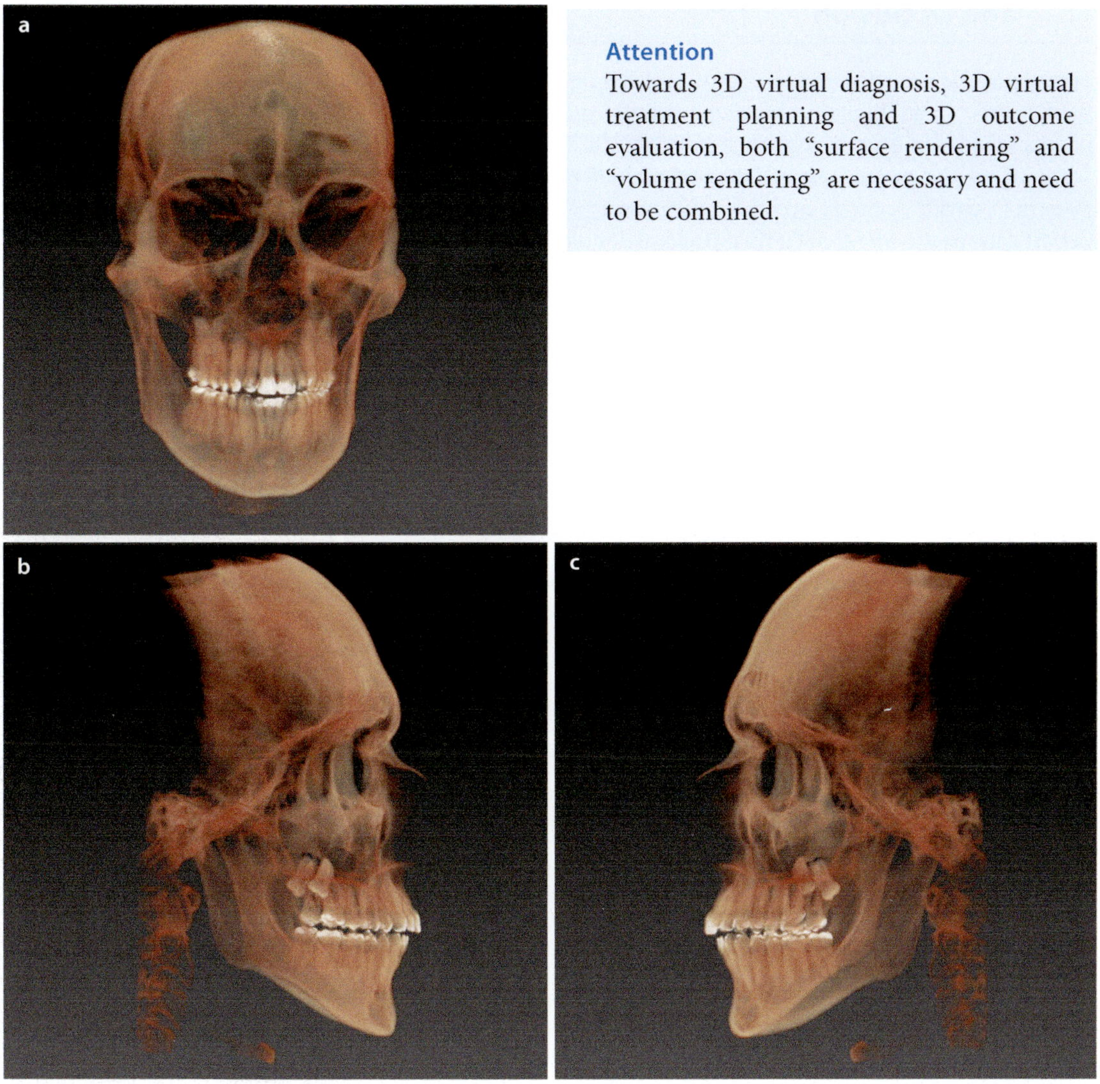

Fig. 1.9 3D "volume-rendered" (IPS CaseDesigner ALPHA version) hard tissue representations of the head of volunteer M.G., as acquired during CBCT image acquisition (i-CAT^{TM}, Imaging Sciences International, Inc., Hatfield, USA). Volunteer M.G. was vertically scanned with a wax-bite wafer in place in a natural seated position using a standardised CBCT scanning protocol ("extended field" modus; FOV, 17 cm diameter – 22 cm height; scan time 2 × 20 s; voxel size 0.4 mm at 120 kV according to DICOM field, 0018,0060 KVP, and 48 mA according to DICOM field, 0018,1151 XRayTubeCurrent) (volunteer M.G.). Frontal (**a**), right profile (**b**) and left (**c**) views. Note that "volume rendering" produces less artefacts and gives more detailed information towards the roots of the teeth and interdental space

1

1.1.2 Additional Image Acquisition of the Patient's Dentition and Occlusion

For proper "3D virtual treatment planning of orthognathic surgery", additional image acquisition of the patient's dentition is necessary, since isolated CBCT scanning of the patient's head (▶ see Sect. 1.1.1) does not provide accurate occlusal and intercuspidation data, necessary for 3D virtual occlusal definition (▶ see also Sect. 3.3) and 3D CAD/CAM splint manufacturing (▶ see also Sect. 4.1.1).

Additional image acquisition of the patient's dentition in order to obtain accurate occlusal and intercuspidation data can be performed by:

1. Direct scanning of the impressions of the patient's dental arches
2. Indirect scanning of the plaster dental models of the patient
3. Intra-oral scanning of the patient's dentition

> "Single CBCT scanning of the patient's head" does not provide accurate occlusal and intercuspidation data which are mandatory for proper 3D virtual orthognathic surgery planning.

1. Direct scanning of the impressions of the patient's dental arches

Direct scanning of the impression(s) of the patient's dental arches can be performed with the same CBCT apparatus that is used for scanning of the patient's head. Either an "all-in-one" impression or separate impressions of the upper and lower dental arches can be CBCT scanned. Laser surface scanning is not recommended for scanning of impressions since undercuts are not imaged correctly due to the fact that the laser light is following a straight path.

Direct CBCT scanning of the impression(s) of the patient's dental arches provides additional accurate occlusal and intercuspidation data data (◘ Figs. 1.10 and 1.11).

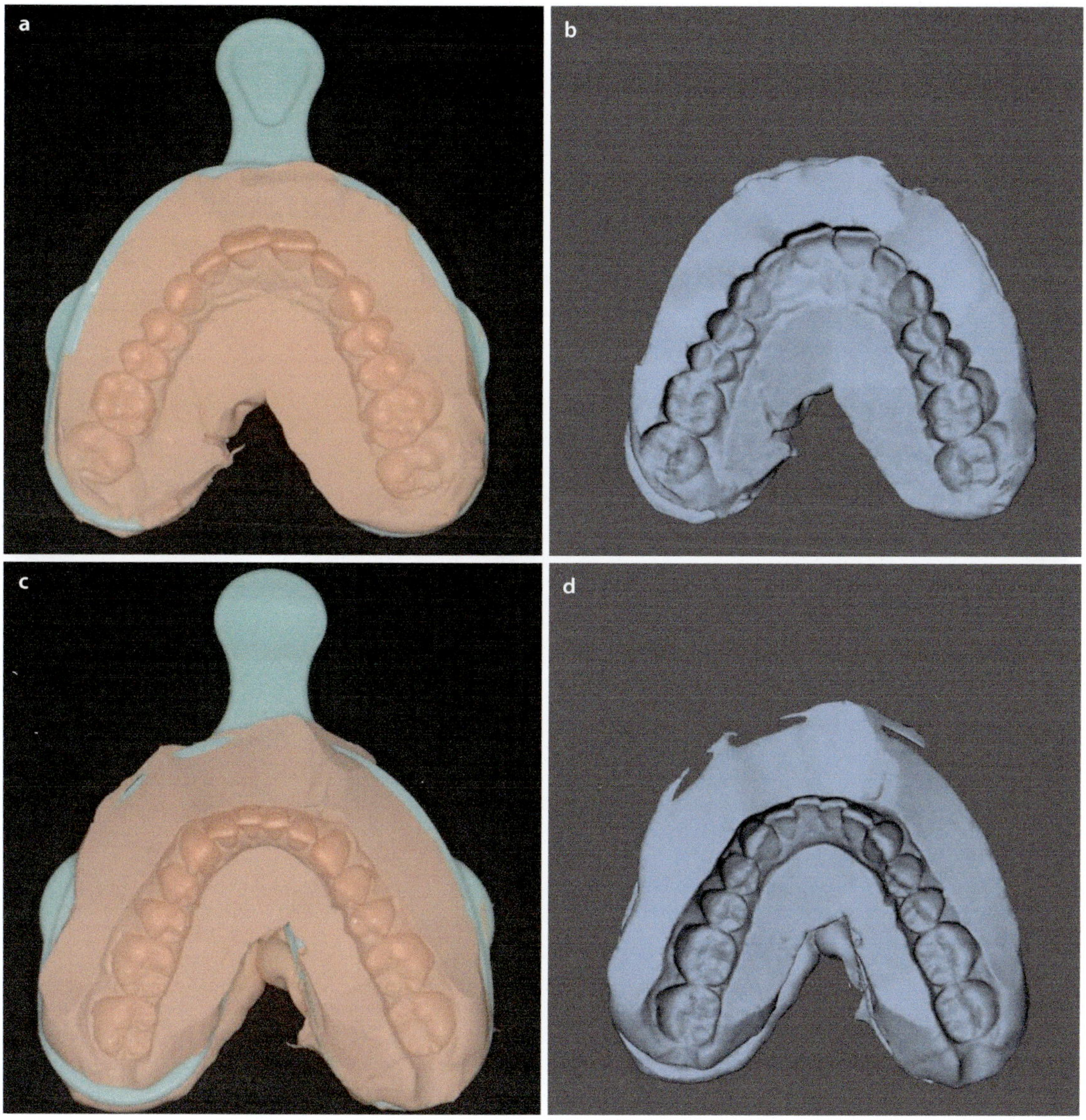

◘ **Fig. 1.10** Clinical photographs of the "all-in-one" impression of the upper and lower dental arches (**a**, **c**, **e**) and 3D "surface-rendered" representations (**b**, **d**, **f**). The Triple Tray® AlgiNot^{TM} impression (► see also Sect. 1.2.2) was scanned using a high-resolution standardised CBCT scanning protocol (i-CAT^{TM}, Imaging Sciences International, Inc., Hatfield, USA, "high-resolution" modus; FOV, 17 cm diameter – 6 cm height; scan time 40 s; voxel size 0.2 mm, at 120 kV according to DICOM field, 0018,0060 KVP, and 47 mA according to DICOM field, 0018,1151 XRayTubeCurrent) (Maxilim v. 2.3.0.3., volunteer M.G.). Note that the plastic Triple Tray® is no longer visible on the 3D surface representations because of its radiolucent nature

Direct Scanning of the Impressions of the Patient's Dental Arches

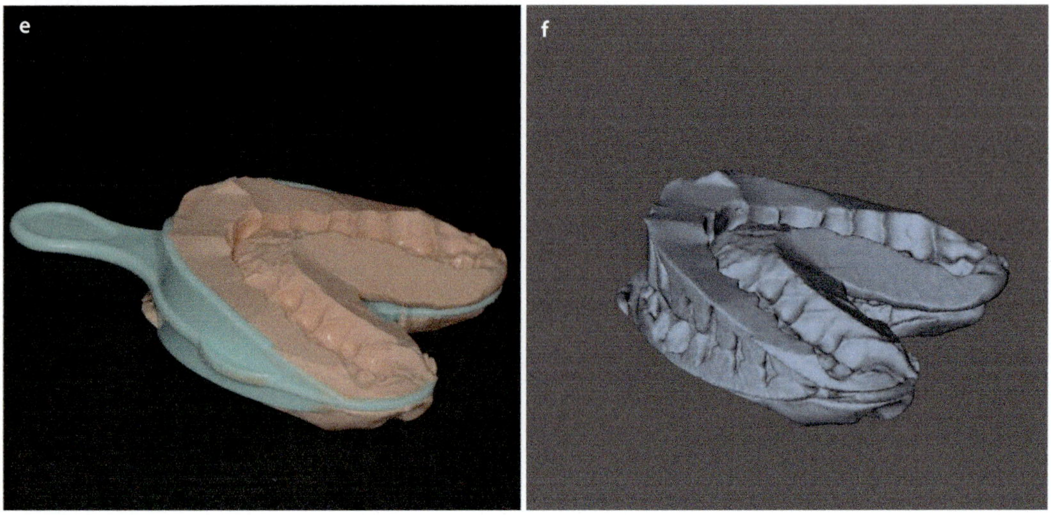

■ **Fig. 1.10** (continued)

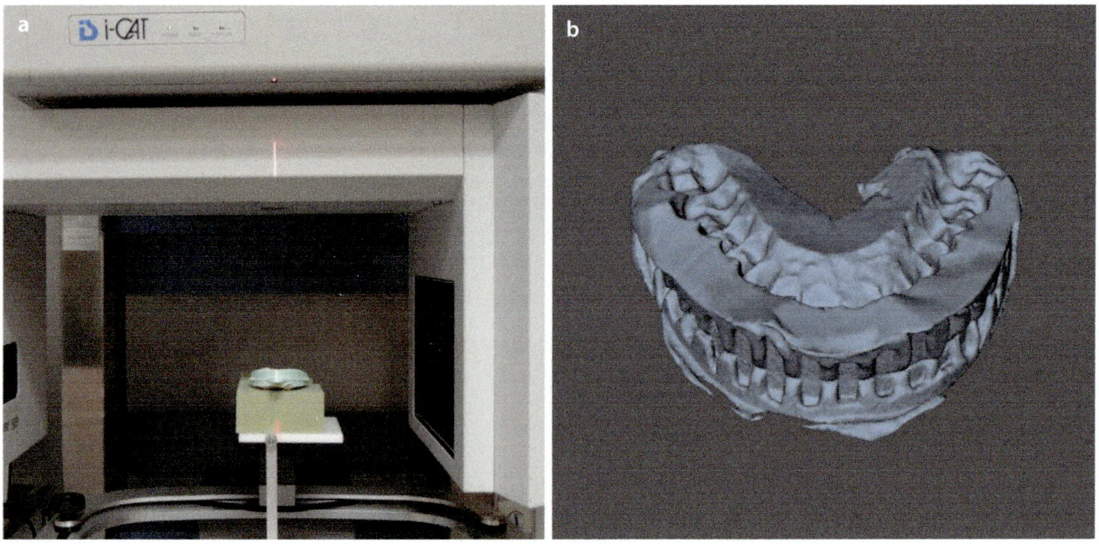

■ **Fig. 1.11** To scan the Triple Tray® AlgiNot^{TM} impression, it was put on a commercially available sponge (**a**) to avoid segmentation problems with the CBCT apparatus table. The Triple Tray® AlgiNot^{TM} impression was scanned using a high-resolution standardised CBCT scanning protocol (i-CAT^{TM}, Imaging Sciences International, Inc., Hatfield, USA, "high-resolution" modus; FOV, 17 cm diameter – 6 cm height; scan time 40 s; voxel size 0.2 mm, at 120 kV according to DICOM field, 0018,0060 KVP, and 47 mA according to DICOM field, 0018,1151 XRayTubeCurrent). 3D "surface-rendered" representation (**b**) (Maxilim v. 2.3.0.3.) (volunteer M.G.)

2. Indirect scanning of the plaster dental models of the patient

Additional accurate occlusal and intercuspidation data can also be obtained "indirectly" by scanning of the plaster dental models of the patient. This can be performed with the same CBCT apparatus (◘ Fig. 1.12) that is used for scanning of the patient's head or by laser surface scanning. Moreover, the actual occlusion of the patient can be scanned (◘ Fig. 1.13).

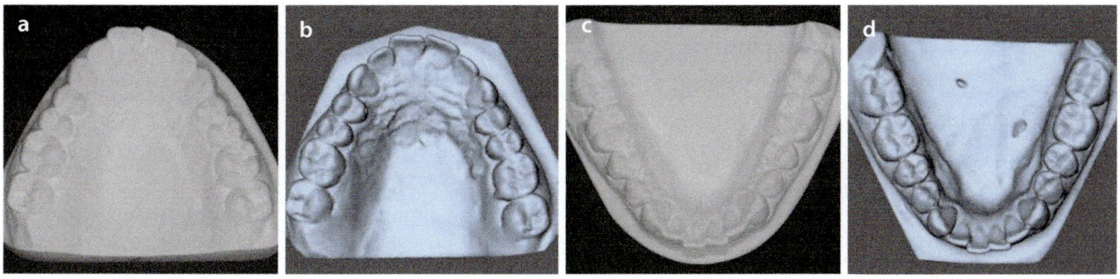

◘ **Fig. 1.12** Additional image acquisition of the dentition by indirect high-resolution standardised CBCT scanning of the upper and lower plaster dental models (**a**, **c**) (i-CAT^{TM}, Imaging Sciences International, Inc., Hatfield, USA, "high-resolution" modus; FOV, 17 cm diameter – 6 cm height; scan time 40 s; voxel size 0.2 mm, at 120 kV according to DICOM field, 0018,0060 KVP, and 47 mA according to DICOM field, 0018,1151 XRayTubeCurrent) and their 3D "surface-rendered" representations (**b**, **d**) (Maxilim v. 2.3.0.3.) (volunteer M.G.)

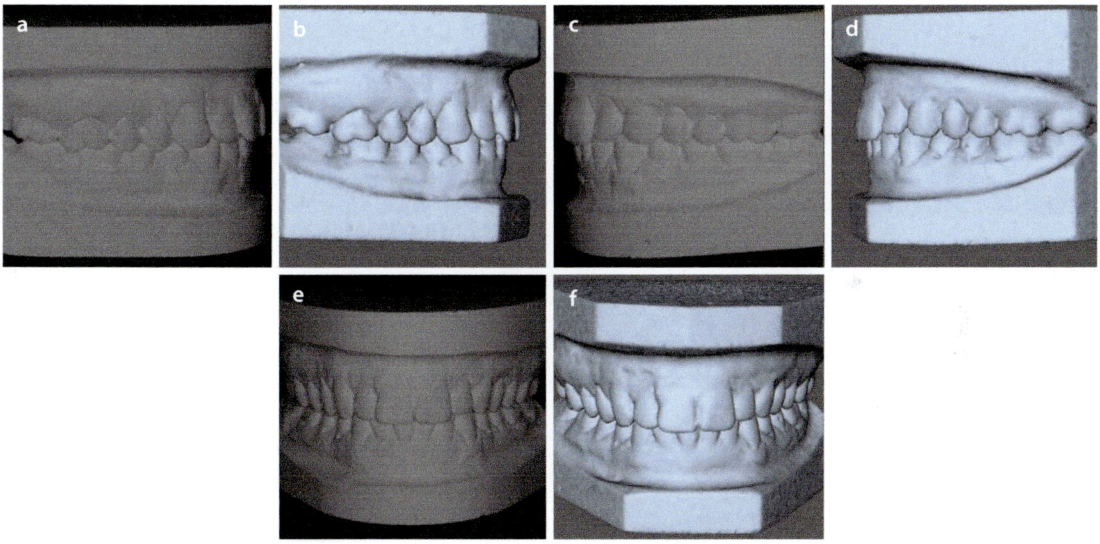

◘ **Fig. 1.13** Additional image acquisition of the occlusion by indirect high-resolution standardised CBCT scanning of the upper and lower plaster dental models, in final occlusion (**a**, **c**, **e**) (i-CAT^{TM}, Imaging Sciences International, Inc., Hatfield, USA, "high-resolution" modus; FOV, 17 cm diameter – 8 cm height; scan time 40 s; voxel size 0.2 mm, at 120 kV according to DICOM field, 0018,0060 KVP, and 47 mA according to DICOM field, 0018,1151 XRayTubeCurrent) and their 3D "surface-rendered" representations (**b**, **d**, **f**) (Maxilim v. 2.3.0.3.) (volunteer M.G.)

3. Intra-oral scanning of the patient's dentition

Intra-oral scanning allows scanning of the patient's upper and lower dental arches with an accuracy of a few microns (► Fig. 1.14a, c). The scanning process is currently still rather slow compared to direct scanning of impressions or indirect scanning of plaster dental models. More-

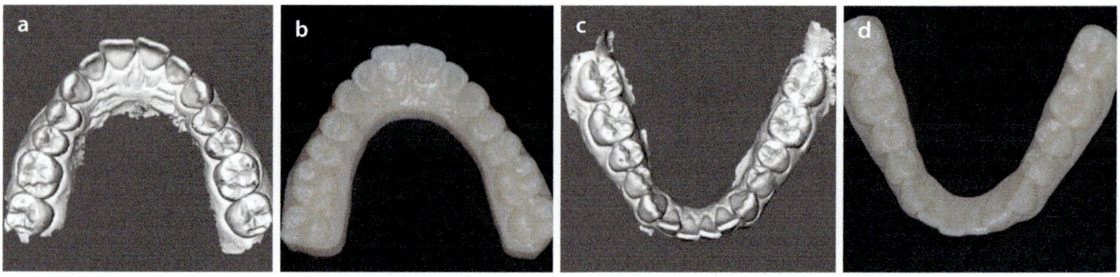

Fig. 1.14 Additional image acquisition of the patient's dentition with direct intra-oral optical scanning (3M^{TM} Lava^{TM} Chairside Oral Scanner) of the upper and lower dental arches. 3D "surface-rendered" representations of the upper (**a**) and (**c**) lower arches (Maxilim v. 2.3.0.3.). The STL files were 3D printed (**b, d**) for educational purposes (volunteer M.G.)

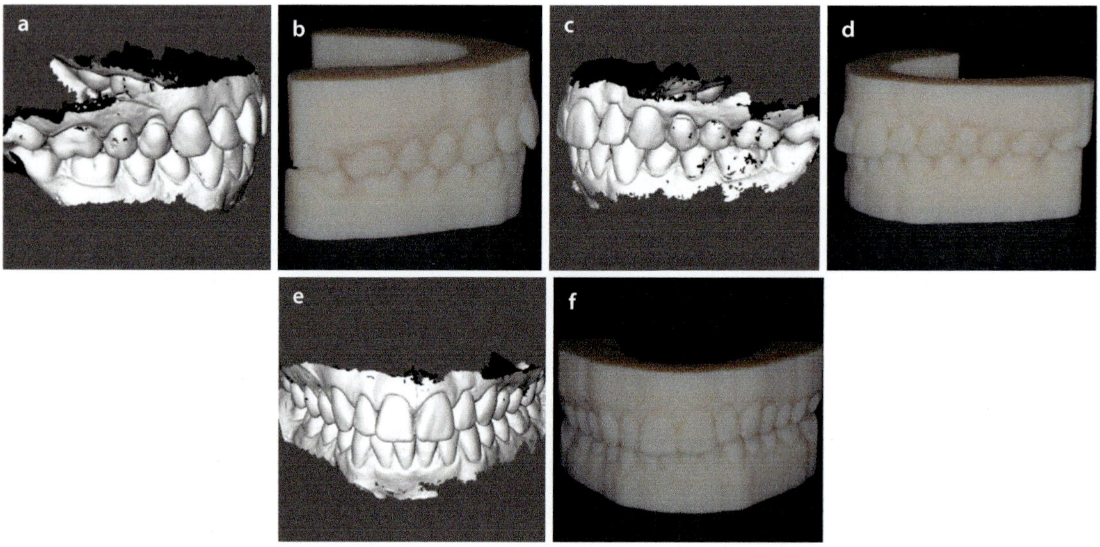

Fig. 1.15 Additional image acquisition of the occlusion with direct intra-oral optical scanning (3M^{TM} Lava^{TM} Chairside Oral Scanner). 3D "surface-rendered" representations (**a, c, e**) (Maxilim v. 2.3.0.3.). The STL files were 3D printed (**b, d, f**) for educational purposes (volunteer M.G.)

over, the actual occlusion of the patient can be scanned (▶ Fig. 1.15a, c, e).

1.1.3 Additional Image Acquisition of the Texture of the Patient's Head

For proper "3D virtual treatment planning of orthognathic surgery", additional image acquisition of the texture of the patient's head in order to augment (▶ see also Sect. 1.2) the CBCT 3D facial soft tissue mask of the patient with texture and colour is not essential and currently still error prone.

Additional image acquisition of the texture of the patient's head can be performed by:

1. Standardised clinical 2D photographs of the patient's head in rest in NHP (▶ Fig. 1.16a, b, c, g, h, i, m)
2. 3D photographs made by 3D surface imaging systems based on active stereo photogrammetry (▶ Fig. 1.16d, e, f, j, k, l, n)

Towards 3D virtual evaluation of orthognathic surgery, 3D photographs offer an important clinical relevant potential and benefit towards longitudinal non-ionising treatment outcome analysis (▶ see also Sect. 5.2.2).

Additional dynamic 4D image acquisition of the texture of the patient's head and the underlying 3D facial soft tissue mask is promising. From a computational point of view, it is currently too time consuming to implement in the clinical daily routine and therefore actually dedicated for research purposes.

Attention
Additional image acquisition of the texture of the patient's head in order to augment the 3D facial soft tissue mask is not essential for proper 3D virtual treatment planning, however, certainly of interest in "Step 9" of 3D-VPS$_5$ "Patient Communication of the Individualised 3D Virtual Treatment Plan".

Additional Image Acquisition of the Texture of the Patient's Head

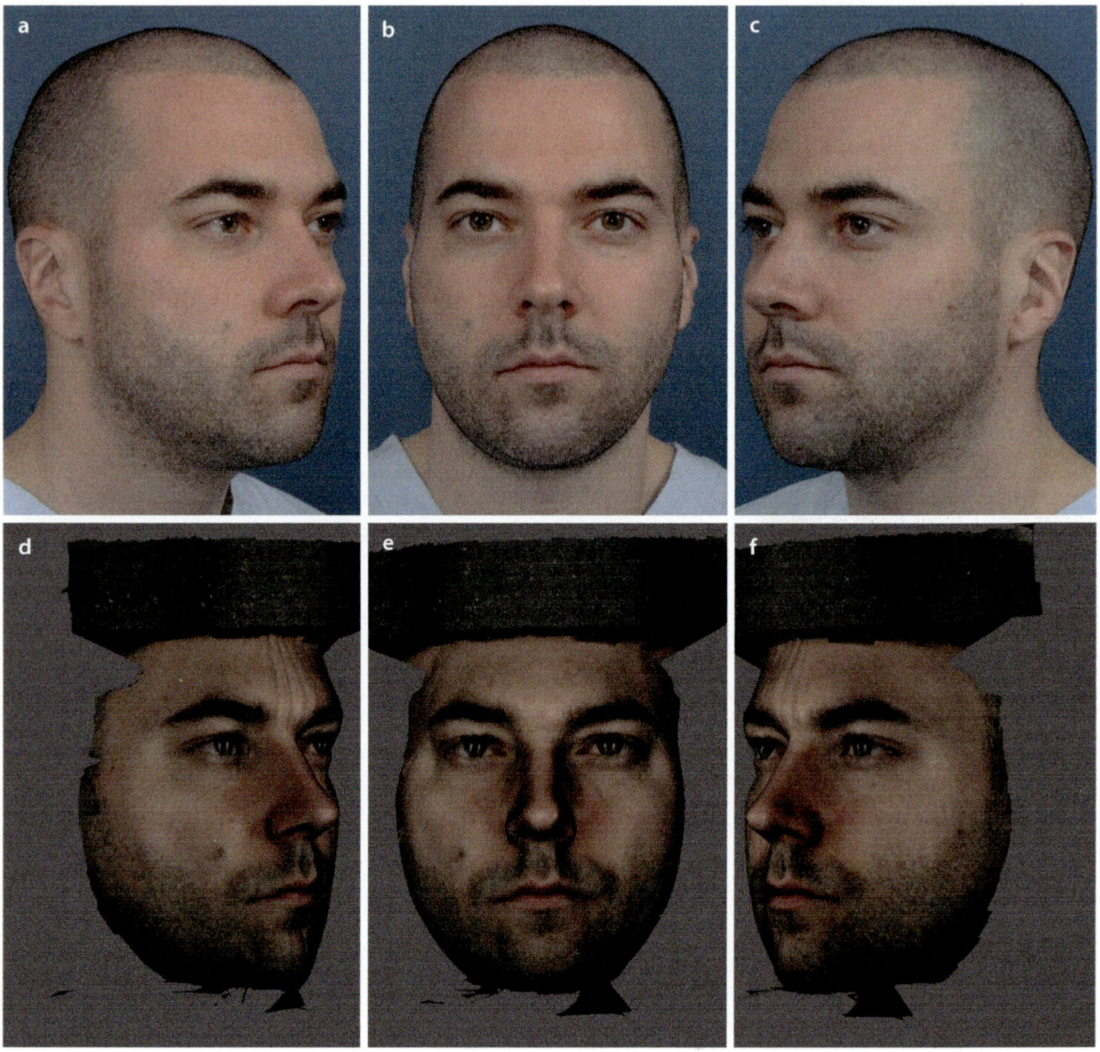

Fig. 1.16 Additional image acquisition of the texture of the head. Standardised 2D clinical photographs (**a**, **b**, **c**, **g**, **h**, **i**, **m**) and 3D photographs of the head (**d**, **e**, **f**, **j**, **k**, **l**, **n**) (Planmeca ProMax® 3D Max, ProFace™, Planmeca Oy, Helsinki, Finland) (volunteer M.G.). Note that 2D clinical photographs still have a higher image quality than 3D photographs

Additional Image Acquisition of the Texture of the Patient's Head

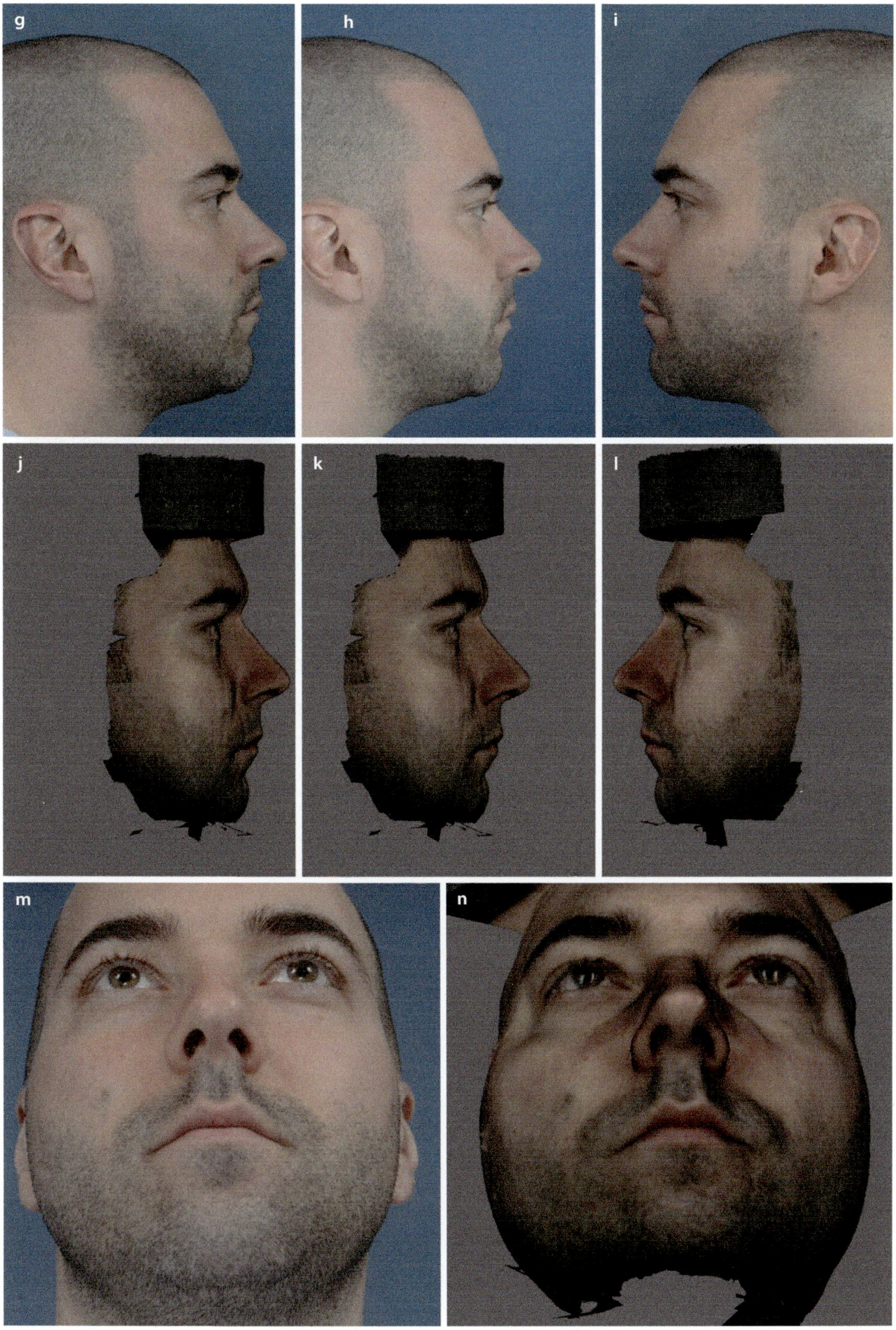

Fig. 1.16 (continued)

1.2 Processing of Acquired Image Data Towards a 3D Virtual Augmented Model of the Patient's Head

1.2.1 Principles of Rigid Registration

Single CBCT image acquisition of the patient's head (▶ Sect. 1.1.1) does not provide a 3D virtual patient model appropriate for 3D virtual treatment planning of orthognathic surgery since it lacks sufficient accuracy at the occlusal and intercuspidation level.

Therefore, additional image acquisition of the patient's dentition (▶ Sect. 1.1.2) is necessary to provide accurate occlusal and intercuspidation data.

Moreover, additional image acquisition of the texture of the patient's head (▶ Sect. 1.1.3) can be performed but is not essential for proper 3D virtual planning of orthognathic surgery.

In order to process the acquired image data towards a "3D virtual augmented model (AUM)" of the patient's head appropriate for 3D virtual treatment planning of orthognathic surgery, accurate "rigid registration" is necessary.

Registration techniques are based on similarity measures between two (e.g. pre- and post-treatment) or more (e.g. pretreatment, 3D virtual treatment plan and post-treatment) datasets (Swennen and Schutyser 2007).

With "rigid registration", a rotation and translation is searched which aligns both or more datasets and therefore increases the similarity of both or more datasets.

Traditionally, different types of "rigid registration" exist: (1) point-based, (2) surface-based and (3) voxel-based rigid registration.

1. **"Point-based rigid registration"** only uses corresponding points to compute the rotation and translation between datasets. The residual distance between the point pairs after registration is minimised.
2. **"Surface-based rigid registration"** uses surface information of two datasets to compute the rotation and translation between datasets. Corresponding points and shapes are searched and the distance after rotation and translation is minimised.
3. **"Voxel-based rigid registration"** uses the grey value information of two datasets to compute the rotation and translation between datasets by maximising the mutual information between both datasets.

A new and innovative rigid registration algorithm, "surface to image registration (STI)" (Nobel Biocare c/o Medicim NV, Mechelen, Belgium) also called "CBCT to image registration" or "smart fusion", was evaluated and validated in 2013 by Swennen and colleagues to obtain a 3D virtual AUM of the patient's head appropriate for orthognathic surgery planning (▶ see also Sects. 1.2.2 and 1.2.3).

"Surface to image registration (STI)" uses a combined surface to voxel approach and registers the image intensities of the surfaces "gradient based" to the corresponding voxels.

To integrate accurate occlusal and intercuspidation data into the 3D patient model, "rigid registration" with or without markers, based on points, surfaces, voxels or a combination, currently still *needs to be performed* of:

1. The CBCT imaging acquisition data of the patient's head (▶ Sect. 1.1.1)
2. Additional image acquisition data of the patient's dentition and occlusal surfaces (▶ Sect. 1.1.2)
   (a) Without the use of plaster dental models
   (b) With the use of plaster dental models

Although different attempts have been reported by different research groups, only few methods have been properly validated and consequently applied in sufficient consecutive clinical patient series in order to provide evidence-based data. Moreover, all existing protocols at the moment still have their limitations and drawbacks towards the daily clinical application.

1.2.2 Without the Use of Plaster Dental Models

In 2009, Swennen and colleagues introduced and validated the "Triple CBCT Scan Protocol" in order to obtain an AUM of the patient appropriate for 3D virtual orthognathic surgery planning without the use of plaster dental models.

1. "CBCT scan N°1": Full face scan of the patient in a vertical natural seated position in CR with a wax-bite in place without deformation of the facial soft tissue mask (► see also Sect. 1.1.1) (◘ Fig. 1.17)
2. "CBCT scan N°2": Limited low-dose scan of the patient with a Triple Tray® AlgiNot™ all-in-one impression in place (◘ Fig. 1.18)
3. "CBCT scan N°3": High-resolution scan of the Triple Tray® AlgiNot™ all-in-one impression (◘ Fig. 1.19)

Following sequential semi-automatical triple "voxel-based rigid registration", the patient's head is augmented with accurate occlusal and intercuspidation data (◘ Fig. 1.20). The "Triple CBCT Scan Protocol" has meanwhile been used in daily clinical routine in the author's department in more than 2250 cases. Although accurate, it requires an important learning curve towards the imaging workflow for both image acquisitions as processing of the acquired image data towards a 3D virtual AUM of the patient. Moreover, the protocol requires two CBCT scans of the patient, which inherently increases the amount of radiation.

In 2013, Swennen and colleagues evaluated and validated "CBCT to image registration (also called Smart Fusion)" in order to obtain an AUM of the patient appropriate for 3D virtual orthognathic surgery planning without the use of plaster dental models.

Following "surface to image registration (STI)", the patient's head is augmented with accurate occlusal and intercuspidation data. Although the "CBCT to image registration protocol" has been validated on 30 orthognathic patients without the use of plaster dental models, it still needs to be integrated in the daily clinical workflow. Compared to the "Triple CBCT Scan Protocol", the imaging workflow for both image acquisitions as processing of the acquired image data towards a 3D virtual AUM of the patient is less time consuming and more user-friendly. Moreover, it requires only one CBCT patient scan in CR without deformation of the patient's facial soft tissue mask (► see also Sect. 1.1.1).

In 2013, Hernandez-Alfaro and Guijarro-Martinez evaluated intra-oral scanning of the patient's dentition to augment the patient's head with accurate occlusal and intercuspidation data in an in vitro (n = 3) and in vivo study (n = 6) based on "surface-based rigid registration". Intra-oral scanning of the dental arches of the patient in order to create an AUM is promising but still needs further validation towards accuracy in large prospective and consecutive patient series.

3D Virtual Augmented Model (AUM) of the Patient's Head "without the Use of Plaster Dental Models"

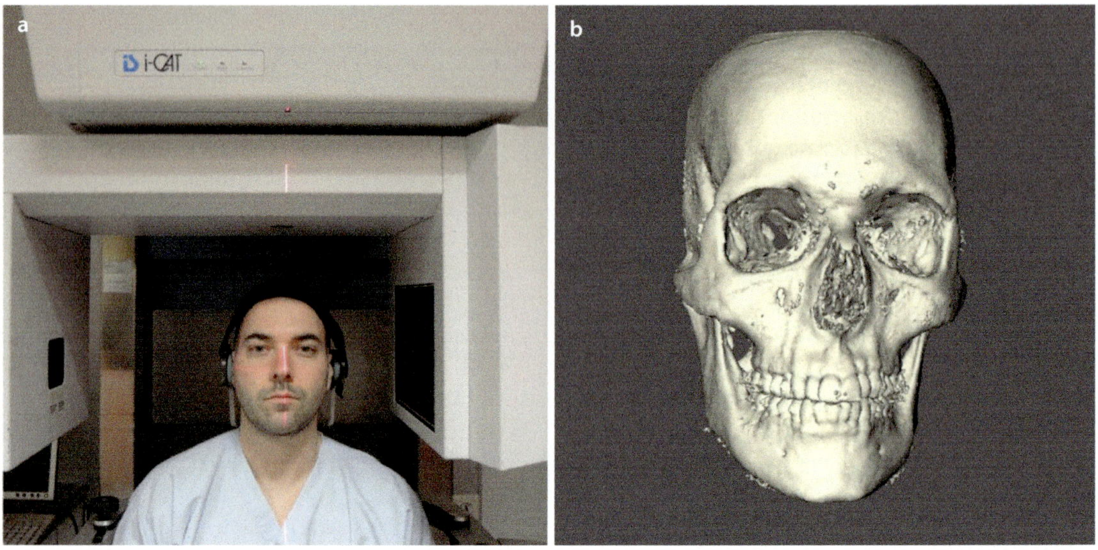

Fig. 1.17 CBCT scan N°1 in CR of the "Triple CBCT Scan Protocol". Volunteer M.G. was vertically scanned with a wax-bite wafer in place in a natural seated position (**a**) using a standardised CBCT scanning protocol ("i-CAT^{TM}, Imaging Sciences International, Inc., Hatfield, USA: extended field" modus; FOV, 17 cm diameter – 22 cm height; scan time 2 × 20 s; voxel size 0.4 mm at 120 kV according to DICOM field, 0018,0060 KVP, and 48 mA according to DICOM field, 0018,1151 XRayTubeCurrent). 3D "surface-rendered" (Maxilim v. 2.3.0.3) hard tissues surface representation (**b**) (volunteer M.G.). Note that there is no distortion of the lips neither of the cheeks

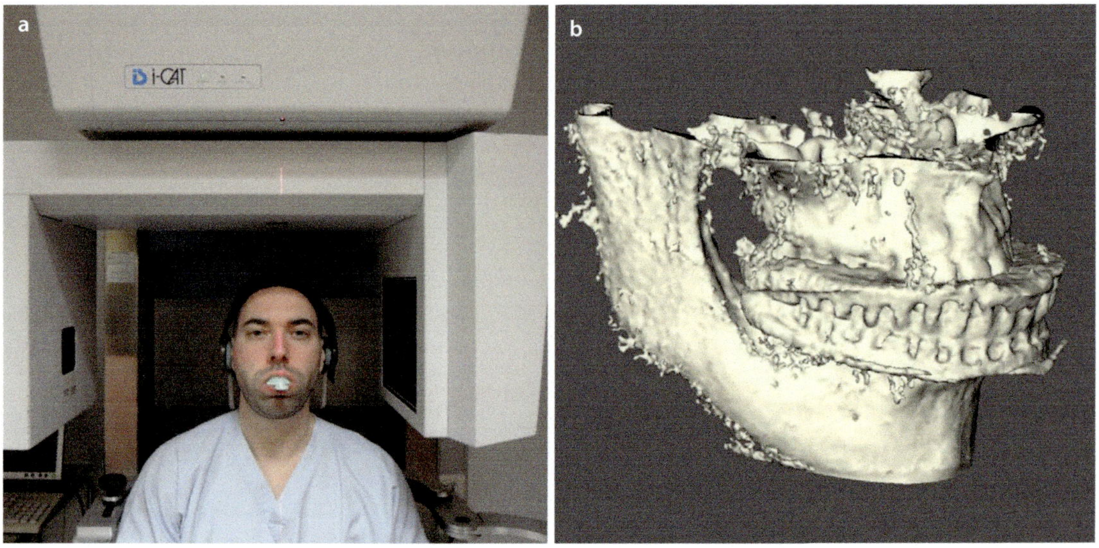

Fig. 1.18 "Low-dose" CBCT scan N°2 of the "Triple CBCT Scan Protocol". Volunteer M.G. was vertically scanned in a seated position with the Triple Tray® AlgiNot^{TM} impression in place (**a**) using a standardised CBCT scanning protocol ("i-CAT^{TM}, Imaging Sciences International, Inc., Hatfield, USA: FOV, 17 cm diameter – 8 cm height; scan time 1 × 10 s; voxel size 0.4 mm at 120 kV according to DICOM field, 0018,0060 KVP, and 48 mA according to DICOM field, 0018,1151 XRayTubeCurrent). 3D "surface-rendered" (Maxilim v. 2.3.0.3) hard tissues surface representation (**b**) (volunteer M.G.). Note the significant distortion of both the lips and the cheeks

3D Virtual Augmented Model (AUM) of the Patient's Head "without the Use of Plaster Dental Models"

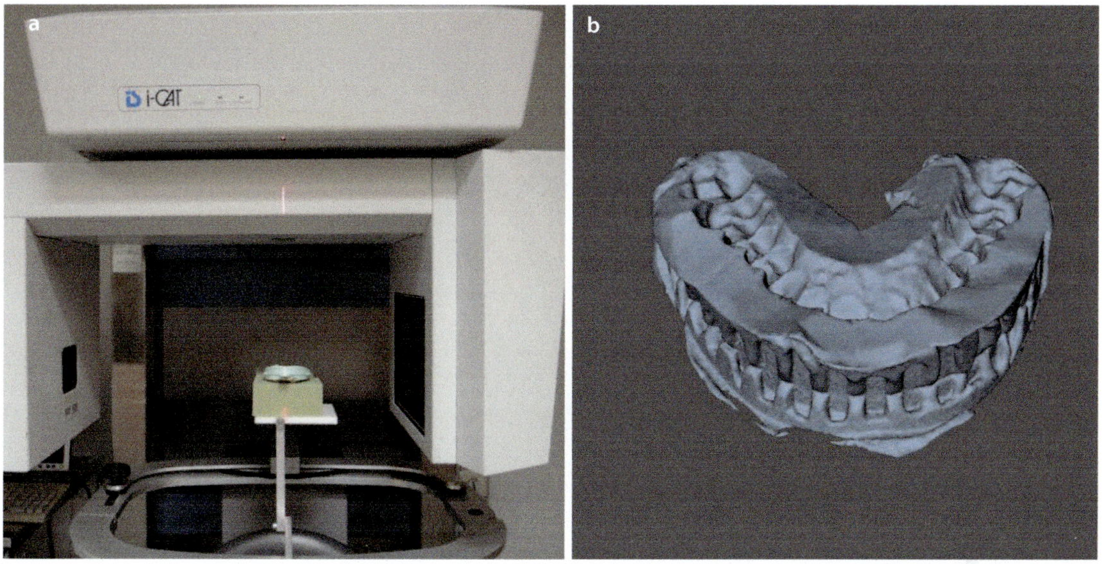

Fig. 1.19 "High-resolution" CBCT scan N°3 of the "Triple CBCT Scan Protocol". The Triple Tray® AlgiNot™ impression is scanned with the same CBCT apparatus (**a**) with high resolution using a standardised CBCT scanning protocol ("i-CAT™, Imaging Sciences International, Inc., Hatfield, USA: "high-resolution" modus; FOV, 17 cm diameter – 6 cm height; scan time 40 s; voxel size 0.2 mm at 120 kV according to DICOM field, 0018,0060 KVP, and 48 mA according to DICOM field, 0018,1151 XRayTubeCurrent). 3D "surface-rendered" (Maxilim v. 2.3.0.3) surface representation (**b**) (volunteer M.G.). Note that the impression is placed on a commercially available sponge instead of directly on the table of the CBCT apparatus to avoid segmentation problems

Rigid Registration

of the CBCT scan of the patient's head (► Sect. 1.1.1) and additional image acquisition of the patient's dentition (► Sect. 1.1.2) are mandatory for proper 3D virtual orthognathic surgery planning.

3D Virtual Augmented Model (AUM) of the Patient's Head "without the Use of Plaster Dental Models"

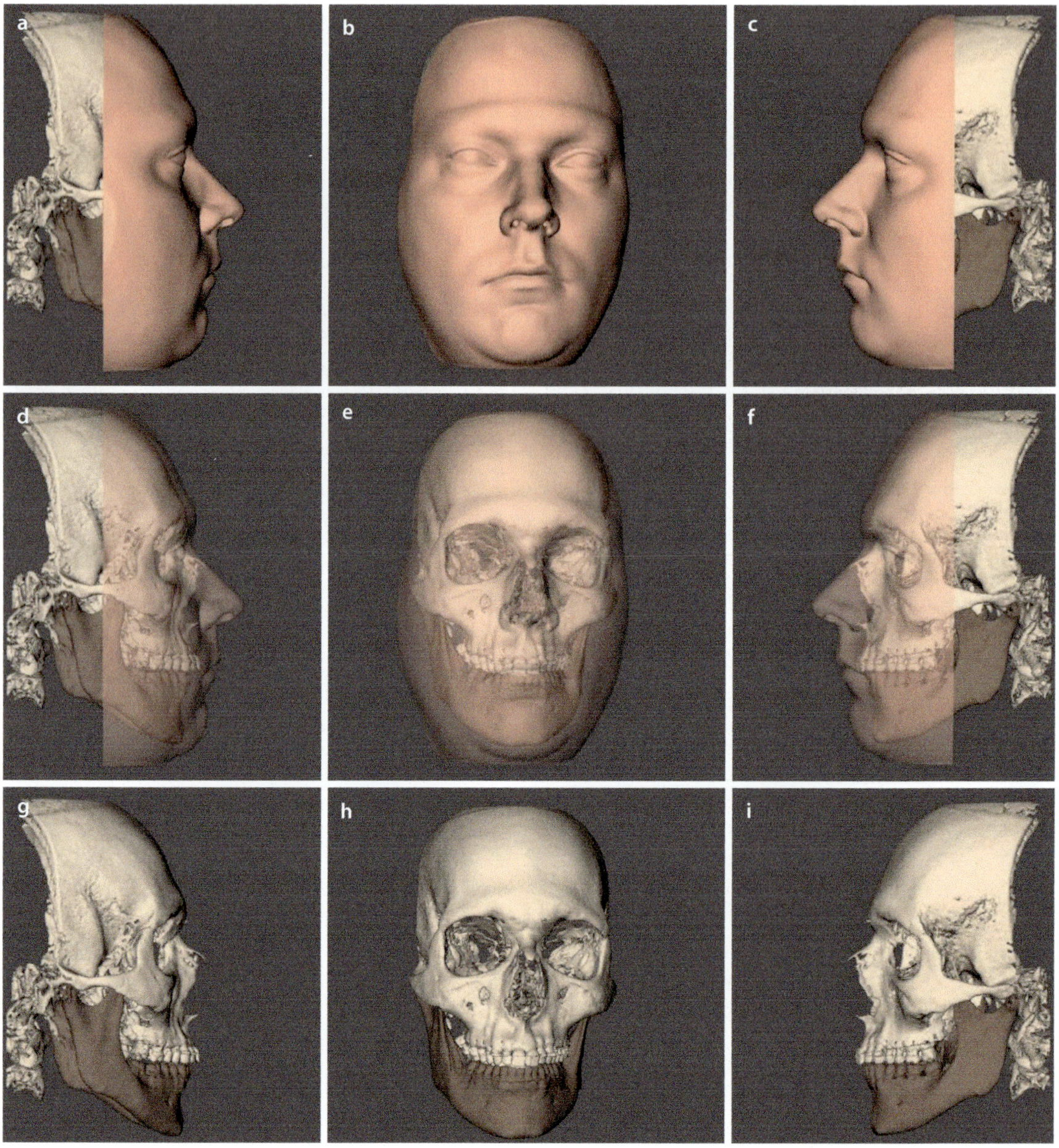

Fig. 1.20 Pre-surgical 3D "surface-rendered" AUM of the head following the "Triple Scan Protocol". Right profile (**a**, **d**, **g**), frontal (**b**, **e**, **h**) and left profile (**c**, **f**, **i**) views (i-CAT, Imaging Sciences International Inc., Maxilim v. 2.3.0.3., volunteer M.G.). Note the integration of accurate occlusal and intercuspidation data compared to Fig. 1.7. Also note the incorrect position and orientation of the patient's head although it was attempted to scan the patient in his correct NHP

3D Virtual Augmented Model (AUM) of the Patient's Head "without the Use of Plaster Dental Models"

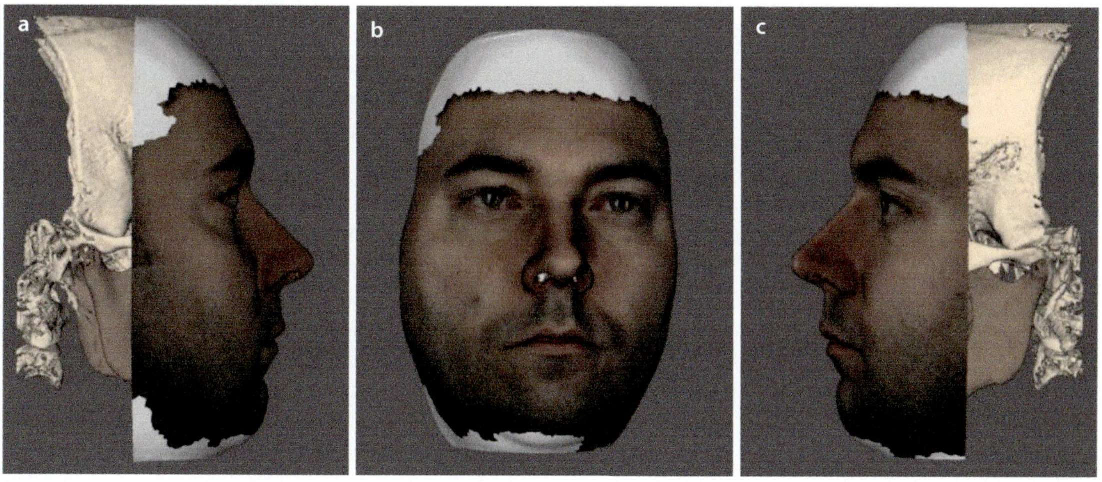

Fig. 1.21 Pre-surgical 3D "surface-rendered" AUM of the head following CBCT image acquisition (i-CAT, Imaging Sciences International Inc.) according to the "Triple Scan Protocol" with additional "surface-based rigid registration" of the 3D photograph (Planmeca ProMax® 3D Max, ProFace™, Planmeca Oy, Helsinki, Finland): right profile (**a**), frontal (**b**) and left profile (**c**) views (Maxilim v. 2.3.0.3., volunteer M.G.). Note the incorrect position and orientation of the head although it was attempted to scan volunteer M.G. in his correct NHP

Additional image acquisition (Sect. 1.1.3) and rigid registration of the texture of the patient's head is not essential for proper 3D virtual planning of orthognathic surgery (Fig. 1.21). Moreover, it is not recommended since it is still too error prone, too time consuming in the daily clinical routine and above can falsify the patient's 3D facial soft tissue mask.

It is therefore advised to use the CBCT 3D facial soft tissue mask for the following 3D virtual planning steps:

1. (3D-VPS_2) Definition of 3D cephalometric landmarks of the patient's soft tissues (► see also Sect. 2.2.3).
2. (3D-VPS_5) "Step-by-step" individualised 3D virtual treatment planning of orthognathic surgery (► see also Sect. 3.5).

However, additional image acquisition and rigid registration of the texture of the patient's head is certainly of interest in "Step 9 of 3D-VPS_5 – Patient Communication of the Individualised 3D Virtual Treatment Plan".

1.2.3 With the Use of Plaster Dental Models

In 2003, Gateno and colleagues were the first to describe a new technique to create a computerised composite patient model by integration of plaster dental models using sphere-type fiducial markers using "surface-based rigid registration". Although accurate, the major drawback of this protocol is the distortion of lip morphology and posture in the 3D AUM of the patient.

"CBCT to image registration" introduced and validated by Swennen and colleagues in 2013 to obtain an AUM of the patient appropriate for 3D virtual orthognathic surgery planning "without the use of plaster dental models" (▶ see also Sect. 1.2.2) can also be used "with the use of plaster dental models":

1. "CBCT Scan N°1": Full face scan of the patient in a vertical natural seated position in CR with a wax-bite in place without deformation of the facial soft tissue mask (▶ see also Sect. 1.1.1) (◘ Fig. 1.22)
2. "CBCT scan N°2": High-resolution scan of the plaster dental models (▶ see also Sect. 1.1.1) (◘ Fig. 1.23)

Following "surface to image rigid registration", the patient's head is augmented with accurate occlusal and intercuspidation data. The advantage compared to the above-mentioned protocol is that there is no distortion of lip morphology and posture (◘ Fig. 1.24).

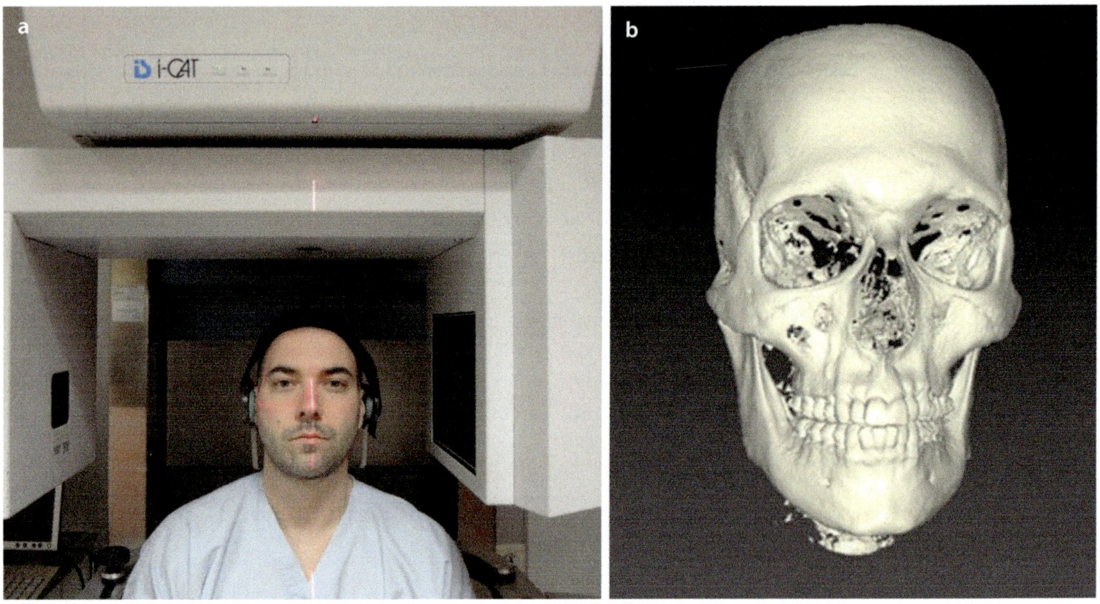

◘ **Fig. 1.22** CBCT scan N°1 in CR. Volunteer M.G. was vertically scanned with a wax-bite wafer in place in a natural seated position (**a**) using a standardised CBCT scanning protocol ("i-CAT™, Imaging Sciences International, Inc., Hatfield, USA: extended field" modus; FOV, 17 cm diameter – 22 cm height; scan time 2 × 20 s; voxel size 0.4 mm at 120 kV according to DICOM field, 0018,0060 KVP, and 48 mA according to DICOM field, 0018,1151 TubeCurrent. 3D. 3D "surface-rendered" (IPS CaseDesigner ALPHA version) hard tissues surface representation (**b**) (volunteer M.G.). Note that CBCT N°1 is the same as CBCT scan N°1 of the "Triple CBCT Scan Protocol" (◘ Fig. 1.17a)

3D Virtual Augmented Model (AUM) of the Patient's Head "with the Use of Plaster Dental Models"

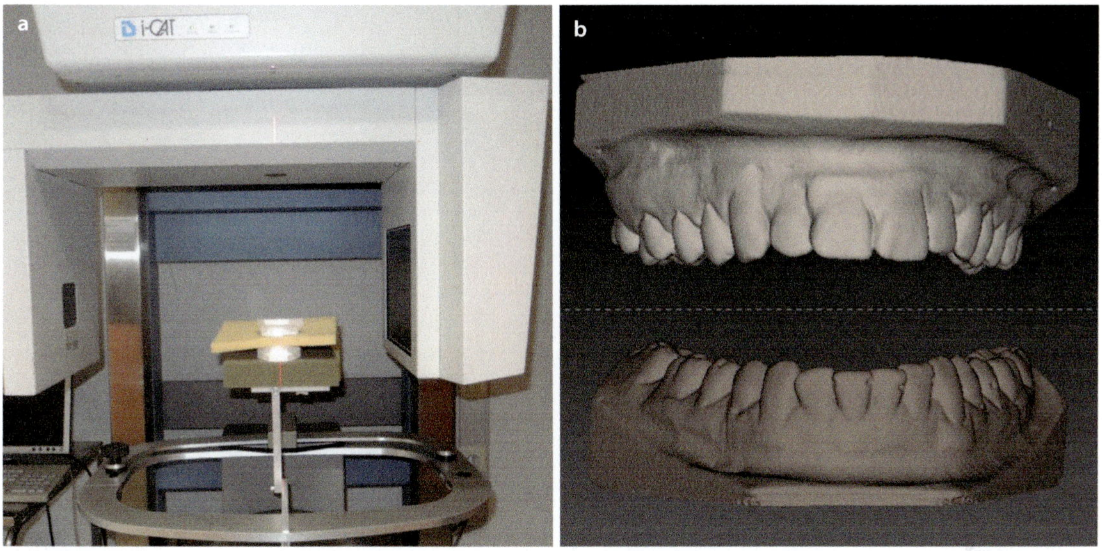

Fig. 1.23 "High-resolution" CBCT scan N°2 of the plaster dental models of the patient with the same CBCT apparatus (**a**) with high resolution using a standardised CBCT scanning protocol ("i-CAT™, Imaging Sciences International, Inc., Hatfield, USA: "high-resolution" modus; FOV, 17 cm diameter – 6 cm height; scan time 40 s; voxel size 0.2 mm at 120 kV according to DICOM field, 0018,0060 KVP, and 48 mA according to DICOM field, 0018,1151 TubeCurrent. 3D "surface-rendered" (IPS CaseDesigner ALPHA version) surface representation (**b**) (volunteer M.G.). Note that the plaster dental models are separated by a commercially available sponge in order to avoid segmentation problems (volunteer M.G.)

3D Virtual Augmented Model (AUM) of the Patient's Head "with the Use of Plaster Dental Models"

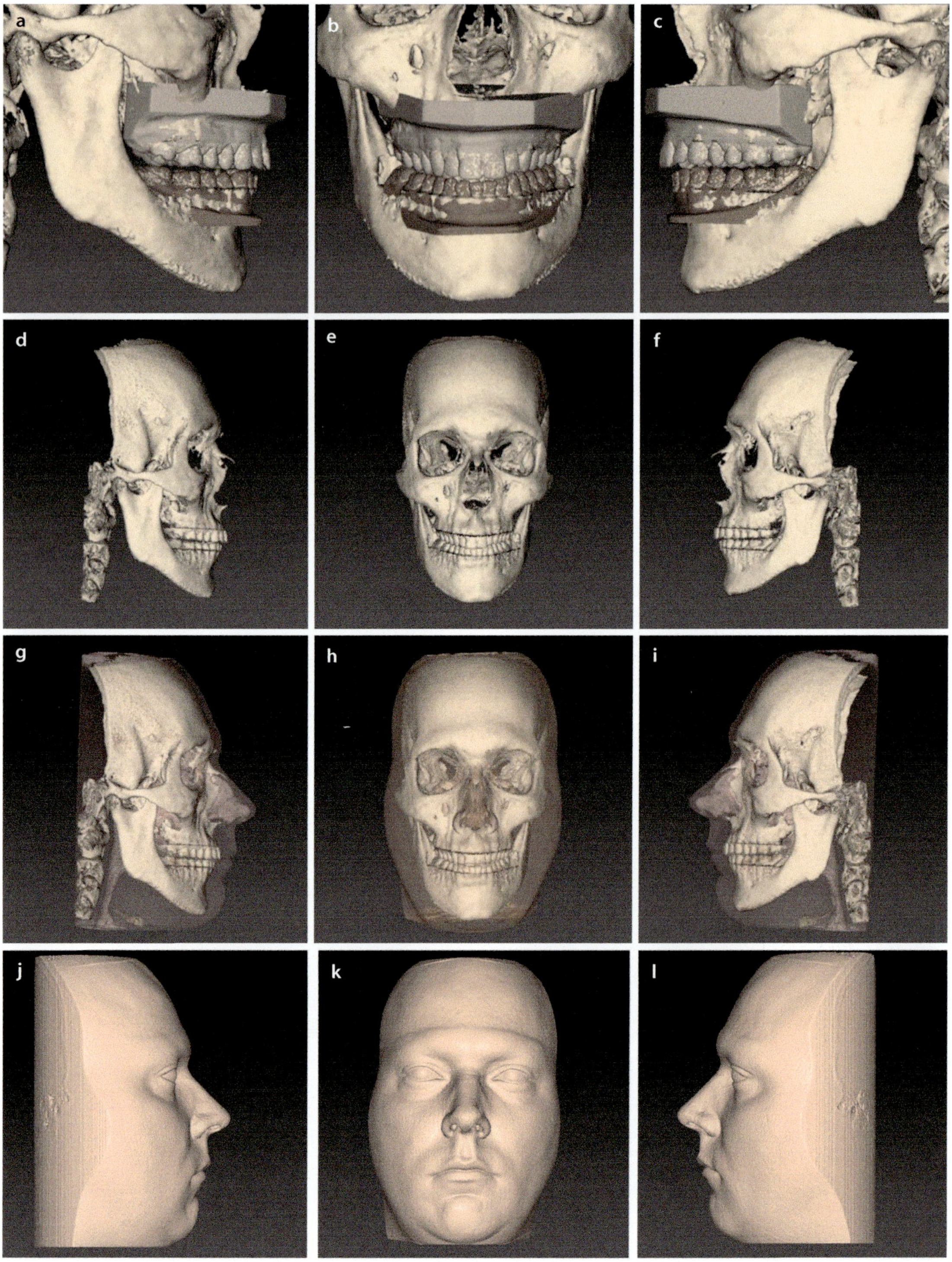

Fig. 1.24 Pre-surgical 3D "surface-rendered" AUM of the head following "CBCT to image registration" (**a**, **b**, **c**, **d**, **e**, **f**). Note the integration of accurate occlusal and intercuspidation data compared to Figs. 1.7 and 1.8. Additionally, 3D "volume-rendered" soft tissues are added: right profile (**g**, **j**), frontal (**h**, **k**) and left profile (**i**, **l**) views (i-CAT, Imaging Sciences International Inc., IPS CaseDesigner ALPHA version) (volunteer M.G.). Note that there is no distortion of lip morphology neither posture

"Step-by-Step" Quality Control of the 3D Virtual Augmented Model (AUM) of the Patient's Head

Whether the "3D virtual AUM of the patient's head" has been made "without the use of plaster dental models", "with the use of plaster dental models" or "which rigid registration process has been used", it is always imperative that the clinician verifies the patient's AUM at this stage before initiating further planning steps.

Therefore, a "Step-by-Step Quality Control Checklist" is provided (see also Addendum 1).

> *Step 1: Verification of the overall AUM of the patient by the clinician*:
> - Accuracy of registration of the upper dental arch
> - Accuracy of registration of the lower dental arch
> - Quality of the 3D rendering of the bone
> - Quality of the 3D rendering of the soft tissues
>
> *Step 2: Verification of the condyle (CR) position in the AUM of the patient by the clinician:*
> - Right condyle well seated in CR
> - Left condyle well seated in CR
>
> *Step 3: Verification of the overall soft tissue quality of the AUM of the patient by the clinician:*
> - Absence of eyebrow distortion (> fixation band during CBCT scanning)
> - Absence of lip distortion (> wax bite)
> - Lips in repose
> - Mentalis muscle relaxed
> - Absence of chin distortion (> chin support during CBCT scanning)

The "step-by-step" quality control of the 3D virtual augmented model of the patient's head is illustrated on volunteer M.G. but also on Case 1 (patient V.E.W.) which will be used throughout this book (► Chaps. 2, 3, 4, 5 and 6).

Step 1: Verification of the Overall AUM of the Patient by the Clinician

In this step, the clinician needs to verify (1) the accuracy of registration of the upper and lower dental arch and (2) the quality of the 3D rendering of the bone and the soft tissues.

Accuracy of Registration of the Upper and Lower Dental Arch

This is verified by evaluation of multiplanar orthogonal slices at molar, canine and incisal level and correlation with standardised clinical photographs (◘ Figs. 1.25, 1.26, 1.27, 1.28, 1.29, 1.30, 1.31).

> **Attention**
> It is the responsibility of the clinician to verify the patient's AUM before initiating further 3D virtual planning steps (3D-$VPS_{1\text{-}5}$).

Verification of the Accuracy of Registration of the Upper and Lower Dental Arch

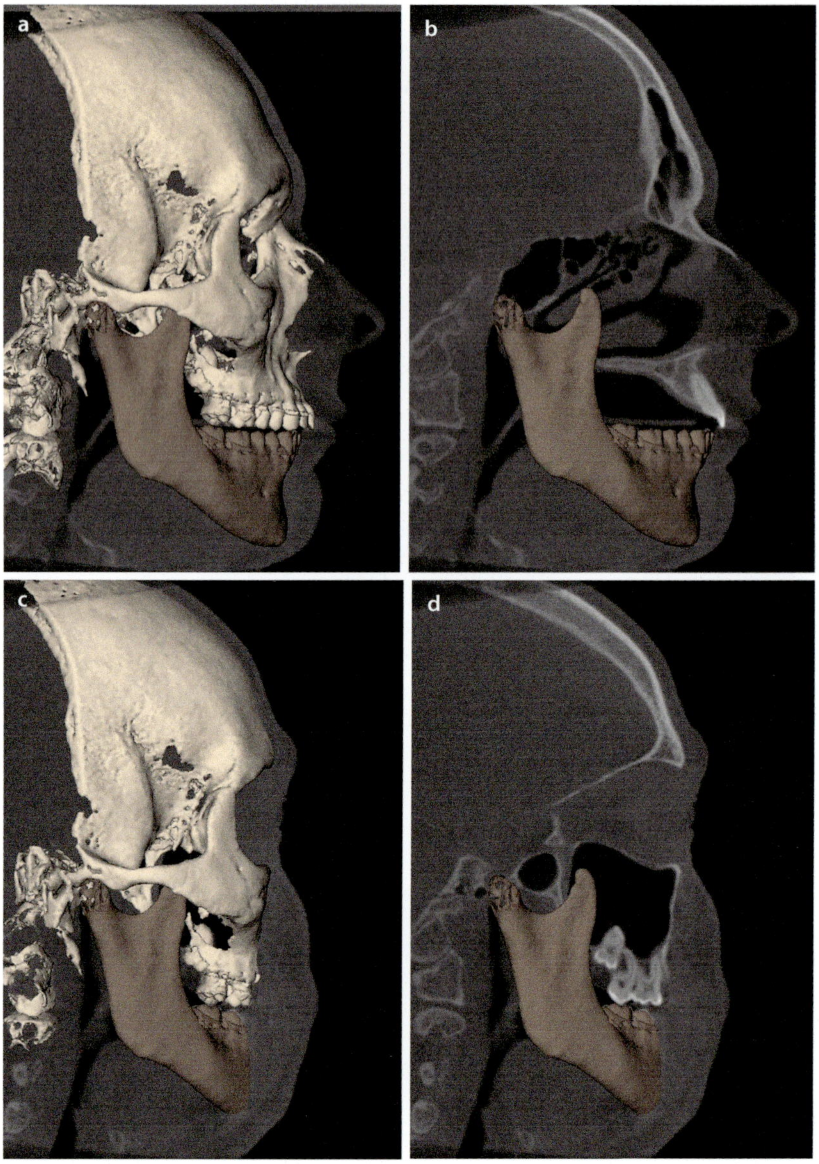

Fig. 1.25 "Step 1" of the "Step-by-Step Quality Control Checklist" of the AUM of the patient's head: accuracy of registration of the occlusal and intercuspidation surfaces of the upper dental arch. Perpendicular multiplanar orthogonal reslices are used to verify the accuracy of the registration at the upper dental midline and molar region: sagittal (**a**–**d**) and coronal (**e**, **f**) reslices (i-CAT, Imaging Sciences International Inc., Maxilim v. 2.3.0.3., volunteer M.G.). Note that triple voxel-based registration according to the "Triple Scan Protocol" (► see also Sect. 1.2.2) was used to register the CBCT scanned all-in-one impression of the dental arches with the CBCT scan of the patient's head

Verification of the Accuracy of Registration of the Upper and Lower Dental Arch

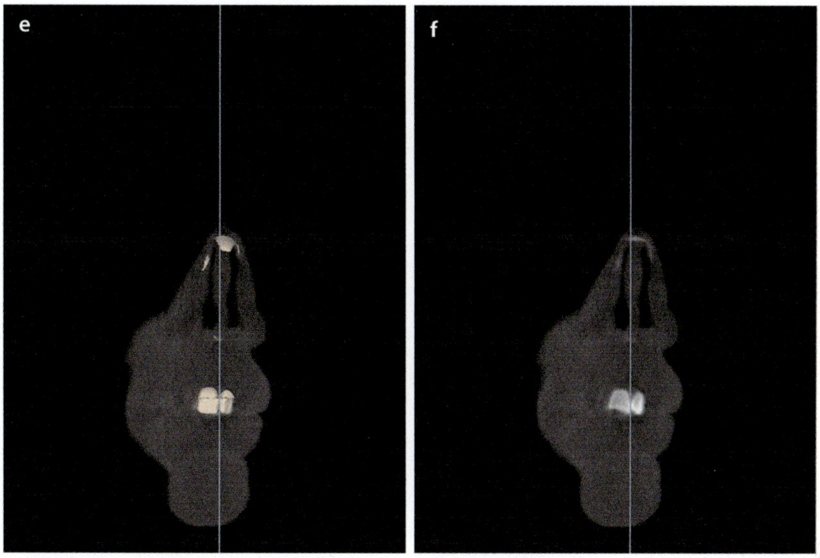

Fig. 1.25 (continued)

Verification of the Accuracy of Registration of the Upper and Lower Dental Arch

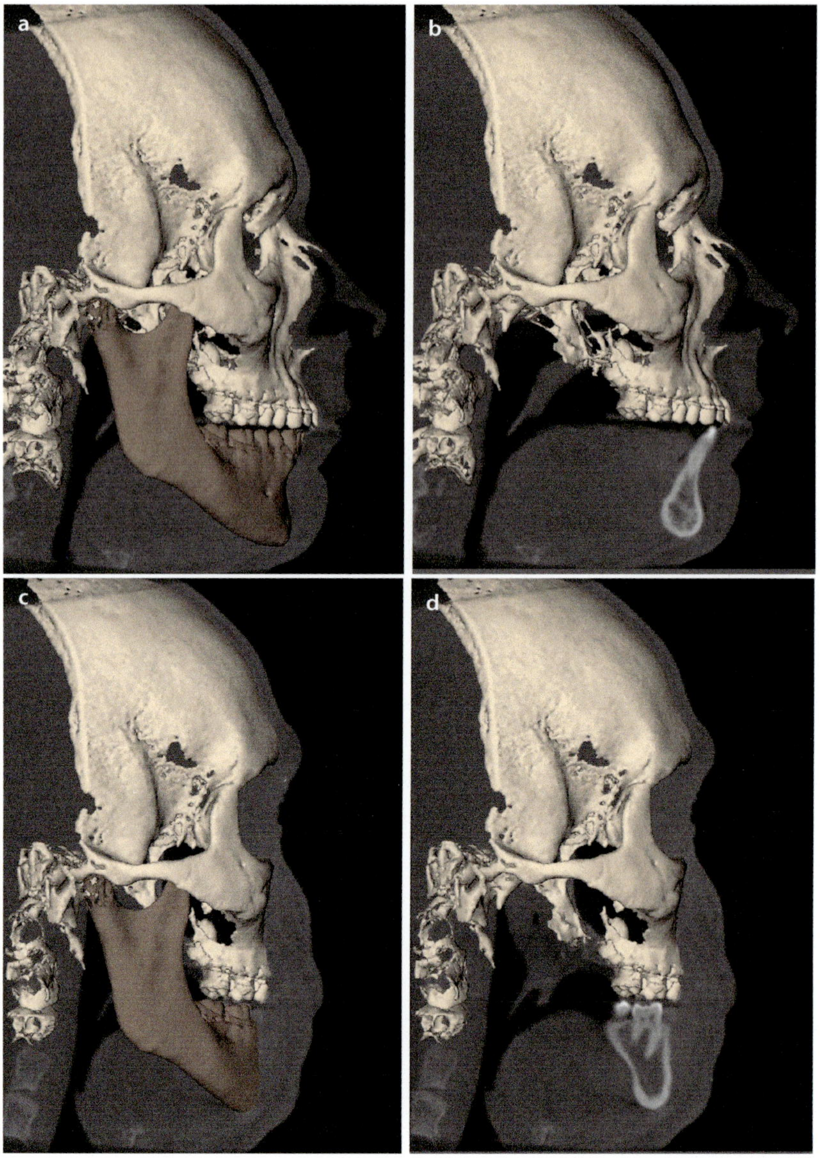

Fig. 1.26 "Step 1" of the "Step-by-Step Quality Control Checklist" of the AUM of the patient's head: accuracy of registration of the occlusal and intercuspidation surfaces of the lower dental arch. Perpendicular multiplanar orthogonal reslices are used to verify the accuracy of the registration at the lower dental midline and molar region: sagittal (**a**–**d**) and coronal (**e**, **f**) reslices (i-CAT, Imaging Sciences International Inc., Maxilim v. 2.3.0.3., volunteer M.G.). Note that triple voxel-based registration according to the "Triple Scan Protocol" (► see also Sect. 1.2.2) was used to register the CBCT scanned all-in-one impression of the dental arches with the CBCT scan of the patient's head

Verification of the Accuracy of Registration of the Upper and Lower Dental Arch

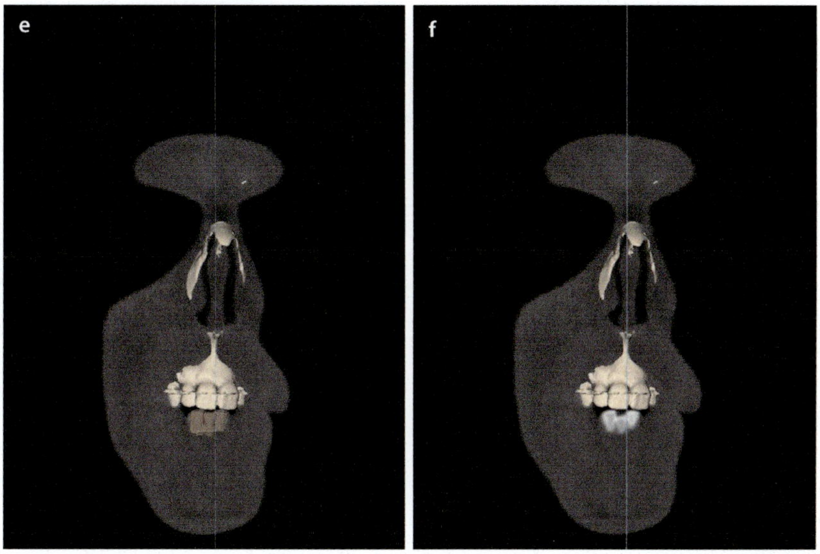

Fig. 1.26 (continued)

Verification of the Accuracy of Registration of the Upper and Lower Dental Arch

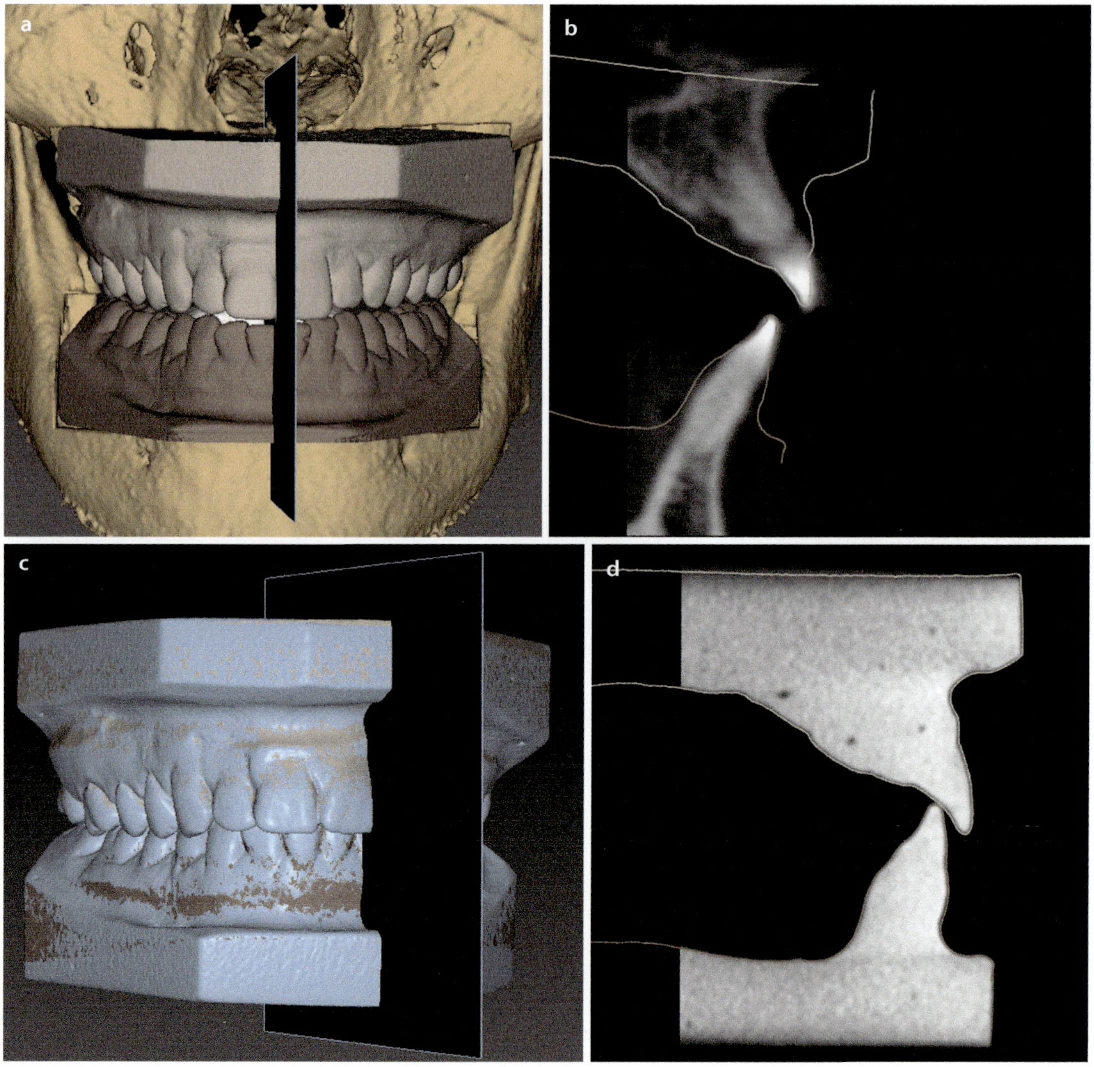

Fig. 1.27 "Step 1" of the "Step-by-Step Quality Control Checklist" of the AUM of the patient's head: accuracy of registration of the occlusal and intercuspidation surfaces of the upper and lower dental arches. Reslices perpendicular to the occlusal curve (**a**, **c**) are semi-automatically reconstructed and dynamically visualised (**b**, **d**) towards the clinician in a more user-friendly way (IPS CaseDesigner ALPHA version) to verify simultaneously the accuracy of registration of both the upper and lower dental arches (i-CAT, Imaging Sciences International Inc., volunteer M.G.). Note that "CBCT to image registration" was used to register the CBCT scanned plaster dental models with the CBCT scan of the patient's head (► see also Sect. 1.2.3)

Verification of the Accuracy of Registration of the Upper and Lower Dental Arch

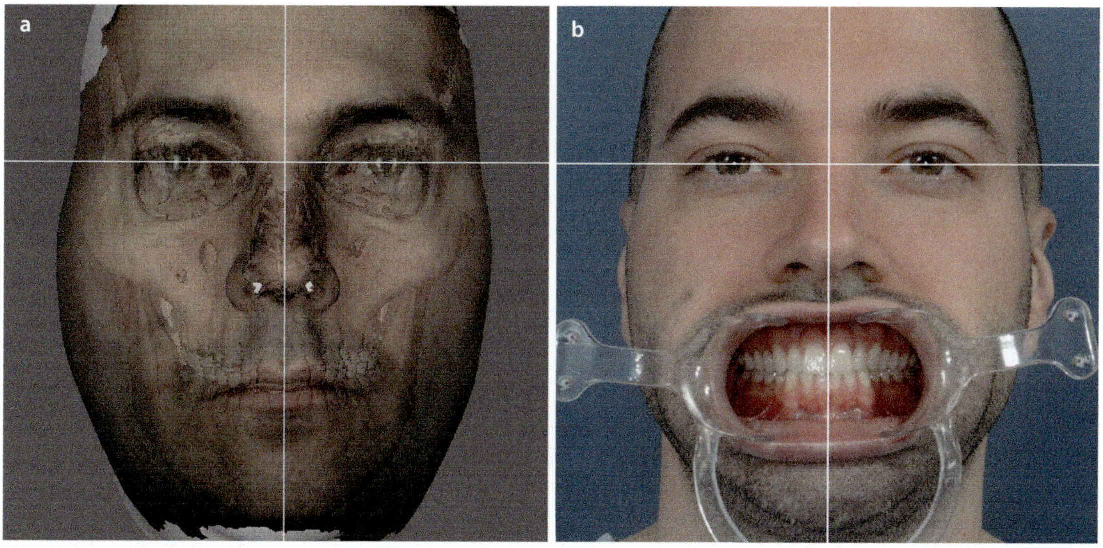

Fig. 1.28 "Step 1" of the "Step-by-Step Quality Control Checklist" of the AUM of the patient's head: correlation and comparison of the dental midlines between the AUM of the patient (**a**) and the standardised clinical frontal photograph (**b**) (i-CAT, Imaging Sciences International Inc., Maxilim v. 2.3.0.3., volunteer M.G.). Note that ideally cheek retractors are used (**b**)

Verification of the Accuracy of Registration of the Upper and Lower Dental Arch

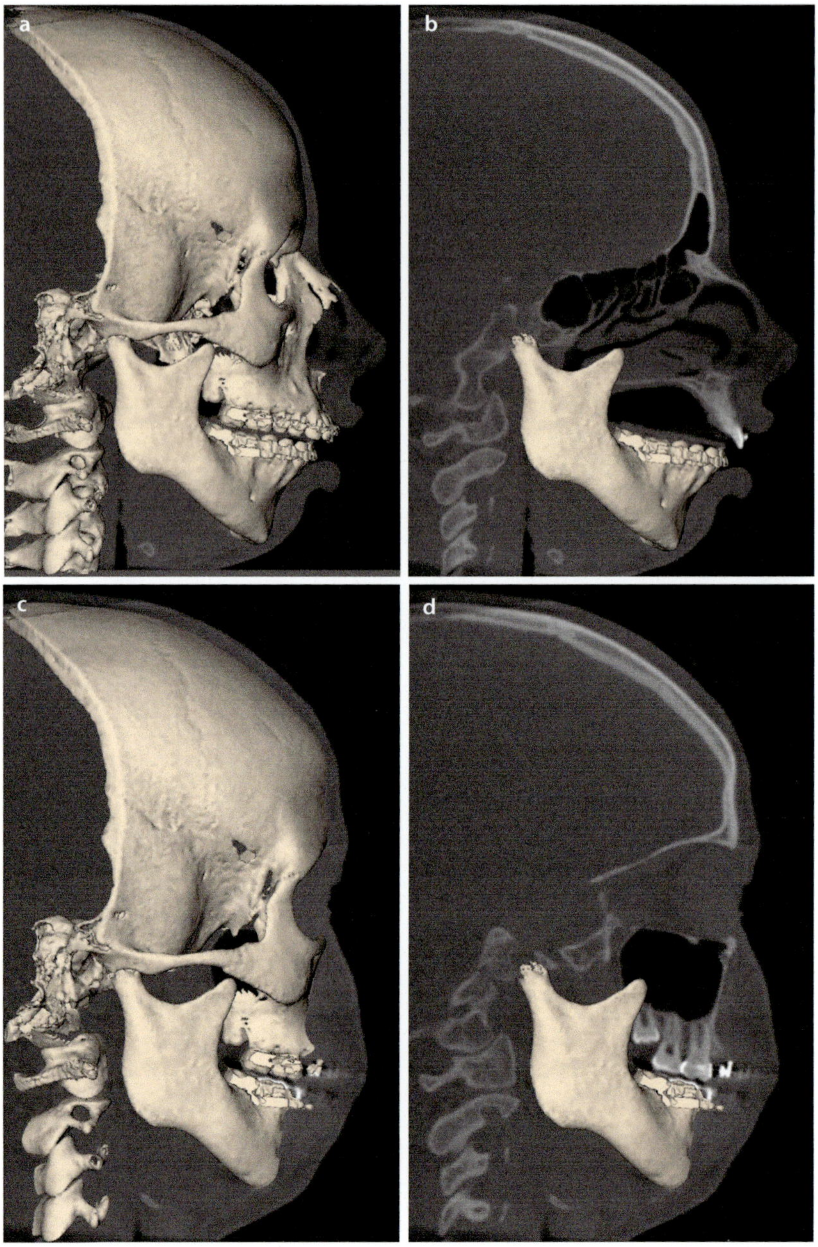

Fig. 1.29 "Step 1" of the "Step-by-Step Quality Control Checklist" of the AUM of the patient's head: accuracy of registration of the occlusal and intercuspidation surfaces of the upper dental arch. Perpendicular multiplanar orthogonal reslices are used to verify the accuracy of the registration at the upper dental midline and molar region: sagittal (**a**–**d**) and coronal (**e**, **f**) reslices (i-CAT, Imaging Sciences International Inc., Maxilim v. 2.3.0.3., patient V.E.W.). Note that triple voxel-based registration according to the "Triple Scan Protocol" (▶ see also Sect. 1.2.2) was used to register the CBCT scanned all-in-one impression of the dental arches with the CBCT scan of the patient's head

Verification of the Accuracy of Registration of the Upper and Lower Dental Arch

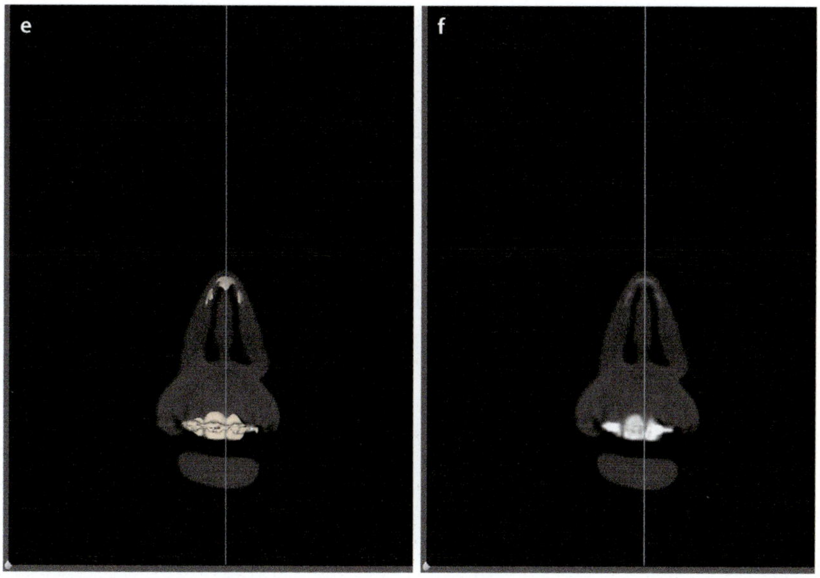

Fig. 1.29 (continued)

Verification of the Accuracy of Registration of the Upper and Lower Dental Arch

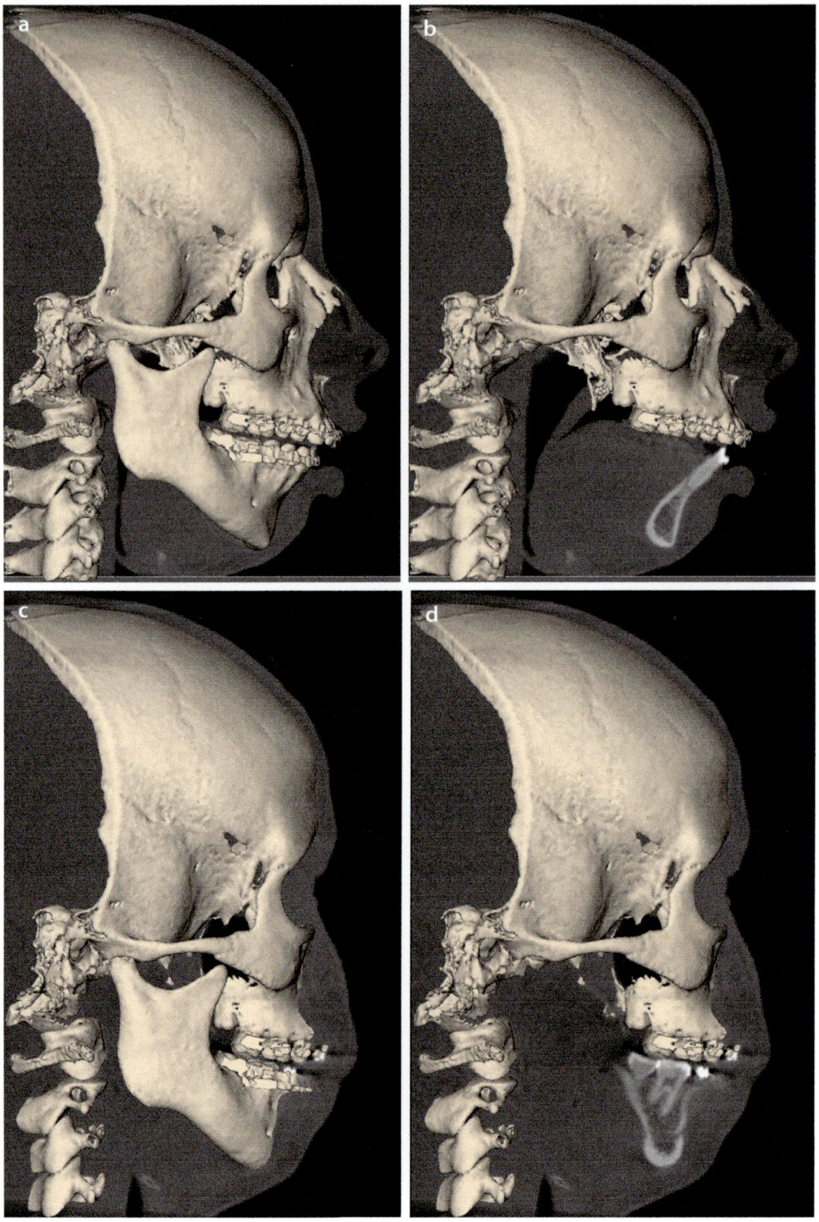

Fig. 1.30 "Step 1" of the "Step-by-Step Quality Control Checklist" of the AUM of the patient's head: accuracy of registration of the occlusal and intercuspidation surfaces of the lower dental arch. Perpendicular multiplanar orthogonal reslices are used to verify the accuracy of the registration at the lower dental midline and molar region: sagittal (**a–d**) and coronal (**e**, **f**) reslices (i-CAT, Imaging Sciences International Inc., Maxilim v. 2.3.0.3., patient V.E.W.). Note that the AUM was made following triple voxel-based registration according to the "Triple Scan Protocol" (▶ see also Sect. 1.2.2)

Verification of the Accuracy of Registration of the Upper and Lower Dental Arch

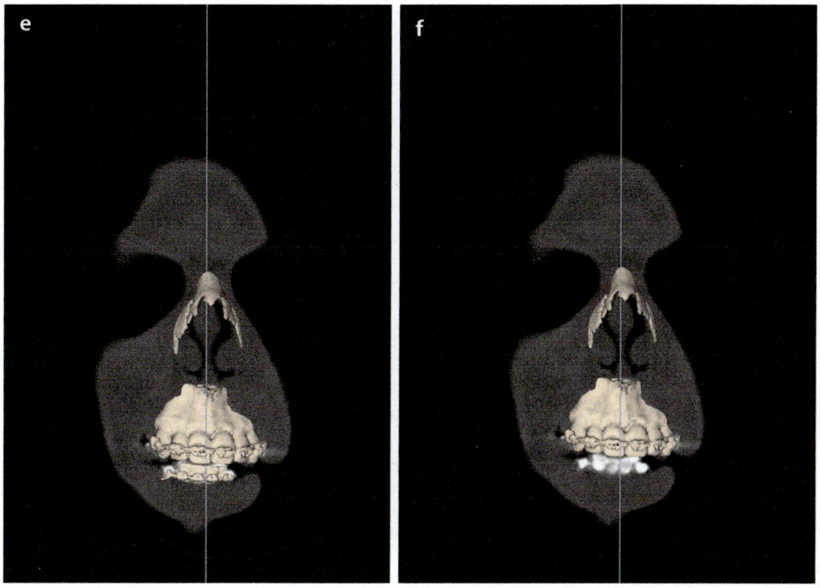

Fig. 1.30 (continued)

Verification of the Accuracy of Registration of the Upper and Lower Dental Arch

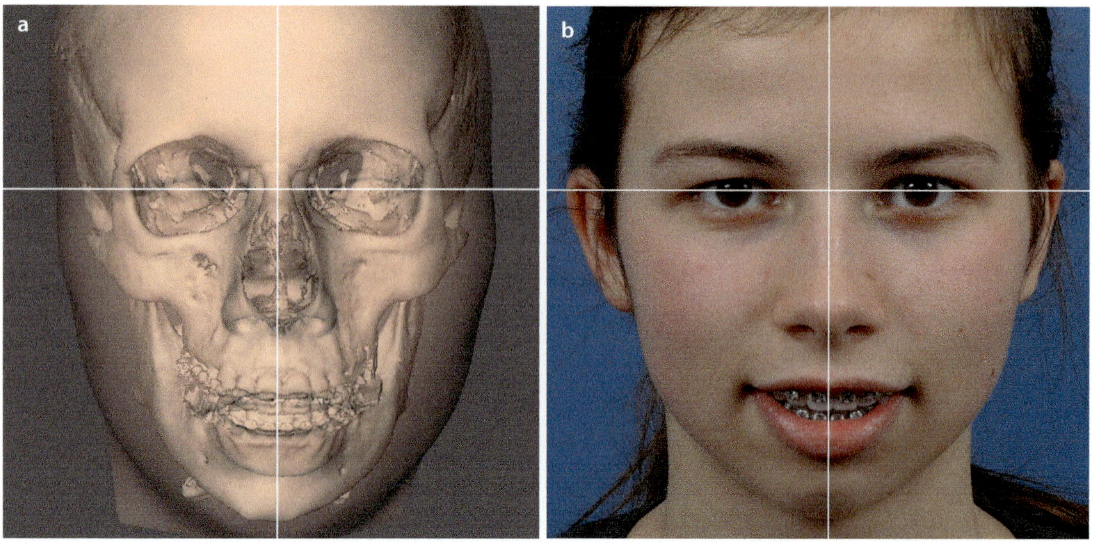

Fig. 1.31 "Step 1" of the "Step-by-Step Quality Control Checklist" of the AUM of the patient's head: correlation and comparison of the dental midlines between the AUM of the patient (**a**) and the standardised clinical frontal photograph (**b**) (i-CAT, Imaging Sciences International Inc., Maxilim v. 2.3.0.3., patient V.E.W.). Note that triple voxel-based registration according to the "Triple Scan Protocol" (▶ see also Sect. 1.2.2) was used to register the CBCT scanned all-in-one impression of the dental arches with the CBCT scan of the patient's head. Note that ideally cheek retractors are used (see Fig. 1.28b)

Trick

Aligning both the AUM of the patient and the standardised clinical frontal photograph based on the exocanthion and pupil landmarks followed by dropping a perpendicular line in the centre of the nasal root allows a clinical correlation of the upper dental midline position … it is crucial that no "Yaw" rotation of the patient's head (3D virtual vs 2D clinical) is present…

Quality of the 3D Rendering of the Bone and the Soft Tissues

The quality of the 3D "surface-rendered" soft (◻ Figs. 1.32a and 1.33a) and hard tissue (◻ Figs. 1.32b and 1.33b) surface representations of the patient's AUM needs to be verified by the clinician prior to all further "3D virtual planning steps (3D-VPS_{1-5})".

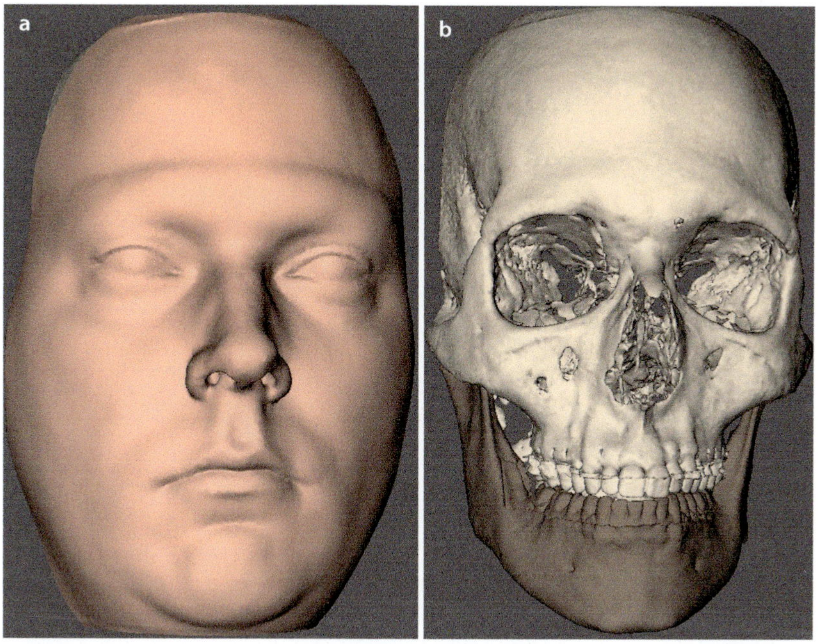

◻ **Fig. 1.32** "Step 1" of the "Step-by-Step Quality Control Checklist" of the AUM of the patient's head: overall appreciation of the quality of the rendering of the soft (**a**) and hard tissue (**b**) prior to 3D virtual planning of orthognathic surgery (i-CAT, Imaging Sciences International Inc., Maxilim v. 2.3.0.3., volunteer M.G.)

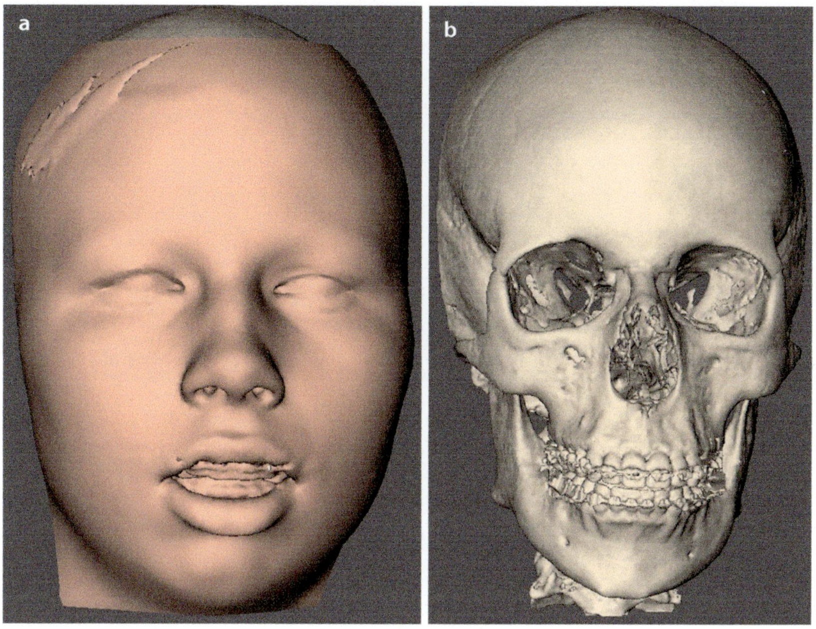

◻ **Fig. 1.33** "Step 1" of the "Step-by-Step Quality Control Checklist" of the AUM of the patient's head: overall appreciation of the quality of the rendering of the soft (**a**) and hard tissue (**b**) prior to 3D virtual planning of orthognathic surgery (i-CAT, Imaging Sciences International Inc., Maxilim v. 2.3.0.3., patient V.E.W.)

▪ Step 2: Verification of the Condyle (CR) Position in the AUM of the Patient by the Clinician

In this step, the clinician needs to verify if both condyles are well seated in CR.

As mentioned in Sect. 1.1.1, it is advised to always perform a CBCT scout view, prior to CBCT scanning of the patient's head. A CBCT scout view, however, remains a 2D representation and therefore does not absolutely exclude inappropriate seating of both condyles. Moreover, in the clinical daily routine, it unfortunately occurs that the CBCT scout view was performed inappropriately by the nursing imaging staff or even forgotten.

The CR position of both condyles in the patient's AUM is easily verified by evaluation of the sagittal and coronal slices (◘ Fig. 1.34 and 1.35).

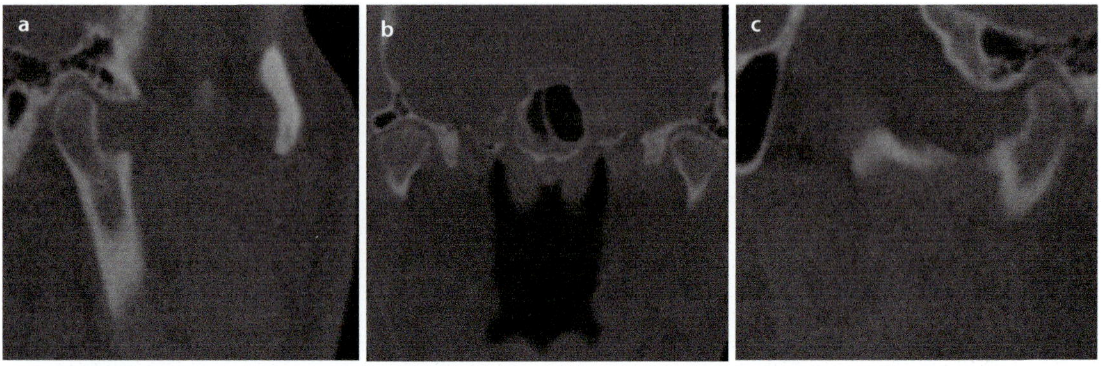

◘ **Fig. 1.34** "Step 2" of the "Step-by-Step Quality Control Checklist" of the AUM of the patient's head: the seating of both condyles in the glenoid fossa is evaluated with multiplanar orthogonal reslices in the sagittal (**a**, **c**) and coronal planes (**b**). Enhanced TMJ imaging and evaluation will be elaborated on in Sect. 2.1.4 (i-CAT, Imaging Sciences International Inc., Maxilim v. 2.3.0.3., volunteer M.G.). Note appropriate seating of both condyles in CR

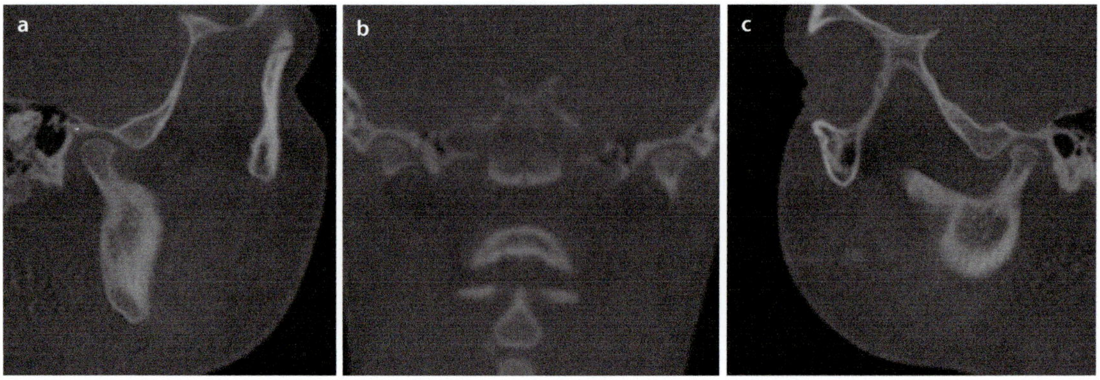

◘ **Fig. 1.35** "Step 2" of the "Step-by-Step Quality Control Checklist" of the AUM of the patient's head: the seating of both condyles in the glenoid fossa is evaluated with multiplanar orthogonal reslices in the sagittal (**a**, **c**) and coronal planes (**b**). Enhanced TMJ imaging and evaluation will be elaborated on in Sect. 2.1.4 (i-CAT, Imaging Sciences International Inc., Maxilim v. 2.3.0.3., patient V.E.W.). Note appropriate seating of both condyles in CR

■ Step 3: Verification of the Overall Soft Tissue Quality of the AUM of the Patient by the Clinician

In this step, the clinician needs to verify the overall soft tissue quality of the AUM of the patient: (1) absence of eyebrow distortion (due to the fixation band during CBCT scanning); (2) absence of lip distortion (due to the wax-bite wafer or registration devices); (3) lips in repose; (4) mentalis muscle relaxed and (5) absence of chin distortion (due to a chin support during CBCT scanning) (◘ Figs. 1.36, 1.37, 1.38, and 1.39).

As mentioned in Sect. 1.1.1, the patient needs to be scanned without deformation of the facial soft tissue mask and with relaxed lips. The clinician, however, is usually not present at the time of image acquisition.

Therefore, it is crucial that the nursing imaging staff is well trained and aware of all potential pitfalls during CBCT image acquisition as in conventional treatment planning. Unfortunately, distortion of an aesthetic unit of the facial mask of the patient can occur in the daily clinical routine. In such a case, the clinician needs to be aware since this will have its implications on soft tissue simulation and patient communication.

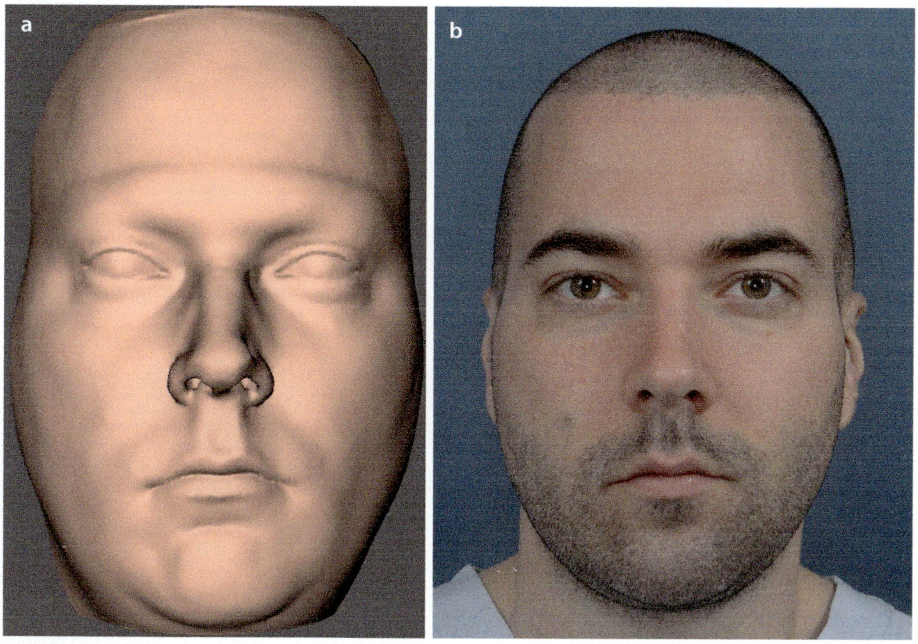

◘ **Fig. 1.36** "Step 3" of the "Step-by-Step Quality Control Checklist" of the AUM of the patient's head. The frontal 3D "surface-rendered" soft tissue representation (**a**) is correlated to the frontal standardised clinical photograph (**b**) (i-CAT, Imaging Sciences International Inc., Maxilim v. 2.3.0.3., volunteer M.G.). Note the distortion of the fronto-temporal soft tissues caused by the head fixation band that was placed too low on the forehead during CBCT scanning

Verification of the Overall Soft Tissue Quality of the AUM of the Patient by the Clinician

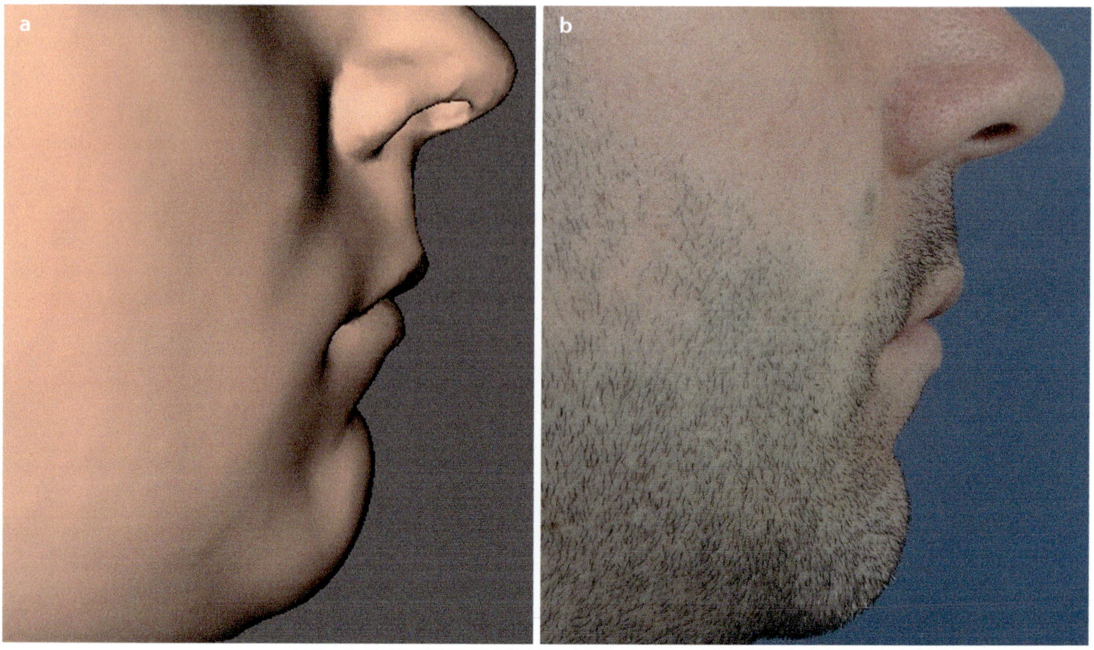

Fig. 1.37 "Step 3" of the "Step-by-Step Quality Control Checklist" of the AUM of the patient's head. The right profile 3D "surface-rendered" surface representation (**a**) is correlated to the right profile standardised clinical photograph (**b**) (i-CAT, Imaging Sciences International Inc., Maxilim v. 2.3.0.3., volunteer M.G.). Note the absence of lip and chin distortion, as well as absence of lip and mentalis muscle contraction

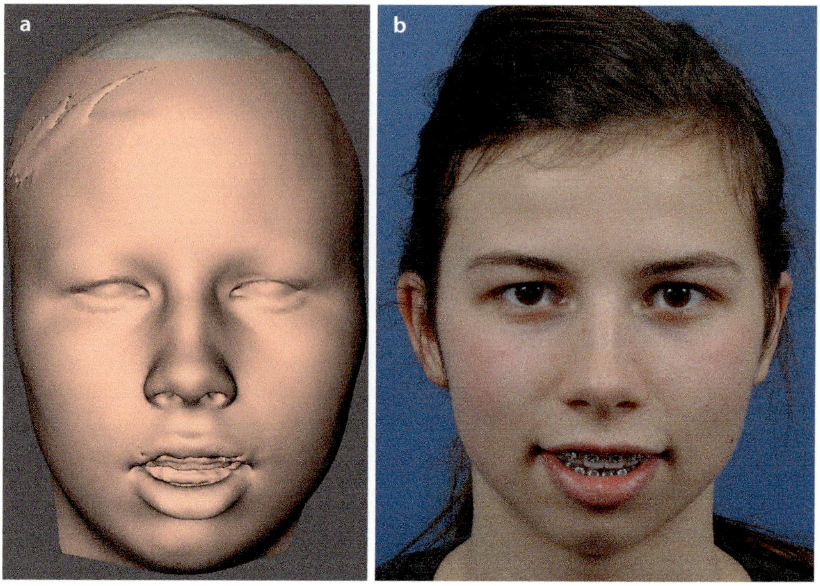

Fig. 1.38 "Step 3" of the "Step-by-Step Quality Control Checklist" of the AUM of the patient's head. The frontal 3D "surface-rendered" soft tissue representation (**a**) is correlated to the frontal standardised clinical photograph (**b**) (i-CAT, Imaging Sciences International Inc., Maxilim v. 2.3.0.3., patient V.E.W.). Note that there is no distortion of the fronto-temporal soft tissues due to proper position of the head fixation band during CBCT scanning

Verification of the Overall Soft Tissue Quality of the AUM of the Patient by the Clinician

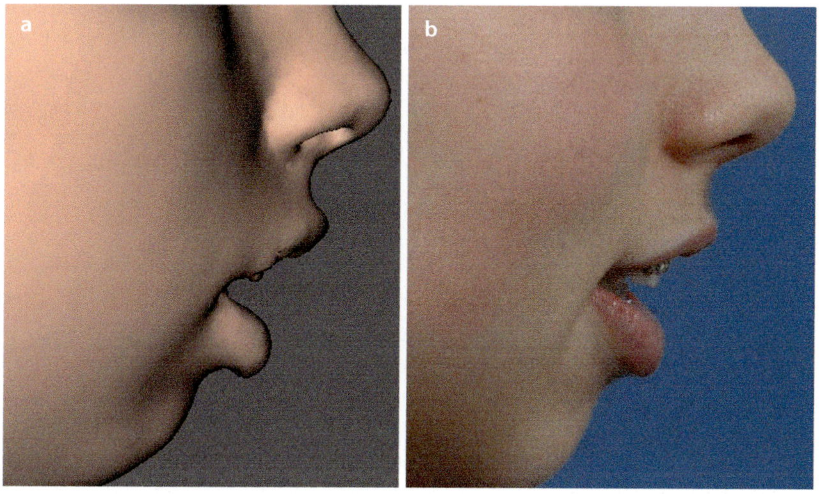

Fig. 1.39 "Step 3" of the "Step-by-Step Quality Control Checklist" of the AUM of the patient's head. The right profile 3D "surface-rendered" surface representation (**a**) is correlated to the right profile standardised clinical photograph (**b**) (i-CAT, Imaging Sciences International Inc., Maxilim v. 2.3.0.3., patient V.E.W.). Note the absence of lip and chin distortion, as well as absence of lip and mentalis muscle contraction

Attention

A prerequisite for proper 3D virtual soft tissue simulation consists of adequate image acquisition of the patient's head (► Sect. 1.1.1.) without deformation of the facial soft tissue mask especially lip morphology and posture.

1.3 Virtual Mandibular Autorotation

The relevance and potential of predicting "mandibular autorotation" in orthognathic surgery have already been discussed in the late 1970s by Bell and Jacobs (1979) and in the beginning of the 1980s by Epker and Fish (1980), Sperry and colleagues (1982) and Wessberg and colleagues (1982). Relative mandibular deficiency can be treated by isolate Le Fort I surgery to reposition the maxilla superiorly to allow forward and upward movement of the retropositioned mandible by autororation Bell and Jacobs 1979). It was initially presumed that during superior repositioning of the maxilla, the mandible autorotates forward and upwards at pogonion with the condyle being the centre of mandibular autorotation (Epker and Fish 1980). Evidence with lateral head films taken in centric occlusion (CO) showed that the centre of mandibular rotation was rather in the mastoid region (Sperry and colleagues 1982). All attempts in the past to calculate the "centre of mandibular autorotation" and "the arc of mandibular autorotation" were inherently biassed because of 2D image acquisition based on lateral cephalograms.

The "3D virtual visualisation paradigm" and "3D Virtual Scene Approach" have the potential to visualise and calculate the "centre of mandibular autorotation" and "the arc of mandibular autorotation" in the 3D virtual scene.

In 2013, Swennen and colleagues evaluated the potential of 3D image acquisition by means of the "CBCT triple scan protocol" (▶ see also Sect. 1.2.2) to calculate the "individual 3D virtual mandibular autorotation" in 50 consecutive prospective orthognathic cases.

1. "CBCT scan N° 1" was performed in CR following the "CBCT triple scan protocol" (▣ Fig. 1.40).
2. "CBCT scan N° 2" was performed with a forced opening of the bite due to the thickness of the Triple Tray® AlgiNot™ all-in-one impression (▣ Fig. 1.41).

In order to evaluate the mandibular displacement, "voxel-based registration" (▶ see also Sect. 5.1.1) of CBCT scan N°2 on CBCT scan N°1 was performed based on the maxillary anatomy. In only 25 % of the cases, no condylar dislocations or translations did occur. This finding could be explained by the fact that CBCT scan N° 2 was not performed in CR in the original "CBCT triple scan protocol".

By modification of the "CBCT triple scan protocol" and performing CBCT scan N°2 also in CR, the "individual 3D virtual mandibular autorotation" can be visualised in the 3D virtual scene (▣ Figs. 1.42, 1.43 and 1.44).

> The "3D Virtual Visualisation Paradigm" and the "3D Virtual Scene Approach" have the potential to visualise the "individual 3D virtual mandibular autorotation" and to calculate the "centre and arc of mandibular autorotation" ... from a computational point of view this is currently still highly demanding...

Case 7: Class III, Midfacial Hypoplasia (Patient B.B.)

To illustrate the concept of visualisation of 3D virtual mandibular autorotation, patient B.B. is used (▶ see also Chap. 6).

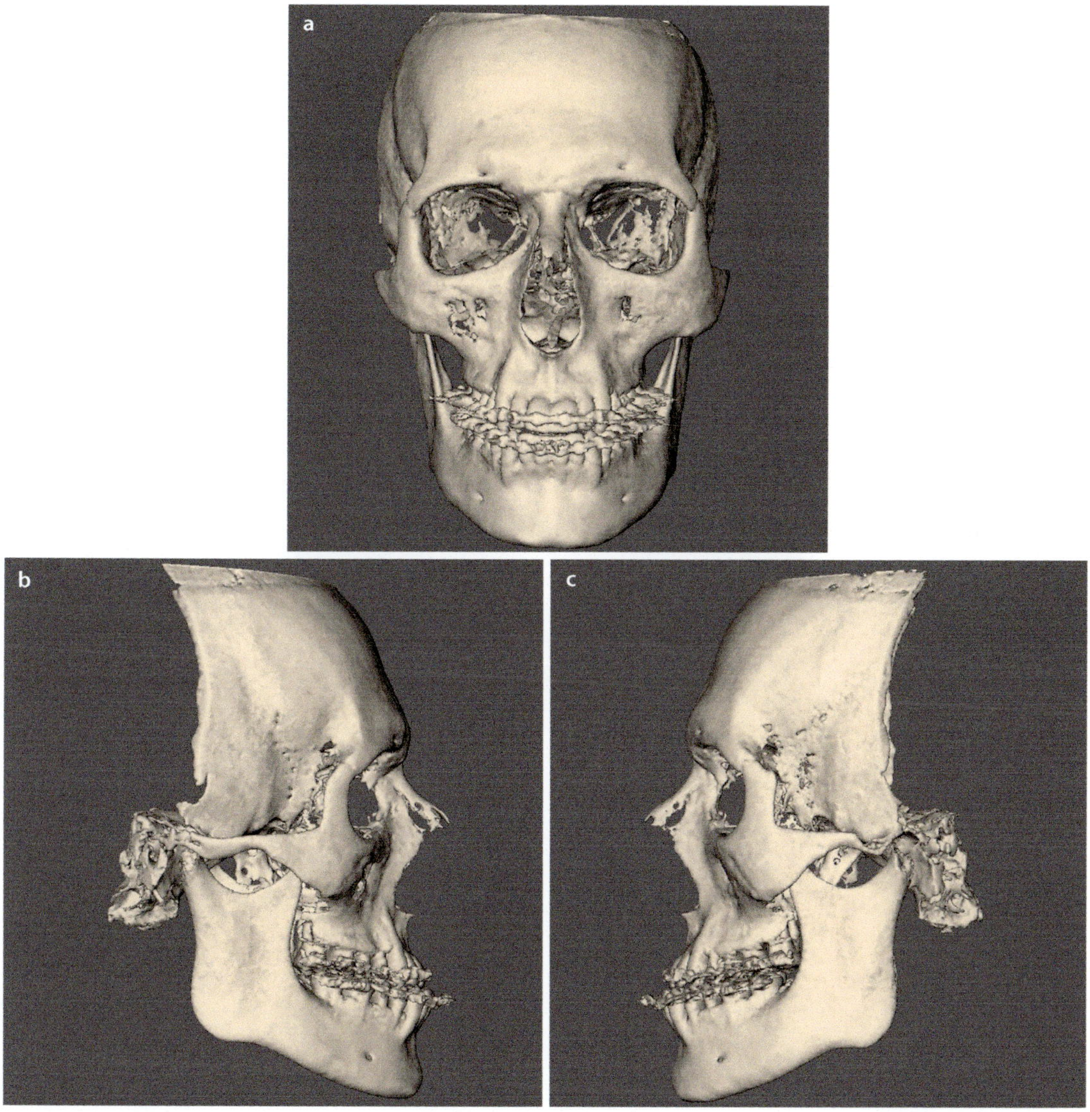

Fig. 1.40 CBCT scan N°1 in CR of the "Triple CBCT Scan Protocol" (▶ see also Sect. 1.2.2). 3D "surface-rendered" (Maxilim v. 2.3.0.3) frontal (**a**), right profile (**b**) and left (**c**) hard tissues surface representations. Patient B.B. was vertically scanned with a wax-bite wafer in place in a natural seated position using a standardised CBCT scanning protocol ("i-CAT^{TM}, Imaging Sciences International, Inc., Hatfield, USA, extended field" modus; FOV, 17 cm diameter – 22 cm height; scan time 2 × 20 s; voxel size 0.4 mm at 120 kV according to DICOM field, 0018,0060 KVP, and 48 mA according to DICOM field, 0018,1151 XRayTubeCurrent) (patient B.B.)

■ Visualisation of 3D Virtual Mandibular Autorotation

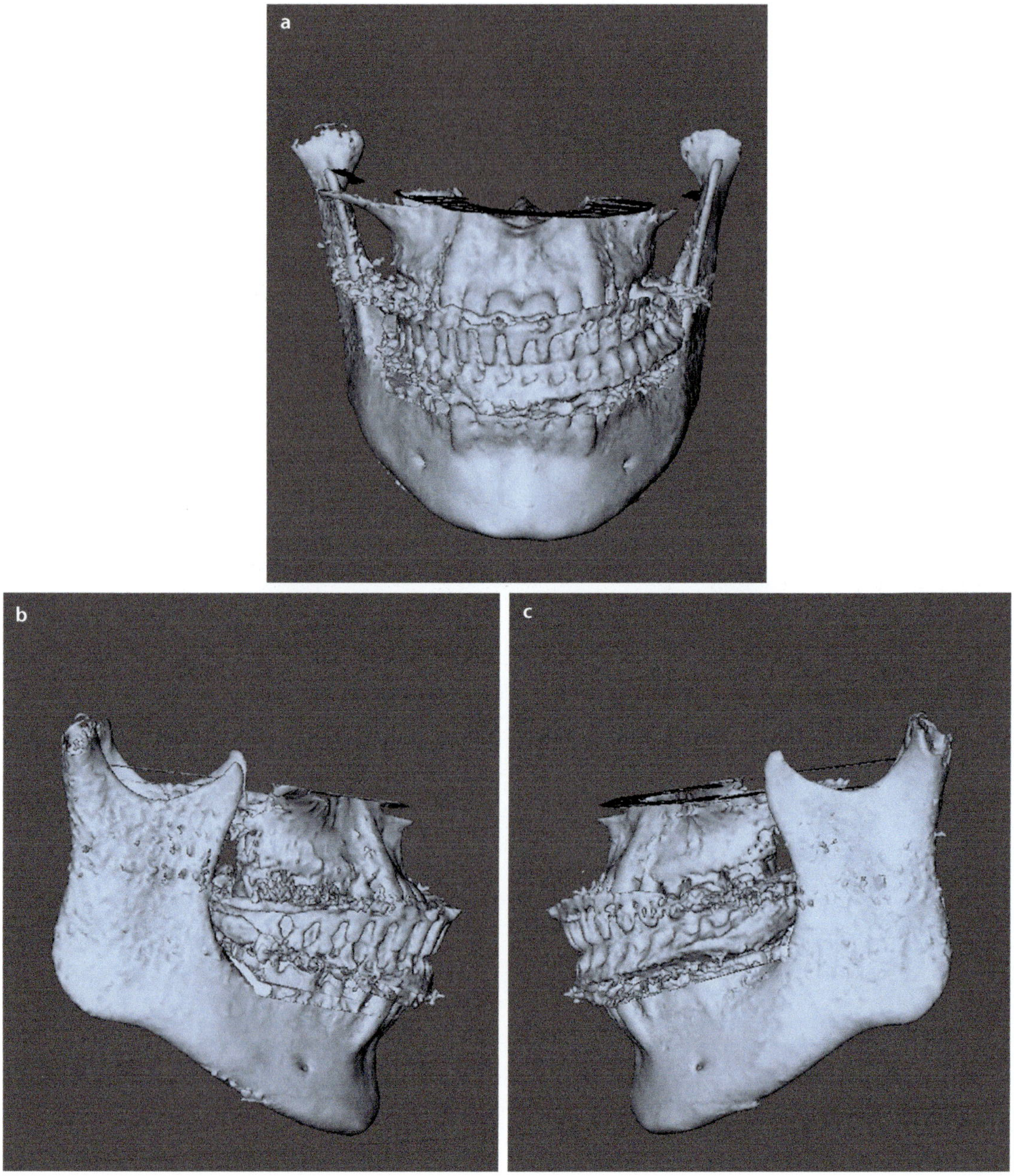

Fig. 1.41 CBCT scan N°2 in CR of the "Triple CBCT Scan Protocol" (▶ see also Sect. 1.2.2) with forced opening of the bite due to the Triple Tray® AlgiNot™ impression in place. 3D "surface-rendered" (Maxilim v. 2.3.0.3) frontal (**a**), right profile (**b**) and left (**c**) hard tissues surface representations ("i-CAT™, Imaging Sciences International, Inc., Hatfield, USA; FOV, 17 cm diameter – 8 cm height; scan time 1 × 10 s; voxel size 0.4 mm at 120 kV according to DICOM field, 0018,0060 KVP, and 48 mA according to DICOM field, 0018,1151 XRayTubeCurrent) (patient B.B.)

Visualisation of 3D Virtual Mandibular Autorotation

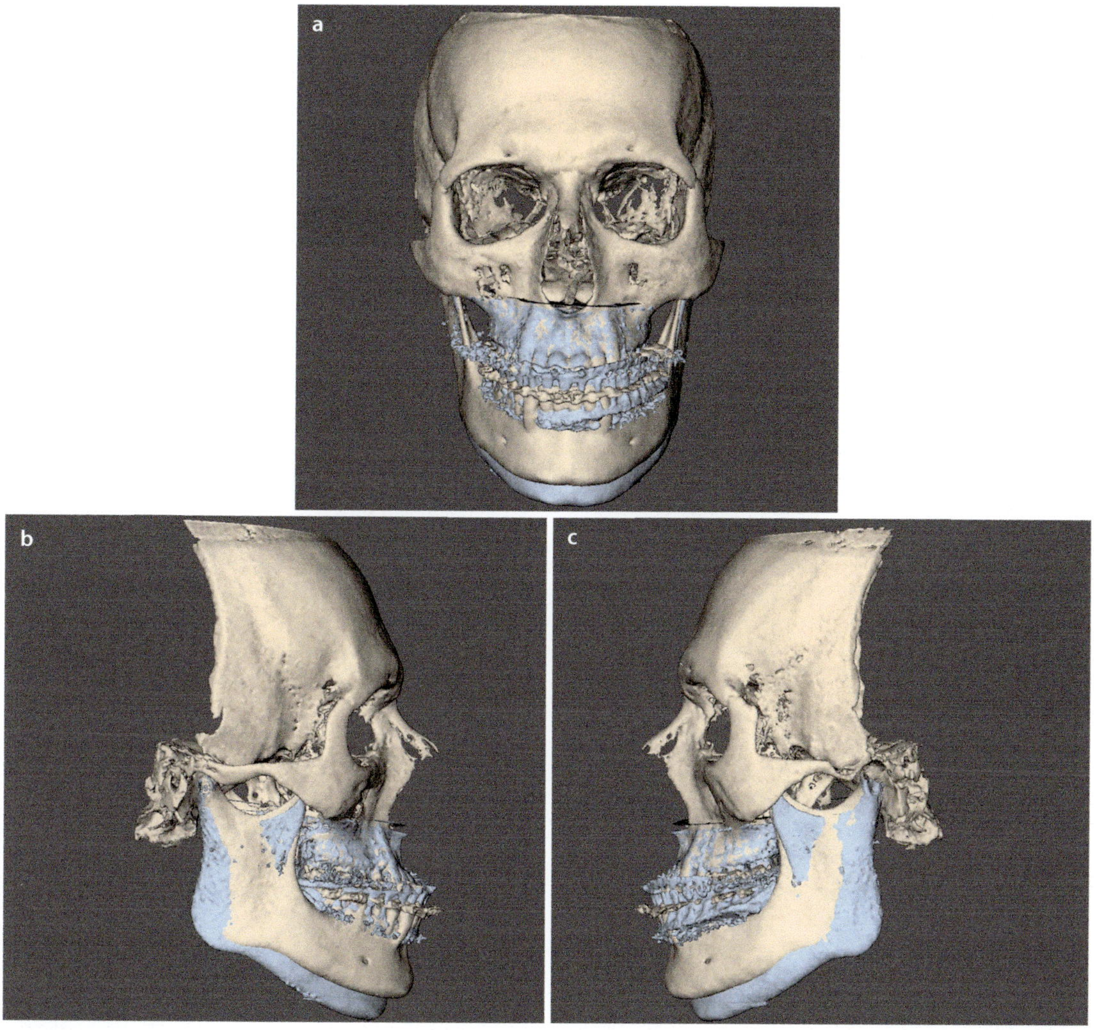

Fig. 1.42 Voxel-based registration of CBCT scan N°2 on CBCT scan N°1 based on the maxillary anatomy. Note the individual CW mandibular autorotation of patient B.B. 3D "surface-rendered" frontal (**a**), right profile (**b**) and left (**c**) hard tissues surface representations ("i-CAT^{TM}, Imaging Sciences International, Inc., Hatfield, USA, Maxilim v. 2.3.0.3) (patient B.B.)

Visualisation of 3D Virtual Mandibular Autorotation

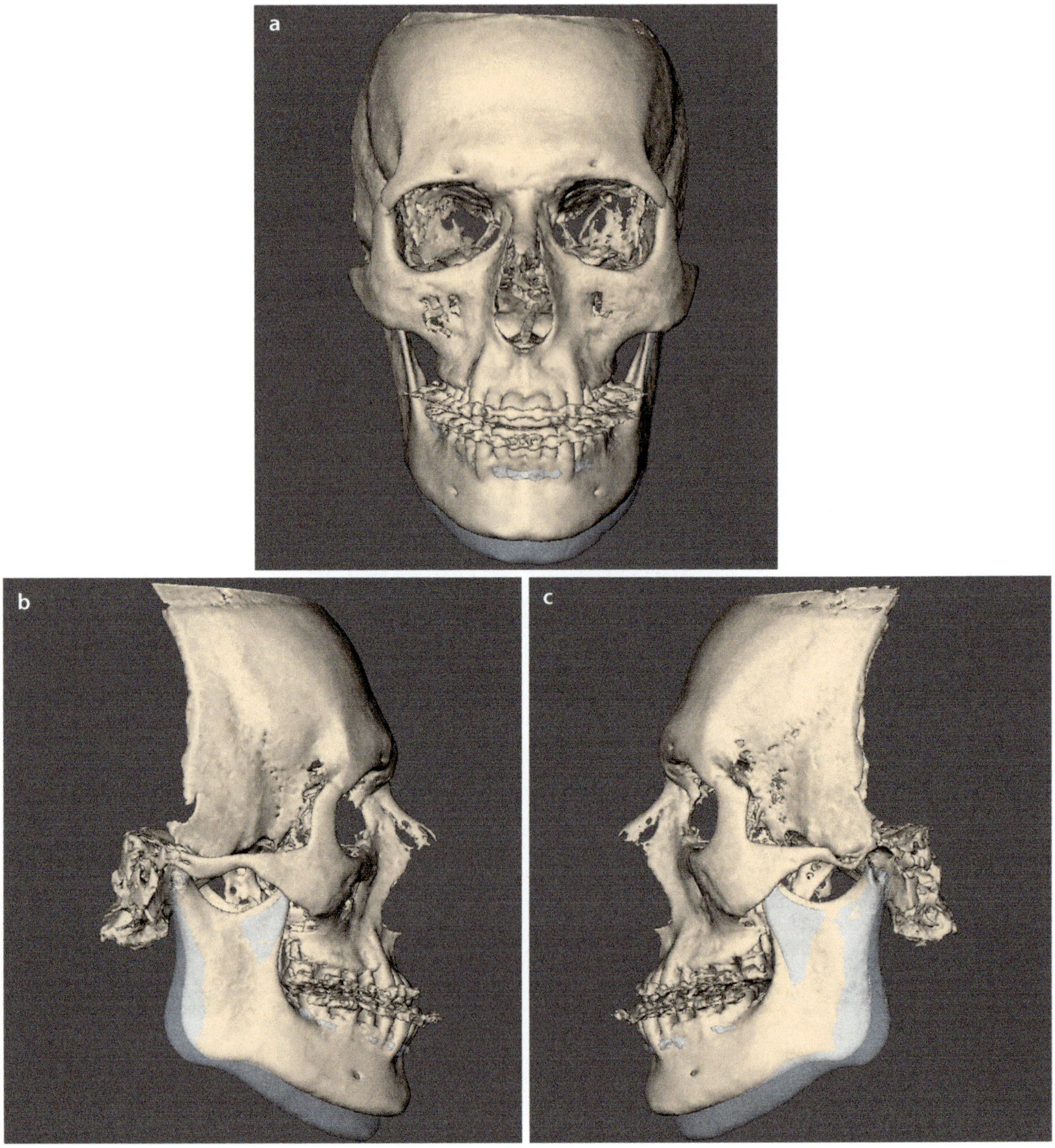

Fig. 1.43 Voxel-based registration of CBCT scan N°2 on CBCT scan N°1 based on the maxillary anatomy. Note the individual CW mandibular autorotation of patient B.B. 3D "surface-rendered" frontal (**a**), right profile (**b**) and left (**c**) hard tissues surface representations ("i-CAT^{TM}, Imaging Sciences International, Inc., Hatfield, USA, Maxilim v. 2.3.0.3) (patient B.B.). Note the arc of CW mandibular autorotation

Visualisation of 3D Virtual Mandibular Autorotation

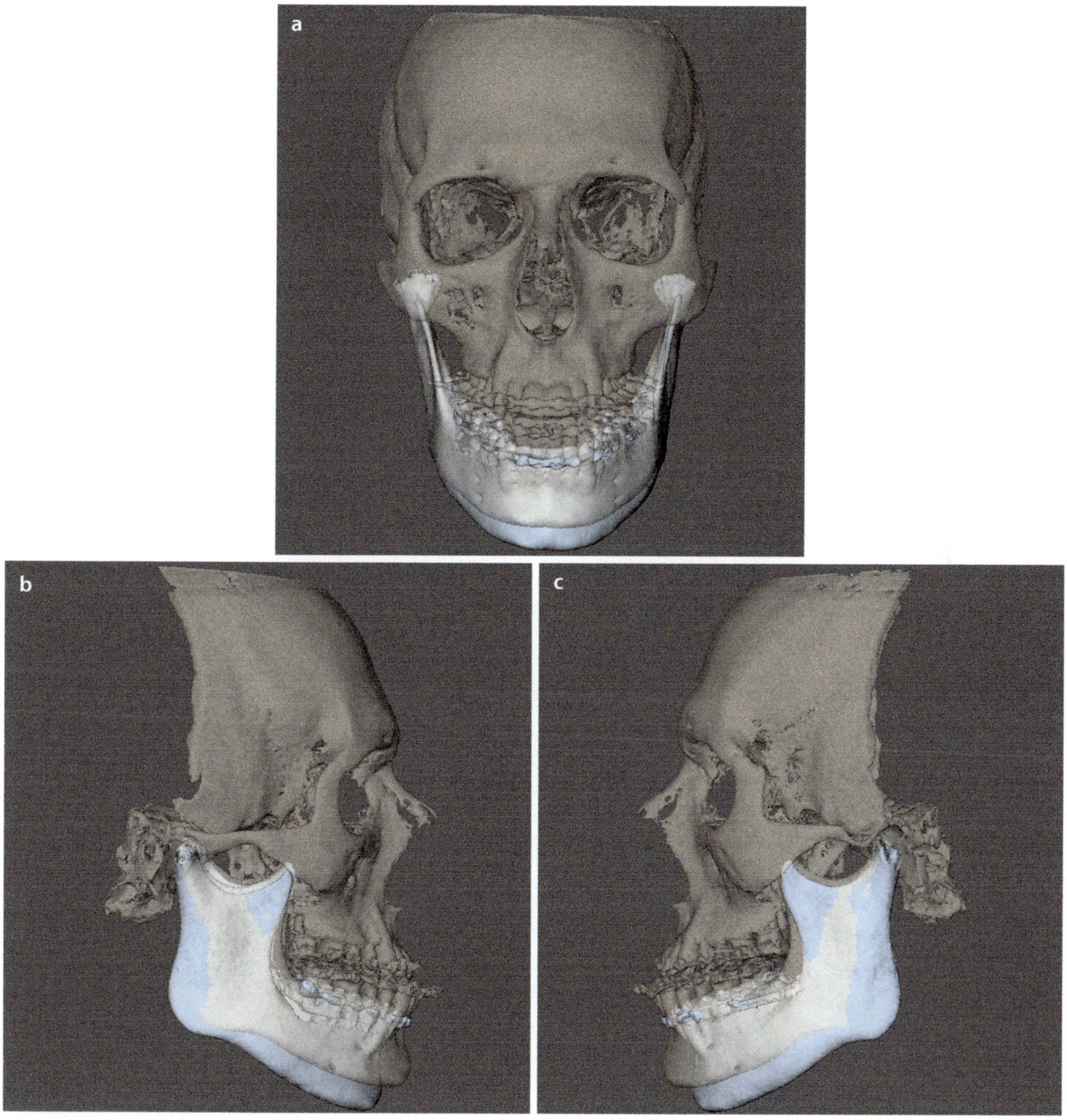

Fig. 1.44 Voxel-based registration of CBCT scan N°2 on CBCT scan N°1 based on the maxillary anatomy visualises the individual CW mandibular autorotation of patient B.B. 3D "surface-rendered" frontal (**a**), right profile (**b**) and left (**c**) hard tissues surface representations ("i-CAT™, Imaging Sciences International, Inc., Hatfield, USA, Maxilim v. 2.3.0.3) (patient B.B.). Note the forced opening of the bite

Additional Recommended Reading

Al-Anezi T, Khambay B, Peng MJ, O'Leary E, Ju X, Ayoub A (2013) A new method for automatic tracking of facial landmarks in 3D motion captured images (4D). Int J Oral Maxillofac Surg 42:9–18

Bell JW, Jacobs JD (1979) Combined orthodontic-surgical correction of moderate mandibular deficiency. Am J Orthod 75:481–506

De Vos W, Casselman J, Swennen GRJ (2009) Cone-beam computerized tomography (CBCT) imaging of the oral and maxillo-facial region: a systematic review of the literature. Int J Oral Maxillofac Surg 38:609–625

Epker BN, Fish LC (1980) Surgical superior repositioning of the maxilla: what to do with the mandible? Am J Orthod 78:164–191

Gateno J, Xia J, Teichgraeber JF et al (2003) A new technique for the creation of a computerized composite skull model. J Oral Maxillofac Surg 61:222–227

Hernández-Alfaro F, Guijarro-Martínez R (2013) New protocol for three-dimensional surgical planning and CAD/CAM splint generation in orthognathic surgery: an in vitro and in vivo study. Int J Oral Maxillofac Surg 42:1547–15556

Plooij JM, Maal TJJ, Haers P, Borstlap WA, Kuijpers-Jagtman AM, Bergé SJ (2011) Digital three-dimensional image fusion processes for planning and evaluating orthodontics and orthognathic surgery. A systematic review. Int J Oral Maxillofac Surg 40:341–352

Schutyser F (2005). From 3-D volumetric computer tomography to 3-D cephalometry. In Swennen GRJ, Schutyser F, Hausamen JE (eds) Three-dimensional cephalometry, vol 1. Springer, Heidelberg, pp 2–11

Sperry TP, Steinberg MJ, Gans BJ (1982) Mandibular movement during autorotation as a result of maxillary impaction surgery. Am J Orthod 81:116–123

Swennen GRJ, Schutyser F (2007) Three-dimensional virtual approach to diagnosis and treatment planning of maxillofacial deformity. In: Bell WH, Guerrero CA (eds) Distraction osteogenesis of the facial skeleton. BC Decker Inc., Hamilton

Swennen GRJ, Mollemans W, De Clercq C, Abeloos J, Lamoral P, Lippens F, Neyt N, Casselman J, Schutyser F (2009a) A cone-beam CT triple scan procedure to obtain a three-dimensional augmented virtual skull model appropriate for orthognathic surgery planning. J Craniofac Surg 20:297–307

Swennen GRJ, Mollemans W, Schutyser F (2009b) Three-dimensional treatment planning of orthognathic surgery in the era of virtual imaging. J Oral Maxillofac Surg 67:2080–2092

Swennen GRJ, Cimen K, Nagy K, Abeloos J, De Clercq C (2013a) Three-dimensional virtual simulation of mandibular autorotation in orthognathic surgery. Int J Oral Maxillofac Surg 42:1338

Swennen GRJ, Van Leemput P, Mollemans W, Schutyser F, De Clercq C (2013b) A new "surface to Cone-Beam CT" registration method to obtain an appropriate 3D virtual patient model for orthognathic surgery planning. Int J Oral Maxillofac Surg 42:1338

Wessberg GA, Washburn MC, Labanc JP, Epker BN (1982) Autorotation of the mandible: effect of surgical superior repositioning of the maxilla on mandibular resting posture. Am J Orthod 81:465–472

3D Virtual Diagnosis of the Orthognathic Patient

Gwen R.J. Swennen and Martin Gaboury

Electronic supplementary material The online version of this chapter (doi:10.1007/978-3-662-47389-4_2) contains supplementary material, which is available to authorized users.

G.R.J. Swennen (ed.), *3D Virtual Treatment Planning of Orthognathic Surgery*,
DOI 10.1007/978-3-662-47389-4_2

2.1 Systematic Virtual Diagnosis of the Patient's Deformity, Anatomy and Pathology

The "3D Virtual Visualisation Paradigm" (Swennen and Schutyser 2007) (► see also Sect. 1.1.1) offers the clinician (both orthodontists and surgeons) a new tool towards virtual diagnosis of the patient's deformity, anatomy and pathology in the daily clinical routine.

In this section, a standardised "step-by-step" approach towards "systematic virtual diagnosis of the patient's deformity, anatomy and pathology" is described based on the "3D Virtual Visualisation Paradigm":

1. Dento-maxillo-facial deformity and bite
2. Individual anatomy and pathology
3. Airway
4. TMJ

The "3D Virtual Scene Approach" allows to visualise 3D virtual images of the patient's head by both "surface rendering" and "volume rendering" from the individual DICOM CBCT data of the patient. The 3D soft and hard tissue representations will especially be used to evaluate the "dento-maxillo-facial deformity and bite" of the patient. In the "3D Virtual Scene Approach", additional axial, sagittal and coronal reslices can be added which are especially valuable for in-depth diagnosis of the "individual anatomy and pathology" of the patient. Finally, multiplanar reslices can be added and more enhanced 3D virtual diagnostics can be performed of the "airway" and "TMJ".

This initial overall radiological CBCT assessment takes place before "3D cephalometric analysis of the patient (► see Sect. 2.2)" and always needs to be related towards the clinical examination of the patient.

2.1.1 Dento-maxillo-facial Deformity and Bite

After appropriate CBCT image acquisition and consecutive 3D rendering (► see also Sect. 1.1.1), the 3D soft and hard tissue surface representations of the patient's head can be systematically evaluated in the "3D virtual scene" towards the patient's individual dento-maxillo-facial deformity and bite.

This initial step makes the crucial bridge between conventional and 3D virtual planning of orthognathic surgery. Once an appropriate full-face CBCT scan of the patient has been taken, no additional lateral or frontal cephalograms, neither orthopanthomographs (OPG's) are necessary anymore. Moreover, all these conventional radiological examinations can be virtually computed from the CBCT data set if desired.

■ **Case 1**

Patient V.E.W. is used to demonstrate the systematic approach towards individualised patient's anatomy assessment, while patient's specific pathology is demonstrated by other clinical cases (► see also Chap. 6).

3D Virtual Patient: Systematic Virtual Evaluation of the Patient's Deformity and Bite

In order to evaluate the patient's deformity and bite, the following views are systematically analysed on the 3D hard and soft tissue surface representations of the patient's head:

1. Frontal view (Fig. 2.1)
2. Profile view right/left (Figs. 2.2 and 2.3)
3. Base view (Fig. 2.4)
4. Cranial view (Fig. 2.5)
5. Posterior view (Fig. 2.6)

In the "3D Virtual Scene Approach", "volume rendering" is more valuable than "surface rendering" for appropriate evaluation of the patient's deformity and bite since it allows a more detailed visualisation of the patient's occlusion and dentition (Figs. 2.7, 2.8 and 2.9).

> 3D volume rendering is more appropriate for virtual evaluation of the patient's deformity and bite.

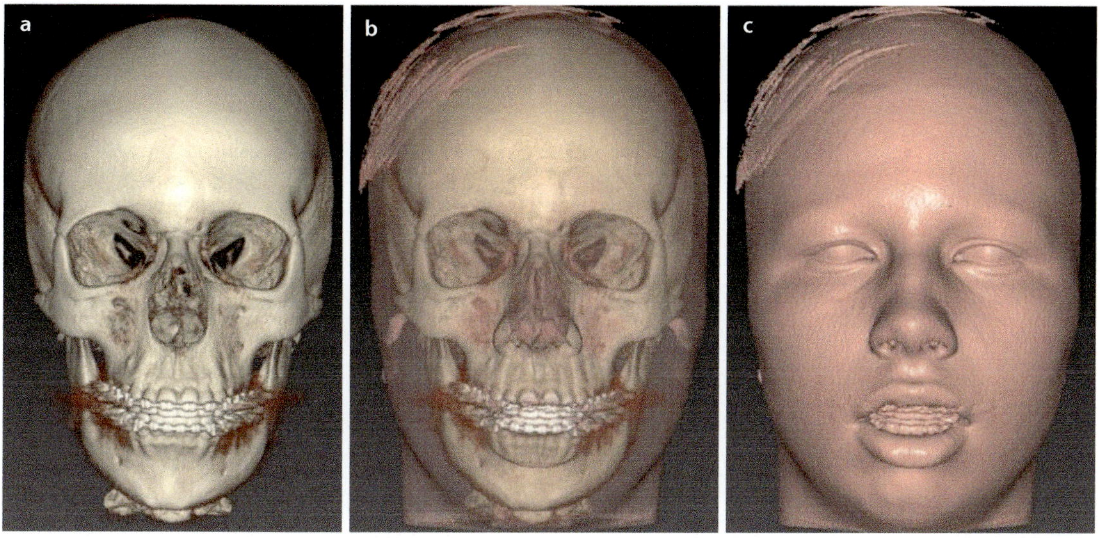

Fig. 2.1 Frontal views of 3D "volume-rendered" hard (**a**) and soft tissue (**b**, **c**) surface representations of the patient's head (i-CAT, Imaging Sciences International Inc, IPS CaseDesigner ALPHA version) (patient V.E.W.). Note the "long-face" pattern, chin deviation to the right, asymmetric gonial angles and increased interlabial distance with lip incompetency

3D Virtual Patient: Systematic Virtual Evaluation of the Patient's Deformity and Bite

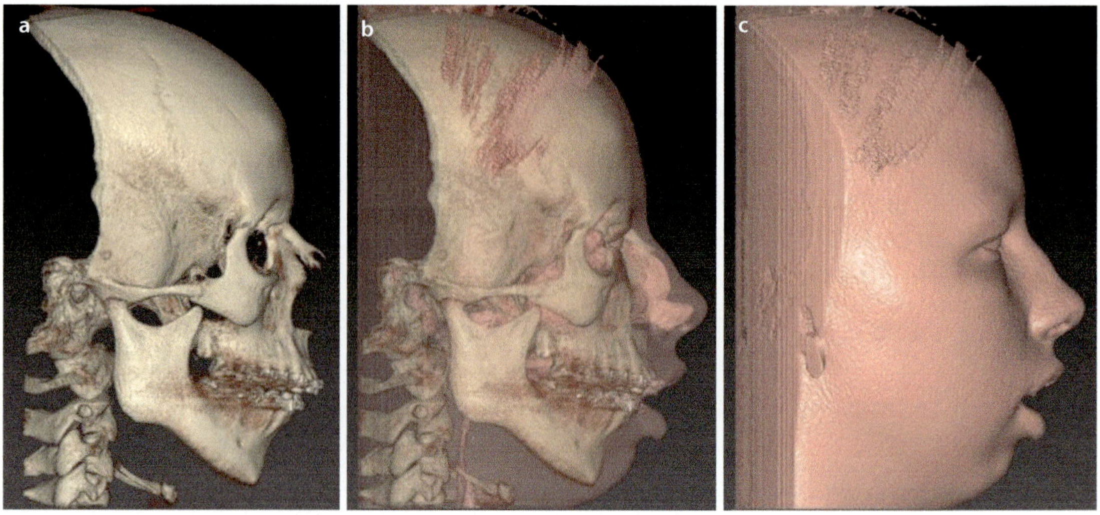

Fig. 2.2 Right profile views of 3D "volume-rendered" hard (**a**) and soft tissue (**b**, **c**) surface representations of the patient's head (i-CAT, Imaging Sciences International Inc, IPS CaseDesigner ALPHA version) (patient V.E.W.). Note the Angle "class II" relationship, the increased sagittal overjet, retruded mandible and chin, dorsal nasal hump, atonic upper and lower lips with increased interlabial distance and lip incompetency

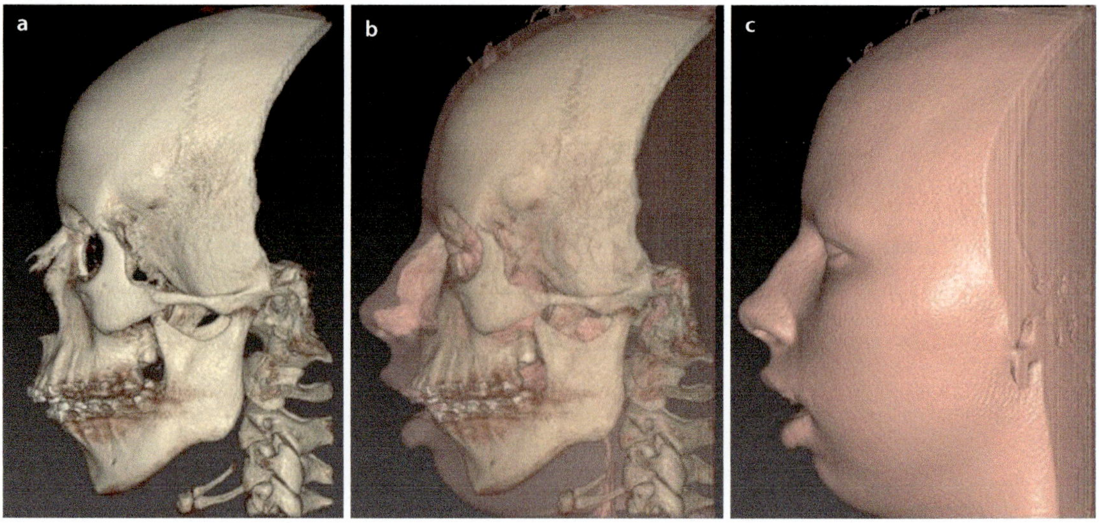

Fig. 2.3 Left profile views of 3D "volume-rendered" hard (**a**) and soft tissue (**b**, **c**) surface representations of the patient's head (i-CAT, Imaging Sciences International Inc, IPS CaseDesigner ALPHA version) (patient V.E.W.). Note the Angle "class II" relationship, the increased sagittal overjet, retruded mandible and chin, dorsal nasal hump, atonic upper and lower lips with increased interlabial distance and lip incompetency

3D Virtual Patient: Systematic Virtual Evaluation of the Patient's Deformity and Bite

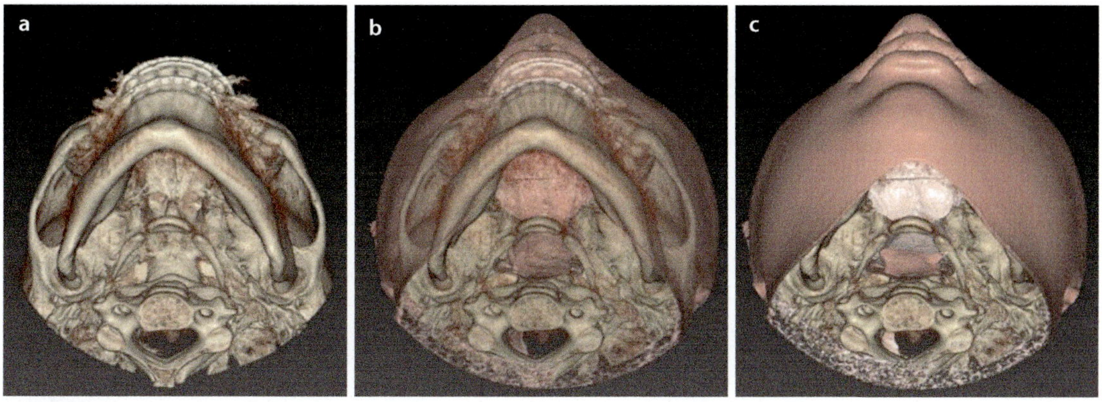

Fig. 2.4 Base views of 3D "volume-rendered" hard (**a**) and soft tissue (**b**, **c**) surface representations of the patient's head (i-CAT, Imaging Sciences International Inc, IPS CaseDesigner ALPHA version) (patient V.E.W.). Note the retruded mandible, increased sagittal overjet, chin deviation to the right and "Yaw" rotation (▶ see also Sect. 3.4) of the mandible

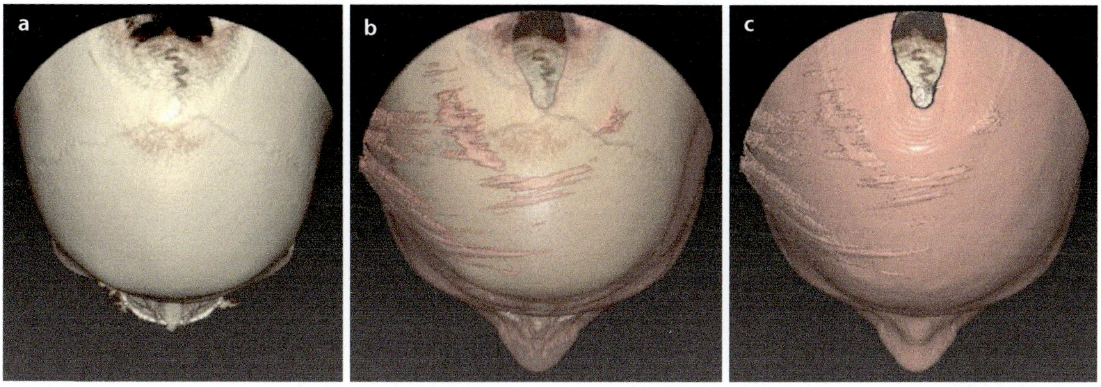

Fig. 2.5 Cranial views of 3D "volume-rendered" hard (**a**) and soft tissue (**b**, **c**) surface representations of the patient's head (i-CAT, Imaging Sciences International Inc, IPS CaseDesigner ALPHA version) (patient V.E.W.). Note the symmetric projection of the frontal and zygomatic bones, while the nasal tip is slightly deviated to the right

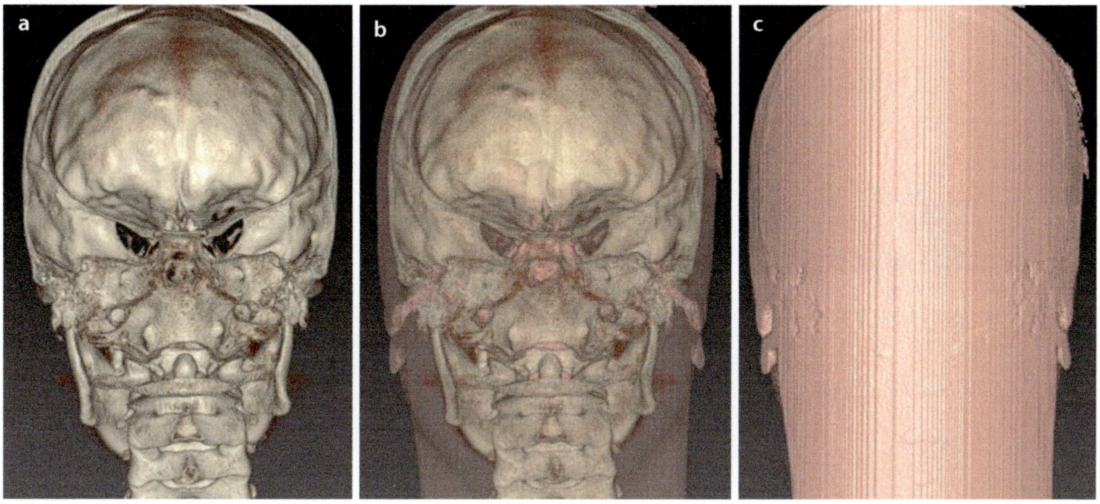

Fig. 2.6 Posterior views of 3D "volume-rendered" hard (**a**) and soft tissue (**b**, **c**) surface representations of the patient's head (i-CAT, Imaging Sciences International Inc, IPS CaseDesigner ALPHA version) (patient V.E.W.). Note the overall symmetric cranial base but discrepancy in vertical ramus height with asymmetric gonial angles

3D Virtual Patient: Systematic Virtual Evaluation of the Patient's Deformity and Bite

2

Attention
The 3D "volume-rendered" surface representations, despite providing additional radiological information, cannot be used for the creation of a 3D Virtual Augmented Model of the patient's head (▶ see also Sect. 1.2).

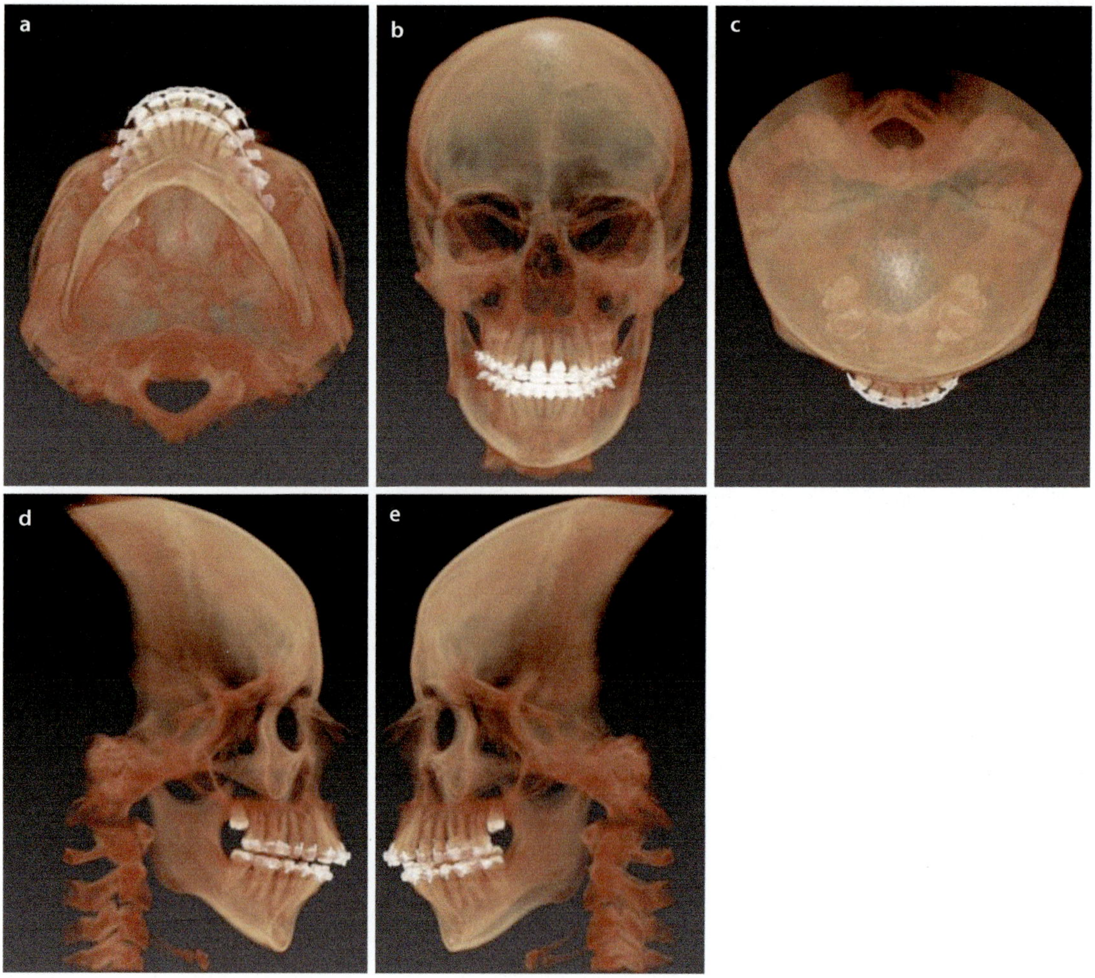

Fig. 2.7 Base (**a**), frontal (**b**), cranial (**c**), profile right (**d**) and left (**e**) views of 3D "volume-rendered" hard tissue surface representations of the patient's head based on a different shading algorithm (i-CAT, Imaging Sciences International Inc, IPS CaseDesigner ALPHA version) (patient V.E.W.). Note the visualisation of the dental roots and more clear presence of two impacted upper wisdom teeth

3D Virtual Patient: Systematic Virtual Evaluation of the Patient's Deformity and Bite

3D Volume rendering using different shading algorithms is beneficial to improve both occlusal and dental assessment.

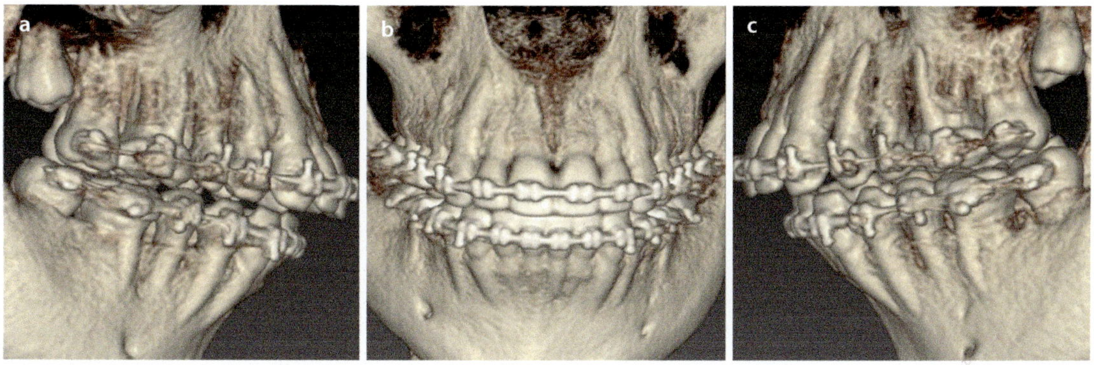

Fig. 2.8 Detailed profile right (**a**), frontal (**b**) and profile left (**c**) views of 3D "volume-rendered" hard tissue surface representations of the patient's dental occlusion and teeth based on a different shading algorithm (i-CAT, Imaging Sciences International Inc, IPS CaseDesigner ALPHA version) (patient V.E.W.). Note the Angle "class II" molar and canine relationship, the inferior midline deviation to the right, the adequate transverse relationship, the increased sagittal overjet and the decreased overbite. Also note the missing upper and lower premolars and impacted upper wisdom teeth

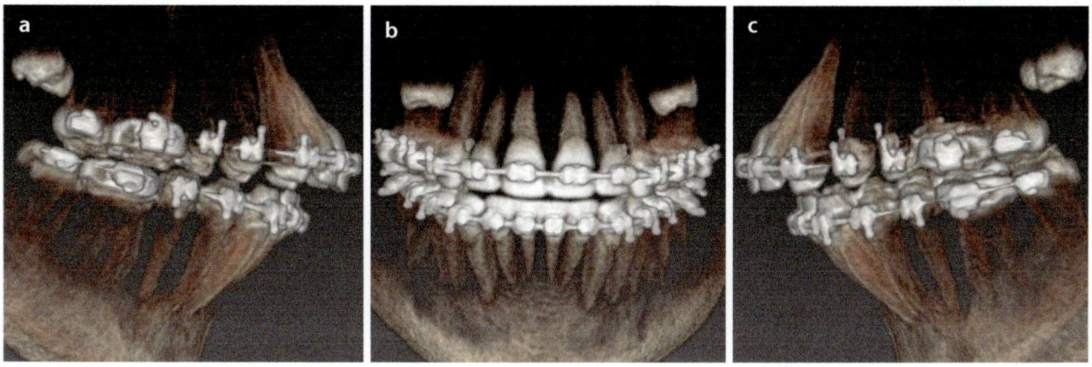

Fig. 2.9 Detailed profile right (**a**), frontal (**b**) and profile left (**c**) views of 3D "volume-rendered" hard tissue surface representations of the patient's dental occlusion and teeth based on a different shading algorithm (i-CAT, Imaging Sciences International Inc, IPS CaseDesigner ALPHA version) (patient V.E.W.). Note the more clear visualisation of the roots of the teeth. This is especially of interest if additional micro-screws are indicated for skeletal anchorage or if segmentation of the jaws is necessary. Also note appropriate dental root angulation, adequate pre-surgical orthodontic preparation and decompensation with accurate levelling of the Spee's curve. Upper and lower dental arch coordination is not evaluated at this stage and will be assessed during "3D virtual occlusal definition (▶ see also Sect. 3.3)"

2.1.2 Individual Anatomy and Pathology

After standardised and individualised virtual evaluation of the 3D hard and soft tissue surface representations of the patient's head, the "3D Virtual Scene Approach" allows to add axial, sagittal and coronal orthogonal reslices to the "3D virtual scene". Moreover, additional multiplanar reslices can be reconstructed and added for enhanced diagnostics (◘ Fig. 2.10).

In this section, a systematic "step-by-step" evaluation of the patient's individual anatomy and pathology is outlined, based on:

1. Baseline *axial* reslices
2. Reconstructed *coronal* reslices
3. Reconstructed *sagittal* reslices

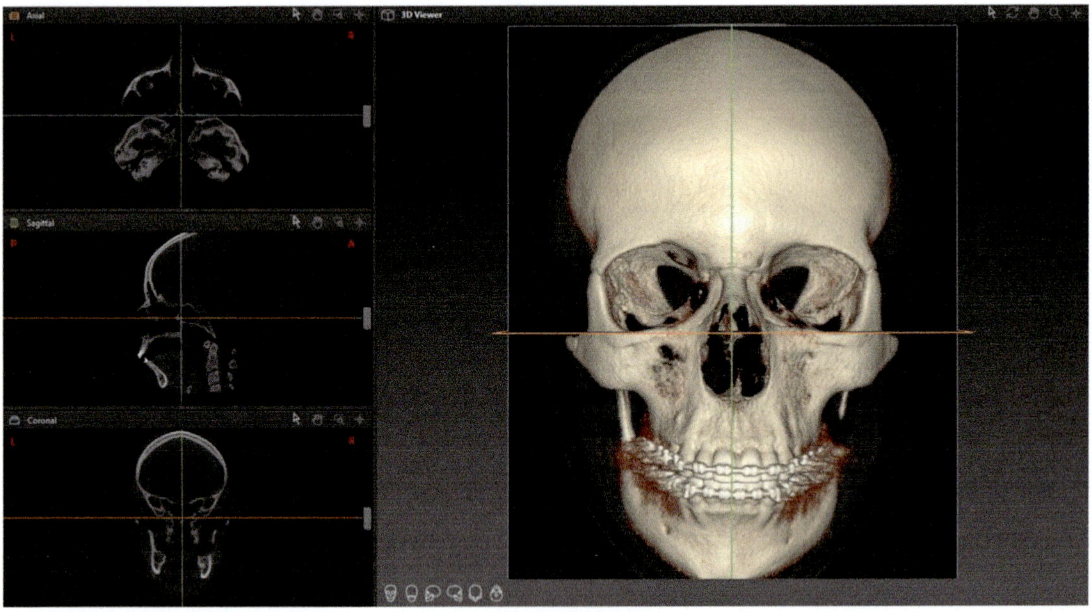

◘ **Fig. 2.10** 3D "volume-rendered" hard tissue surface representation with axial, sagittal and coronal reconstructed orthogonal reslices (i-CAT, Imaging Sciences International Inc, IPS CaseDesigner ALPHA version) (patient V.E.W.)

Axial Slices: Systematic Virtual Evaluation of the Patient's Anatomy and Pathology

The following clinical features relevant to combined orthodontic-surgical treatment planning are systematically analysed on the baseline axial slices by scrolling through the individual patient's DICOM data set.

A standardised checklist for systematic virtual evaluation of the patient's individual anatomy and pathology, based on the axial slices, is hereby provided:

1. Upper face contour (Fig. 2.11)
2. Frontal sinuses (Fig. 2.12)
3. Orbits and bulbus position (Fig. 2.13)
4. Ethmoid sinuses (Fig. 2.14)
5. Midface contour (Fig. 2.15)
6. Maxillary sinuses (Figs. 2.16 and 2.17)
7. Nasal septum (Fig. 2.18)
8. Nasal turbinates (Fig. 2.19)
9. Condylar morphology (Fig. 2.20)
10. Mandibular vertical ramus thickness above the lingula (Figs. 2.21, 2.22 and 2.23)
11. Maxillary dento-alveolar width (Fig. 2.24)
12. Mandibular dento-alveolar width (Fig. 2.25)
13. Lower face contour (Fig. 2.26)
14. Airway (Fig. 2.27)
15. Patient's specific pathology

It needs to be emphasised that standardised virtual evaluation of the axial slices is of major clinical importance and needs to be performed dynamically by the clinician (orthodontist and/or surgeon). Moreover, by using the hereby proposed systematic approach, it is not time consuming.

Case 1

(Patient V.E.W.) is used to demonstrate the systematic approach towards individualised patient's anatomy assessment, while patient's specific pathology is demonstrated by other clinical cases (▶ see also Chap. 6).

Axial Slices: Upper Face Contour

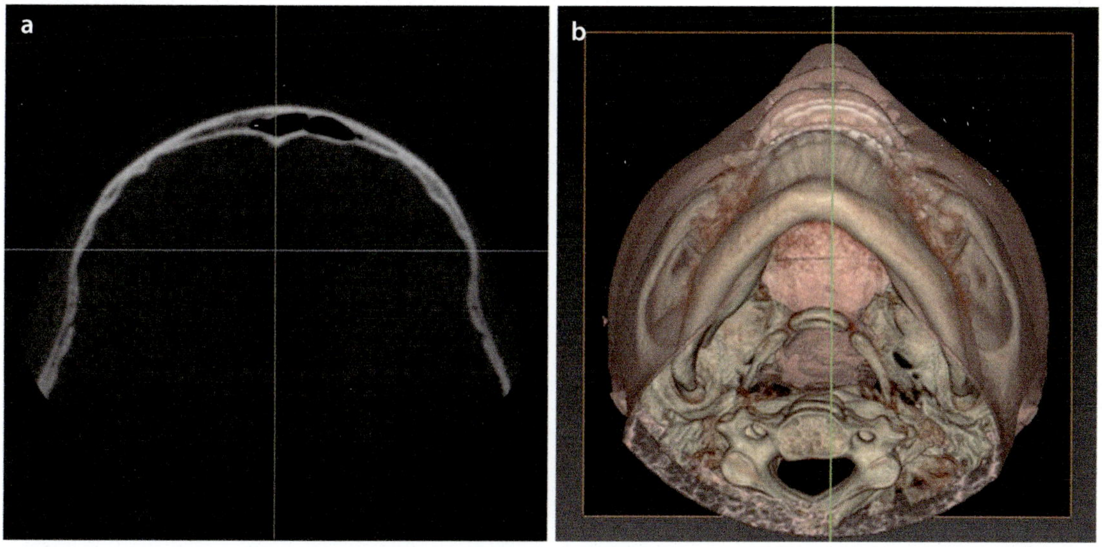

Fig. 2.11 Axial slices through the forehead allow to evaluate the upper face contour at the soft and bony tissue level (**a**). In this case, the patient is displaying normal anatomy. The clinician should look for soft tissue irregularities, frontal bossing, exostosis and diverse pathologies like osteomas. (**b**) visualises the level of the axial reconstructed reslice on the 3D "volume-rendered" patient model (i-CAT, Imaging Sciences International Inc, IPS CaseDesigner ALPHA version) (patient V.E.W.)

Axial Slices: Frontal Sinuses

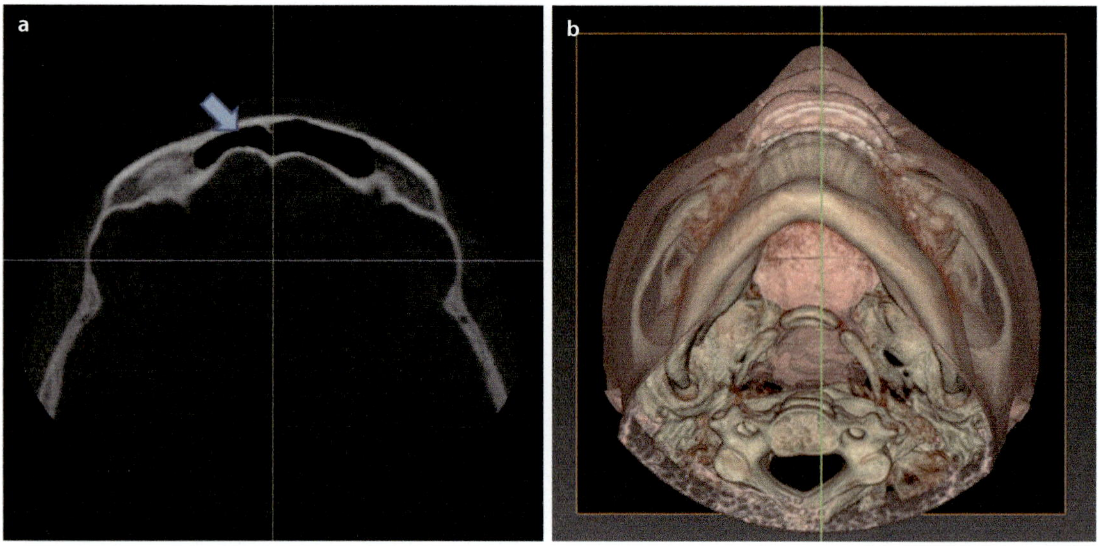

Fig. 2.12 Axial slice through the frontal sinus (*arrow*) (**a**). The clinician should look for signs of sinusitis, drainage obstruction and diverse pathologies. (**b**) visualises the level of the axial reconstructed reslice on the 3D "volume-rendered" patient model (i-CAT, Imaging Sciences International Inc, IPS CaseDesigner ALPHA version) (patient V.E.W.)

Axial Slices: Orbits and Bulbus Position

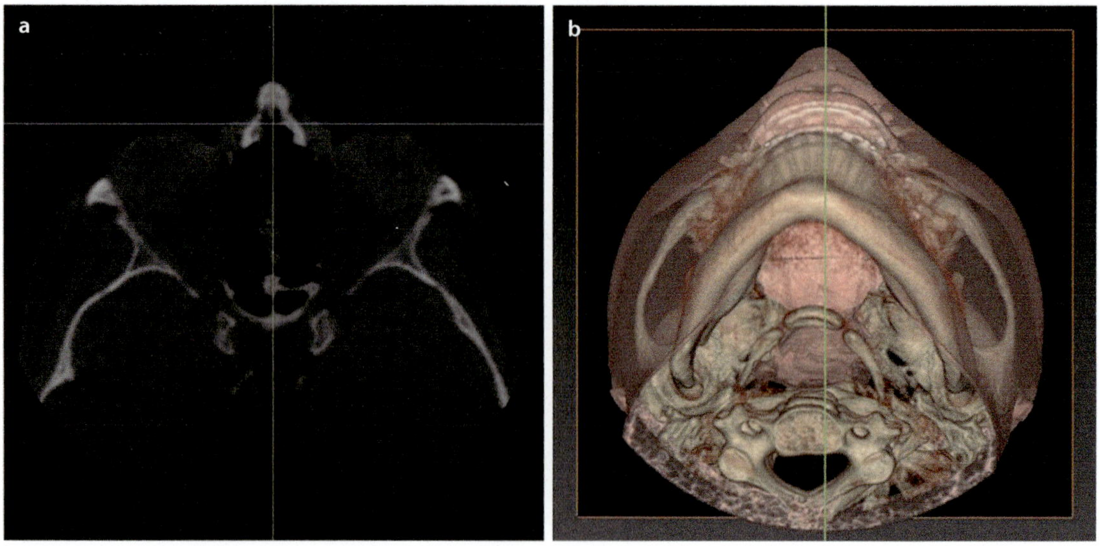

Fig. 2.13 Axial slice at the level of the greater axis of the bulbus (**a**). The anteroposterior position (enophthalmos or exophthalmos) of the globes can be evaluated by adding a horizontal line tangential to the anterior surface of the cornea (*blue line*). (**b**) visualises the level of the axial reconstructed reslice on the 3D "volume-rendered" patient model (i-CAT, Imaging Sciences International Inc, IPS CaseDesigner ALPHA version) (patient V.E.W.)

Axial Slices: Ethmoid Sinuses

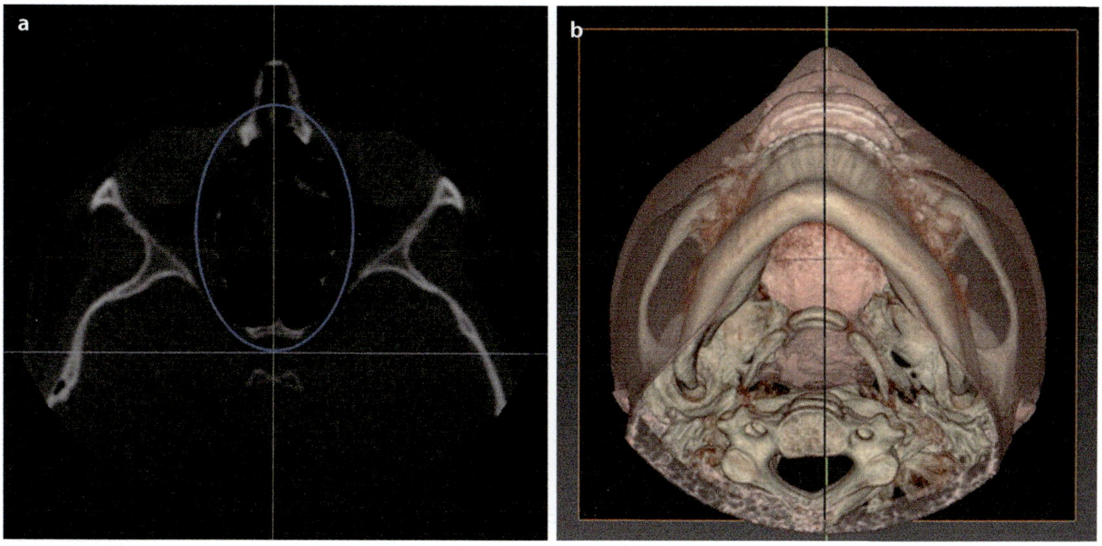

Fig. 2.14 Axial slice through the ethmoidal sinus (**a**). A blue circle delineates the region to be examined. In this case, early signs of mucosal thickening are seen in the ethmoidal air cells. (**b**) visualises the level of the axial reconstructed reslice on the 3D "volume-rendered" patient model (i-CAT, Imaging Sciences International Inc, IPS CaseDesigner ALPHA version) (patient V.E.W.)

Axial Slices: Midfacial Contour

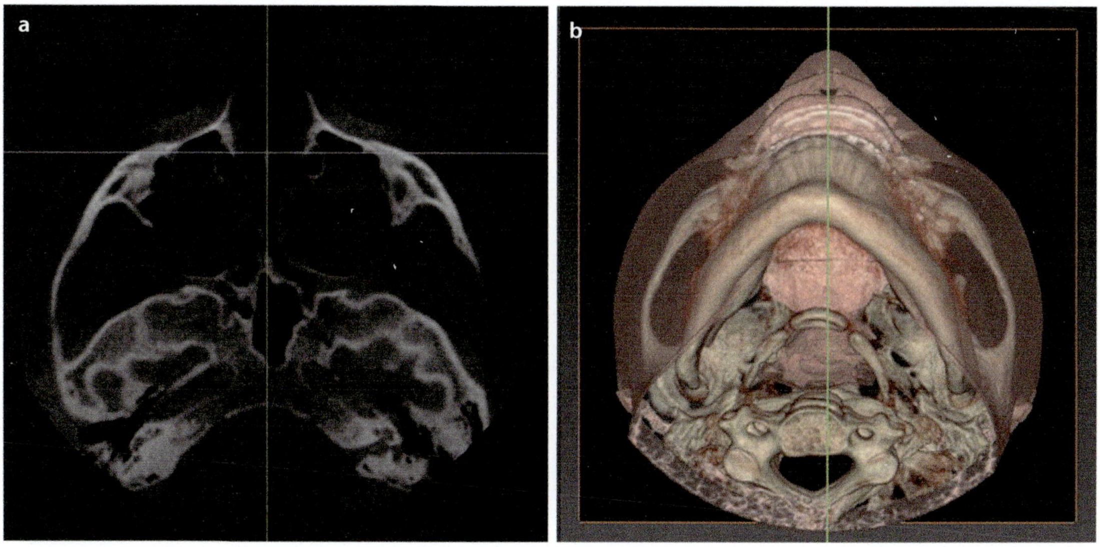

Fig. 2.15 Axial slice at the level of the most projecting point of the malar prominence (**a**). Both soft and bony tissues can be evaluated for asymmetry and malar hypoplasia. In this case, the patient is displaying normal malar and zygomatic arch anatomy. (**b**) visualises the level of the axial reconstructed reslice on the 3D "volume-rendered" patient model (i-CAT, Imaging Sciences International Inc, IPS CaseDesigner ALPHA version) (patient V.E.W.)

Axial Slices: Maxillary Sinuses

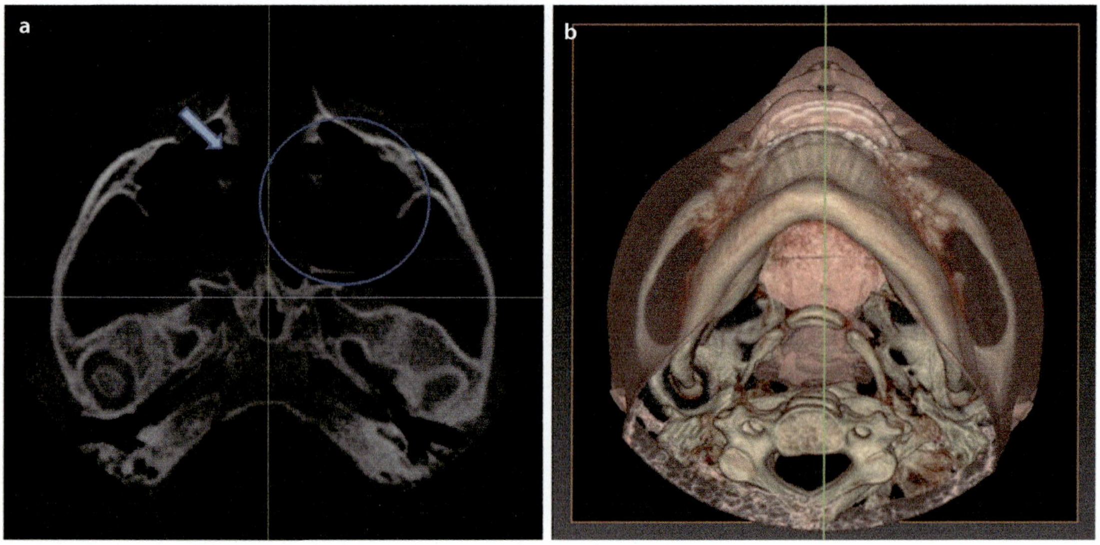

Fig. 2.16 Axial slice through the maxillary sinuses (**a**). The left maxillary sinus is delineated with a *blue circle*, while the *arrow* demonstrates the right nasolacrimal duct. (**b**) visualises the level of the axial reconstructed reslice on the 3D "volume-rendered" patient model (i-CAT, Imaging Sciences International Inc, IPS CaseDesigner ALPHA version) (patient V.E.W.)

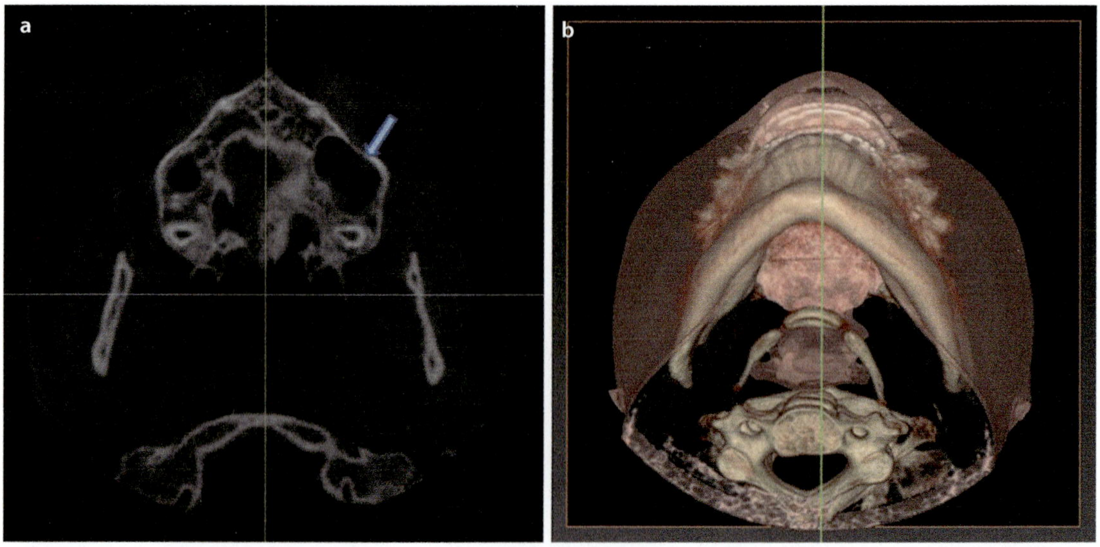

Fig. 2.17 Another axial slice through the maxillary sinuses, at a more inferior level (**a**). The *arrow* demonstrates a small mucous retention cyst of the left maxillary sinus. (**b**) visualises the level of the axial reconstructed reslice on the 3D "volume-rendered" patient model (i-CAT, Imaging Sciences International Inc, IPS CaseDesigner ALPHA version) (patient V.E.W.)

Axial Slices: Nasal Septum

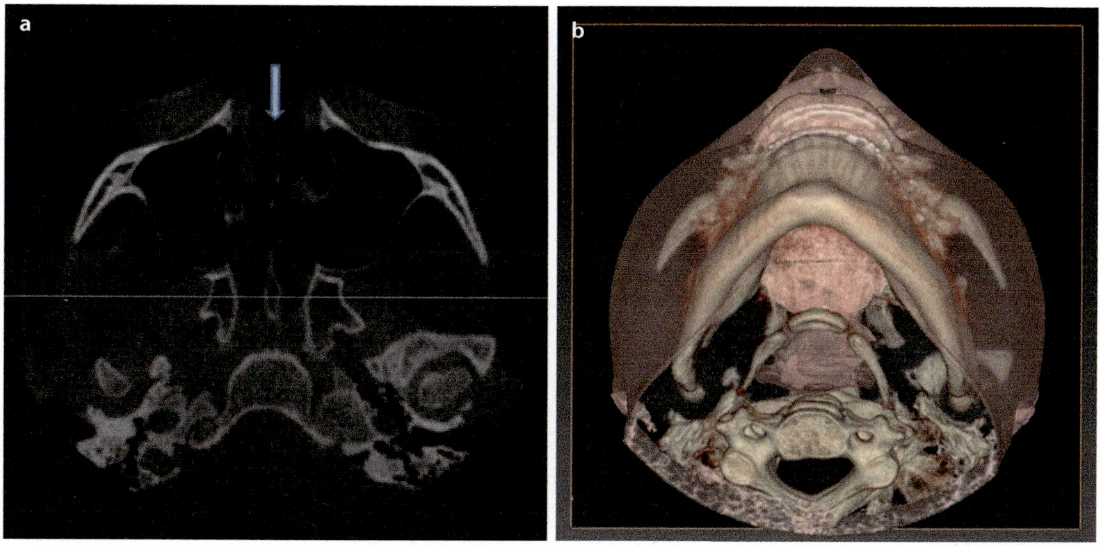

Fig. 2.18 Axial slice at the level of the bony nasal septum (*arrow*), which is formed by the septal crest of the maxilla, the vomer and the perpendicular plate of the ethmoidal bone (**a**). The anterior cartilaginous septum is more difficult to visualise with MSCT and CBCT imaging. In this case, a slight septal deviation is observed. (**b**) demonstrates the virtual orientation of the patient for orthogonal axial slice reconstruction (i-CAT, Imaging Sciences International Inc, IPS CaseDesigner ALPHA version) (patient V.E.W.)

Axial Slices: Nasal Turbinates

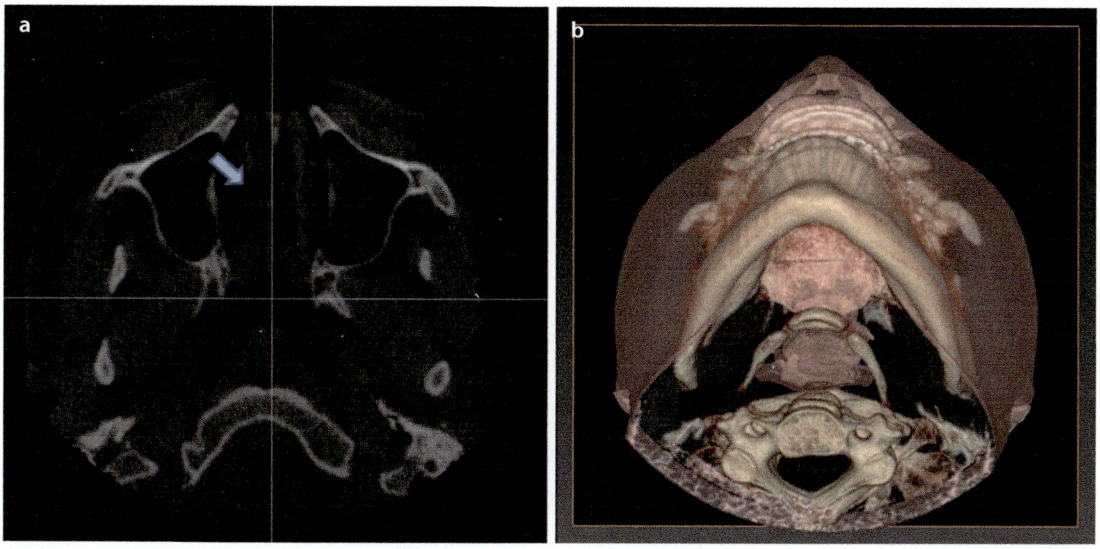

Fig. 2.19 Axial slice through the inferior nasal turbinates (*arrow*) (**a**). Especially in cases of maxillary impaction, the presence of inferior nasal turbinate hypertrophy should be evaluated. In this case, the inferior nasal turbinates are normal. (**b**) visualises the level of the axial reconstructed reslice on the 3D "volume-rendered" patient model (i-CAT, Imaging Sciences International Inc, IPS CaseDesigner ALPHA version) (patient V.E.W.)

Axial Slices: Condylar Morphology

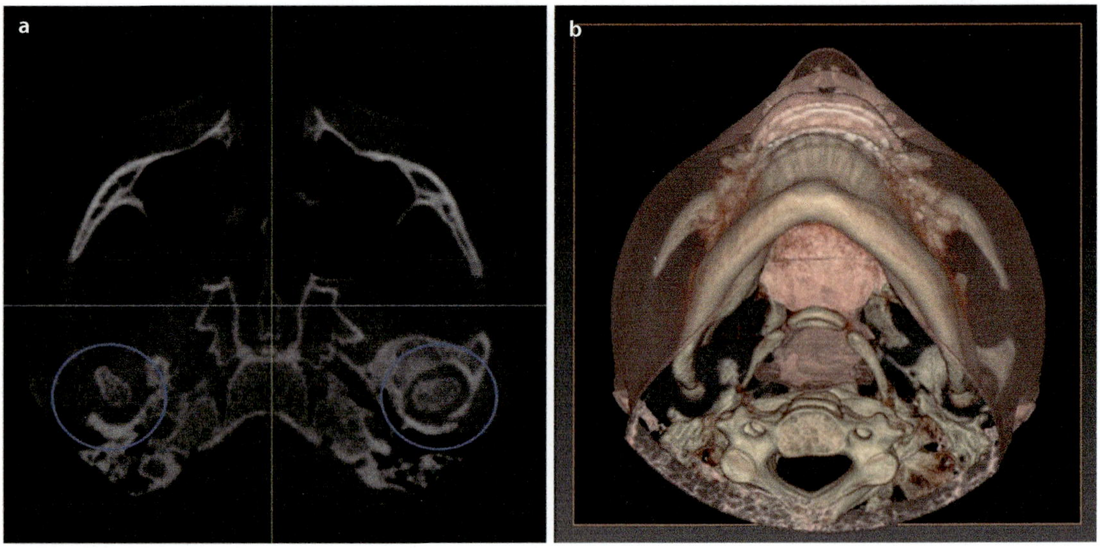

Fig. 2.20 Axial slice at the level of the mandibular condyles, delineated with *blue circles* (**a**). Note a discrete asymmetry at the cranial base, despite proper axial reslice reconstruction. An intact cortical layer is seen, without any significant pathology. Enhanced TMJ imaging and evaluation will be discussed in (► Sect. 2.1.4). (**b**) visualises the level of the axial reconstructed reslice on the 3D "volume-rendered" patient model (i-CAT, Imaging Sciences International Inc, IPS CaseDesigner ALPHA version version) (patient V.E.W.)

Axial Slices: Mandibular Vertical Ramus Thickness Above the Lingula

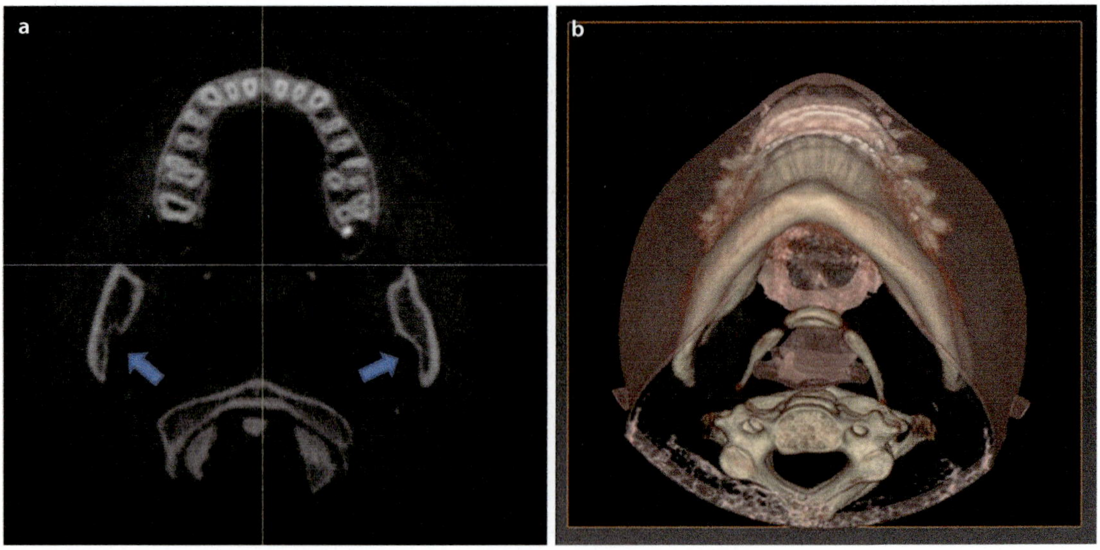

Fig. 2.21 Axial slice at the level of the mandibular lingula (*arrows*) (**a**). On the left side, the concavity posterior to the lingual is noticed, while on the right side, the opening of the mandibular foramen can be observed. (**b**) visualises the level of the axial reconstructed reslice on the 3D "volume-rendered" patient model (i-CAT, Imaging Sciences International Inc, IPS CaseDesigner ALPHA version) (patient V.E.W.)

Axial Slices: Mandibular Vertical Ramus Thickness Above the Lingula

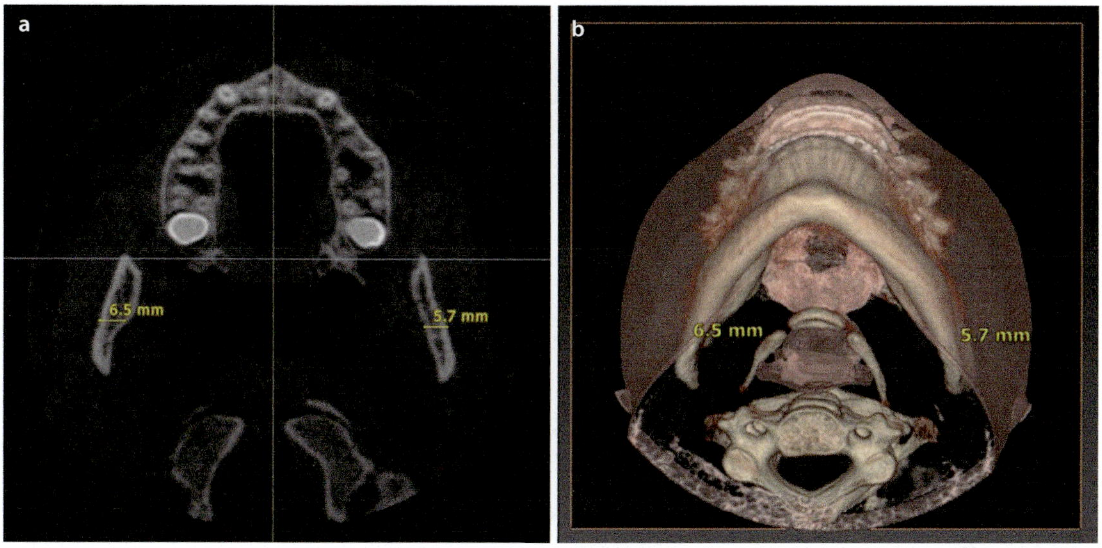

Fig. 2.22 Another axial slice, just superior to the lingula (**a**). The width of the mandibular vertical ramus can be measured at both sides, where the horizontal corticotomy of the bilateral sagittal split osteotomy (BSSO) will be made. (**b**) visualises the level of the axial reconstructed reslice on the 3D "volume-rendered" patient model (i-CAT, Imaging Sciences International Inc, IPS CaseDesigner ALPHA version) (patient V.E.W.)

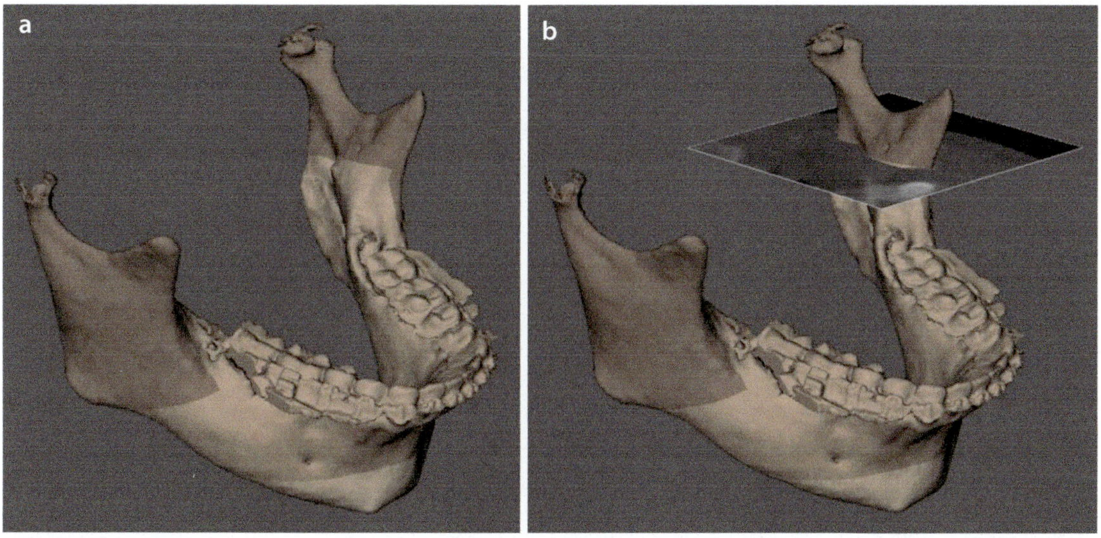

Fig. 2.23 3D "surface-rendered" representation of the mandible with a virtual bilateral sagittal split osteotomy (▶ see also Sect. 3.2.2) (BSSO) (**a**). The individual anatomy of the vertical mandibular ramus at the level of the horizontal corticotomy can be evaluated on an additional multiplanar reslice (**b**) (i-CAT, Imaging Sciences International Inc, Maxilim v. 2.3.0.3.) (patient V.E.W.)

Axial Slices: Maxillary Dento-Alveolar Width

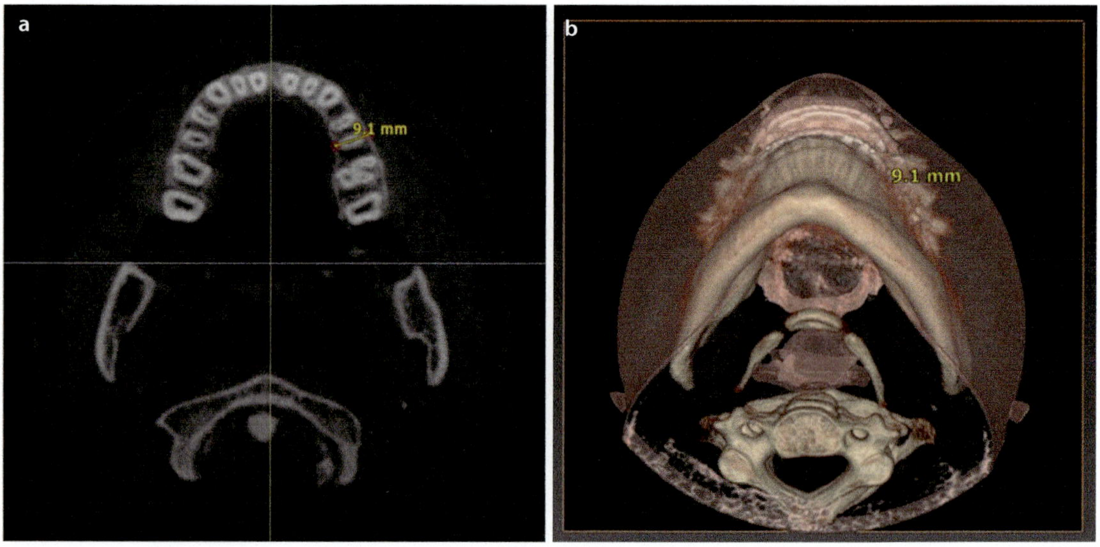

Fig. 2.24 Axial slice through the maxillary dento-alveolar process (**a**). The width of the maxillary dento-alveolar process can be evaluated from an orthodontic and eventual preprosthetic implant point of view. In cases of agenesis or tooth loss, the width of the dento-alveolar crest can be evaluated and measured. The position of maxillary teeth within the dento-alveolar bone and presence of buccal bony fenestrations can be assessed. (**b**) visualises the level of the axial reconstructed reslice on the 3D "volume-rendered" patient model (i-CAT, Imaging Sciences International Inc, IPS CaseDesigner ALPHA version) (patient V.E.W.)

Axial Slices: Mandibular Dento-Alveolar Width

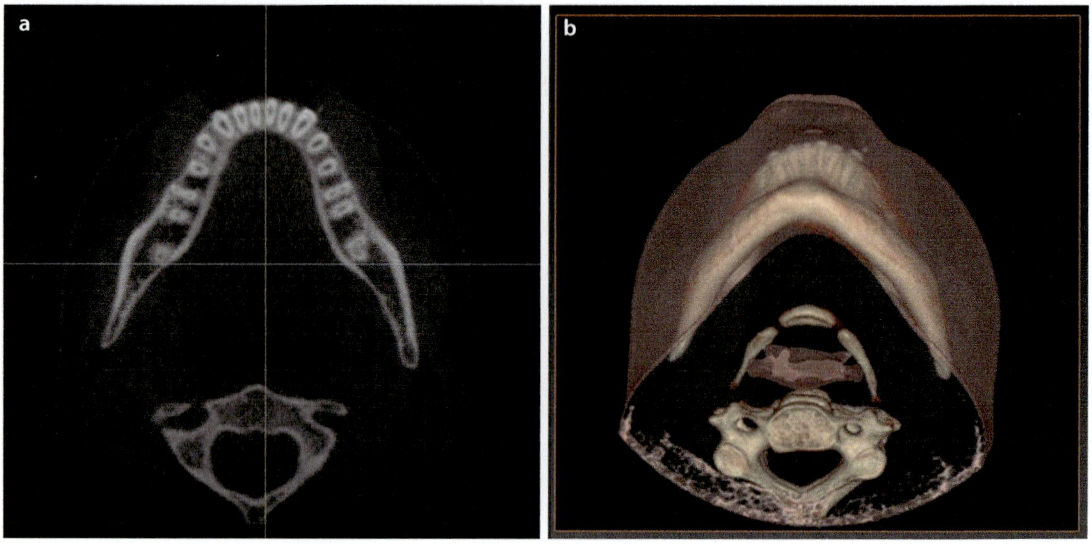

Fig. 2.25 Axial slice through the mandibular dento-alveolar process (**a**). The width of the mandibular dento-alveolar process can be evaluated from an orthodontic and eventual preprosthetic implant point of view. In cases of agenesis or tooth loss, the width of the dento-alveolar crest can be evaluated and measured. The position of mandibular teeth within the dento-alveolar bone and presence of buccal bony fenestrations can be assessed. (**b**) visualises the level of the axial reconstructed reslice on the 3D "volume-rendered" patient model (i-CAT, Imaging Sciences International Inc, IPS CaseDesigner ALPHA version) (patient V.E.W.)

Axial Slices: Lower Face Contour

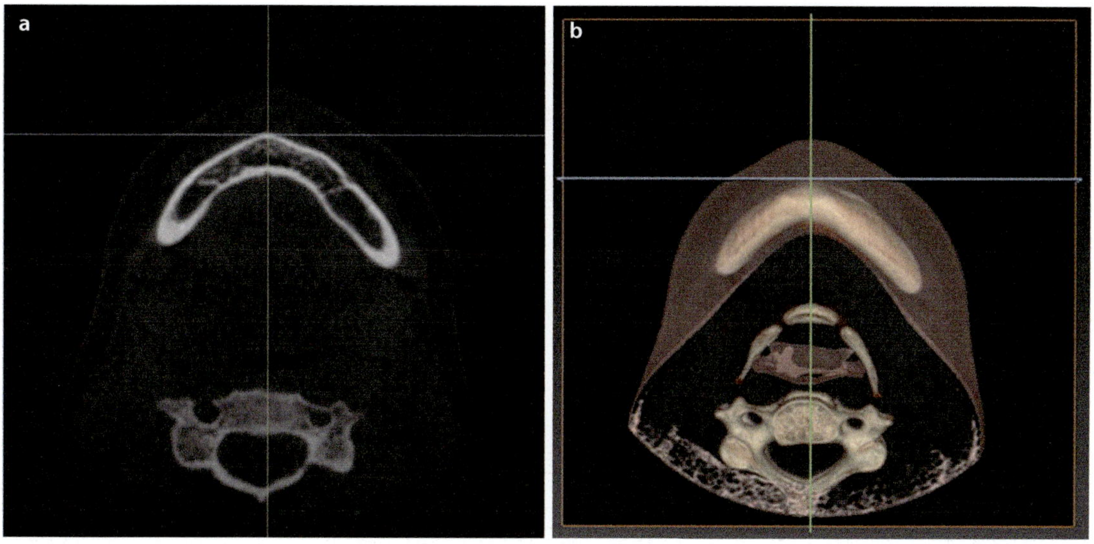

Fig. 2.26 An axial slice through the inferior third of the face (**a**). In this case, a discrete soft tissue and bony asymmetry is visible. (**b**) visualises the level of the axial reconstructed reslice on the 3D "volume-rendered" patient model (i-CAT, Imaging Sciences International Inc, IPS CaseDesigner ALPHA version) (patient V.E.W.)

Axial Slices: Airway

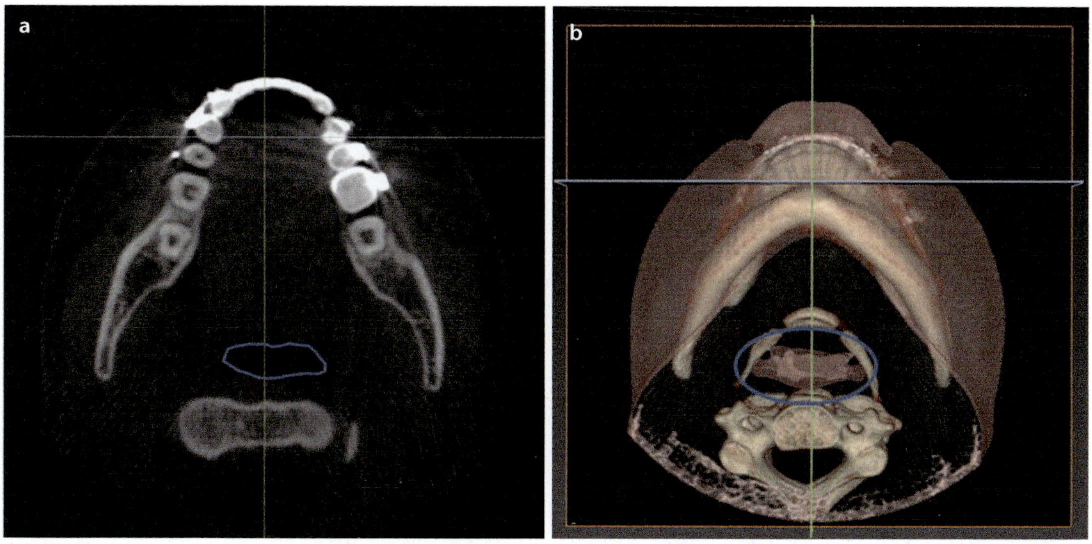

Fig. 2.27 Axial slice at the level of the tongue base demonstrates the oropharyngeal airway, delineated in blue (**a**). Enhanced 3D airway imaging and evaluation will be discussed in (▶ Sect. 2.1.3). (**b**) visualises the level of the axial reconstructed reslice on the 3D "volume-rendered" patient model, where the airway is outlined with a *blue circle* (i-CAT, Imaging Sciences International Inc, IPS CaseDesigner ALPHA version) (patient V.E.W.)

Coronal Slices: Systematic Virtual Evaluation of the Patient's Anatomy and Pathology

The following clinical features relevant to combined orthodontic-surgical treatment planning are systematically analysed on the coronal slices by scrolling through the individual patient's DICOM data set.

A standardised checklist for systematic virtual evaluation of the patient's individual anatomy and pathology, based on the coronal slices, is hereby provided:

1. Nasal airway (◘ Fig. 2.28)
2. Maxillary and mandibular interdental space in the frontal region (◘ Fig. 2.29)
3. Frontal sinuses (◘ Fig. 2.30)
4. Orbits and bulbus position (◘ Fig. 2.31)
5. Maxillary sinuses (◘ Fig. 2.32)
6. Nasal septum (◘ Fig. 2.33)
7. Nasal turbinates (◘ Fig. 2.34)
8. Ethmoidal sinuses (◘ Fig. 2.35)
9. Upper and lower molar/premolar inclination in regard to the alveolar ridge (◘ Fig. 2.36)
10. Tranversal occlusal relationship (◘ Fig. 2.37)
11. Course of the inferior alveolar nerve (IAN) (◘ Figs. 2.38, 2.39 and 2.40)
12. Condylar morphology (◘ Fig. 2.41)
13. Posterior airway (◘ Fig. 2.42)
14. Cervical spine (◘ Fig. 2.43)
15. Patient's specific pathology

It needs to be emphasised that standardised virtual evaluation of the coronal slices is of major clinical importance and needs to be performed dynamically by the clinician (orthodontist and/or surgeon). Moreover, by using the hereby proposed systematic approach, it is not time consuming.

Case 1

Patient V.E.W. is used to demonstrate the systematic approach towards individualised patient's anatomy assessment, while patient's specific pathology is demonstrated by other clinical cases (▶ see also Chap. 6).

Coronal Slices: Nasal Airway

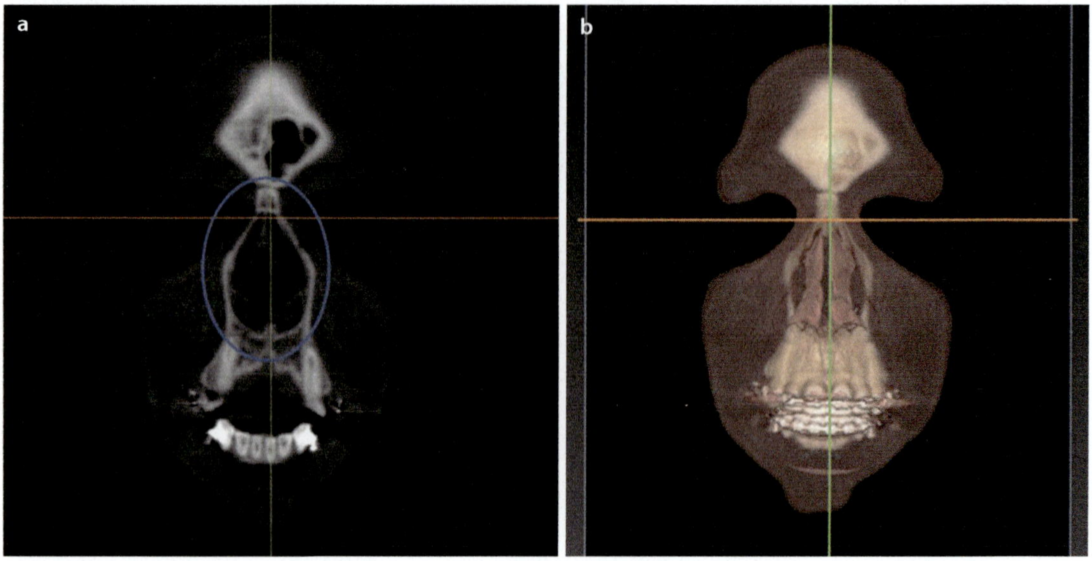

◘ **Fig. 2.28** Coronal slice at the level of the anterior nasal airway, outlined by a *blue circle* (**a**). The nasal airway is evaluated from anterior to posterior for possible obstruction caused by a septal deviation, inferior nasal turbinate hypertrophy or nasal bony pyramid asymmetry. (**b**) visualises the level of the coronal reconstructed reslice on the 3D "volume-rendered" patient model (i-CAT, Imaging Sciences International Inc, IPS CaseDesigner ALPHA version) (patient V.E.W.). Note the visualisation of the upper and lower lateral cartilages on the "volume-rendered" 3D image

Coronal Slices: Maxillary and Mandibular Interdental Space in the Frontal Region

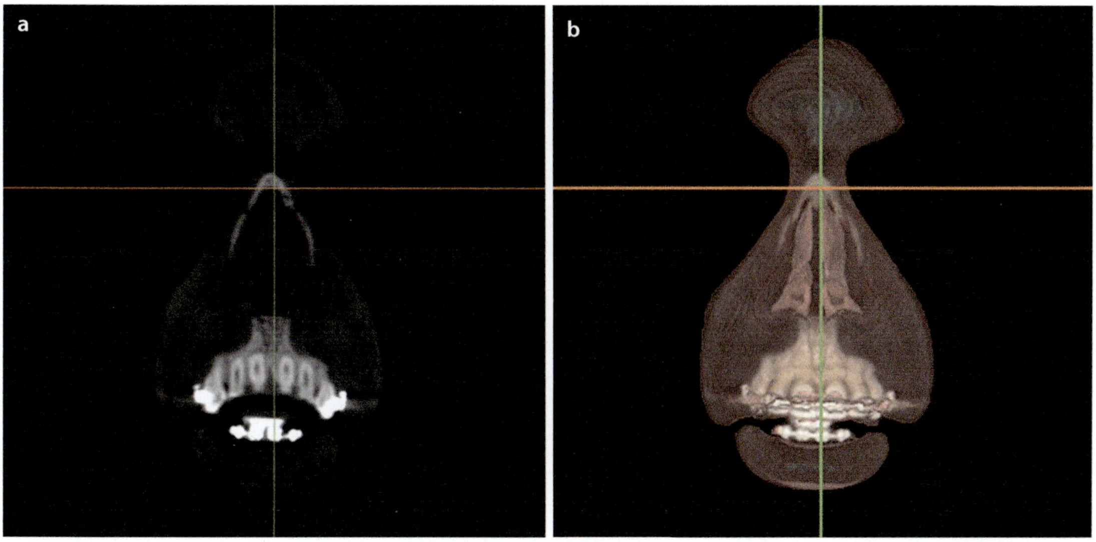

Fig. 2.29 Coronal slice at the level of the upper dental midline (**a**). Note the adequate interdental space for segmental maxillary surgery between the upper central incisors. (**b**) visualises the level of the coronal reconstructed reslice on the 3D "volume-rendered" patient model (i-CAT, Imaging Sciences International Inc, IPS CaseDesigner ALPHA version) (patient V.E.W.)

Coronal Slices: Frontal Sinuses

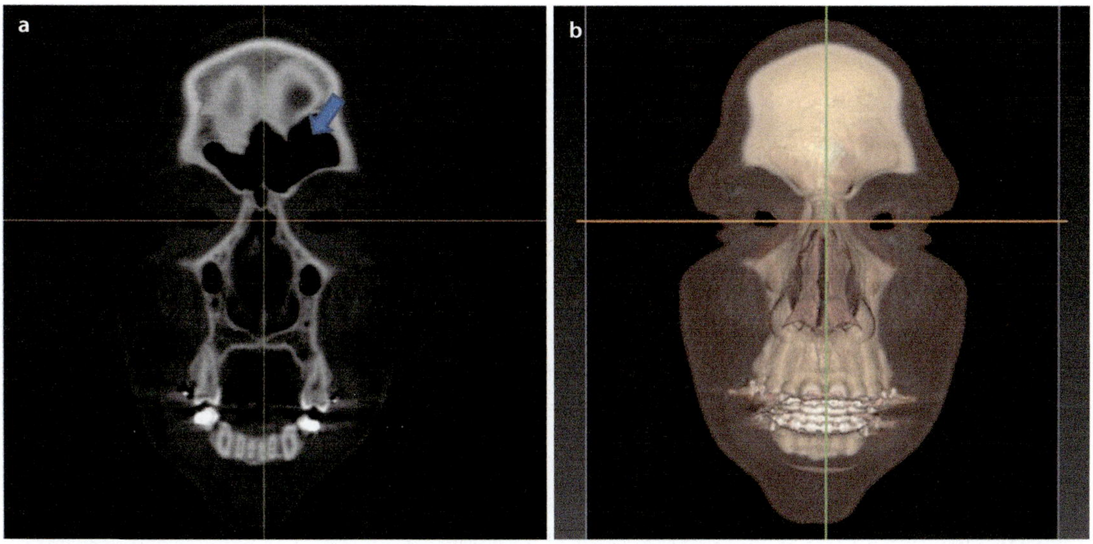

Fig. 2.30 Coronal slice through the frontal sinus (*arrow*) (**a**). In this case, the sinus is well aerated without any significant pathology. (**b**) visualises the level of the coronal reconstructed reslice on the 3D "volume-rendered" patient model (i-CAT, Imaging Sciences International Inc, IPS CaseDesigner ALPHA version) (patient V.E.W.). Note the visible outline of the frontal sinus by transparency on the "volume-rendered" 3D image

Coronal Slices: Orbits and Bulbus Position

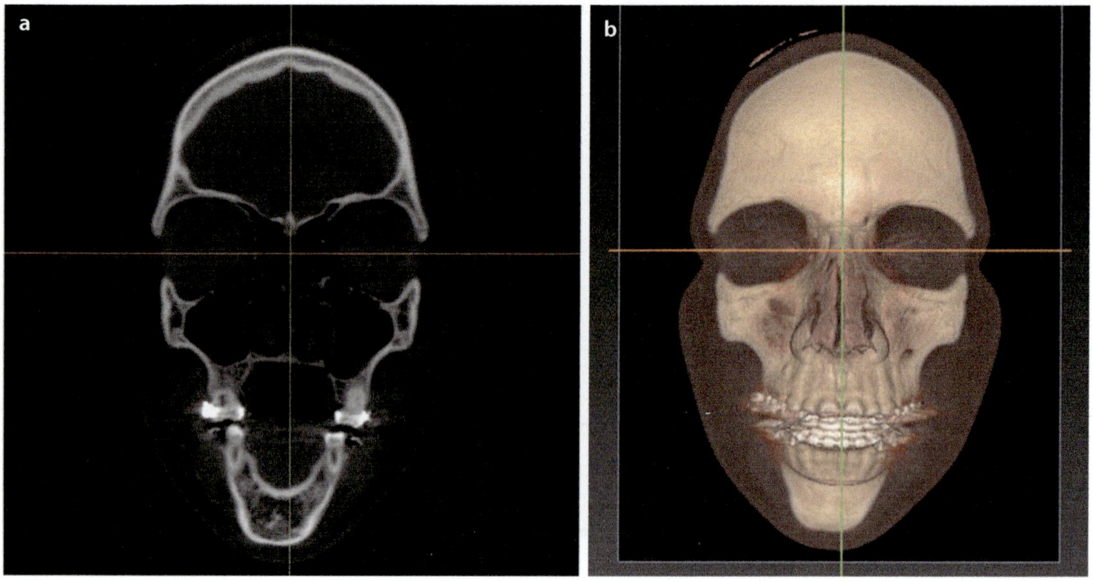

Fig. 2.31 Coronal slice through the greater axis of the globes (**a**). A horizontal plane (*orange line*) is added at the bi-pupillary level to evaluate bulbous position (vertical dystopia). In this case, the patient displays normal bulbus anatomy. (**b**) visualises the level of the coronal reconstructed reslice on the 3D "volume-rendered" patient model (i-CAT, Imaging Sciences International Inc, IPS CaseDesigner ALPHA version) (patient V.E.W.)

Coronal Slices: Maxillary Sinuses

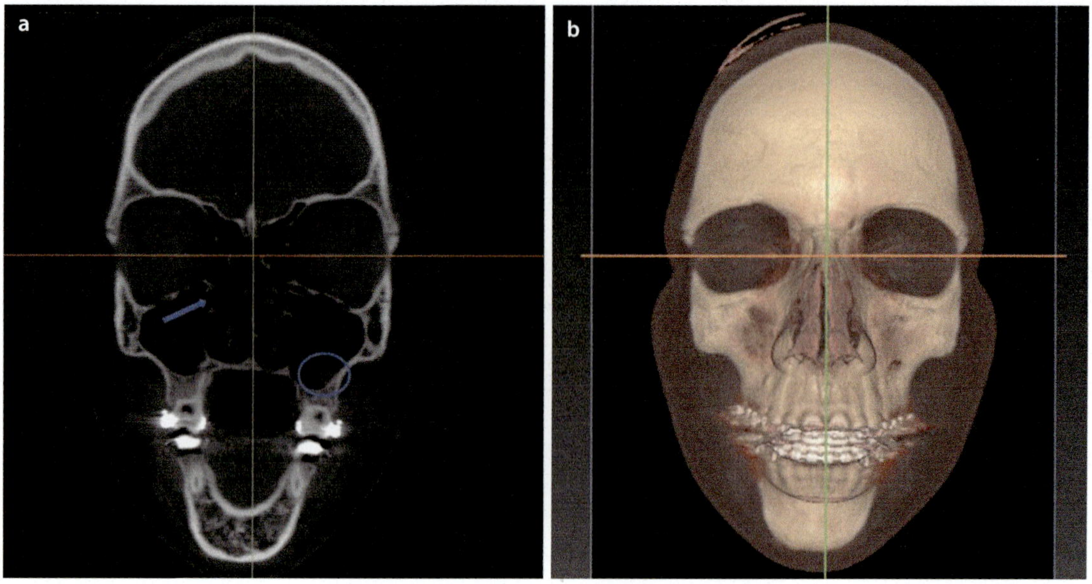

Fig. 2.32 Coronal slice through the maxillary sinuses (**a**). The *arrow* demonstrates the opening of the right maxillary sinus in the middle nasal meatus, while the *circle* delineates a small mucus retention cyst, as seen on the previous axial slices (Fig. 2.17). (**b**) visualises the level of the coronal reconstructed reslice on the 3D "volume-rendered" patient model (i-CAT, Imaging Sciences International Inc, IPS CaseDesigner ALPHA version) (patient V.E.W.)

Coronal Slices: Nasal Septum

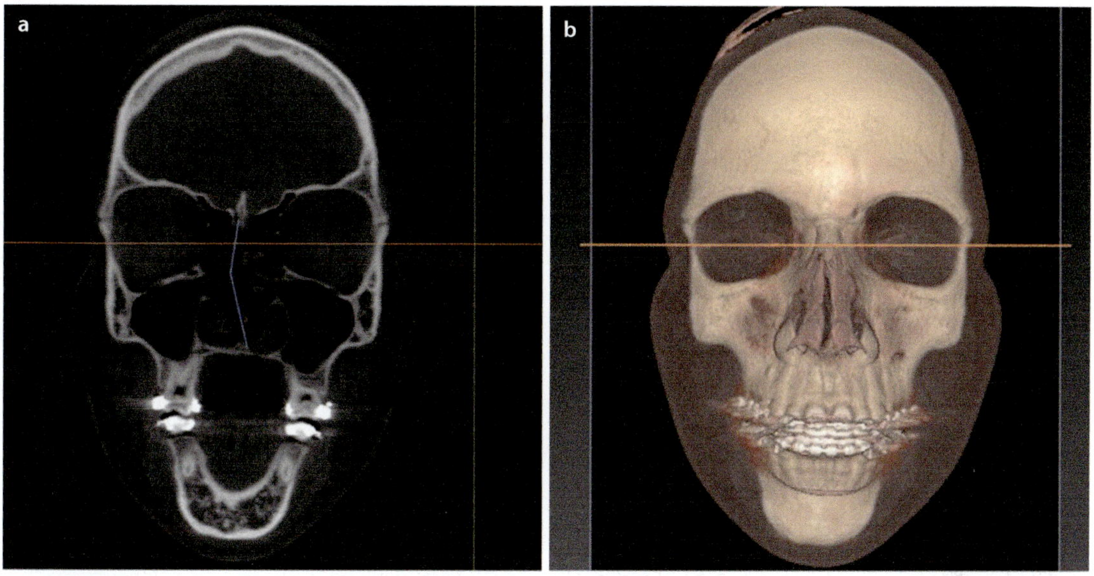

Fig. 2.33 Coronal slice at the level of the bony septum, demonstrating a mild deviation of the posterior bony nasal septum to the right (*blue line*) (**a**). (**b**) visualises the level of the coronal reconstructed reslice on the 3D "volume-rendered" patient model (i-CAT, Imaging Sciences International Inc, IPS CaseDesigner ALPHA version) (patient V.E.W.)

Coronal Slices: Nasal Turbinates

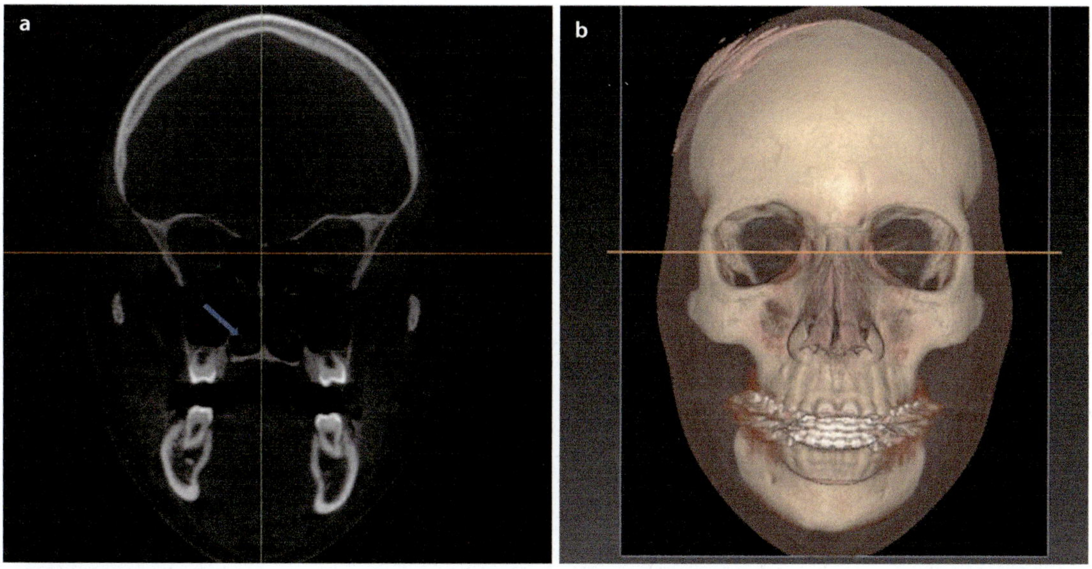

Fig. 2.34 A more posterior coronal slice, to demonstrate the inferior nasal turbinates (*arrow*) (**a**). Note the absence of posterior nasal septal deviation. (**b**) visualises the level of the coronal reconstructed reslice on the 3D "volume-rendered" patient model (i-CAT, Imaging Sciences International Inc, IPS CaseDesigner ALPHA version) (patient V.E.W.)

Coronal Slices: Ethmoidal Sinuses

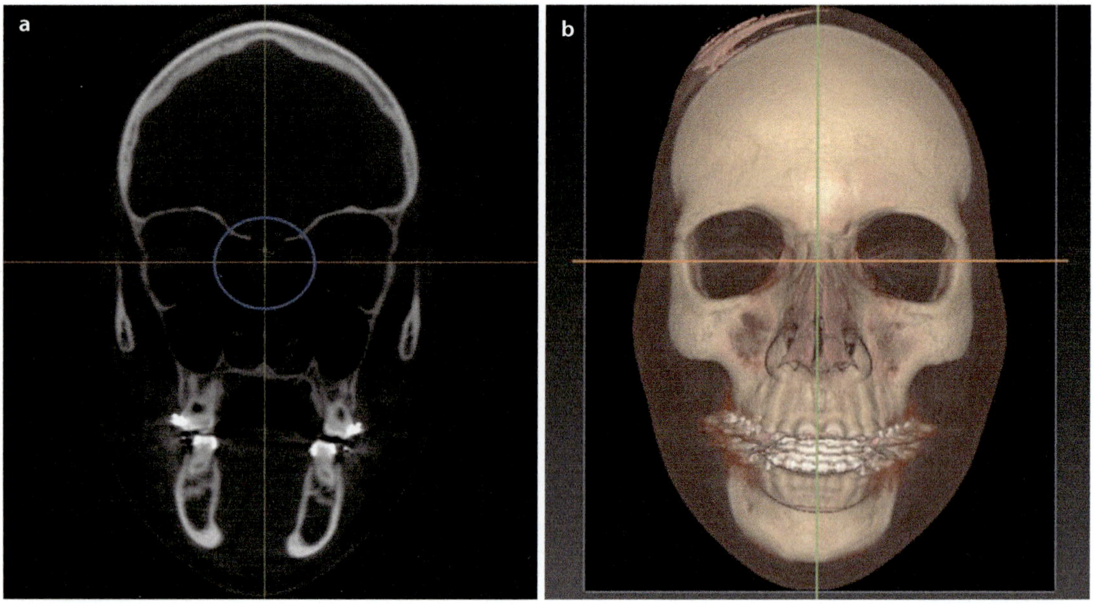

Fig. 2.35 Coronal slice through the etmoid sinus, outlined by a *blue circle* (**a**). Note the discrete opacification of the ethmoidal air cells. (**b**) visualises the level of the coronal reconstructed reslice on the 3D "volume-rendered" patient model (i-CAT, Imaging Sciences International Inc, IPS CaseDesigner ALPHA version) (patient V.E.W.)

Coronal Slices: Upper and Lower Molar/Premolar Inclination in Regard to the Alveolar Ridge

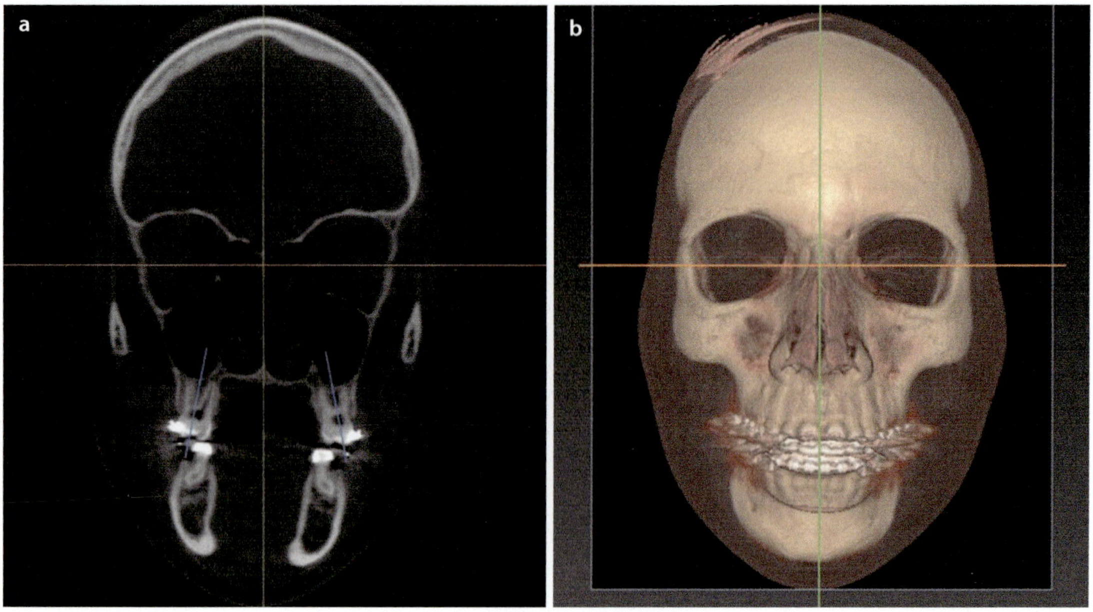

Fig. 2.36 Coronal slice through the posterior alveolar process, at the second upper molar level (**a**). The evaluation of the upper (*blue lines*) and lower Wilson's curve is of paramount importance in maxillary transverse insufficiency cases. (**b**) visualises the level of the coronal reconstructed reslice on the 3D "volume-rendered" patient model (i-CAT, Imaging Sciences International Inc, IPS CaseDesigner ALPHA version) (patient V.E.W.)

Coronal Slices: Transversal Occlusal Relationship

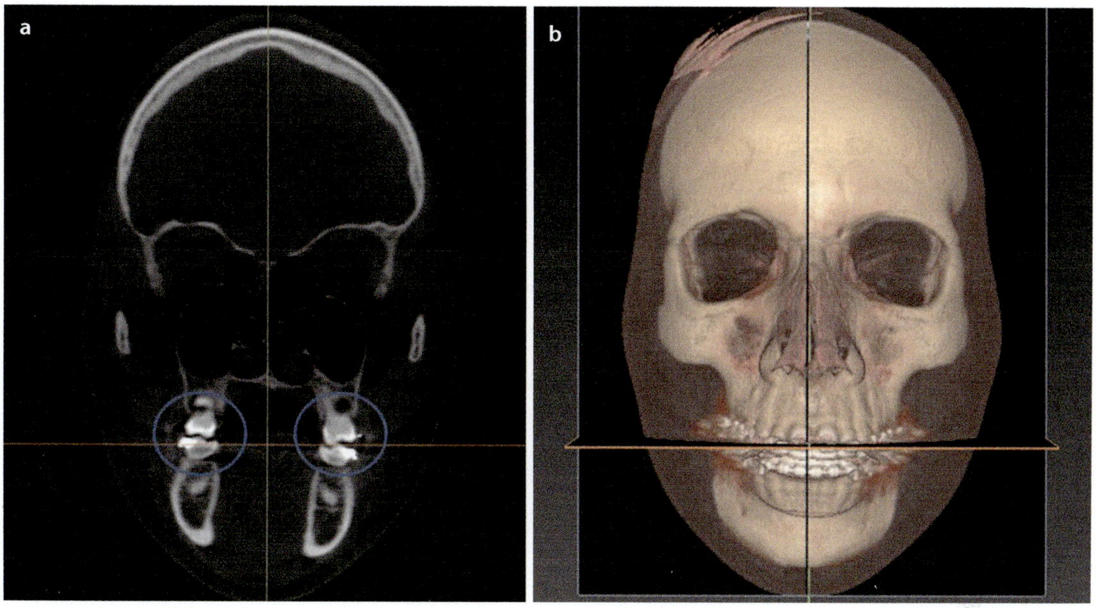

Fig. 2.37 Coronal slice at the level of the first molars (*blue circles*) (**a**). Note the relatively adequate transverse relationship between the upper and lower dental arches. The true transverse relation of the upper and lower dentition must however be evaluated in Angle "class I" relationship. The upper and lower arch coordination is not evaluated at this stage and will be assessed during "3D virtual occlusal definition (► see also Sect. 3.3)". (**b**) visualises the level of the coronal reconstructed reslice on the 3D "volume-rendered" patient model (i-CAT, Imaging Sciences International Inc, IPS CaseDesigner ALPHA version) (patient V.E.W.)

Coronal Slices: Course of the Inferior Alveolar Nerve (IAN)

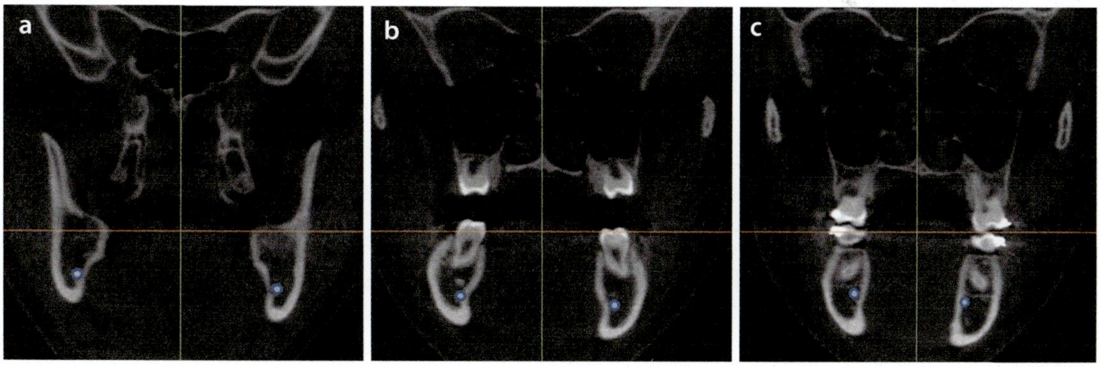

Fig. 2.38 Multiple coronal slices, at the gonial angle notch (**a**), distally to the second lower molar (**b**) and between the first and second lower molar (**c**) show the location of the IAN in the mandible, outlined in blue (i-CAT, Imaging Sciences International Inc, IPS CaseDesigner ALPHA version) (patient V.E.W.)

Coronal Slices: Course of the Inferior Alveolar Nerve (IAN)

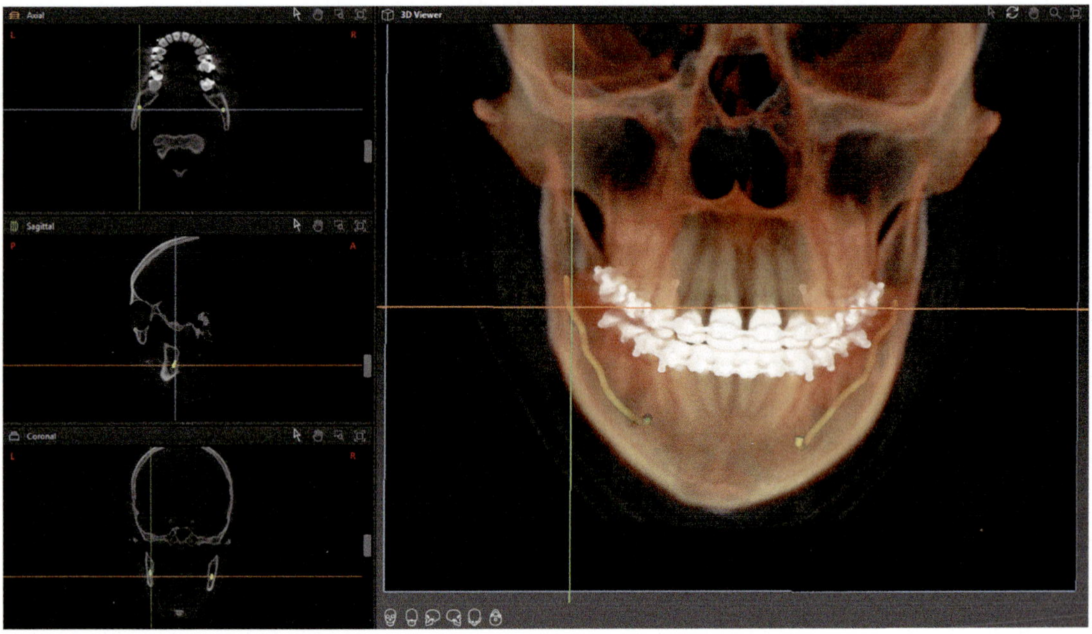

Fig. 2.39 More enhanced diagnostic features show the bilateral course of the IAN visualised on the "volume-rendered" patient model in dynamic relation towards the axial, sagittal and coronal reconstructed slices (i-CAT, Imaging Sciences International Inc, IPS CaseDesigner ALPHA version) (patient V.E.W.)

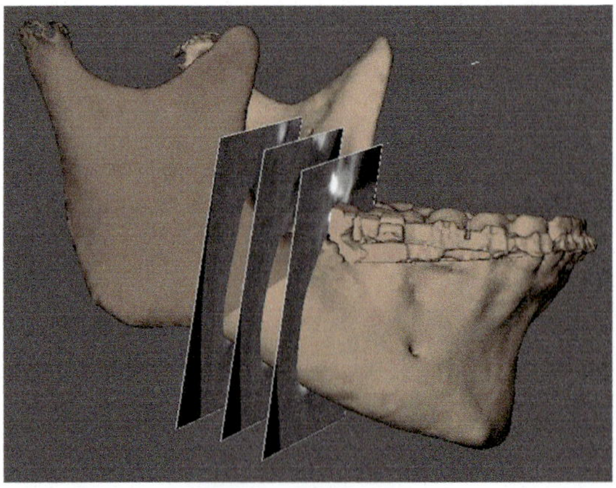

Fig. 2.40 3D "surface-rendered" representation of the mandible with a virtual bilateral sagittal split osteotomy (▶ see also Sect. 3.2.2) (BSSO). Multiplanar reslices can be reconstructed at different levels (such at the gonial angle notch, distally to the second lower molar and between the first and second lower molar) to identify the position of the IAN at the level of the BSSO (i-CAT, Imaging Sciences International Inc, Maxilim v. 2.3.0.3.) (patient V.E.W.)

Coronal Slices: Condylar Morphology

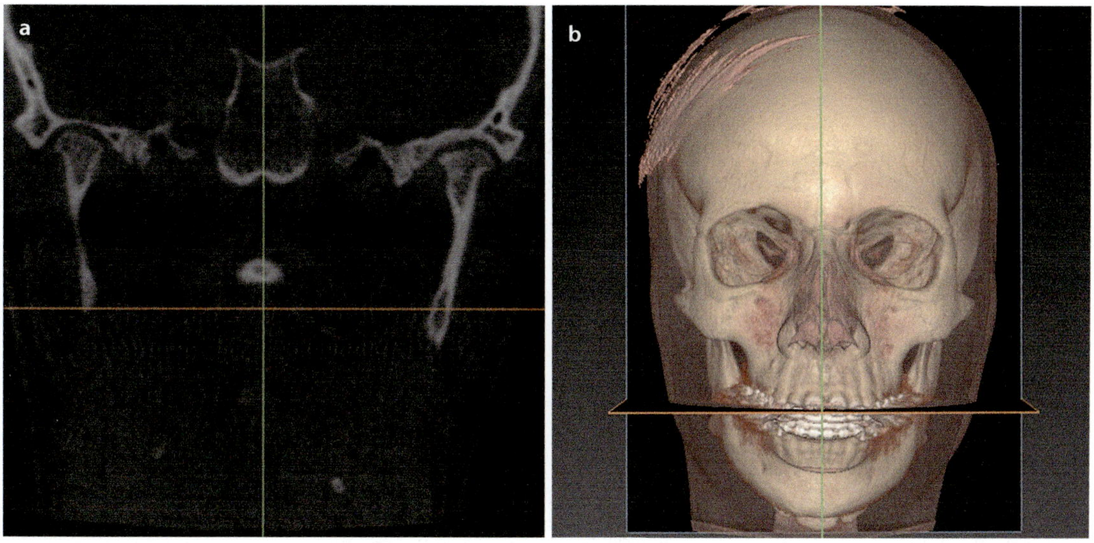

Fig. 2.41 Coronal slice at the level of the mandibular condyles (**a**). Note the proper position of the condyles in the glenoid fossa. Advanced TMJ 3D imaging and evaluation will be discussed in (▶ Sect. 2.1.4). (**b**) visualises the level of the coronal reconstructed reslice on the 3D "volume-rendered" patient model (i-CAT, Imaging Sciences International Inc, IPS CaseDesigner ALPHA version) (patient V.E.W.)

Coronal Slices: Posterior Airway

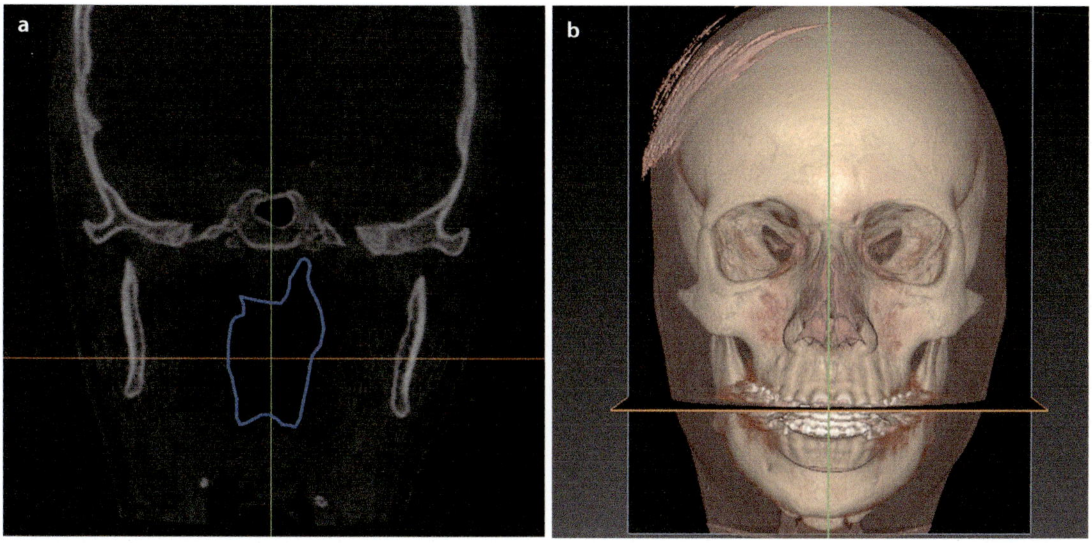

Fig. 2.42 Coronal slice through the nasopharyngeal and oropharyngeal airway, outlined in blue, at the level of the tongue base (**a**). Enhanced 3D airway imaging and evaluation will be discussed in (▶ Sect. 2.1.3). (**b**) visualises the level of the coronal reconstructed reslice on the 3D "volume-rendered" patient model (i-CAT, Imaging Sciences International Inc, IPS CaseDesigner ALPHA version) (patient V.E.W.)

Coronal Slices: Cervical Spine

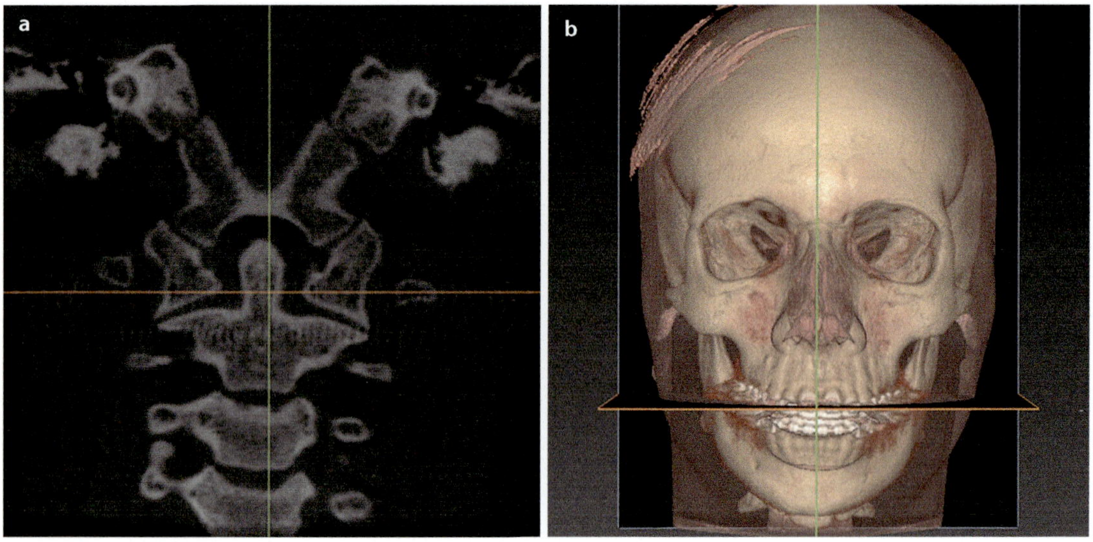

Fig. 2.43 Coronal slice through the cervical spine (**a**). Orthognathic patients can display a cervical scoliosis or even cervical spine anomalies in case of trauma or associated syndromes. In this case, no abnormalities can be diagnosed. (**b**) visualises the level of the coronal reconstructed reslice on the 3D "volume-rendered" patient model (i-CAT, Imaging Sciences International Inc, IPS CaseDesigner ALPHA version) (patient V.E.W.)

Sagittal Slices: Systematic Virtual Evaluation of the Patient's Anatomy and Pathology

The following clinical features relevant to combined orthodontic-surgical treatment planning are systematically analysed on the baseline sagittal slices by scrolling through the individual patient's DICOM data set.

A standardised checklist for systematic virtual evaluation of the patient's individual anatomy and pathology, based on the sagittal slices, is hereby provided:

1. Right condylar morphology and seating (◘ Fig. 2.44)
2. Right vertical level of entrance (lingula) of the inferior alveolar nerve (IAN) (◘ Figs. 2.45 and 2.46)
3. Right maxillary sinus (◘ Fig. 2.47)
4. Right orbit and bulbus position (◘ Fig. 2.48)
5. Right sagittal occlusal relationship (◘ Fig. 2.49)
6. Ethmoidal sinuses (◘ Fig. 2.50)
7. Frontal sinuses (◘ Fig. 2.51)
8. Incisal inclination in regard to the alveolar ridge (◘ Fig. 2.52)
9. Airway and cranio-cervical inclination (◘ Fig. 2.53)
10. Left sagittal occlusal relationship (◘ Fig. 2.54)
11. Left orbit and bulbus position (◘ Fig. 2.55)
12. Left maxillary sinus (◘ Fig. 2.56)
13. Left vertical level of entrance (lingula) of the inferior alveolar nerve (IAN) (◘ Figs. 2.57 and 2.58)
14. Left condylar morphology and seating (◘ Fig. 2.59)
15. Patient's specific pathology

It needs to be emphasised that standardised virtual evaluation of the sagittal slices is of major clinical importance and needs to be performed dynamically by the clinician (orthodontist and/or surgeon). Moreover, by using the hereby proposed systematic approach, it is not time consuming.

Case 1

Patient V.E.W. is used to demonstrate the systematic approach towards individualised patient's anatomy assessment, while patient's specific pathology is demonstrated by other clinical cases (▶ see also Chap. 6).

Sagittal Slices: Right Condylar Morphology and Seating

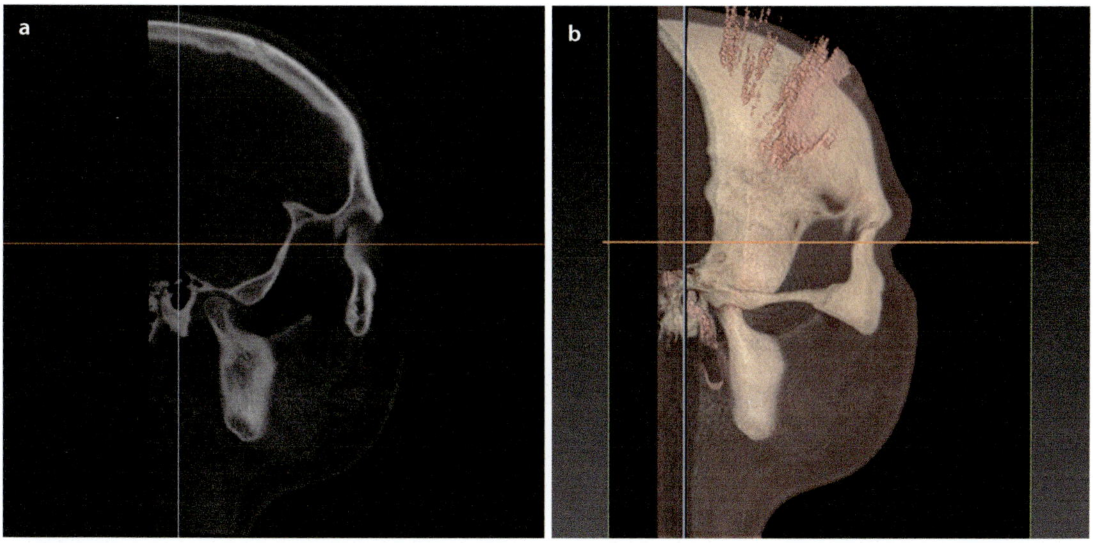

◘ **Fig. 2.44** Sagittal slice through the right mandibular condyle (**a**). Note adequate seating of the right condyle in the glenoid fossa and absence of significant pathology. Enhanced TMJ 3D imaging and evaluation will be discussed in (▶ Sect. 2.1.4). (**b**) visualises the level of the sagittal reconstructed reslice on the 3D "volume-rendered" patient model (i-CAT, Imaging Sciences International Inc, IPS CaseDesigner ALPHA version) (patient V.E.W.)

Sagittal Slices: Right Vertical Level of Entrance (Lingula) of the Inferior Alveolar Nerve (IAN)

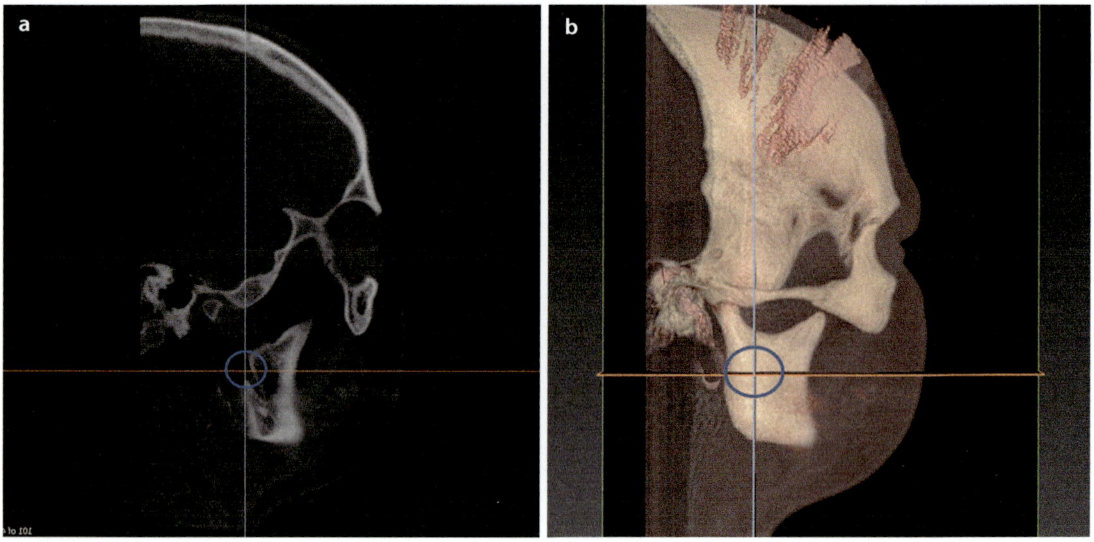

Fig. 2.45 Sagittal slice through the opening of the right mandibular foramen (*blue circle*) (**a**). The vertical and sagittal level of entrance of the right IAN at the lingula provides important anatomical information towards identification of this important landmark during surgery. (**b**) visualises the level of the sagittal reconstructed reslice on the 3D "volume-rendered" patient model, where the location of the mandibular foramen is outlined in blue. (i-CAT, Imaging Sciences International Inc, IPS CaseDesigner ALPHA version) (patient V.E.W.)

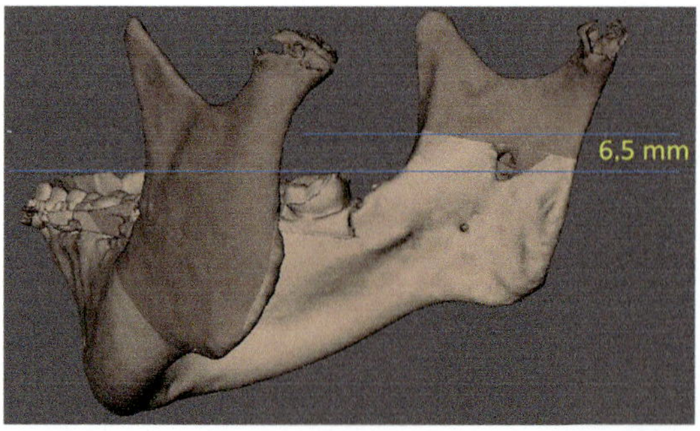

Fig. 2.46 3D "surface-rendered" representation of the mandible with a virtual bilateral sagittal split osteotomy (▶ see also Sect. 3.2.2) (BSSO). The individual anatomy of the right mandibular vertical ramus at the level of the horizontal corticotomy of the virtually planned BSSO can be evaluated. Moreover, the vertical distance between the lingula and the lower occlusal plane (*blue lines*) can be measured to facilitate identification of this important landmark during actual surgery. Especially in patients with abnormal anatomy of the vertical mandibular ramus such as post-traumatic and congenital cases, this can be helpful (i-CAT, Imaging Sciences International Inc, Maxilim v. 2.3.0.3.) (patient V.E.W.)

Sagittal Slices: Right Maxillary Sinus

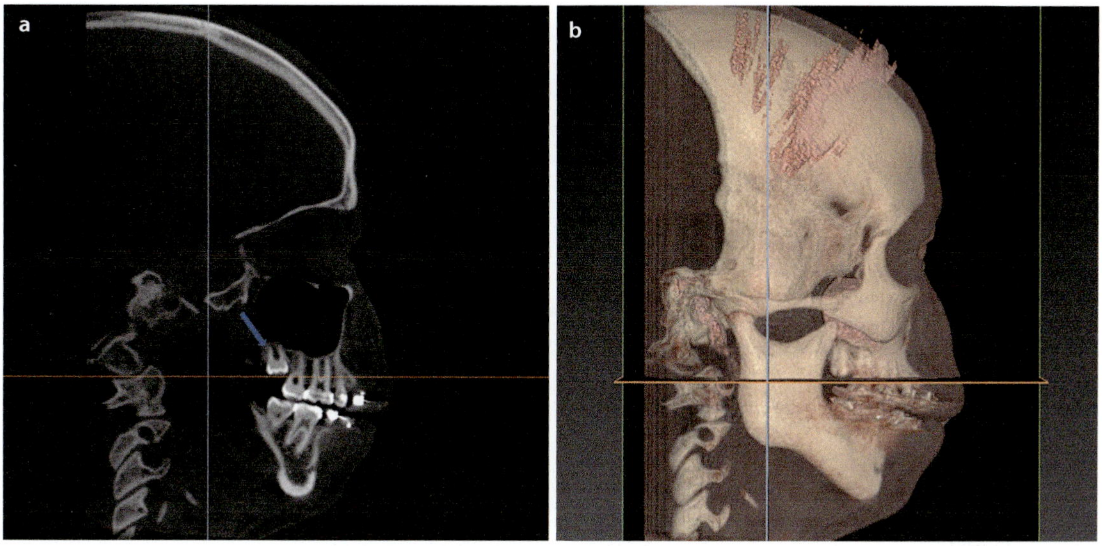

Fig. 2.47 Sagittal slice through the right maxillary sinus (**a**). Note the mesio-angulated upper right wisdom tooth (*arrow*). No abnormalities of the right maxillary sinus can be diagnosed in this patient. (**b**) visualises the level of the sagittal reconstructed reslice on the 3D "volume-rendered" patient model (i-CAT, Imaging Sciences International Inc, IPS CaseDesigner ALPHA version) (patient V.E.W.)

Sagittal Slices: Right Orbit and Bulbus Position

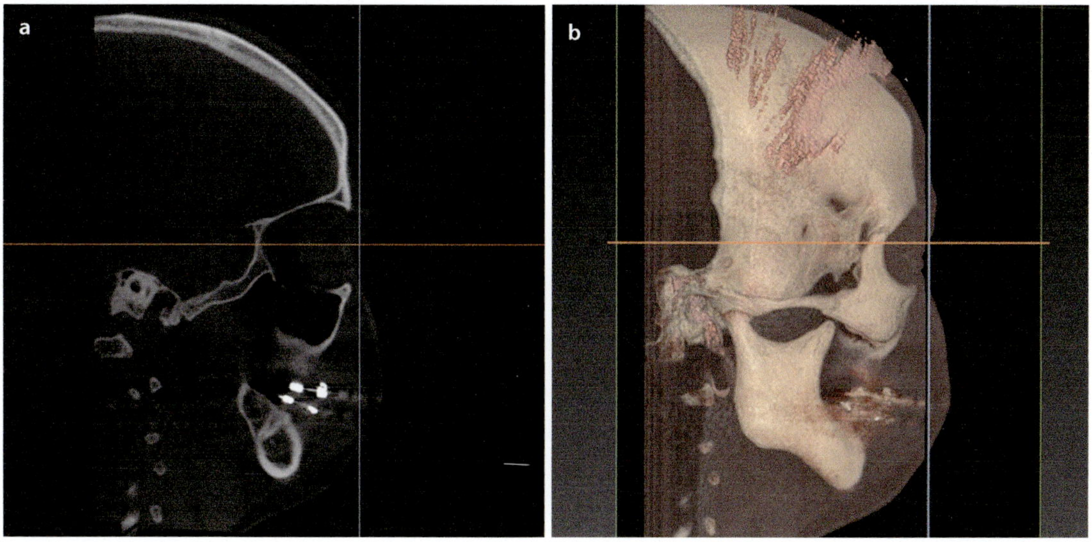

Fig. 2.48 Sagittal slice through the right orbital cavity and bulbus (**a**). In this case, no significant pathology can be observed. (**b**) visualises the level of the sagittal reconstructed reslice on the 3D "volume-rendered" patient model (i-CAT, Imaging Sciences International Inc, IPS CaseDesigner ALPHA version) (patient V.E.W.)

Sagittal Slices: Right Sagittal Occlusal Relationship

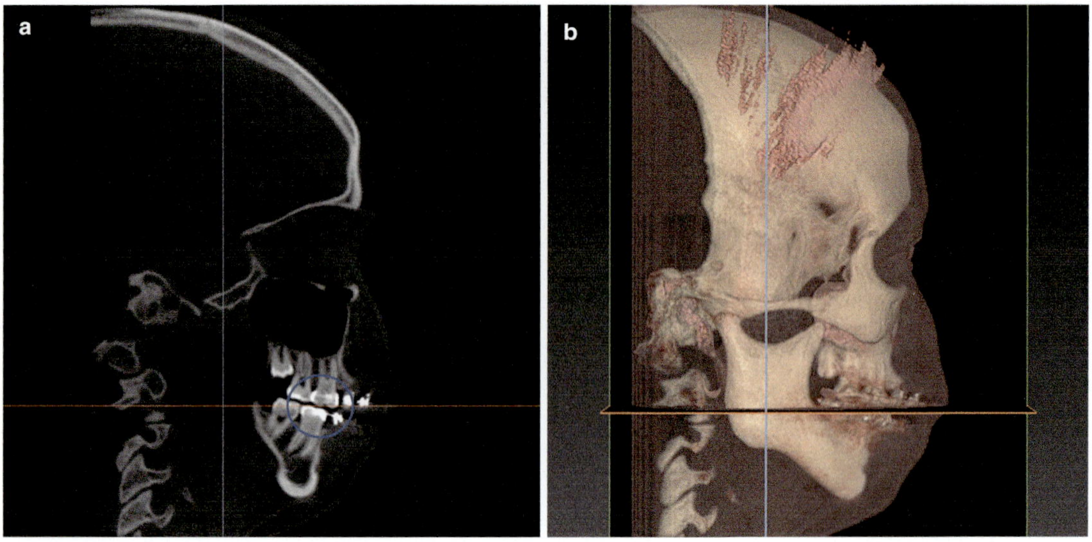

Fig. 2.49 Sagittal slice at the level of the right first upper and lower molars (*blue circle*) (**a**). Note a molar Angle "Class II" malocclusion in this patient. (**b**) visualises the level of the sagittal reconstructed reslice on the 3D "volume-rendered" patient model (i-CAT, Imaging Sciences International Inc, IPS CaseDesigner ALPHA version) (patient V.E.W.)

Sagittal Slices: Ethmoidal Sinuses

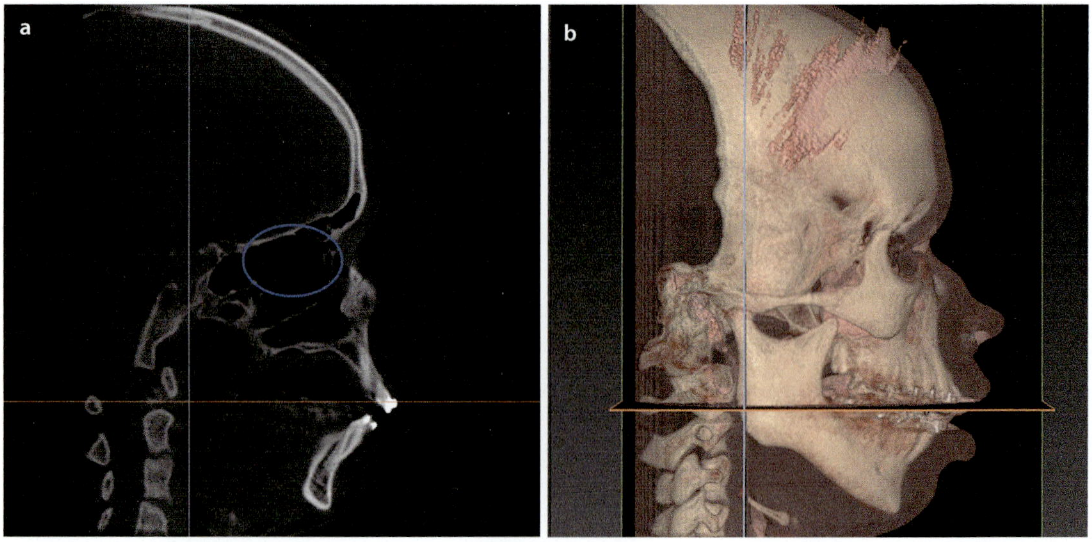

Fig. 2.50 Sagittal slice at the level of the right ethmoidal air cells, outlined with a *blue circle* (**a**). Note the absence of pathology in this particular orthogonal slice in this patient. (**b**) visualises the level of the sagittal reconstructed reslice on the 3D "volume-rendered" patient model (i-CAT, Imaging Sciences International Inc, IPS CaseDesigner ALPHA version) (patient V.E.W.)

Sagittal Slices: Frontal Sinuses

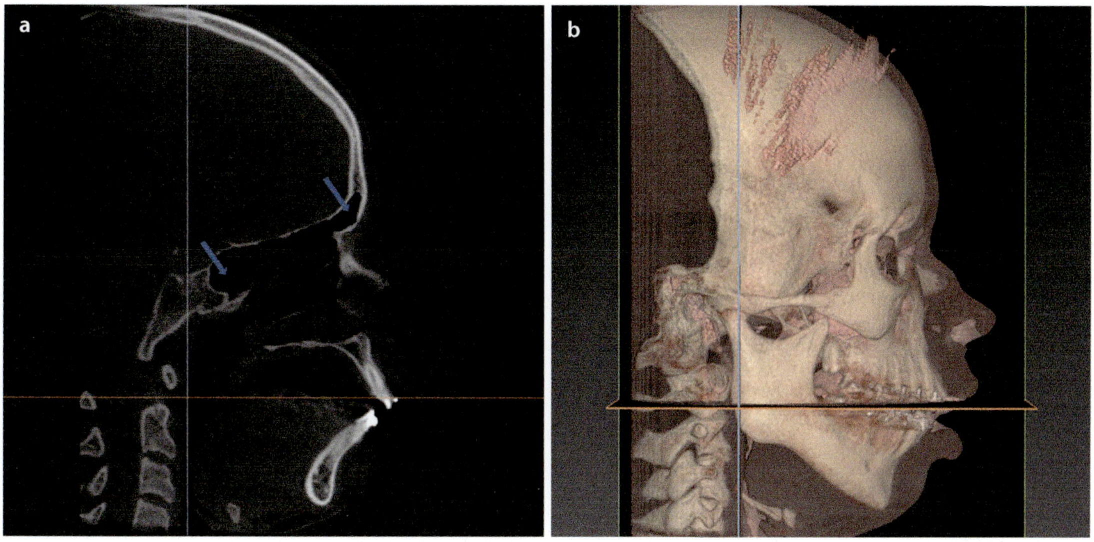

Fig. 2.51 Sagittal slice through the frontal sinus (*right arrow*) (**a**). The sphenoidal sinus is also visualised (*left arrow*). Both sinuses are well aerated. (**b**) visualises the level of the sagittal reconstructed reslice on the 3D "volume-rendered" patient model (i-CAT, Imaging Sciences International Inc, IPS CaseDesigner ALPHA version) (patient V.E.W.)

Sagittal Slices: Incisal Inclination in Regard to the Alveolar Ridge

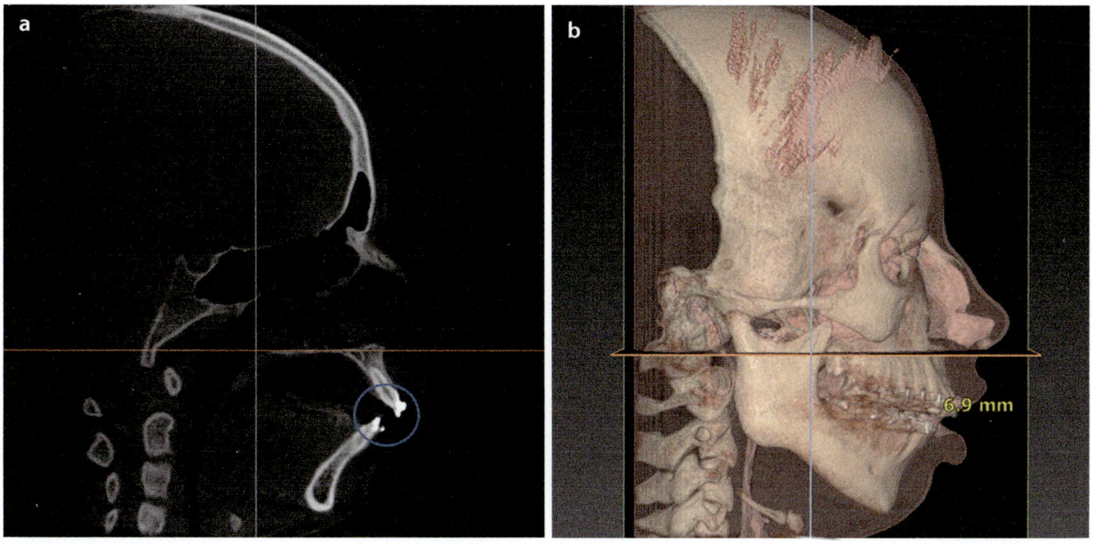

Fig. 2.52 Sagittal slice at the level of the right upper central incisor (*blue circle*) (**a**). Note the increased sagittal overjet of 6.9 mm. (**b**) visualises the level of the sagittal reconstructed reslice on the 3D "volume-rendered" patient model (i-CAT, Imaging Sciences International Inc, IPS CaseDesigner ALPHA version) (patient V.E.W.)

Sagittal Slices: Airway and Cranio-cervical Inclination

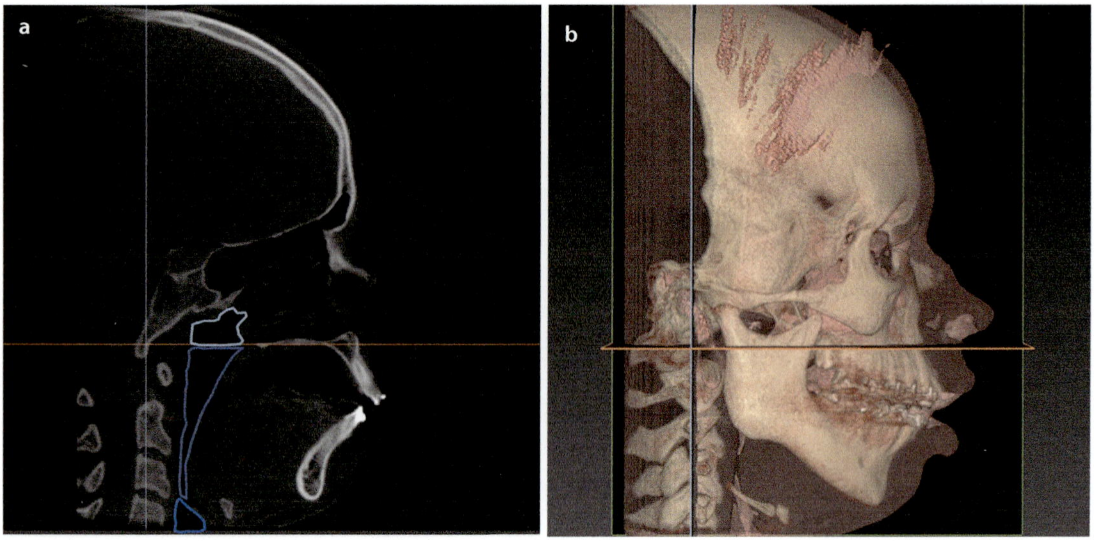

Fig. 2.53 Sagittal slice through the posterior upper airway (**a**). The nasopharyngeal, oropharyngeal and hypopharyngeal subregions of the upper airway delineated according to the radiological limits published by Guijarro-Martinez and Swennen (2013). Enhanced 3D airway imaging, evaluation and cranio-cervical inclination will be discussed in (► Sect. 2.1.3.) (**b**) visualises the level of the sagittal reconstructed reslice on the 3D "volume-rendered" patient model (i-CAT, Imaging Sciences International Inc, IPS CaseDesigner ALPHA version) (patient V.E.W.)

Sagittal Slices: Left Sagittal Occlusal Relationship

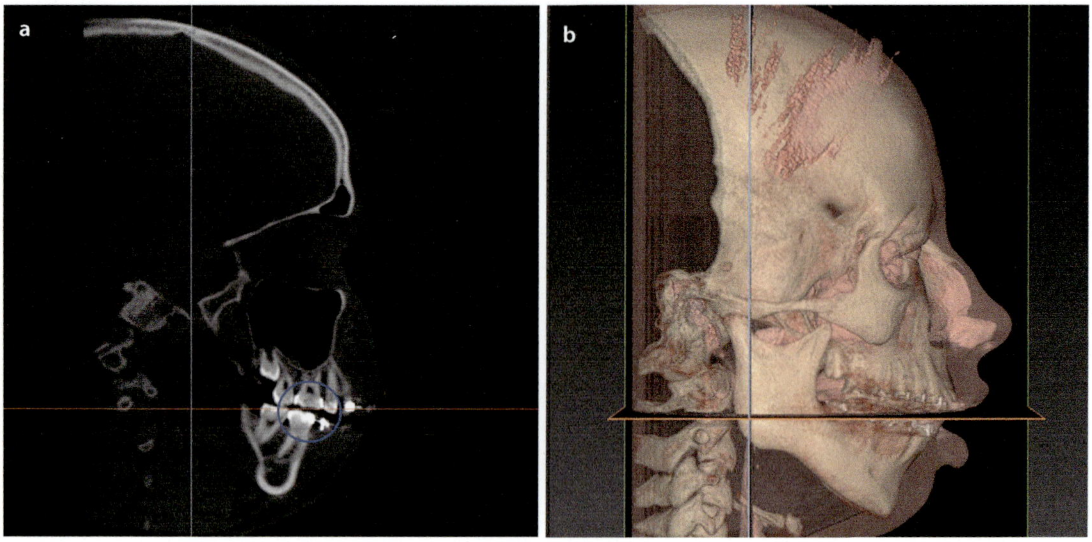

Fig. 2.54 Sagittal slice at the level of the left first upper and lower molars (*blue circle*) (**a**). Note a molar Angle "Class II" malocclusion in this patient. (**b**) visualises the level of the sagittal reconstructed reslice on the 3D "volume-rendered" patient model (i-CAT, Imaging Sciences International Inc, IPS CaseDesigner ALPHA version) (patient V.E.W.)

Sagittal Slices: Left Orbit and Bulbus Position

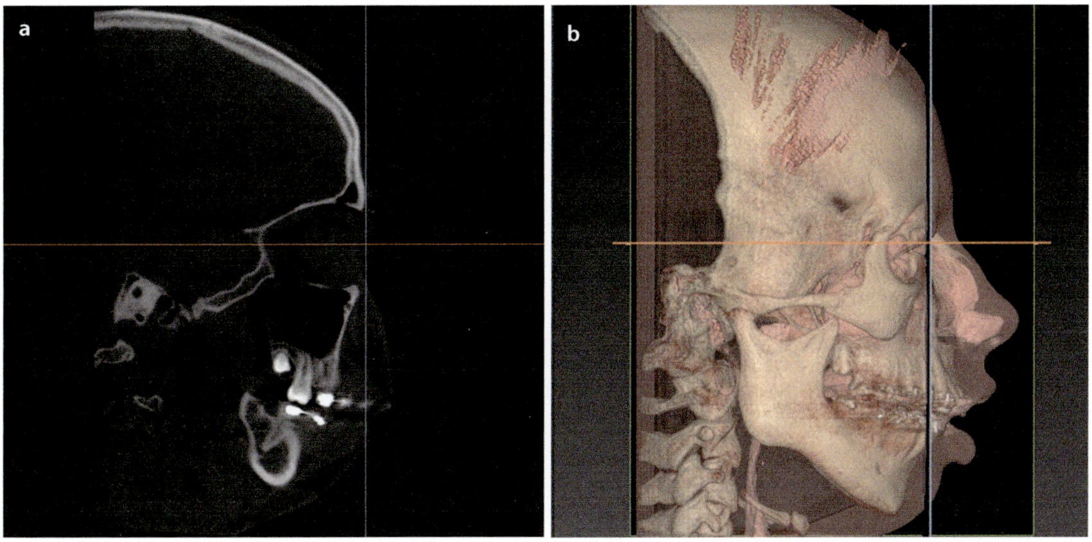

Fig. 2.55 Sagittal slice through the left orbital cavity and bulbus (**a**). In this case, no significant pathology can be observed. (**b**) visualises the level of the sagittal reconstructed reslice on the 3D "volume-rendered" patient model (i-CAT, Imaging Sciences International Inc, IPS CaseDesigner ALPHA version) (patient V.E.W.)

Sagittal Slices: Left Maxillary Sinus

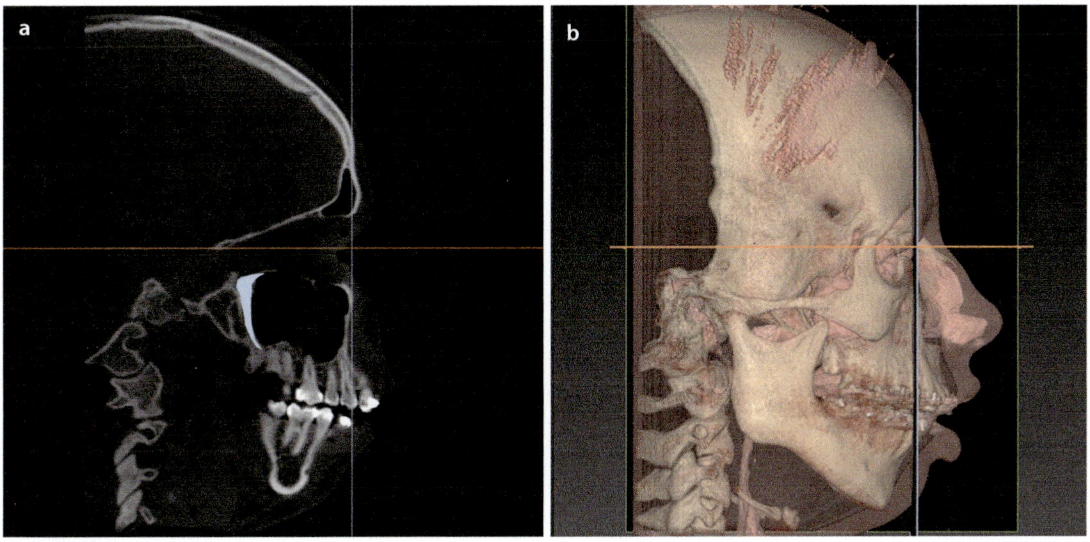

Fig. 2.56 Sagittal slice through the left maxillary sinus (**a**). The left pterygomaxillary (PTM) fissure is outlined in light blue for educational purposes. A small mucous retention cyst can be diagnosed in the left maxillary sinus. (**b**) visualises the level of the sagittal reconstructed reslice on the 3D "volume-rendered" patient model (i-CAT, Imaging Sciences International Inc, IPS CaseDesigner ALPHA version) (patient V.E.W.)

Sagittal Slices: Left Vertical Level of Entrance (Lingula) of the Inferior Alveolar Nerve (IAN)

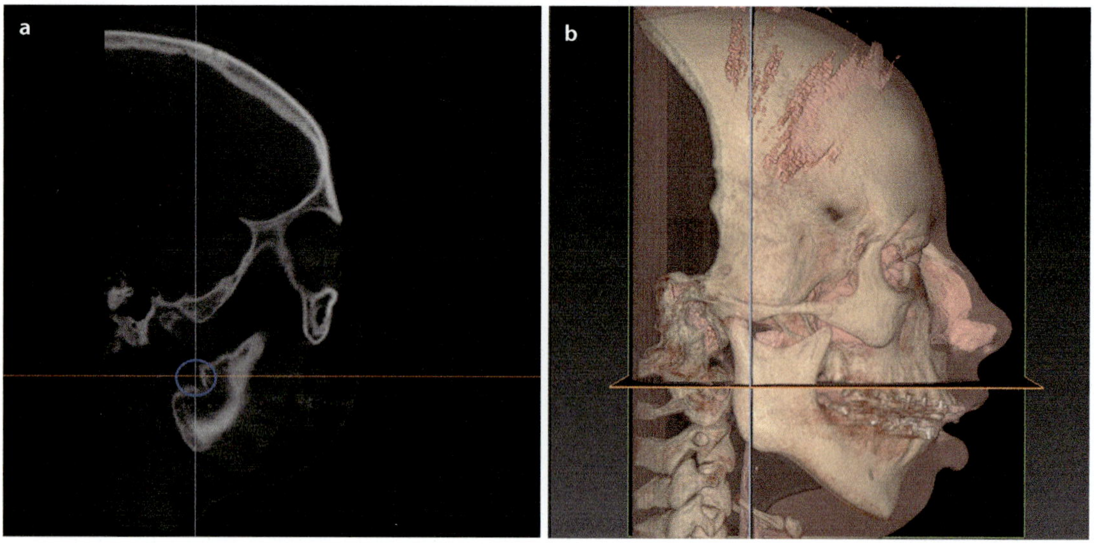

Fig. 2.57 Sagittal slice through the opening of the right mandibular foramen (*blue circle*) (**a**). The vertical and sagittal level of entrance of the left IAN at the lingula provides important anatomical information towards identification of this important landmark during surgery. (**b**) visualises the level of the sagittal reconstructed reslice on the 3D "volume-rendered" patient model (i-CAT, Imaging Sciences International Inc, IPS CaseDesigner ALPHA version) (patient V.E.W.)

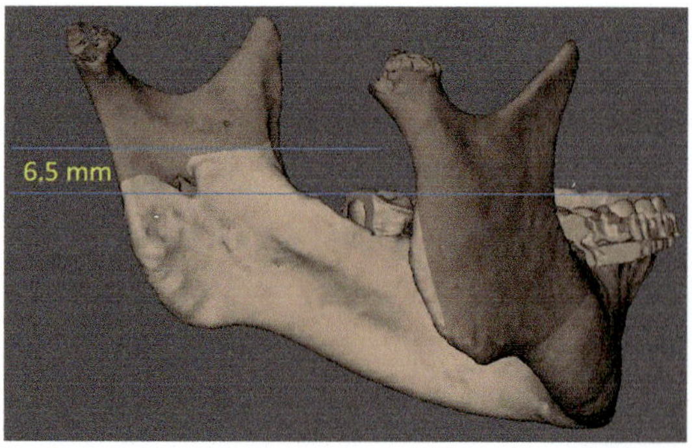

Fig. 2.58 3D "surface-rendered" representation of the mandible with a virtual bilateral sagittal split osteotomy (▶ see also Sect. 3.2.2) (BSSO). The individual anatomy of the left mandibular vertical ramus at the level of the horizontal corticotomy of the virtually planned BSSO can be evaluated. Moreover, the vertical distance between the lingula and the lower occlusal plane (*blue lines*) can be measured to facilitate identification of this important landmark during actual surgery. Especially in patients with abnormal anatomy of the vertical mandibular ramus such as post-traumatic and congenital cases, this can be helpful (i-CAT, Imaging Sciences International Inc, Maxilim v. 2.3.0.3.) (patient V.E.W.)

Sagittal Slices: Left Condylar Morphology and Seating

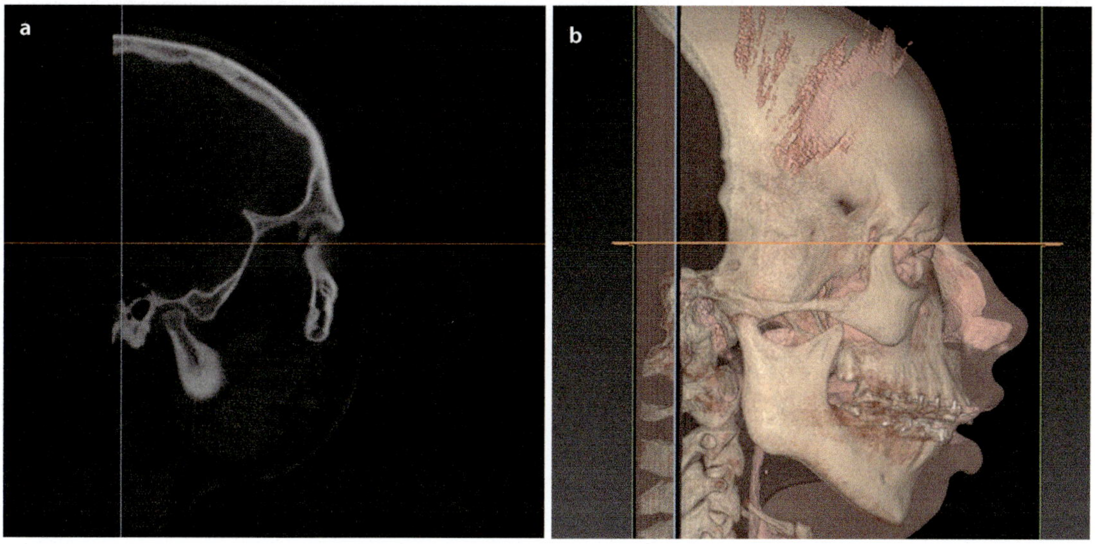

Fig. 2.59 Sagittal slice through the left mandibular condyle (**a**). Note adequate seating of the left condyle in the glenoid fossa and absence of significant pathology. Enhanced TMJ 3D imaging and evaluation will be discussed in (▶ Sect. 2.1.4). (**b**) visualises the level of the sagittal reconstructed reslice on the 3D "volume-rendered" patient model (i-CAT, Imaging Sciences International Inc, IPS CaseDesigner ALPHA version) (patient V.E.W.)

2.1.3 Airway

After standardised "step-by-step" systematic virtual evaluation of the patient's individual "deformity and bite (▶ Sect. 2.1.1)" and "anatomy and pathology (▶ Sect. 2.1.2)", the "3D Virtual Visualisation Paradigm" allows more enhanced diagnostics of the patient's upper airway in the "3D virtual scene".

A systematic review (SR) of the literature (Guijarro-Martínez and Swennen 2011) showed that 3D analysis of the upper airway using CBCT could be performed in an accurate and reliable manner but also identified some important issues that still need to be taken into account:

1. The impact of the respiration phase
2. The influence of the tongue position
3. The morphology and position of the mandible
4. The need for standardisation towards longitudinal and cross-sectional 3D CBCT upper airway evaluation
5. The importance of 3D CBCT definition of the anatomical boundaries of the upper pharyngeal airway and its subregions

In 2013, Guijarro-Martinez and Swennen validated a systematised protocol to define in an accurate and reliable way the upper pharyngeal airway and its subregions: the "nasopharyngeal", "oropharyngeal" and "hypopharyngeal" airway (◘ Figs. 2.68, 2.69 and 2.70).

The standardised protocol consists of:

1. Standardised CBCT scanning of the patient's head in NHP (▶ see also Sect. 1.1.1)
   (a) The patient is scanned in a vertical seated or standing position and instructed to avoid any movement during CBCT scanning.
   (b) The patient is instructed to avoid deglutition and to breath lightly during CBCT scanning, with the tongue in a relaxed position.
   (c) The patient is CBCT scanned with the mandible in a reproducible position which can be "centric occlusion (CO)" with maximal intercuspidation or "centric relation (CR)". In case a wax-bite wafer is used, it should be trimmed in order to avoid distortion of the position of the tongue.
2. Verification of the patient's head position by measuring the "cranio-cervical inclination" in the sagittal plane
3. Virtual reorientation of the patient's head with the set-up of an "Upper Airway 3D Coordinate System"
4. Segmentation of the upper pharyngeal airway by "thresholding" (between 70 and 75 depending on the individual CBCT apparatus scanning parameters) (▶ see also Sect. 1.2.1)
5. 3D CBCT definition of the anatomical boundaries of the upper pharyngeal airway and its subregions using 3D cephalometric hard tissue landmarks and planes (▶ see also Sect. 2.2)

■ Verification of the Patient's Head Position

In order to evaluate the homogenity of head inclination towards longitudinal and cross-sectional 3D CBCT upper airway evaluation, the patient's head position can be verified in the sagittal plane by measuring the "cranio-cervical inclination" (◘ Fig. 2.60). The "cranial base angle" (◘ Fig. 2.61) measures the basicranial flexure and allows to distinct between dolichocephalic (so-called long-face) and brachycephalic (so-called short-face) head forms.

The cranio-cervical inclination is measured as the angle between the line formed by connecting C2od (tangent point at the most superior-posterior point of the odontoid process of C2) and C2ip (the most inferior-posterior point of the body of C2) and the SN line (*Sella-Nasion*).

The cranial base angle is measured between Nasion, Sella and Basion as described by Enlow.

The cranio-cervical inclination and cranial base angle are "angular projective measurements" (▶ see also Sect. 2.2).

> Homogenity in the patient's head orientation is mandatory for precise and reproducible cross-sectional and longitudinal 3D CBCT upper airway analysis.

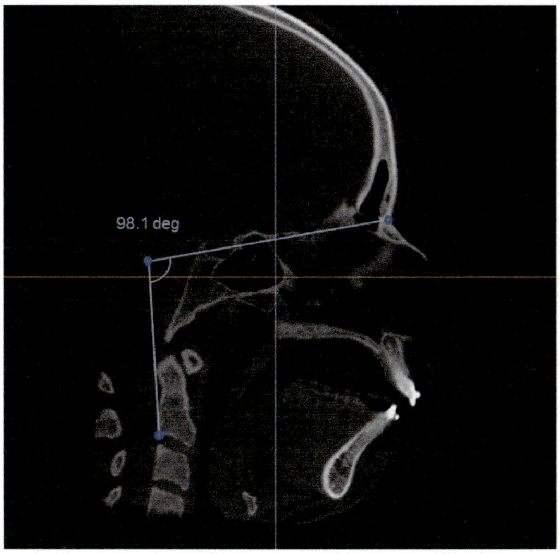

◘ **Fig. 2.60** Sagittal slice illustrating the "cranio-cervical inclination" (i-CAT, Imaging Sciences International Inc, IPS CaseDesigner ALPHA version) (patient V.E.W.)

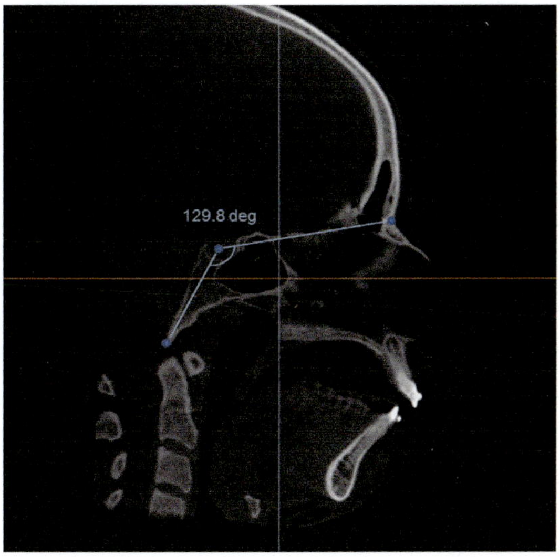

◘ **Fig. 2.61** Sagittal slice illustrating the "cranial base angle" (i-CAT, Imaging Sciences International Inc, IPS CaseDesigner ALPHA version) (patient V.E.W.)

■ Virtual Reorientation and Set-Up of an "Upper Airway 3D Coordinate System"

Once the patient's head position during CBCT scanning has been verified by measuring the cranio-cervical inclination, "virtual head reorientation" with the set-up of an "Upper Airway 3D Coordinate System" is essential for accurate and reproducible analysis of the total upper pharyngeal airway and its subregions.

The patient's head is reoriented towards the Frankfort horizontal (FH) in the frontal and right profile plane (◘ Fig. 2.62) (► see also Sect. 2.2)

The "Upper Airway 3D Coordinate System" is based on the geometric position of the patient's head after virtual reorientation with the axial (x) plane passing through *Orbitale inferior* ($Or(i)_r$), *Orbitale inferior* ($Or(i)_l$) and *Porion* (Po_r). The coronal (y) plane is set-up perpendicular to the axial (x) plane, through C2od (◘ Fig. 2.63), while the sagittal (z) plane is defined perpendicular on the axial and coronal planes through ANS (◘ Fig. 2.64).

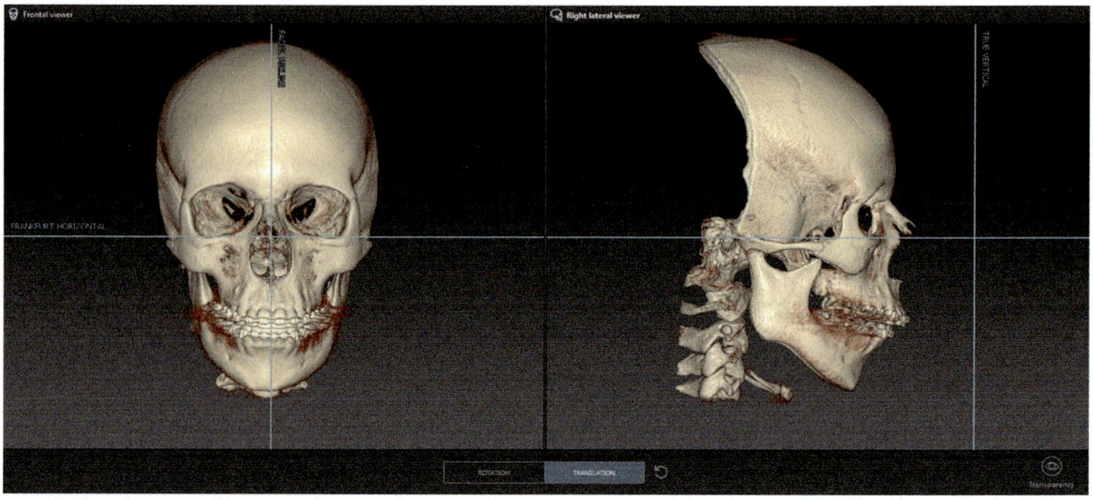

◘ **Fig. 2.62** The 3D "volume-rendered" hard tissue surface representation of the patient is reoriented to the FH plane in the frontal view using the right and left *Orbitale inferior* (*Or*(*i*)) and in the right profile view using the right *Porion* (Po_r) and *Orbitale inferior* ($Or(i)_r$) 3D hard tissue cephalometric landmarks (► see also Sect. 2.2) (i-CAT, Imaging Sciences International Inc, IPS CaseDesigner ALPHA version) (patient V.E.W.)

Virtual Reorientation and Set-Up of an "Upper Airway 3D Coordinate System"

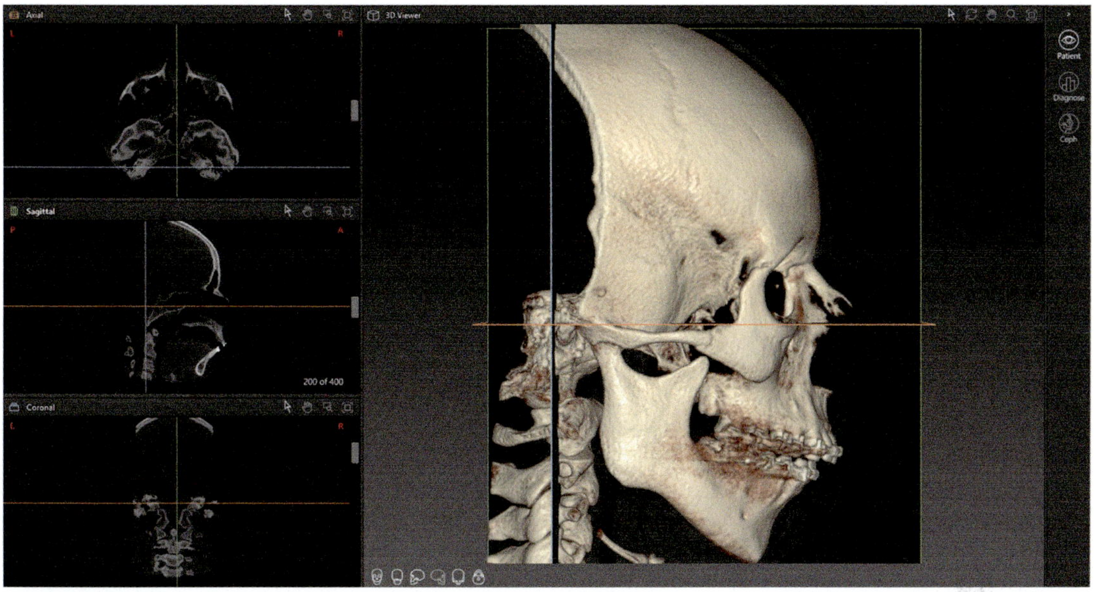

Fig. 2.63 Visualisation of the axial, coronal and sagittal 3D planes of the "Upper Airway 3D Coordinate System" on the 3D "volume-rendered" hard tissue surface representation in the right profile view (i-CAT, Imaging Sciences International Inc, IPS CaseDesigner ALPHA version) (patient V.E.W.)

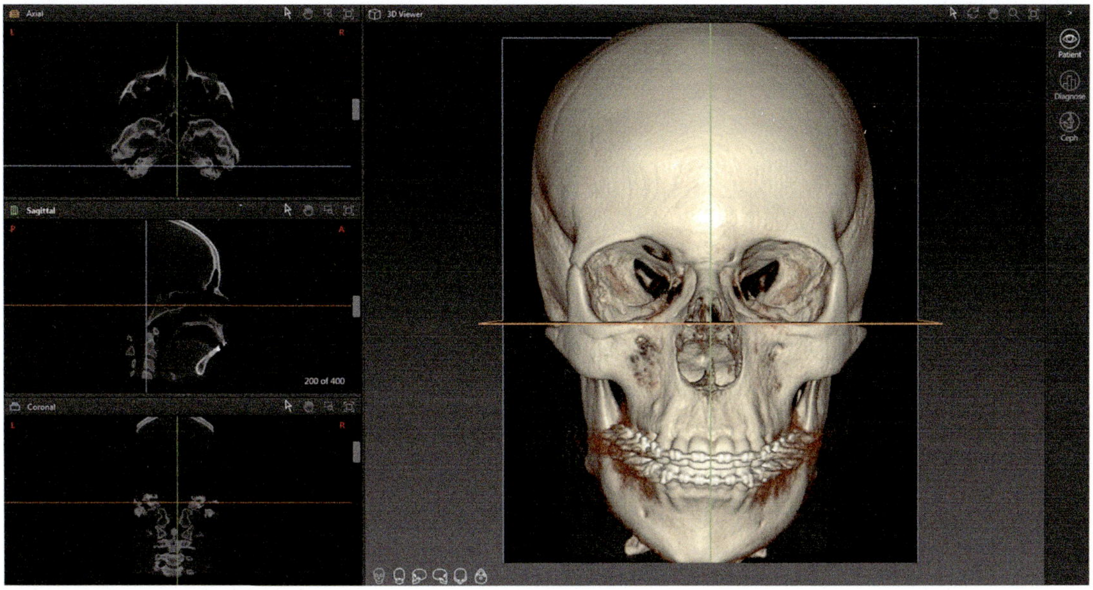

Fig. 2.64 Visualisation of the axial, coronal and sagittal 3D planes of the "Upper Airway 3D Coordinate System" on the 3D "volume -rendered" hard tissue surface representation in the frontal view (i-CAT, Imaging Sciences International Inc, IPS CaseDesigner ALPHA version) (patient V.E.W.)

3D Nasopharyngeal Upper Airway Subregion

The anatomical and technical 3D boundaries of the "nasopharyngeal airway" as a subregion of the upper pharyngeal airway have been described and validated by Guijarro-Martinez and Swennen (2013)" as follows (Fig. 2.65):

Anterior limit: Coronal plane perpendicular to FH (x-plane) passing through PNS

Posterior limit: Soft tissue contour of the pharyngeal wall, technically defined by a coronal plane perpendicular to FH (x-plane) passing through C2sp

Upper limit: Soft tissue contour of the pharyngeal wall, technically defined by an axial plane parallel to FH (x-plane) through the root of the clivus

Lower limit: Plane parallel to FH (x-plane), passing through PNS and extended to the posterior wall of the pharynx

Lateral limit: Soft tissue contour of the pharyngeal lateral walls, technically defined by sagittal planes perpendicular to FH (x-plane), passing the lateral walls of the maxillary sinus

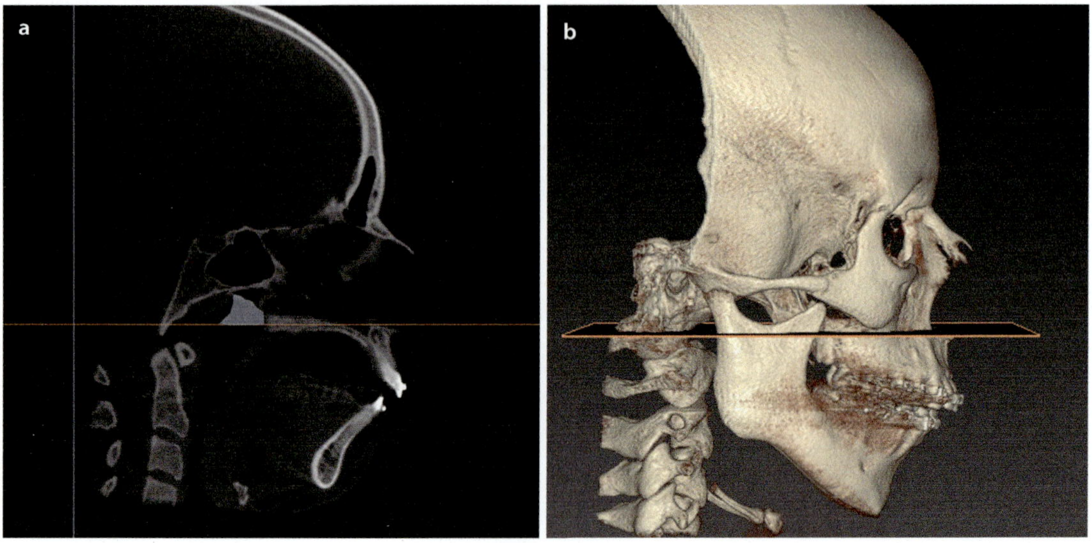

Fig. 2.65 The nasopharyngeal subregion of the upper (pharyngeal) airway, delineated on a sagittal view (**a**). Note the definition of the inferior limit of this subregion, by a 3D plane (*orange line*) parallel to the x-plane through PNS (**b**) (i-CAT, Imaging Sciences International Inc, IPS CaseDesigner ALPHA version) (patient V.E.W.)

▪ 3D Oropharyngeal Upper Airway Subregion

The anatomical 3D boundaries of the "oropharyngeal airway" as a subregion of the upper (pharyngeal) airway have been described and validated by Guijarro-Martinez and Swennen (2013) after setting up an "Upper Airway 3D Coordinate System" as follows (▫ Fig. 2.66):

Anterior limit: Coronal plane perpendicular to FH (x-plane) passing through PNS

Posterior limit: Soft tissue contour of the pharyngeal wall, technically defined by a coronal plane perpendicular to FH (x-plane) passing through C2sp

Upper limit: Plane parallel to FH (x-plane) passing through PNS and extended to the posterior wall of the pharynx

Lower limit: Plane parallel to FH (x-plane) passing through C3ai

Lateral limit: Soft tissue contour of the pharyngeal lateral walls, technically defined by sagittal planes perpendicular to FH (x-plane), passing the lateral walls of the maxillary sinus

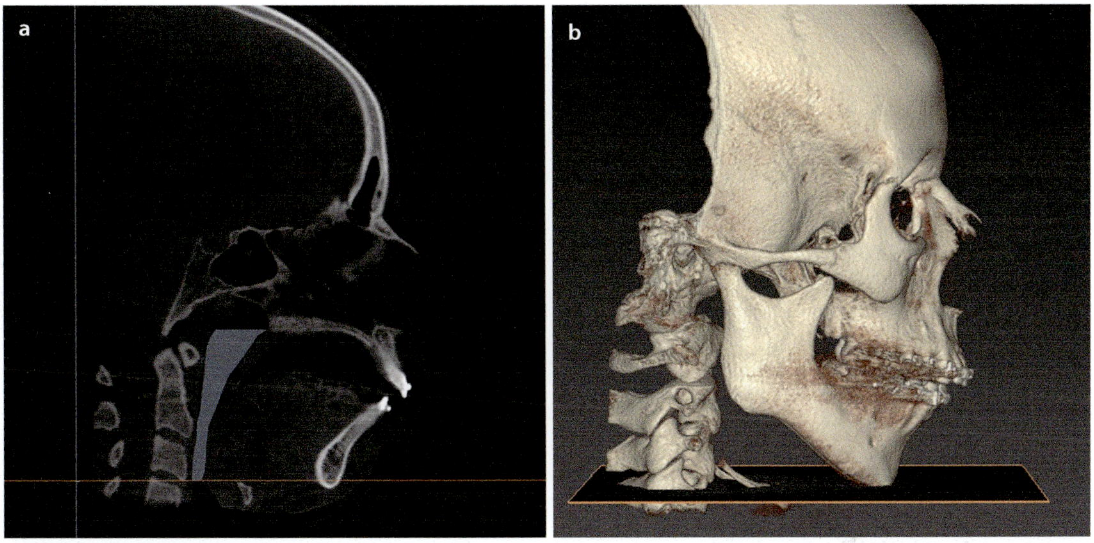

▫ **Fig. 2.66** The oropharyngeal subregion of the upper (pharyngeal) airway, delineated on a sagittal view (**a**). Note the definition of the inferior limit of this subregion, by a 3D plane (*orange line*) parallel to the x-plane through C3ai (**b**) (i-CAT, Imaging Sciences International Inc, IPS CaseDesigner ALPHA version (patient V.E.W.)

3D Hypopharyngeal Upper Airway Subregion

The anatomical 3D boundaries of the "hypopharyngeal airway" as a subregion of the upper (pharyngeal) airway have been described and validated by Guijarro-Martinez and Swennen (2013) after setting up an "Upper Airway 3D Coordinate System" as follows (Fig. 2.67):

Anterior limit: Coronal plane perpendicular to FH (x-plane) passing through PNS

Posterior limit: Soft tissue contour of the pharyngeal wall, technically defined by a coronal plane perpendicular to FH (x-plane) passing through C2sp

Upper limit: Plane parallel to FH (x-plane) passing through C3ai

Lower limit: Plane parallel to FH (x-plane) connecting the base of the epiglottis to the entrance of the oesophagus passing through C4ai

Lateral limit: Soft tissue contour of the pharyngeal lateral walls, technically defined by sagittal planes perpendicular to FH (x-plane), passing the lateral walls of the maxillary sinus

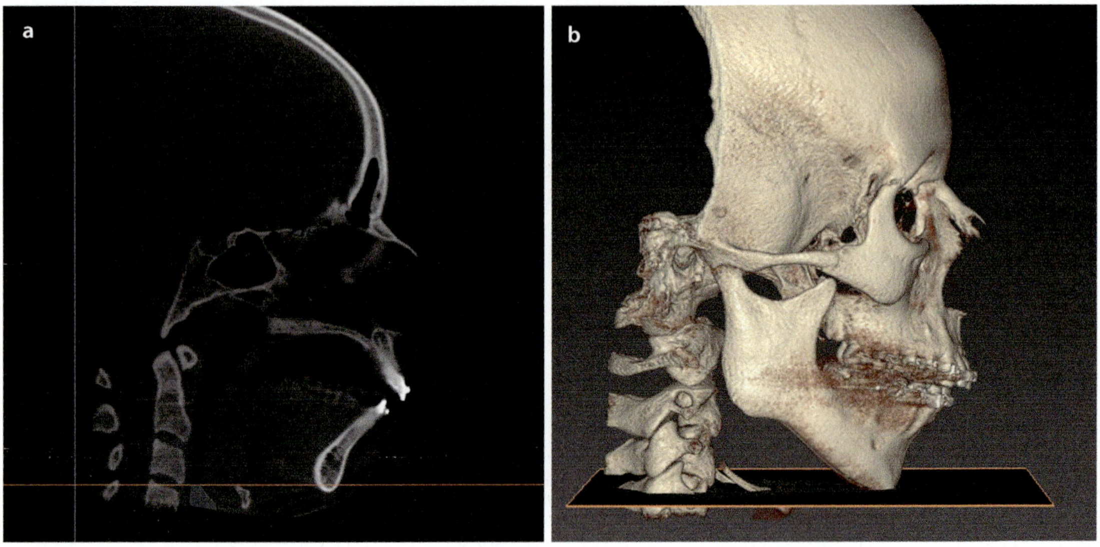

Fig. 2.67 The hypopharyngeal subregion of the upper (pharyngeal) airway, delineated on a sagittal view (**a**). Note the definition of the upper limit of this subregion, by a 3D plane (*orange line*) parallel to the x-plane through C3ai (**b**) (i-CAT, Imaging Sciences International Inc, IPS CaseDesigner ALPHA version) (patient V.E.W.)

▪ 3D Upper Pharyngeal Airway Subregions

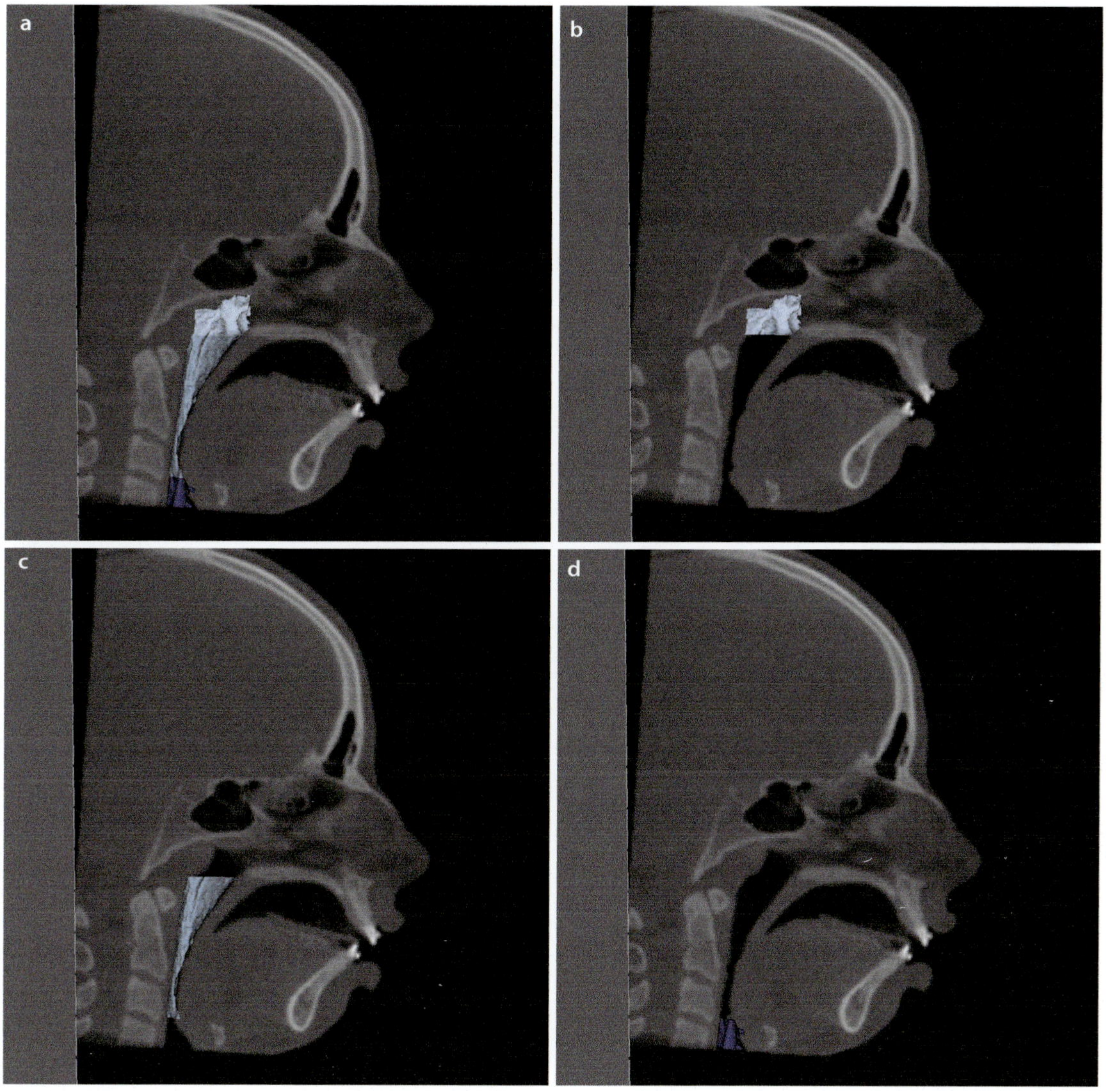

Fig. 2.68 Visualisation of the total volume of the 3D upper pharyngeal airway (18156,28 mm^3) (**a**), the 3D nasopharyngeal (7801,96 mm^3) (**b**), the 3D oropharyngeal (8675,88 mm^3) (**c**) and 3D hypopharygneal (1678,44 mm^3) (**d**) subvolumes of the upper pharyngeal airway on a sagittal reslice through ANS (i-CAT, Imaging Sciences International Inc, Maxilim v. 2.3.0.3.) (patient V.E.W.)

3D Upper Pharyngeal Airway Subregions

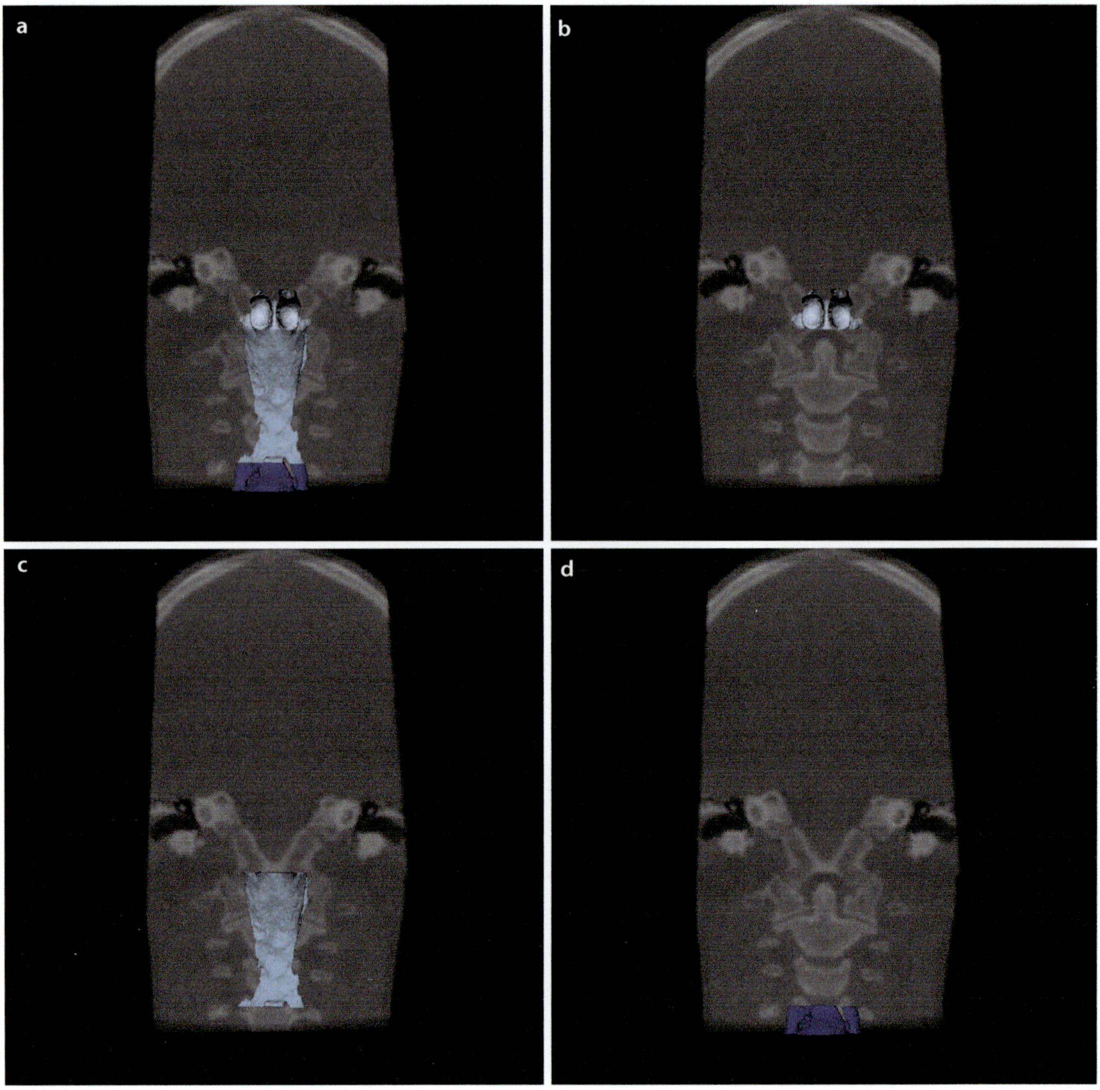

Fig. 2.69 Visualisation of the total volume of the 3D upper pharyngeal airway (18156,28 mm^3) (**a**), the 3D nasopharyngeal (7801,96 mm^3) (**b**), the 3D oropharyngeal (8675,88 mm^3) (**c**) and 3D hypopharyngeal (1678,44 mm^3) (**d**) subvolumes of the upper pharyngeal airway on a coronal reslice through C2sp (i-CAT, Imaging Sciences International Inc, Maxilim v. 2.3.0.3.) (patient V.E.W.)

3D Upper Pharyngeal Airway Subregions

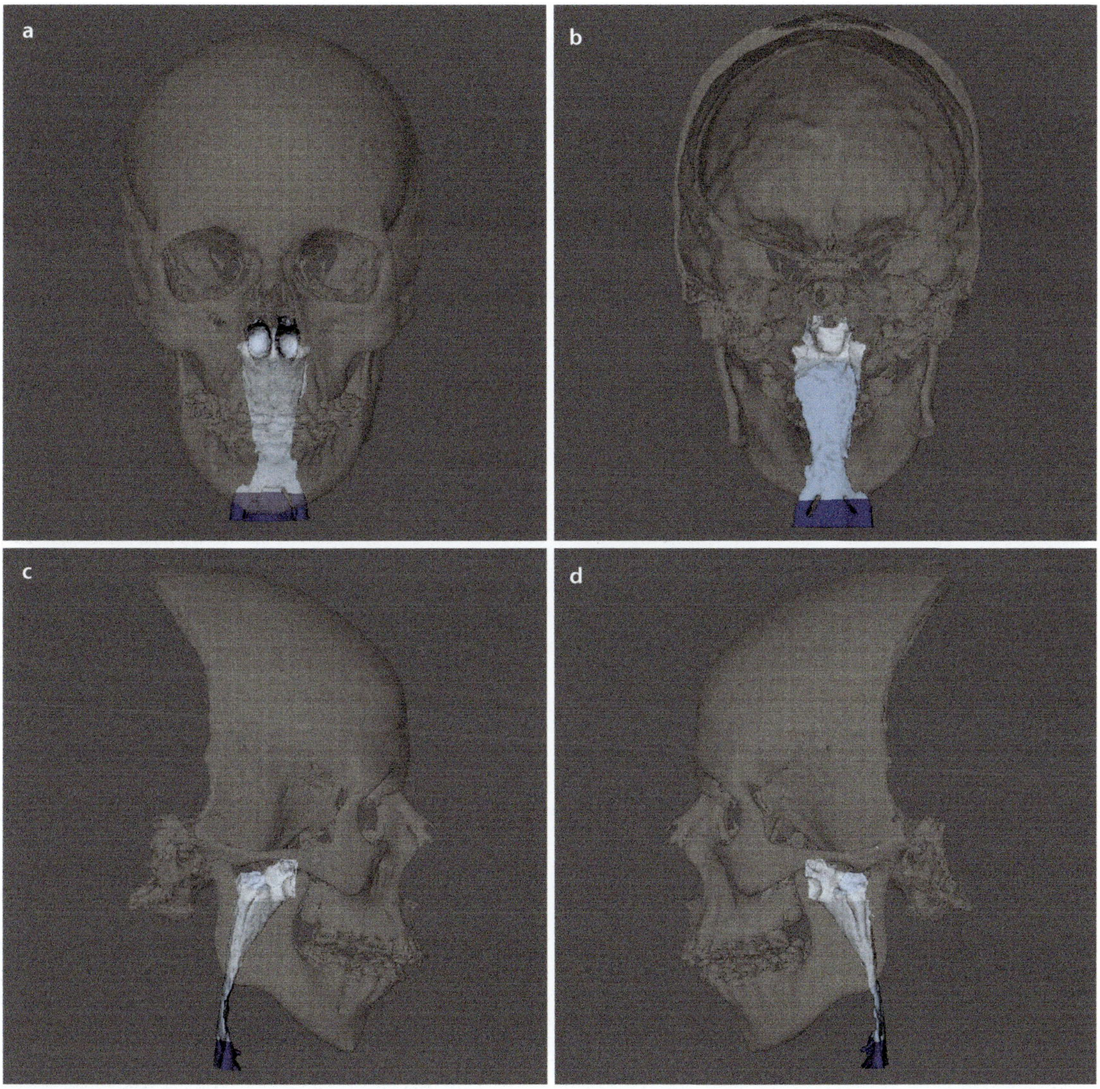

Fig. 2.70 Visualisation of the 3D nasopharyngeal (7801,96 mm^3), the 3D oropharyngeal (8675,88 mm^3) and 3D hypopharyngeal (1678,44 mm^3) subvolumes of the upper pharyngeal airway on semi-transparent "surface-rendered" hard tissue surface representations of the patient's head: (**a**) frontal view, (**b**) posterior view, (**c**) profile view right and (**d**) profile view left (i-CAT, Imaging Sciences International Inc, Maxilim v. 2.3.0.3.) (patient V.E.W.)

2.1.4 TMJ

Finally, after standardised "step-by-step" systematic virtual evaluation of the patient's individual "deformity and bite (▶ Sect. 2.1.1)", "anatomy and pathology (▶ Sect. 2.1.2)" and "upper airway (▶ Sect. 2.1.3)", the "3D Virtual Visualisation Paradigm" allows more enhanced diagnostics of the patient's TMJ in the "3D virtual scene".

Additional multiplanar reslices can be reconstructed and added to the "3D virtual scene" for evaluation of the condyle-fossa units. Most commonly, these multiplanar reslices are calculated based on an individual 2D coordinate system determined by the long axis of the individual condyles in the axial plane (◘ Figs. 2.71 and 2.72).

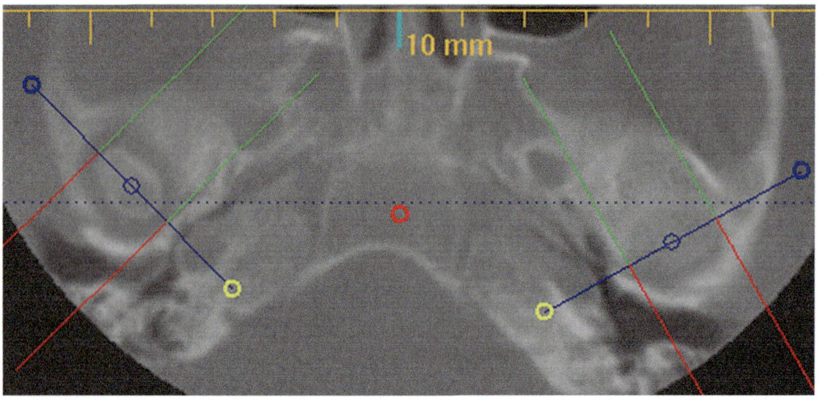

◘ **Fig. 2.71** Axial view at the level of the condyles demonstrating the individual set-up of a 2D coordinate system for generation of multiplanar coronal and sagittal slices, using the CBCT apparatus software (i-CAT, Imaging Sciences International Inc, i-CAT Vision™ software) (patient V.E.W.)

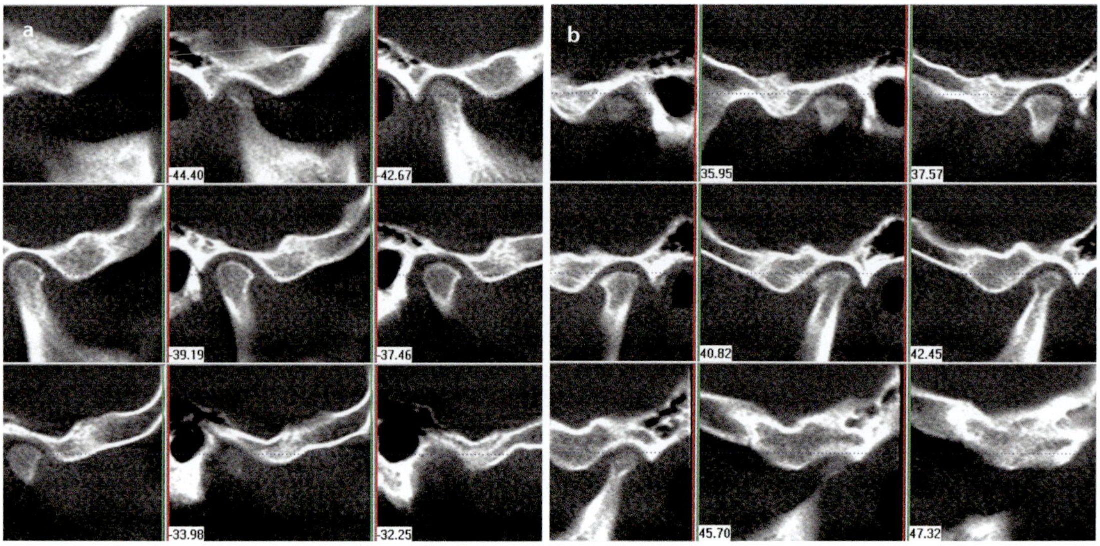

◘ **Fig. 2.72** Multiple reconstructed sagittal views of the right (**a**) and left (**b**) condyle/fossa units using the CBCT apparatus software based on an "individual condylar 2D coordinate system" (i-CAT, Imaging Sciences International Inc, i-CAT Vision™ software) (patient V.E.W.)

▪ Individual Condylar 3D Coordinate System

Multiplanar reslices of the "condyle-fossa unit", reconstructed based on an "individual condylar 2D coordinate system" (▫ Figs. 2.71 and 2.72), certainly already provide more objective and comparable information than axial, coronal and sagittal reslices (▶ see also Sect. 2.1.2) reconstructed from the initial position of the patient's head during CBCT scanning (▶ see also Sect. 1.1.1) or after virtual modification of the patient's NHP (▶ see also Sect. 3.1).

For ideal and objective CBCT TMJ assessment, the authors propose the set-up of a new "Individual Condylar 3D Coordinate System" based on the individual anatomy of the "ramus-condyle-fossa unit" to generate multiplanar orthogonal reslices (▫ Fig. 2.73).

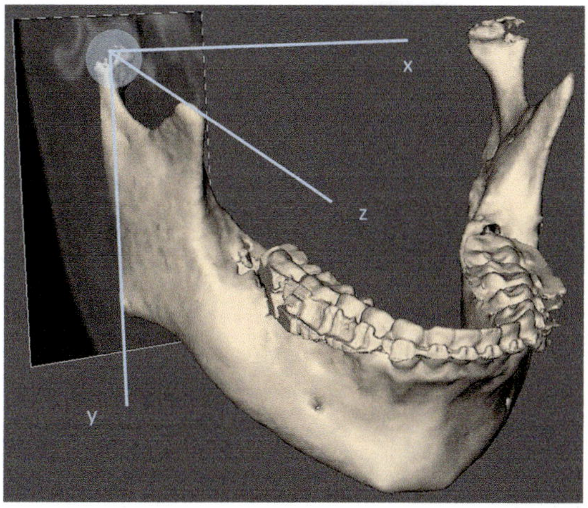

▫ **Fig. 2.73** An "Individual Condylar 3D Coordinate System" based on the individual anatomy of the right "ramus-condyle-fossa unit" to generate multiplanar reslices that allow adequate and objective evaluation (i-CAT, Imaging Sciences International Inc, Maxilim v. 2.3.0.3.) (patient V.E.W.)

Attention

An "Individual Condylar 3D Coordinate System" for multiplanar reconstruction must be generated based on the individual anatomy of each "ramus-condyle-fossa" unit.

Individual Condylar 3D Coordinate System

The "Individual Condylar 3D Coordinate System" is based on the individual angulation of each "ramus-condyle unit" in the sagittal plane (y-axis) and on the individual angulation of each "condylar head" in the axial plane which determines the coronal plane (z-axis). The third plane (x-axis) is finally automatically calculated by the software perpendicularly to the sagittal and coronal planes (Figs. 2.74, 2.75, 2.76 and 2.77).

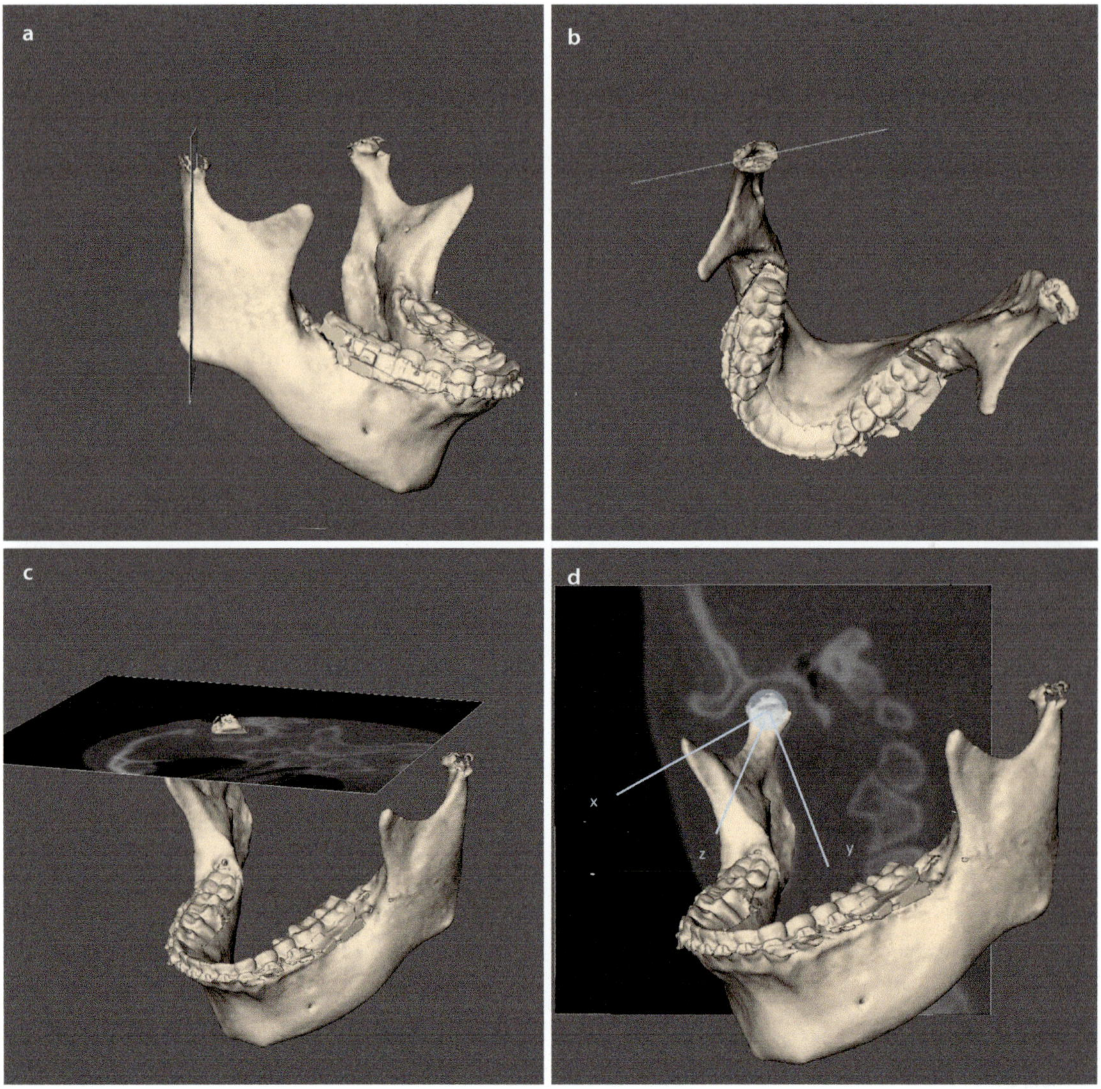

Fig. 2.74 Based on the individual angulation of each "ramus-condyle unit" (**a**), the individual angulation of each "condylar head" (**b**), a perpendicular axial plane (**c**) and an ultimate "Individual Condylar 3D Coordinate System" (**d**) is set up for multiplanar reconstructions of the individual "ramus-condyle-fossa unit" (i-CAT, Imaging Sciences International Inc, Maxilim v. 2.3.0.3.) (patient V.E.W.)

Multiplanar Reslices Based on an "Individual Condylar 3D Coordinate System"

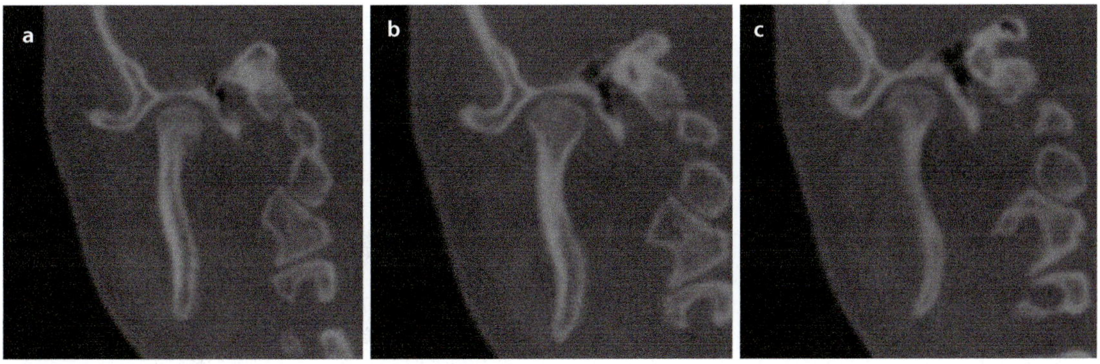

Fig. 2.75 Coronal slices (**a, b, c**) of the right ramus-condyle-fossa unit generated from the "Individual Condylar 3D Coordinate System" (patient V.E.W., i-CAT, Imaging Sciences International Inc, Maxilim v. 2.3.0.3.)

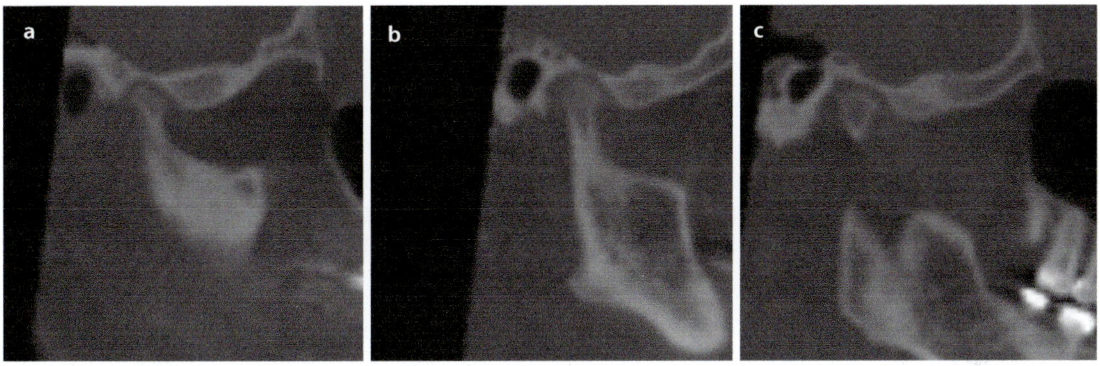

Fig. 2.76 Sagittal slices (**a, b, c**) of the right ramus-condyle-fossa unit generated from the "Individual Condylar 3D Coordinate System" (patient V.E.W., i-CAT, Imaging Sciences International Inc, Maxilim v. 2.3.0.3.)

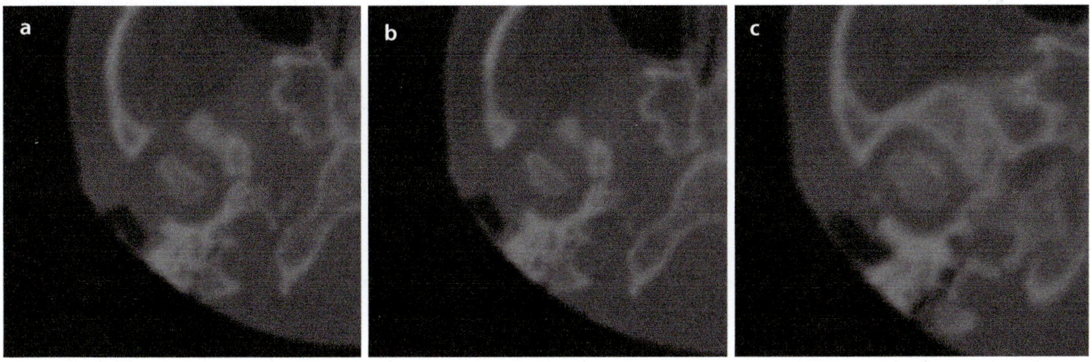

Fig. 2.77 Axial slices (**a, b, c**) of the right ramus-condyle-fossa unit generated from the "Individual Condylar 3D Coordinate System" (patient V.E.W., i-CAT, Imaging Sciences International Inc, Maxilim v. 2.3.0.3.)

2.2 3D Cephalometric Analysis of the Patient

After systematic virtual diagnosis of the patient's individual deformity, anatomy and pathology (▶ Sect. 2.1), 3D cephalometric analysis of the patient is now performed.

In 2005, Swennen, Schutyser and Hausamen made the bridge between conventional 2D and 3D cephalometric analysis by introducing an innovative concept of "3D cephalometry" using a "3D Virtual Scene Approach" that could be used for both clinical and research purposes.

Towards "integrated 3D virtual treatment planning of orthognathic surgery", "3D cephalometry" is an essential part of:

1. 3D virtual diagnosis (▶ see also Sect. 2.1)
2. 3D virtual treatment planning (▶ see also Sect. 3.5)
3. 3D virtual treatment planning transfer (▶ see also Sect. 4.1.2)
4. 3D virtual evaluation of treatment outcome (▶ see also Sect. 5.2.1)

In this chapter, a standardised "step-by-step" approach towards "3D cephalometric analysis" of the patient is described which consists of:

1. Set-up of a 3D cephalometric reference frame
2. Virtual definition of 3D cephalometric hard, soft tissue and teeth landmarks
3. Automated set-up of 3D cephalometric planes
4. 3D cephalometry of the patient's hard tissues and teeth (3D-VPS$_1$) and soft tissues (3D-VPS$_2$)

The "3D Virtual Visualisation Paradigm" allows to virtually define 3D cephalometric landmarks in the "3D virtual scene" on both bony and soft tissue 3D surface representations of the patient's head, which can be visualised by either "surface rendering" or "volume rendering" (▶ see also Sect. 1.1.1). On rare occasion, some 3D cephalometric landmarks are not defined on a 3D surface representation but are rather floating landmarks (e.g. sella, upper and lower incisor apex) (▶ see also Sect. 2.2.2). Additional reslices can then be incorporated in the "3D virtual scene" for precise and reliable 3D cephalometric landmark identification and definition.

The "10 Step-by-Step" Integrated Virtual Planning Approach", described in this atlas (▶ Sect. 3.5), is not based on any particular cephalometric analysis described in the literature but necessitates 3D virtual definition of some cephalometric landmarks. The planning approach is essentially based on "clinical decision-making", starting from the individual patient's "Planning Head Position (PHP)" (▶ see Sect. 3.1).

The authors do not want to dogmatise but push forward clinicians (orthodontists and surgeons) to make the bridge between their own clinical routine conventional 2D cephalometric analysis and 3D cephalometry, towards an individualised 3D virtual treatment planning approach.

The 3D cephalometric approach outlined in this chapter is illustrated on Case 1 Patient V.E.W. which is used throughout this book (▶ Chaps. 1, 3, 4, 5, and 6).

2.2.1 Set-Up of a 3D Cephalometry Reference Frame

The set-up of a "3D Cephalometry Reference Frame", which is an anatomic Cartesian 3D coordinate system, is the basis for 3D cephalometric analysis of the patient's head.

Other types of 3D coordinate systems have been outlined and shown in this atlas for 3D upper airway and TMJ analysis:

1. Upper Airway 3D Coordinate System (▶ see Sect. 2.1.3)
2. Individual Condylar 3D Coordinate System (▶ see Sect. 2.1.4)

In conventional treatment planning of orthognathic surgery, 2D cephalometric reference frames have been mostly based on the Frankfort horizontal (FH) or cranial base (e.g. Profitt and co-workers 1991) or on the true vertical line (TVL) related to the natural head position (NHP) (Arnett and McLaughlin 2004).

In 2005, Swennen introduced and validated an anatomic Cartesian 3D cephalometric reference system based on the 2D cephalometric reference system described by Profitt and co-workers (1991) that at that time truly made the bridge between conventional and 3D cephalometry.

Treatment planning of orthognathic surgery, however, needs to be based on the individual natural head position (NHP) of the patient, which is determined by the clinician and is independent of intracranial reference planes.

In Sect. 3.1, a new concept is introduced and outlined "step-by-step" to virtually modify the CBCT scanned patient's head position towards its *c*-NHP ("clinical natural head position"), which results in the *v*-NHP ("virtual modified natural head position"), or final individual patient's PHP ("Planning Head Position").

A "3D Cephalometry Reference Frame" for treatment planning needs to be set up based on the "patient's individual PHP" which is determined by the clinician.

▪ Set-Up of the 3D PHP Cephalometric Reference Frame

Step 1: Virtual modification of the patient's head position towards its individual PHP (▶ see also Sect. 3.1) (◘ Fig. 2.78)

Step 2: Virtual definition of the 3D PHP cephalometric landmarks ($PHP_{frontal}$ and $PHP_{profile}$) (◘ Figs. 2.79 and 2.80)

Step 3: Automated set-up of the "3D PHP Cephalometric Reference Frame" (◘ Figs. 2.81, 2.82, and 2.83).

Moreover, the "3D Virtual Visualisation Paradigm" allows to simultaneously set up a "cranial-based 3D cephalometric reference frame" (e.g. Swennen 2005, 2006) in the "3D virtual scene" if desired by the clinician (e.g. for research purposes).

3D PHP Cephalometric Reference Frame

- Step 1: Virtual modification of the patient's head position towards its individual PHP

In "Step 1", the patient's head position is virtually modified towards its individual PHP, which is defined by the clinician and outlined in detail in (► Sect. 3.1). After "Step 1", the geometric information is available for automated generation of a 3D reference system as an anatomic Cartesian coordinate system in the "3D virtual scene" (Fig. 2.78).

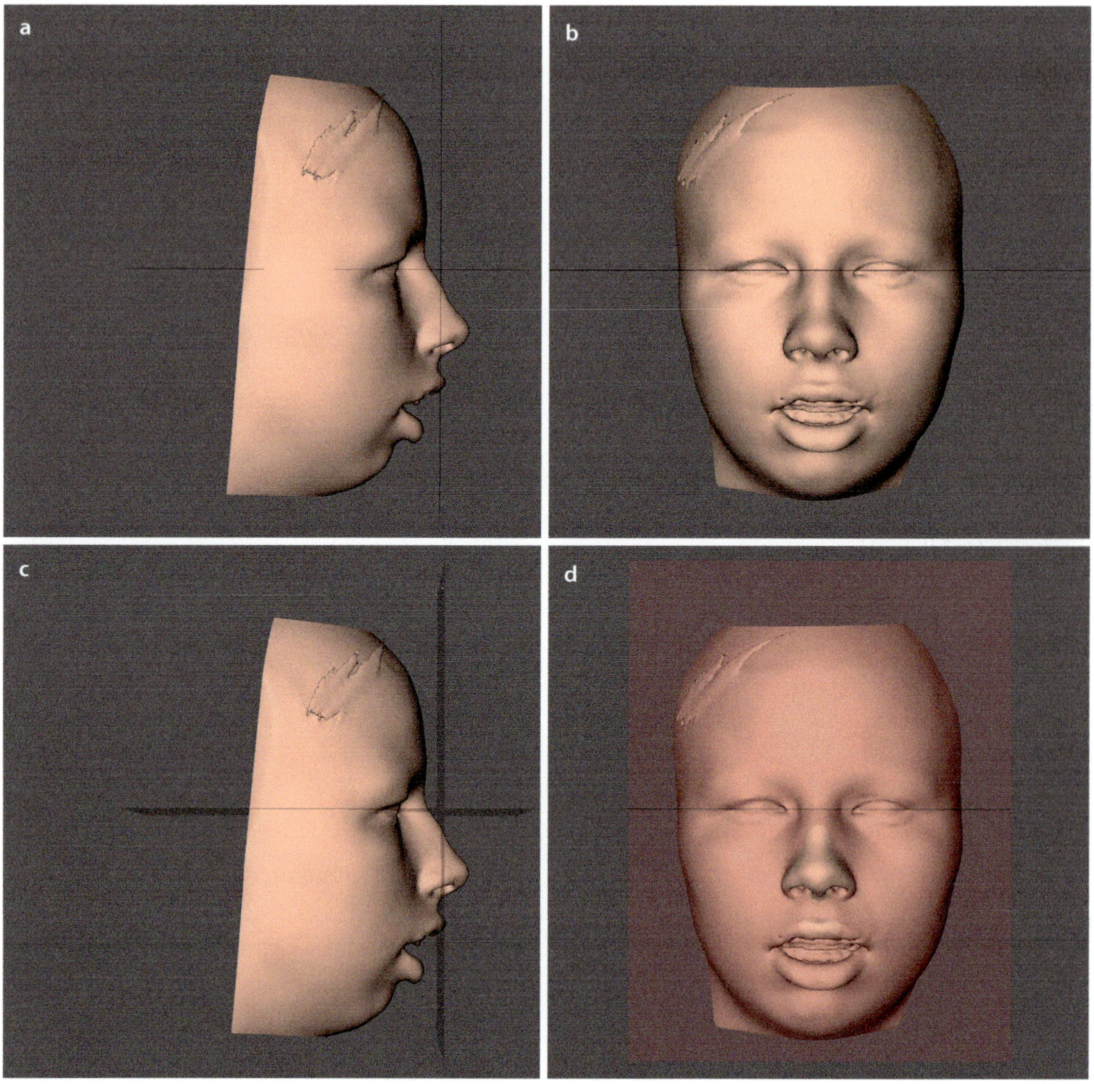

Fig. 2.78 "Step 1". Virtual modification of the patient's head position towards its individual PHP. 3D "surface-rendered" soft tissue representations of the patient's head. Profile view right (**a**), frontal view (**b**), profile view right visualising the TVP (**c**) and frontal view visualising the TVP (**d**) (i-CAT, Imaging Sciences International Inc, Maxilim v. 2.3.0.3., patient V.E.W.)

3D PHP Cephalometric Reference Frame

▪ Step 2: Virtual definition of the 3D PHP cephalometric landmarks

In order to virtually position the 3D reference frame in the "3D virtual scene" towards the patient's head, the 3D PHP cephalometric landmarks ($PHP_{frontal}$ and $PHP_{profile}$) are virtually defined in "Step 2".

The $PHP_{frontal}$ landmark is identified to position the centre of the 3D reference frame in the median (z)- and vertical (y)-axis at the midpoint of the nasal root (Fig. 2.79).

The $PHP_{profile}$ landmark is identified to position the centre of the 3D reference frame in the horizontal (x)-axis at the midpoint of the sella turcica (Fig. 2.80).

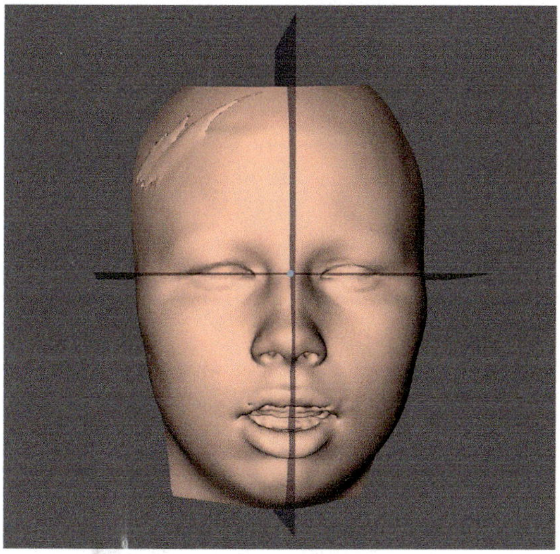

Fig. 2.79 "Step 2". Virtual definition of the $PHP_{frontal}$ landmark. 3D "surface-rendered" soft tissue representation of the patient's head. Frontal view (i-CAT, Imaging Sciences International Inc, Maxilim v. 2.3.0.3., patient V.E.W.)

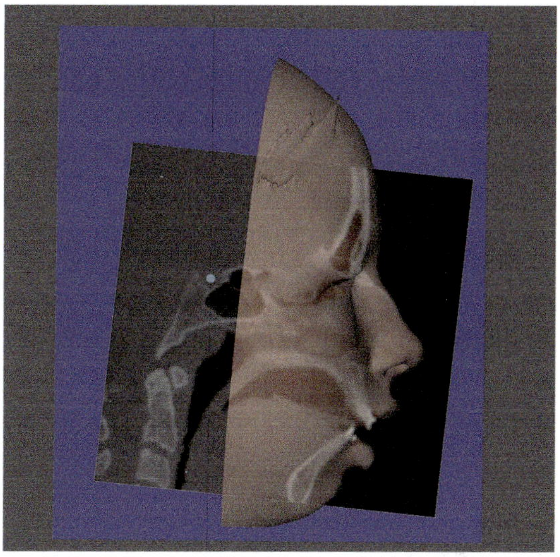

Fig. 2.80 "Step 2". Virtual definition of the $PHP_{profile}$ landmark on the midsagittal reslice. 3D "surface-rendered" transparent soft tissue representation of the patient's head. Profile view right (i-CAT, Imaging Sciences International Inc, Maxilim v. 2.3.0.3., patient V.E.W.)

2

3D PHP Cephalometric Reference Frame

- Step 3: Automated set-up of the 3D PHP Cephalometric Reference frame

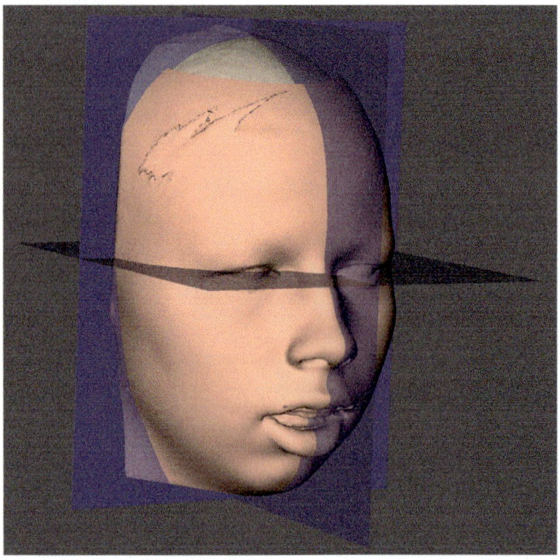

Fig. 2.81 "Step 3". Automated set-up of the 3D PHP cephalometric reference frame. 3D "surface-rendered" soft tissue representation of the patient's head (i-CAT, Imaging Sciences International Inc, Maxilim v. 2.3.0.3.) (patient V.E.W.)

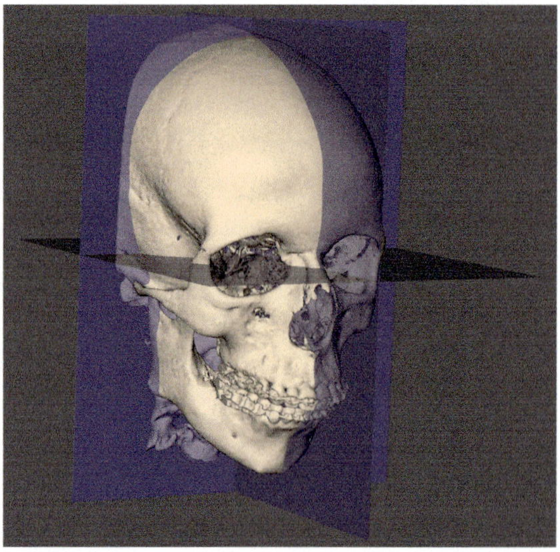

Fig. 2.82 "Step 3". Automated set-up of the 3D PHP cephalometric reference frame. 3D "surface-rendered" hard tissue representation of the patient's head (i-CAT, Imaging Sciences International Inc, Maxilim v. 2.3.0.3., patient V.E.W.)

3D PHP Cephalometric Reference Frame

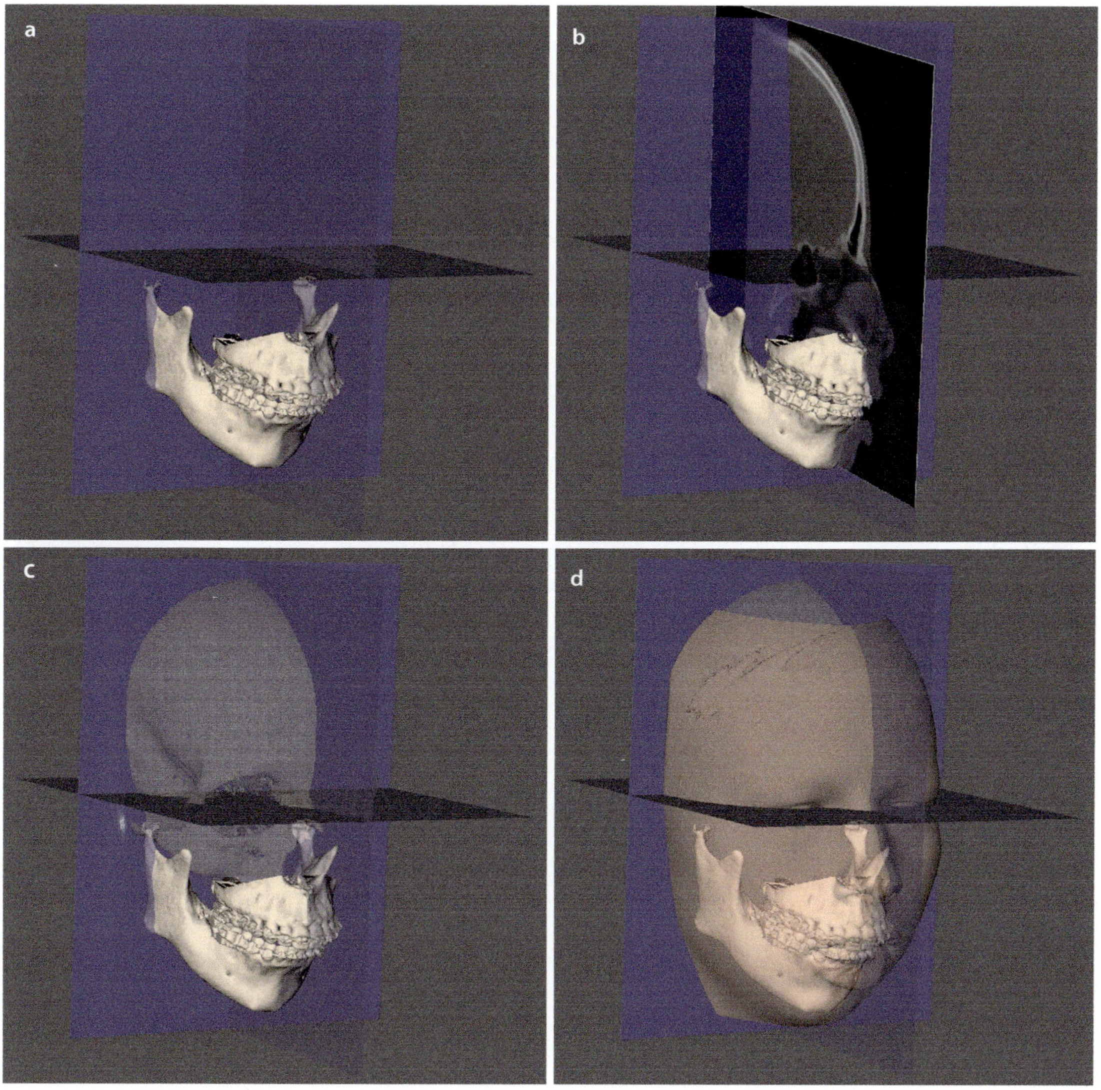

Fig. 2.83 "Step 3". Automated set-up of the 3D PHP cephalometric reference frame (**a**–**d**). 3D "surface-rendered" hard and soft tissue representation of the patient's head (i-CAT, Imaging Sciences International Inc, Maxilim v. 2.3.0.3., patient V.E.W.)

2.2.2 3D Cephalometry of the Patient's Hard Tissues and Teeth (3D-VPS_1)

"3D Cephalometry of the patient's hard tissues and teeth" (3D-VPS_1) can be compared with conventional 2D cephalometric tracing.

Many different cephalometric analyses have been developed and are currently worldwide used for diagnosis of dento-maxillo-facial and cranio-facial deformity, planning of orthodontic treatment and orthognathic, orthofacial and cranio-facial surgery, as well as long-term evaluation of treatment outcome.

Therefore, this section does not intend to promote a specific 3D cephalometric analysis but instead provide:

1. "Step-by-step" 3D virtual definition of common hard tissues and teeth cephalometric landmarks (◘ Figs. 2.146, 2.147, 2.148 and 2.149)
2. Principles of setting up 3D cephalometric planes
3. Principles of creating 3D cephalometric measurements
4. The "Bruges Target Facial Mask" 3D cephalometric analysis as an example

Accurate and reliable identification of 3D cephalometric landmarks requires anatomic knowledge and experience in landmark definition. Moreover, compared to 2D cephalometry, the third dimension needs to be integrated in the virtual definition of 3D cephalometric landmarks.

In this section, 3D cephalometric hard tissue and teeth landmarks are illustrated on a cadaver skull followed by "step-by-step" guidelines for precise and reliable 3D virtual landmark definition illustrated on Case 1 (Patient V.E.W.), which is used throughout this book (► Chaps. 1, 3, 4, 5, and 6).

The clinician (orthodontist or surgeon) can make the bridge between "conventional 2D planning" and "3D virtual treatment planning" of orthognathic surgery by modifying his clinical routine 2D cephalometric tracing towards 3D cephalometric analysis of the patient's head.

▪ Nasion (N)

Definition of Nasion (N)

"Nasion (N)" is the midpoint of the frontonasal suture (▫ Fig. 2.84).

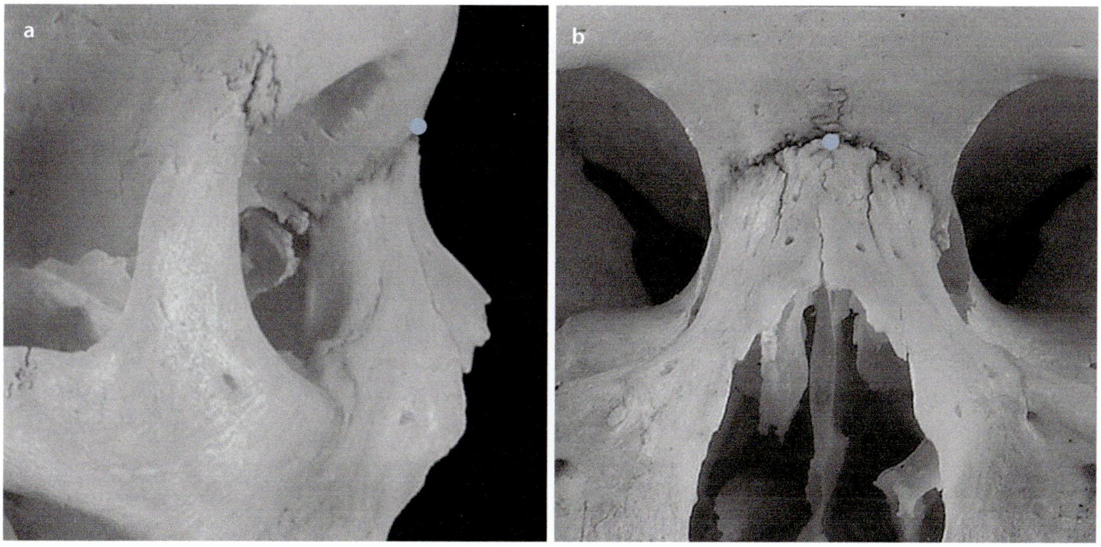

▫ **Fig. 2.84** *Nasion*. Profile right (**a**) and frontal (**b**) views (cadaver skull)

3D virtual definition of the Nasion (N) landmark

Step 1: Define *Nasion* on the right profile view of the 3D hard tissue surface representation (▫ Fig. 2.85a). Eventually *Nasion* can also be defined on a midsagittal reslice (▫ Fig. 2.85b).

Step 2: Verify and eventually correct the median position of the *Nasion* landmark on the frontal view of the 3D hard tissue surface representation (▫ Fig. 2.86a).

Step 3: The position of the *Nasion* landmark is verified on the left (▫ Fig. 2.86b) and right 3D profile views of the 3D hard tissue surface representations.

Nasion (N)

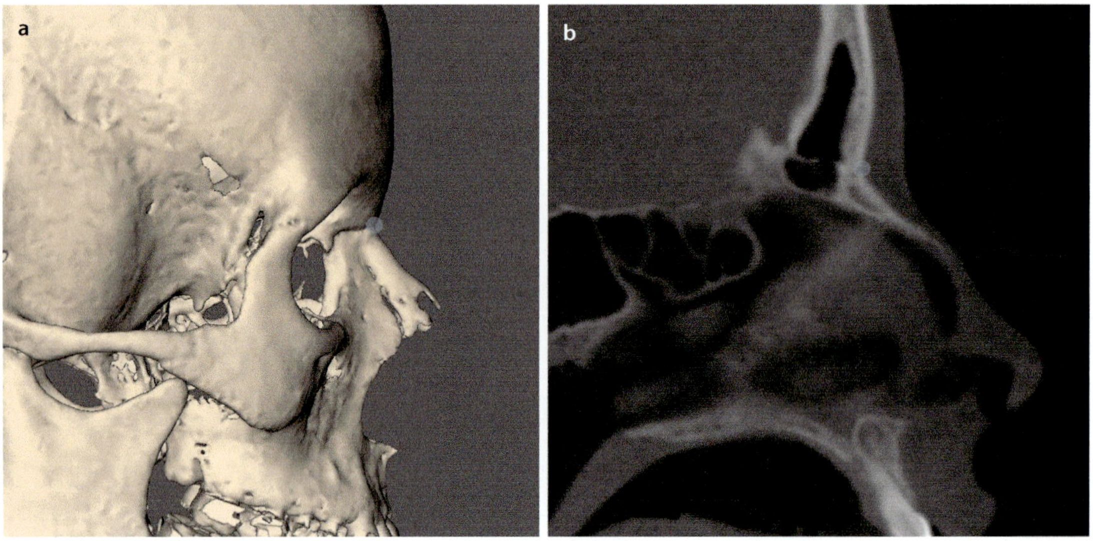

Fig. 2.85 *Nasion*. Profile view right (**a**) of the 3D "surface-rendered" representation of the patient's head and midsagittal reslice (**b**) (i-CAT, Imaging Sciences International Inc, Maxilim v. 2.3.0.3., patient V.E.W.)

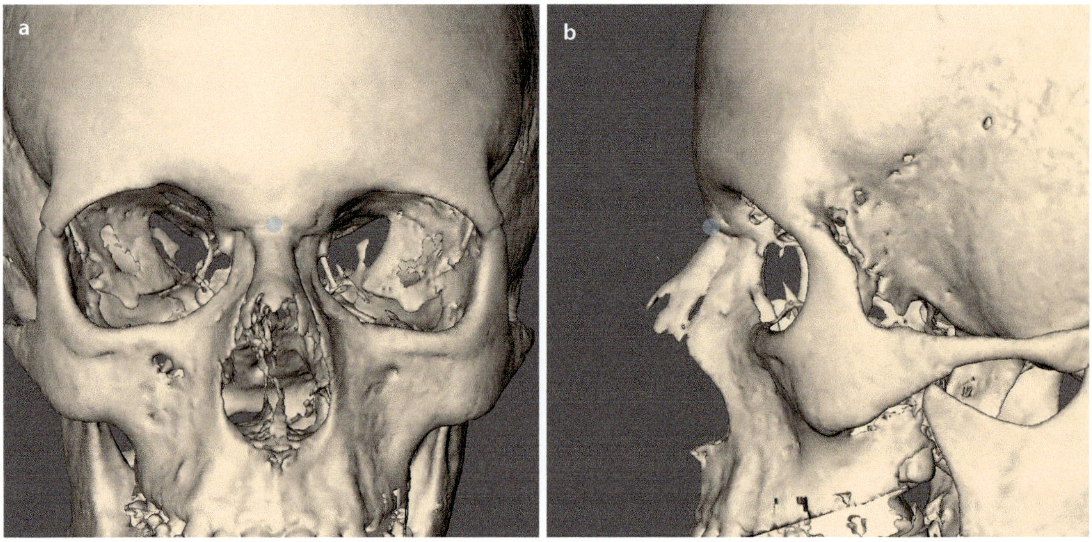

Fig. 2.86 *Nasion*. Frontal (**a**) and profile view left (**b**) of the 3D "surface-rendered" representation of the patient's head (i-CAT, Imaging Sciences International Inc, Maxilim v. 2.3.0.3., patient V.E.W.)

▪ Sella (S)

Definition of Sella (S)

“Sella (S)” is the centre of the hypophyseal fossa (◘ Fig. 2.87).

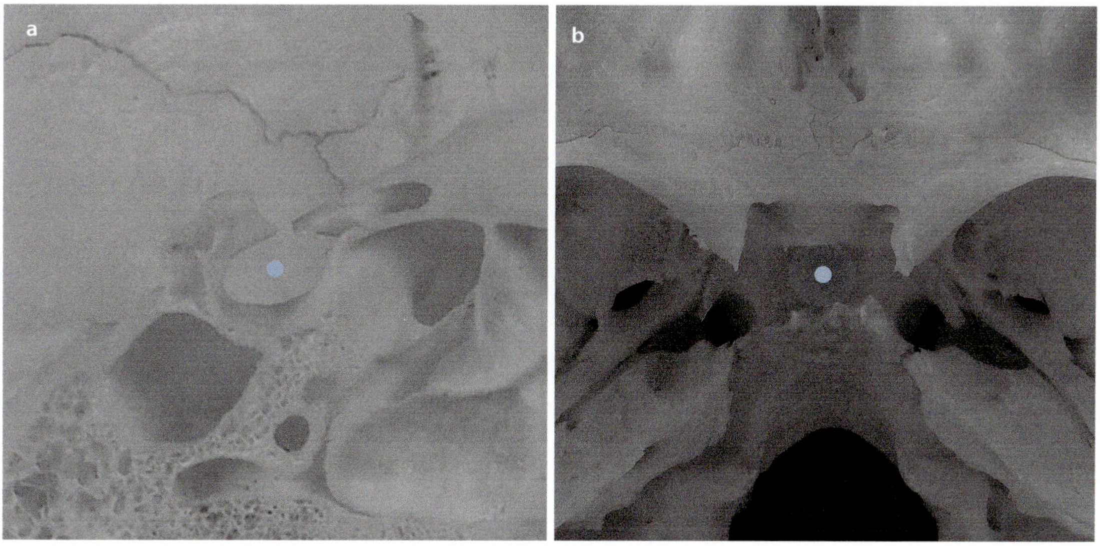

◘ **Fig. 2.87** *Sella*. Paramedian (**a**) and endocranial skull base (**b**) views (cadaver skull)

3D virtual definition of the Sella (S) landmark

Step 1: Define *Sella* on a midsagittal reslice (◘ Fig. 2.88a).

Step 2: Verify and correct the median position of the *Sella* landmark on an axial reslice through the hypophyseal fossa (◘ Fig. 2.88b).

Step 3: Verify and eventually correct the median position of the *Sella* landmark on the endocranial skull base view of the 3D hard tissue surface representation (◘ Fig. 2.89).

Sella (S)

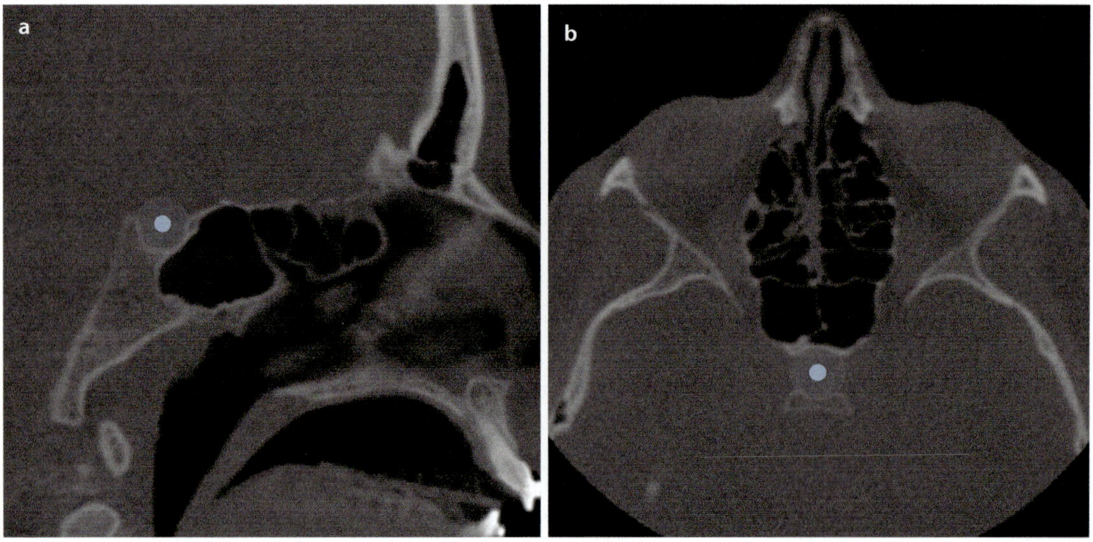

■ **Fig. 2.88** *Sella*. Midsaggital (**a**) and axial (**b**) reslices (i-CAT, Imaging Sciences International Inc, Maxilim v. 2.3.0.3.) (patient V.E.W.)

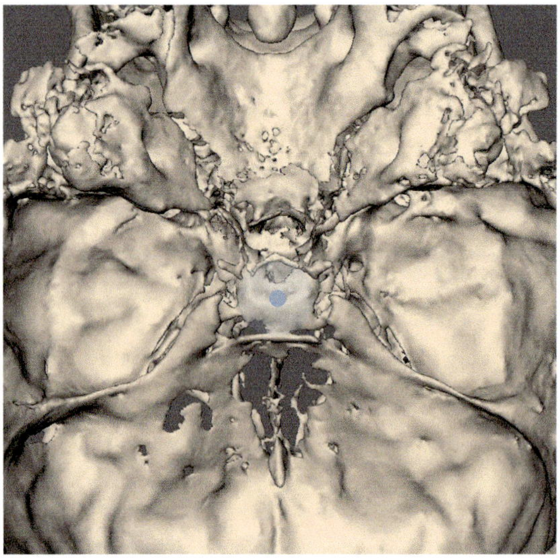

■ **Fig. 2.89** *Sella*. Endocranial skull base view of the 3D "surface-rendered" representation of the patient's head (i-CAT, Imaging Sciences International Inc, Maxilim v. 2.3.0.3., patient V.E.W.)

■ Porion (Po_r-Po_l)

Definition of Porion (Po)

"Porion (Po)" is the most superior point of the external acoustic meatus (◘ Fig. 2.90).

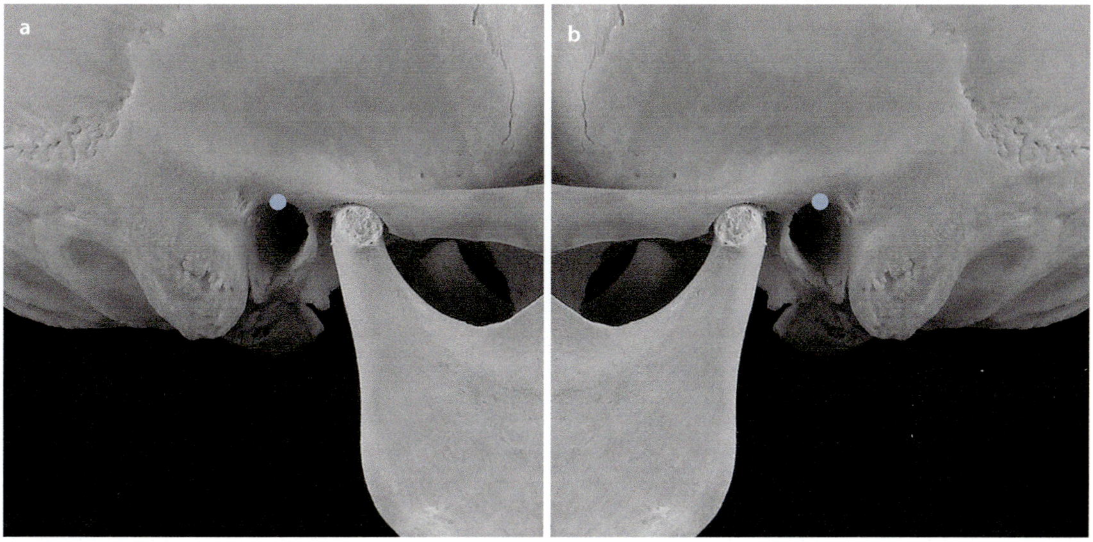

◘ **Fig. 2.90** *Porion*$_r$ and *Porion*$_l$. Profile right (**a**) and left (**b**) views (cadaver skull)

3D virtual definition of the Porion (Po) landmarks

Define *Porion*$_r$ and *Porion*$_l$ on the right (◘ Fig. 2.91a) and left (◘ Fig. 2.91b) profile views of the 3D hard tissue surface representations.

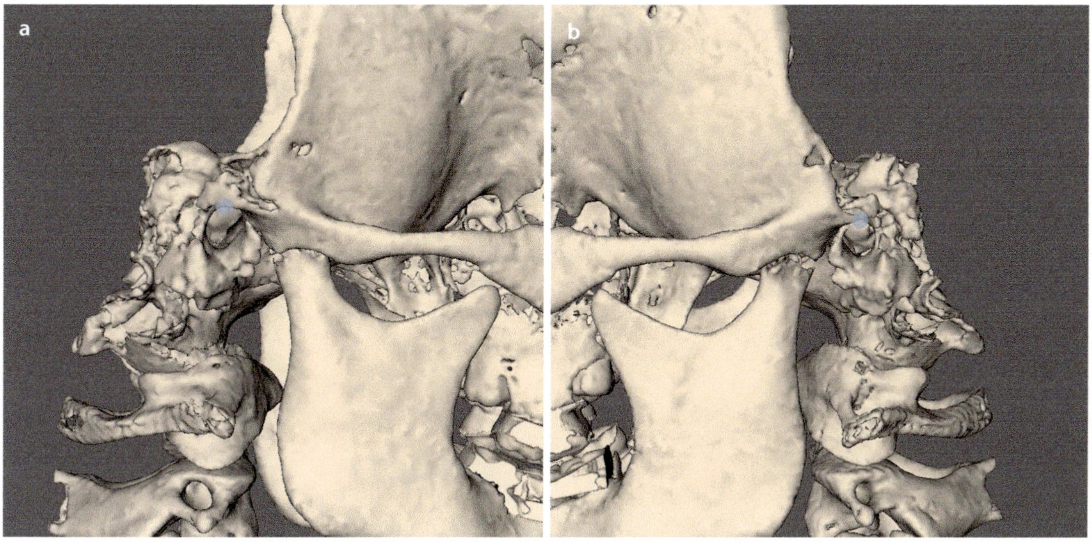

◘ **Fig. 2.91** *Porion*$_r$ and *Porion*$_l$. Profile right (**a**) and left (**b**) views of the 3D "surface-rendered" hard tissue representation of the patient's head (i-CAT, Imaging Sciences International Inc, Maxilim v. 2.3.0.3., patient V.E.W.)

▪ Orbitale (Or_r-Or_l)

Definition of the Orbitale (Or)

"Orbitale (Or)" is the most inferior point of the infraorbital rim (Fig. 2.92).

3D virtual definition of the Orbitale (Or) landmarks

Define *Orbita*$_r$ and *Orbita*$_l$ on the frontal view of the 3D hard tissue surface representation (Fig. 2.93).

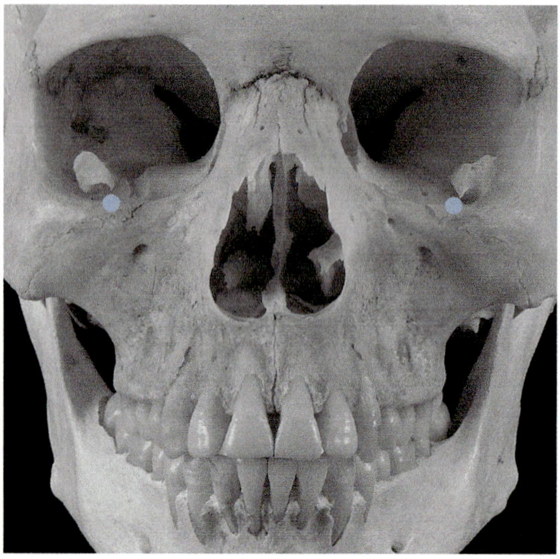

Fig. 2.92 *Orbita*$_r$ and *Orbita*$_l$. Frontal view (cadaver skull)

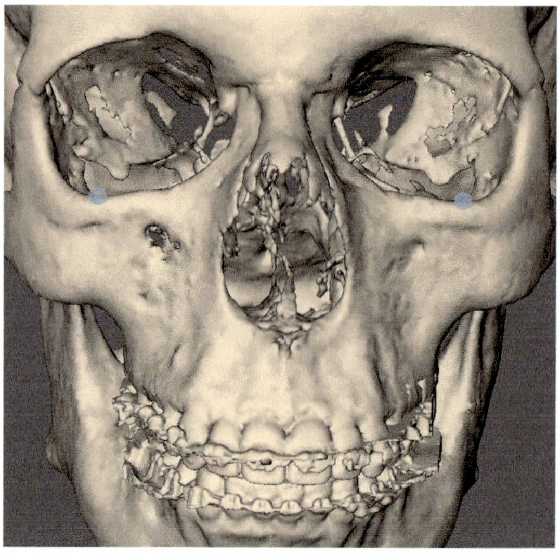

Fig. 2.93 *Orbita*$_r$ and *Orbita*$_l$. Frontal view of the 3D "surface-rendered" hard tissue representation of the patient's head (i-CAT, Imaging Sciences International Inc, Maxilim v. 2.3.0.3., patient V.E.W.)

Anterior Nasal Spine (ANS)

Definition of the Anterior Nasal Spine (ANS)

"Anterior Nasal Spine (ANS)" is the most anterior midpoint of the anterior nasal spine of the maxilla (◘ Fig. 2.94).

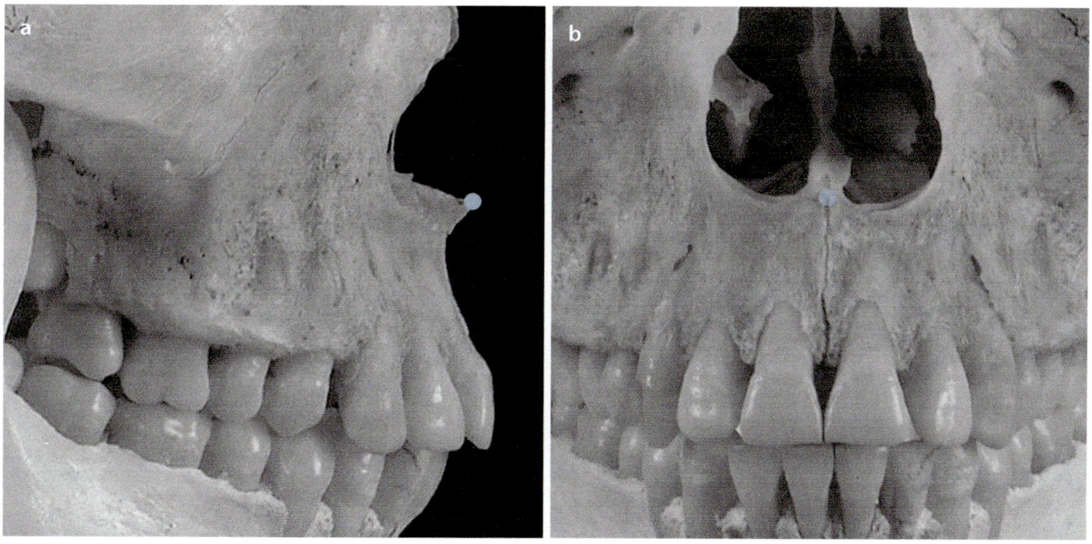

◘ **Fig. 2.94** *Anterior Nasal Spine*. Profile right (**a**) and frontal (**b**) views (cadaver skull)

3D virtual definition of the Anterior Nasal Spine (ANS) landmark

Step 1: Define *Anterior Nasal Spine* on the right profile view of the 3D hard tissue surface representation (◘ Fig. 2.95a).

Step 2: Verify and correct the median position of the *Anterior Nasal Spine* landmark on the frontal view of the 3D hard tissue surface representation (◘ Fig. 2.95b).

Step 3: Verify and correct the position of the *Anterior Nasal Spine* landmark on the left profile view of the 3D hard tissue surface representation (◘ Fig. 2.95c).

Anterior Nasal Spine (ANS)

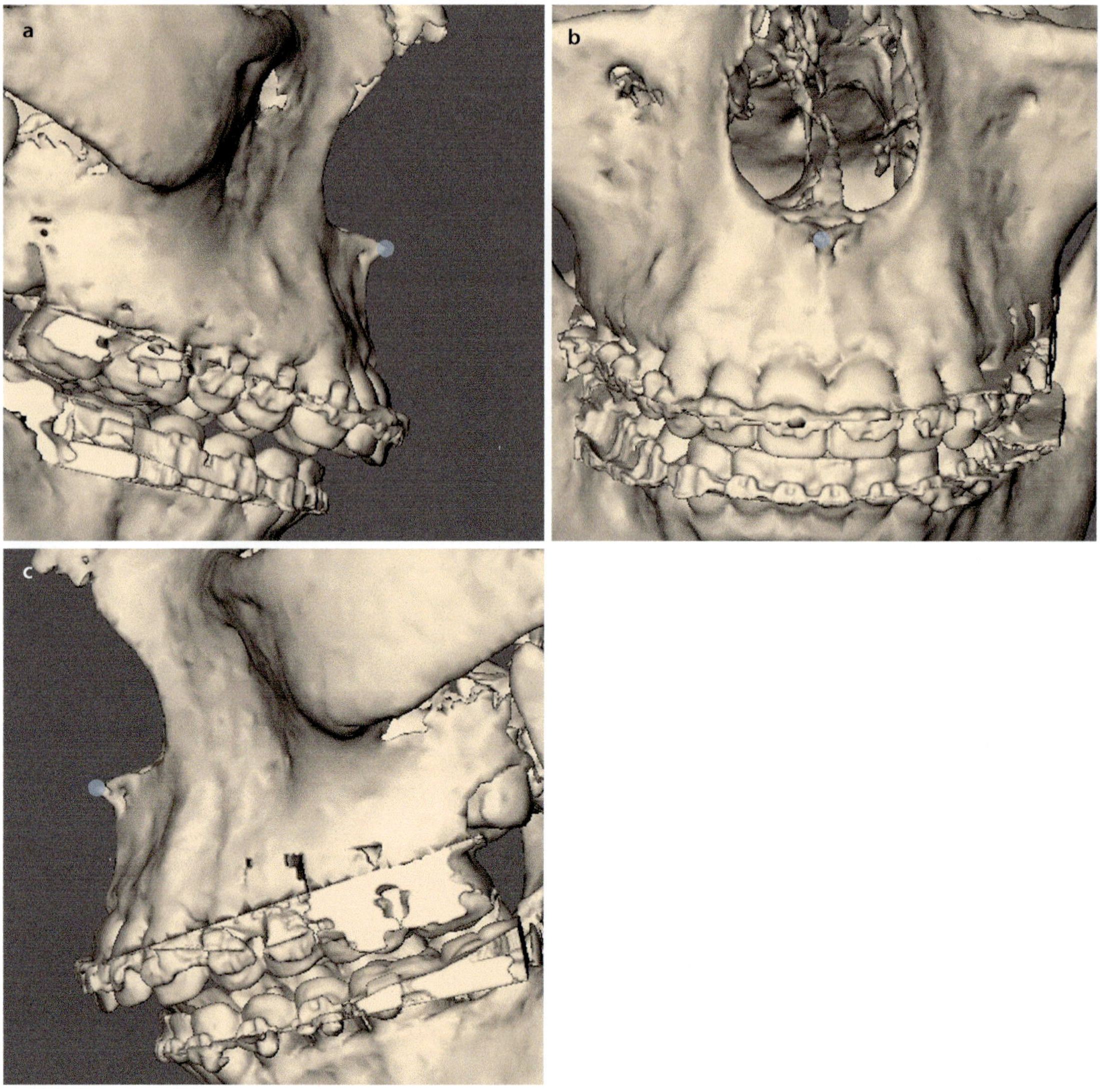

Fig. 2.95 *Anterior Nasal Spine*. Profile right (**a**), frontal (**b**) and profile left (**c**) views of the 3D "surface-rendered" hard tissue representation of the patient's head (i-CAT, Imaging Sciences International Inc, Maxilim v. 2.3.0.3., patient V.E.W.)

▪ Posterior Nasal Spine (PNS)

Definition of the Posterior Nasal Spine (PNS) landmark

"Posterior Nasal Spine (PNS)" is the most posterior midpoint of the posterior nasal spine of the palatine bone (◘ Fig. 2.96).

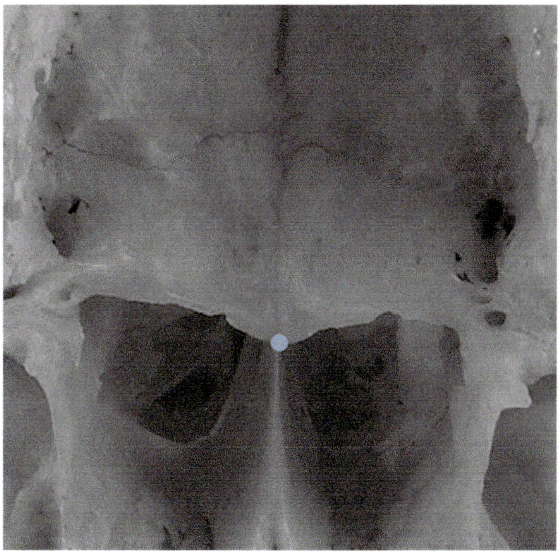

◘ **Fig. 2.96** *Posterior Nasal Spine.* Exocranial skull base view (cadaver skull)

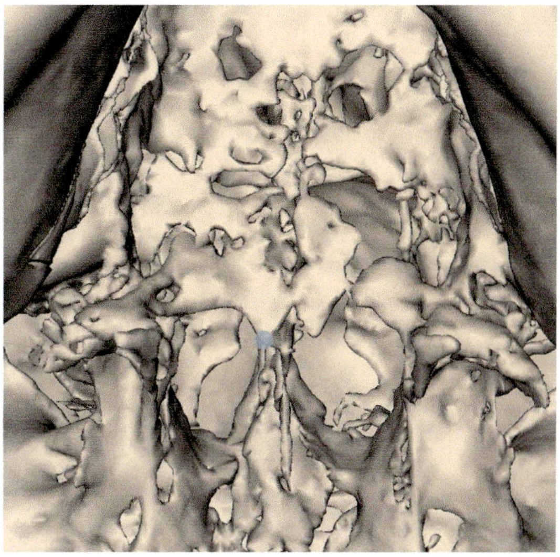

◘ **Fig. 2.97** *Posterior Nasal Spine.* Exocranial skull base view of the 3D "surface-rendered" hard tissue representation of the patient's head (i-CAT, Imaging Sciences International Inc, Maxilim v. 2.3.0.3., patient V.E.W.). Note the posterior spina bifida. In such a case, the PNS is defined at the most posterior spine

3D virtual definition of the Posterior Nasal Spine (PNS) landmark

Step 1: Define *Posterior Nasal Spine* on the exocranial skull base view of the 3D hard tissue surface representation (◘ Fig. 2.97).

Step 2: Verify and eventually correct the position of the *Posterior Nasal Spine* landmark on the sagittal reslices (◘ Fig. 2.98).

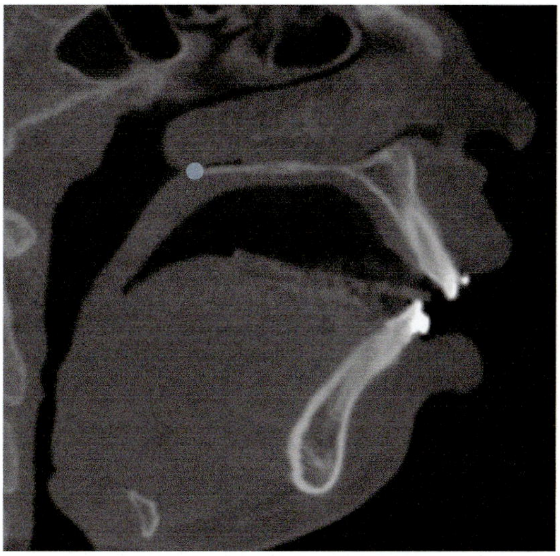

◘ **Fig. 2.98** *Posterior Nasal Spine.* Sagittal reslice (i-CAT, Imaging Sciences International Inc, Maxilim v. 2.3.0.3., patient V.E.W.)

Upper Incisor (UI_r-UI_l)

Definition of Upper Incisor (UI)

"Upper Incisor (UI)" is the most mesial point of the tip of the crown of the upper central incisor (Fig. 2.99).

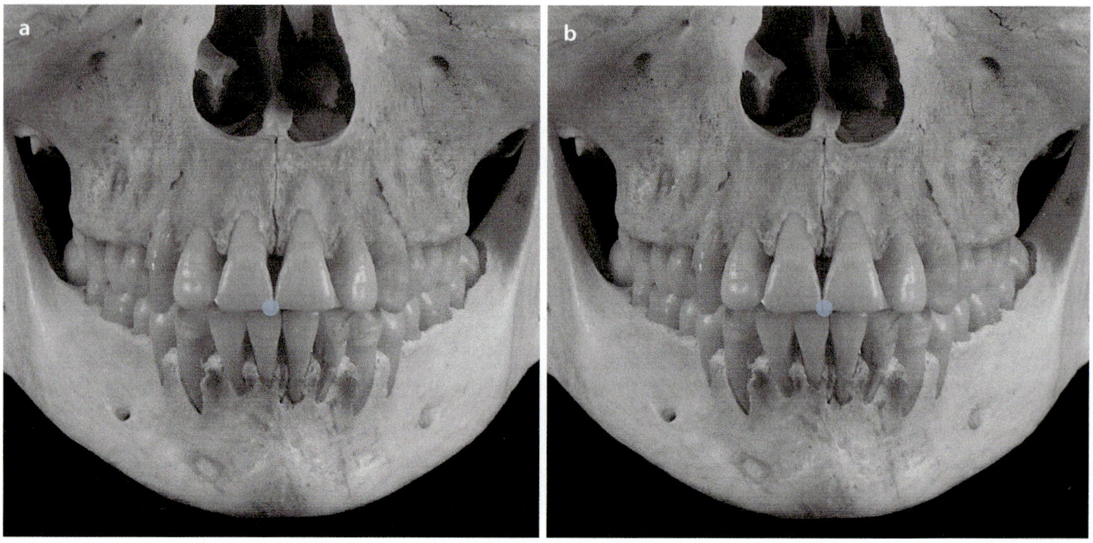

Fig. 2.99 *Upper Incisor$_r$* (**a**) and *Upper Incisor$_l$* (**b**). Frontal views (cadaver skull)

3D virtual definition of the Upper Incisor (UI) landmarks

Step 1: Define both *Upper Incisor$_r$* and *Upper Incisor$_l$* landmarks on the frontal views of the 3D hard tissue surface representations (Figs. 2.100a and 2.101a).

Step 2: Verify and eventually correct the position of the *Upper Incisor$_r$* and *Upper Incisor$_l$* landmarks on the sagittal reslices (Figs. 2.100b and 2.101b).

Upper Incisor (UI_r-UI_l)

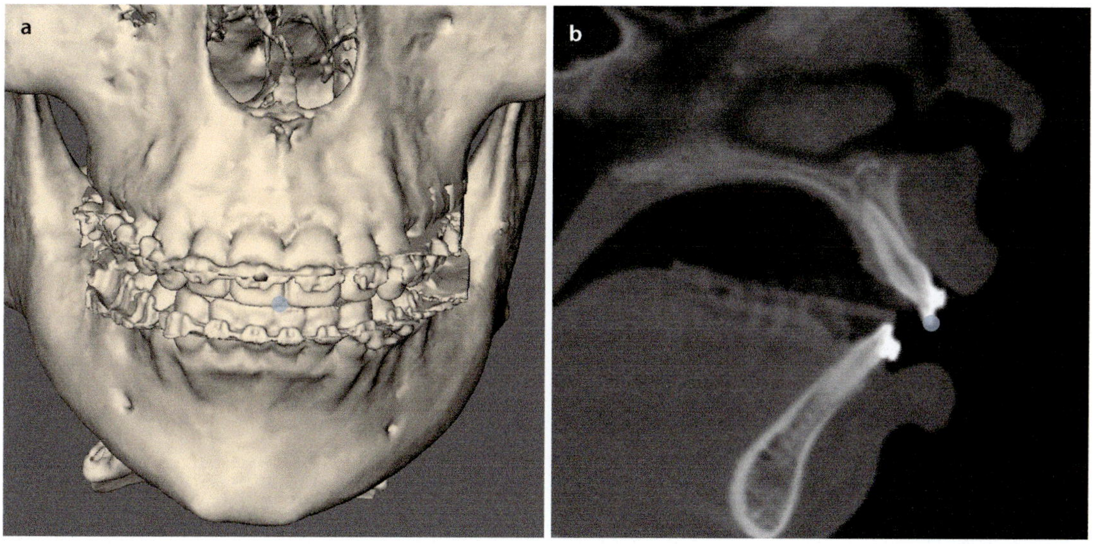

Fig. 2.100 *Upper Incisor$_r$*. Frontal view (**a**) of the 3D "surface-rendered" hard tissue representation of the patient's head and sagittal reslice (**b**) (i-CAT, Imaging Sciences International Inc, Maxilim v. 2.3.0.3., patient V.E.W.)

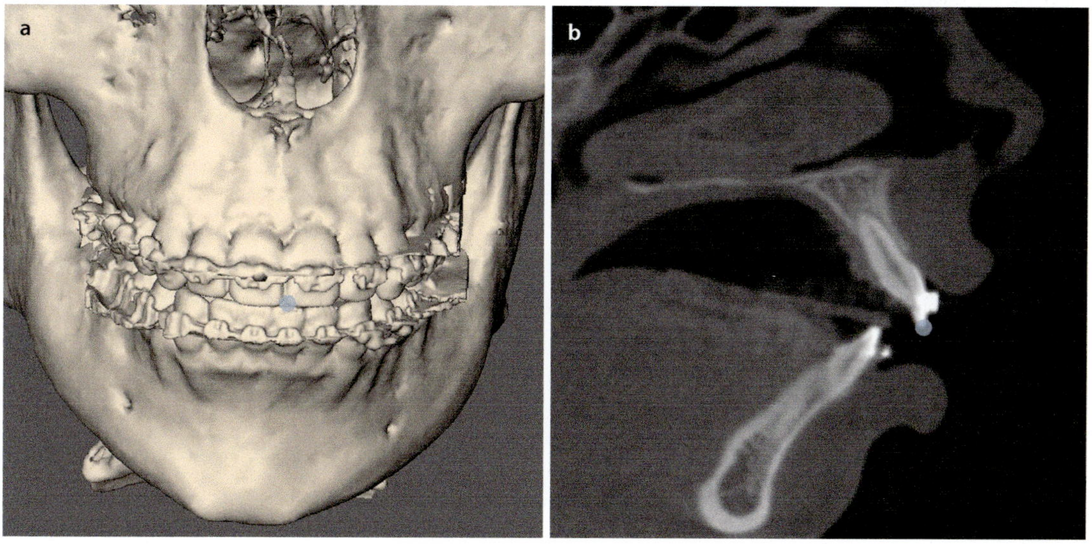

Fig. 2.101 *Upper Incisor$_r$*. Frontal view (**a**) of the 3D "surface-rendered" hard tissue representation of the patient's head and sagittal reslice (**b**) (i-CAT, Imaging Sciences International Inc, Maxilim v. 2.3.0.3., patient V.E.W.)

Lower Incisor (LI_r-LI_l)

Definition of the Lower Incisor (UI) landmark

"Lower incisor (LI)" is the most mesial point of the tip of the crown of the lower central incisor (Fig. 2.102).

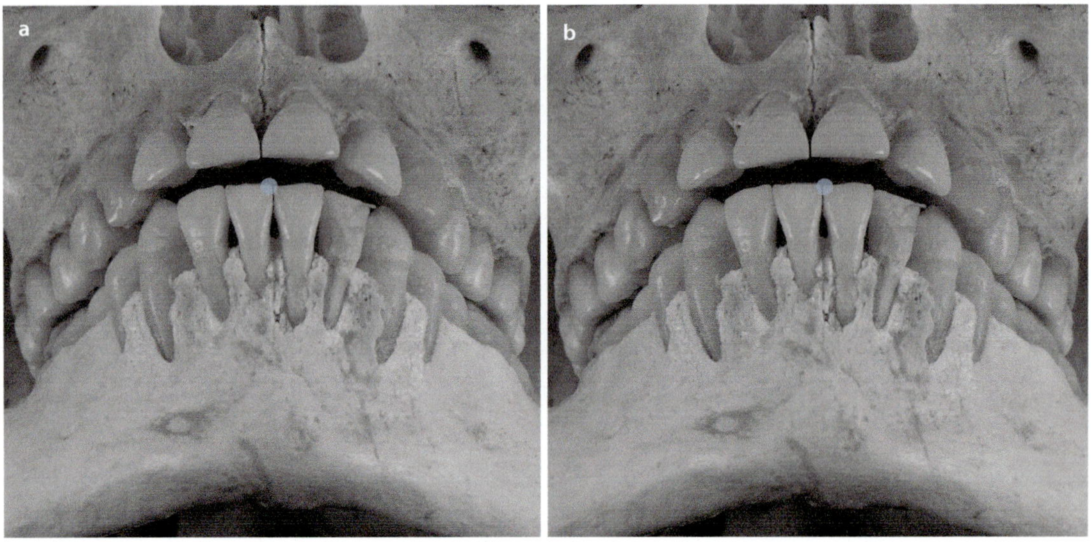

Fig. 2.102 *Lower Incisor$_r$* (**a**) and *Lower Incisor$_l$* (**b**). Submental views (cadaver skull)

Virtual definition of the *Lower Incisor* (LI) landmarks

Step 1: Define both *Lower Incisor$_r$* and *Lower Incisor$_l$* landmarks on the submental views of the 3D hard tissue surface representations (Figs. 2.103a and 2.104a).

Step 2: Verify and eventually correct the position of the *Lower Incisor$_r$* and *Lower Incisor$_l$* landmarks on the sagittal reslices (Figs. 2.103b and 2.104b).

> Especially in deep bite cases, it can be helpful to hide the maxilla during 3D virtual definition of the *Lower Incisor* landmarks.

Lower Incisor (LI_r-LI_l)

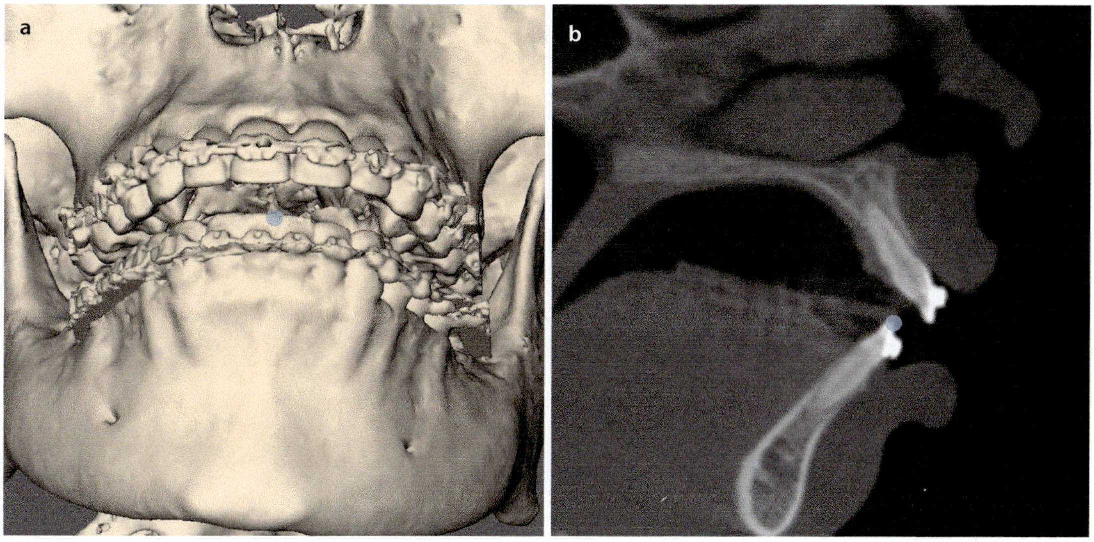

Fig. 2.103 *Lower Incisor$_r$*. Submental view (**a**) of the 3D "surface-rendered" hard tissue representation of the patient's head and sagittal reslice (**b**) (i-CAT, Imaging Sciences International Inc, Maxilim v. 2.3.0.3., patient V.E.W.)

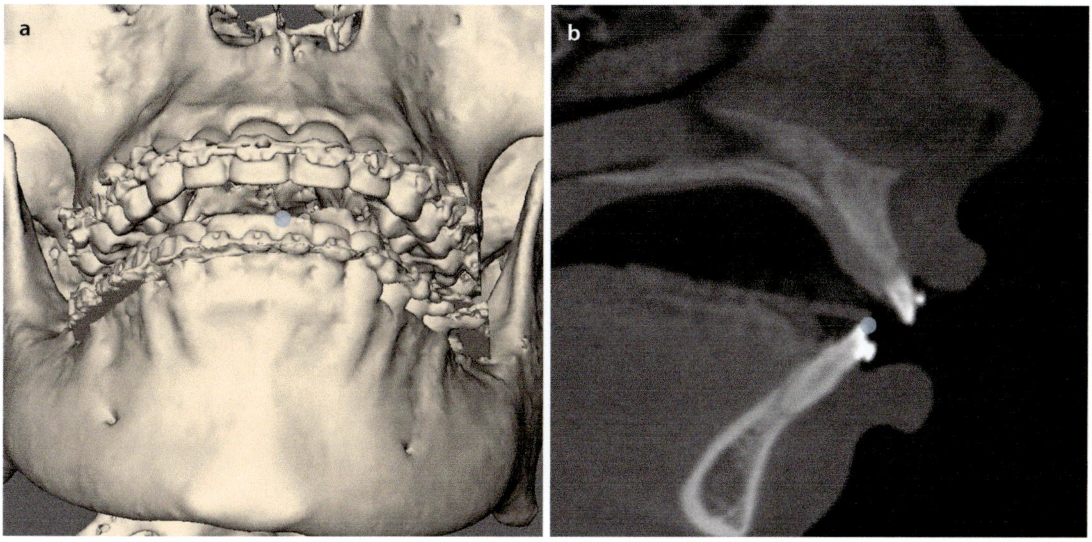

Fig. 2.104 *Lower Incisor$_l$*. Submental view (**a**) of the 3D "surface-rendered" hard tissue representation of the patient's head and sagittal reslice (**b**) (i-CAT, Imaging Sciences International Inc, Maxilim v. 2.3.0.3., patient V.E.W.)

▪ Upper Incisor apex ($UIapex_r$-$UIapex_l$)

Definition of Upper Incisor apex (UIapex)

"Upper Incisor (UIapex)" is the superior tip of the root of the upper central incisor.

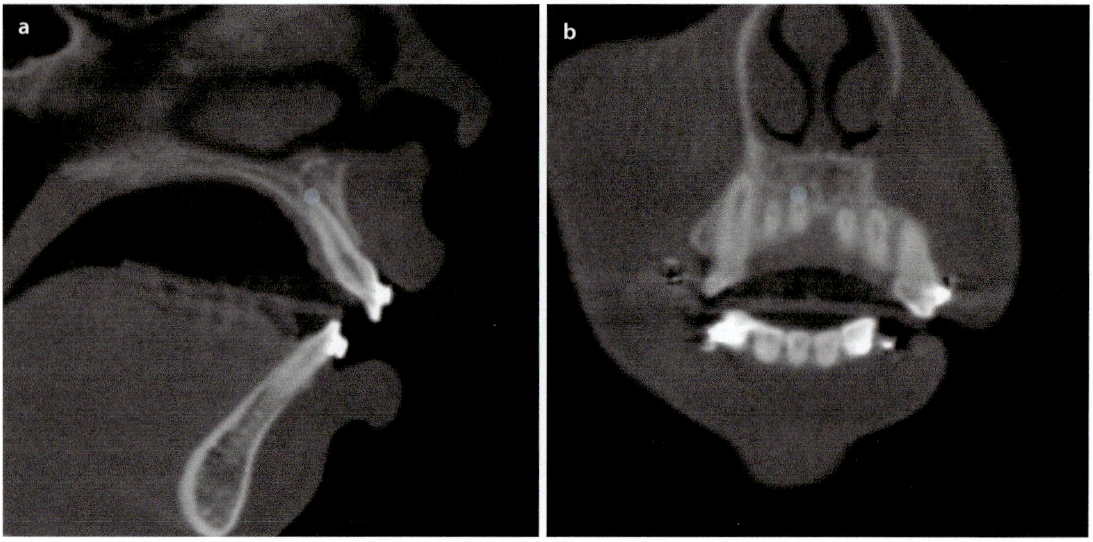

Fig. 2.105 *Upper Incisor apex$_r$*. Sagittal (**a**) and coronal (**b**) reslices of the patient's head (i-CAT, Imaging Sciences International Inc, Maxilim v. 2.3.0.3., patient V.E.W.)

3D virtual definition of the Upper Incisor apex (UIapex) landmarks

Step 1: Define both *Upper Incisor apex$_r$* and *Upper Incisor apex$_l$* landmarks on the sagittal reslices (Fig. 2.105a and 2.106a).

Step 2: Verify and correct the position of the *Upper Incisor apex$_r$* and *Upper Incisor apex$_l$* landmarks on the coronal reslices (Figs. 2.105b and 2.106b).

Upper Incisor apex ($UIapex_r$-$UIapex_l$)

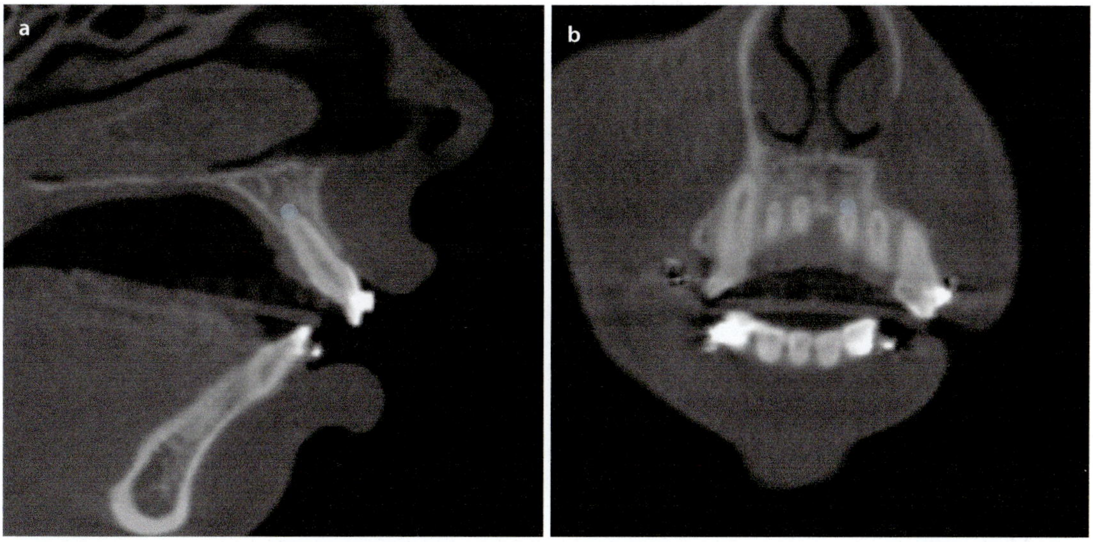

Fig. 2.106 *Upper Incisor apex$_l$*. Sagittal (**a**) and coronal (**b**) reslices of the patient's head (i-CAT, Imaging Sciences International Inc, Maxilim v. 2.3.0.3., patient V.E.W.)

▪ Lower Incisor apex (LIapex$_r$-LIapex$_l$)

Definition of Lower Incisor apex (LIapex)

"Lower Incisor (LIapex)" is the inferior tip of the root of the lower central incisor.

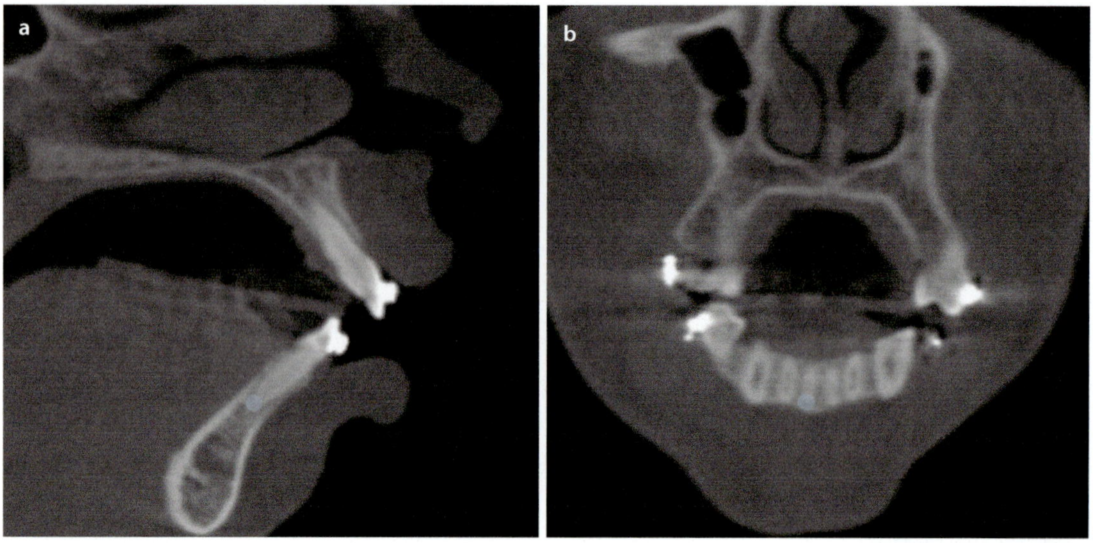

Fig. 2.107 *Lower Incisor apex$_r$*. Sagittal (**a**) and coronal (**b**) reslices of the patient's head (i-CAT, Imaging Sciences International Inc, Maxilim v. 2.3.0.3., patient V.E.W.)

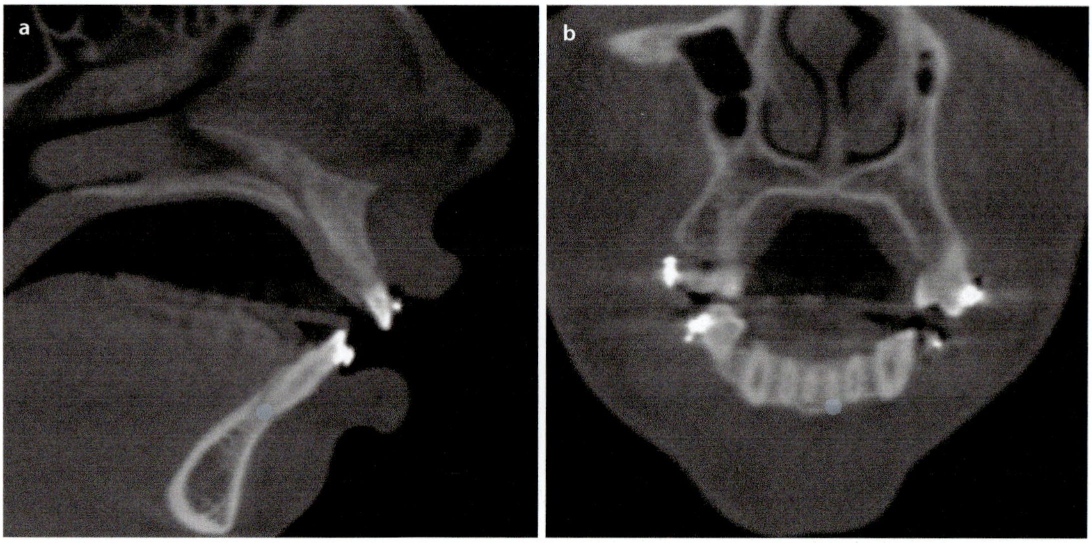

Fig. 2.108 *Lower Incisor apex$_l$*. Sagittal (**a**) and coronal (**b**) reslices of the patient's head (i-CAT, Imaging Sciences International Inc, Maxilim v. 2.3.0.3., patient V.E.W.)

3D virtual definition of the Lower Incisor apex (LIapex) landmarks

Step 1: Define both *Lower Incisor apex$_r$* and *Lower Incisor apex$_l$* landmarks on the sagittal reslices (Figs. 2.107a and 2.108a).

Step 2: Verify and correct the position of the *Lower Incisor apex$_r$* and *Lower Incisor apex$_l$* landmarks on the coronal reslices (Figs. 2.107b and 2.108b).

▪ Upper Canine (UC_r-UC_l)

Definition of the Upper Canine (UC) landmark

"Upper Canine (UC)" is the most inferior point of the tip of the crown of the upper canine (◘ Fig. 2.109).

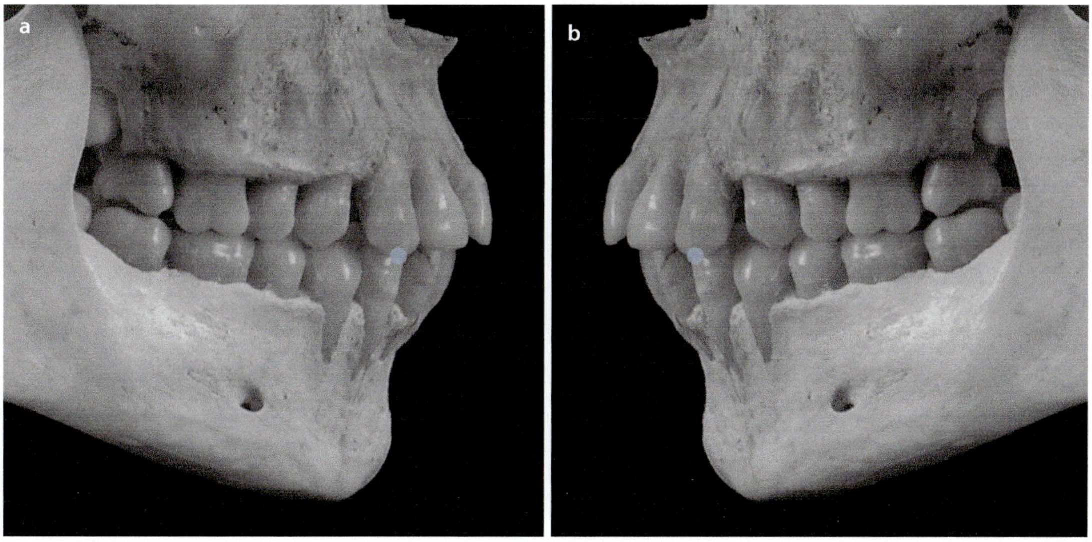

◘ **Fig. 2.109** *Upper Canine$_r$* (**a**) and *Upper Canine$_l$* (**b**). Profile views (cadaver skull)

Virtual definition of the *Upper Canine* (UC) landmarks

Define the *Upper Canine$_r$* and *Upper Canine$_l$* landmarks on the profile views of the 3D hard tissue surface representation (◘ Fig. 2.110).

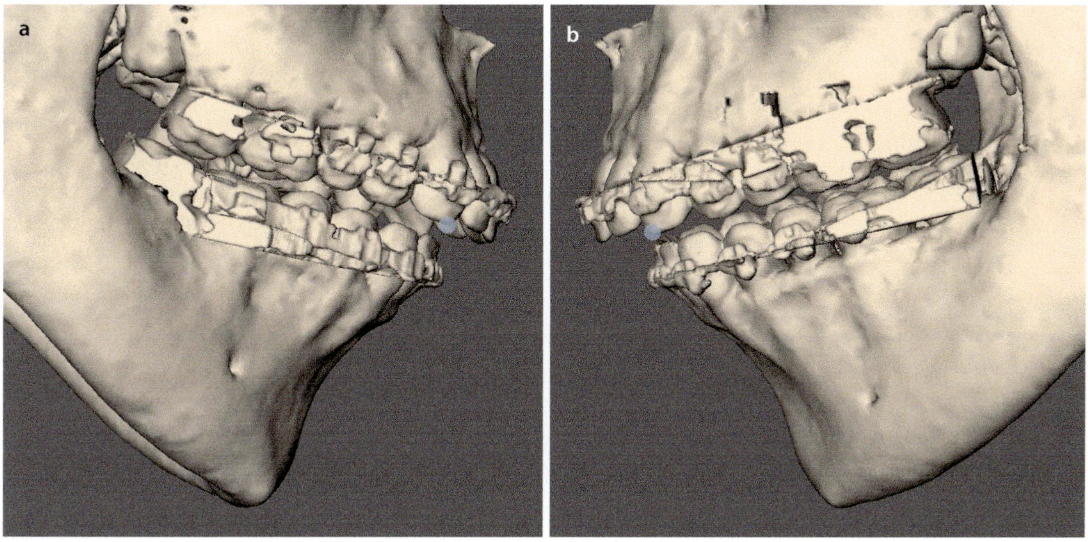

◘ **Fig. 2.110** *Upper Canine$_r$* (**a**) and *Upper Canine$_l$* (**b**). Profile views of the 3D "surface-rendered" hard tissue representation of the patient's head (**a**) and sagittal reslice (**b**) (i-CAT, Imaging Sciences International Inc, Maxilim v. 2.3.0.3., patient V.E.W.)

▪ Upper Molar Cusp ($UMcusp_r$-UM-$cusp_l$)

Definition of the Upper Molar Cusp (UMcusp) landmark

"Upper Molar cusp (UMcusp)" is the most inferior point of the mesial cusp of the crown of the first upper molar in the profile plane (▫ Fig. 2.111).

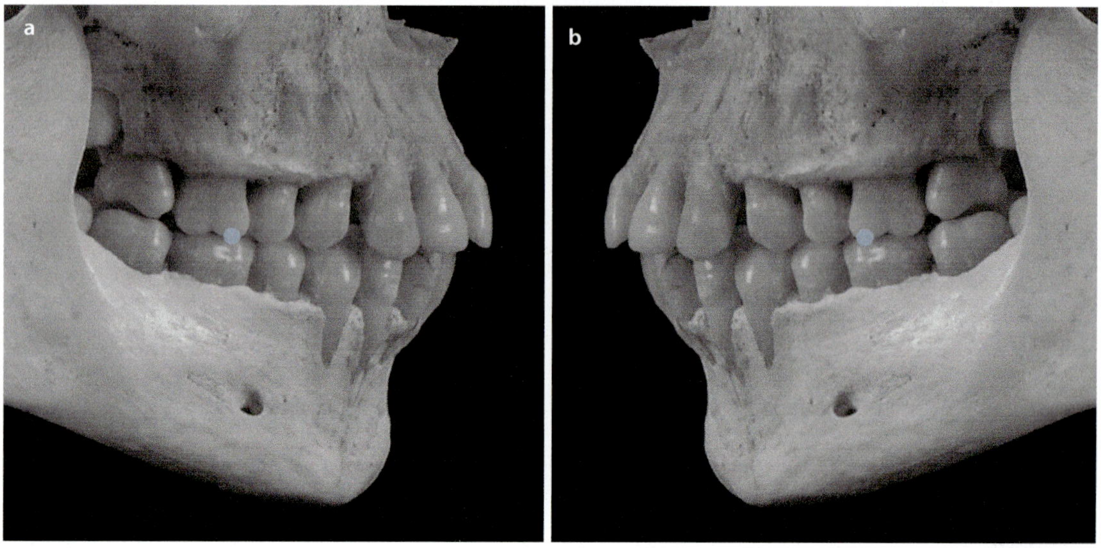

▫ **Fig. 2.111** *Upper Molar Cusp$_r$* (**a**) and *Upper Molar Cusp$_r$* (**b**). Profile views (cadaver skull)

Virtual definition of the *Upper Molar Cusp* (UMcusp) landmarks

Step 1: Define the *Upper Molar Cusp$_r$* and *Upper Molar Cusp$_l$* landmarks on the profile views of the 3D hard tissue surface representation (▫ Figs. 2.112a and 2.113a).

Step 2: Verify and eventually correct the position of the *Upper Molar Cusp$_r$* and *Upper Molar Cusp$_l$* landmarks on the sagittal reslices (▫ Figs. 2.112b and 2.113b).

Step 2: Verify and eventually correct the position of the *Upper Molar Cusp$_r$* and *Upper Molar Cusp$_l$* landmarks on the base view of the 3D hard tissue surface representation (▫ Figs. 2.114 and 2.115).

Upper Molar Cusp ($UMcusp_r$-UM-$cusp_l$)

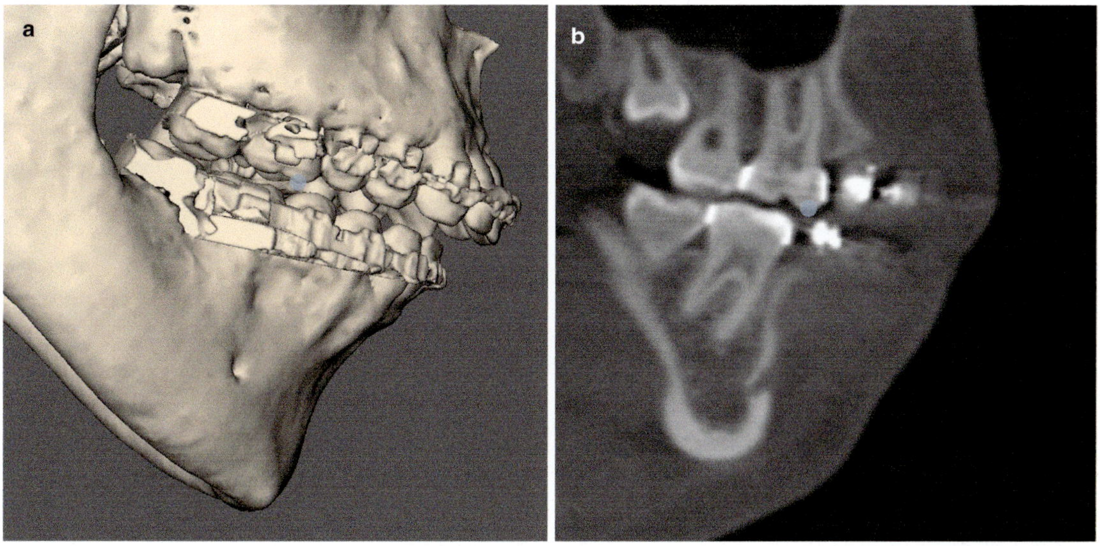

Fig. 2.112 *Upper Molar Cusp$_r$*. Profile view right (**a**) of the 3D "surface-rendered" hard tissue representation of the patient's head and sagittal reslice (**b**) (i-CAT, Imaging Sciences International Inc, Maxilim v. 2.3.0.3., patient V.E.W.)

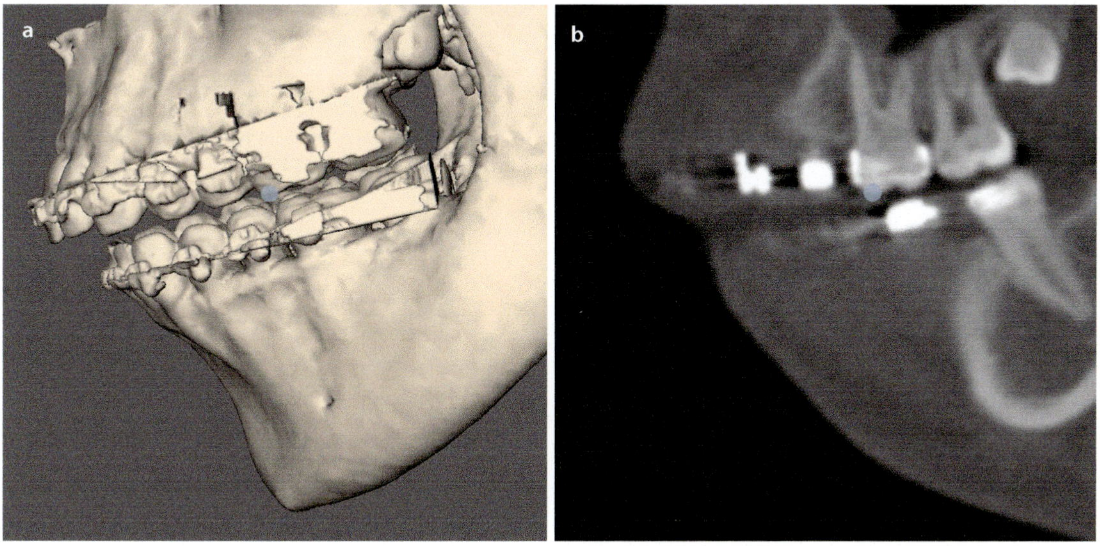

Fig. 2.113 *Upper Molar Cusp$_l$*. Profile view left (**a**) of the 3D "surface-rendered" hard tissue representation of the patient's head and sagittal reslice (**b**) (i-CAT, Imaging Sciences International Inc, Maxilim v. 2.3.0.3., patient V.E.W.)

Upper Molar Cusp (UMcusp$_r$-UM-cusp$_l$)

2

It can be helpful to hide the mandible during 3D virtual definition of the *Upper Molar Cusp* landmarks.

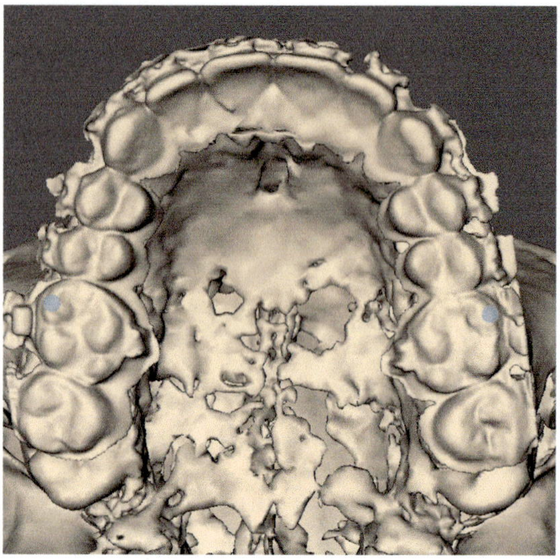

Fig. 2.114 *Upper Molar Cusp$_r$.* and *Upper Molar Cusp$_l$.* Base view of the 3D "surface-rendered" hard tissue representation of the patient's head (i-CAT, Imaging Sciences International Inc, Maxilim v. 2.3.0.3., patient V.E.W.)

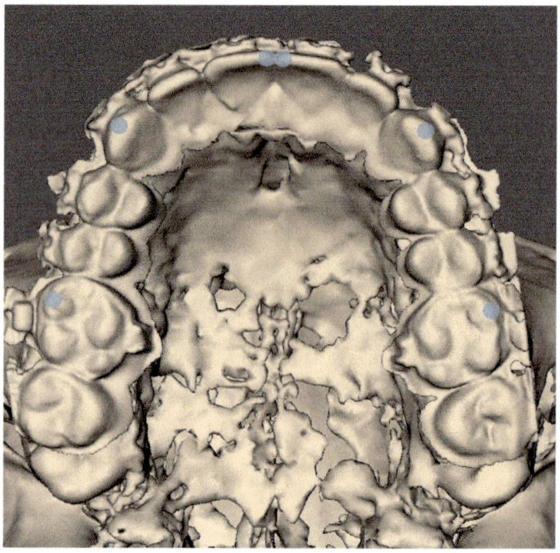

Fig. 2.115 *Upper Molar Cusp$_r$, Upper Canine$_r$, Upper Incisor$_r$, Upper Incisor$_l$, Upper Canine$_l$* and *Upper Molar Cusp$_l$.* Base view of the 3D "surface-rendered" hard tissue representation of the patient's head (i-CAT, Imaging Sciences International Inc, Maxilim v. 2.3.0.3., patient V.E.W.)

▪ Lower Molar Cusp (LMcusp$_r$-LM-cusp$_{l)}$

Definition of the Lower Molar Cusp (UMcusp) landmark

"Lower Molar Cusp (LMcusp)" is the most superior point of the mesial cusp of the crown of the first lower molar in the profile plane (▫ Fig. 2.116).

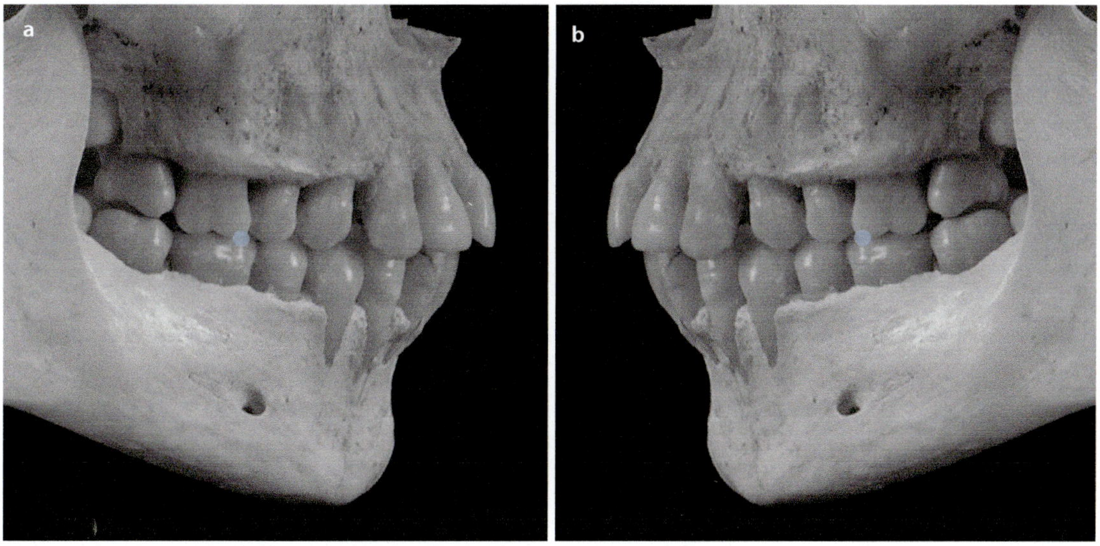

▫ **Fig. 2.116** *Lower Molar Cusp$_r$* (**a**) and *Lower Molar Cusp$_r$* (**b**). Profile views (cadaver skull)

Virtual definition of the *Lower Molar Cusp* (LMcusp) landmarks

Step 1: Define the *Lower Molar Cusp$_r$* and *Lower Molar Cusp$_l$* landmarks on the profile views of the 3D hard tissue surface representation (▫ Figs. 2.117a and 2.118a).

Step 2: Verify and eventually correct the position of the *Lower Molar Cusp$_r$* and *Lower Molar Cusp$_l$* landmarks on the sagittal reslices (▫ Figs. 2.117b and 2.118b).

Step 3: Verify and eventually correct the position of the *Lower Molar Cusp$_r$* and *Lower Molar Cusp$_l$* landmarks on the base view of the 3D hard tissue surface representation (▫ Figs. 2.119 and 2.120).

Lower Molar Cusp ($LMcusp_r$-LM-$cusp_l$)

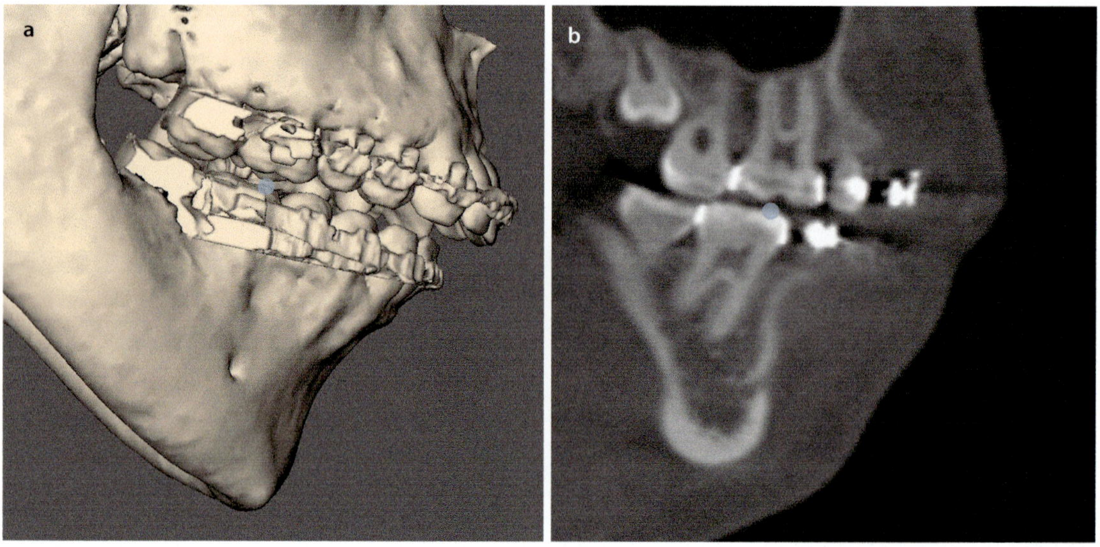

Fig. 2.117 (**a**) *Lower Molar Cusp*$_r$. Profile view right (**a**) of the 3D "surface-rendered" hard tissue representation of the patient's head and sagittal reslice (**b**) (i-CAT, Imaging Sciences International Inc, Maxilim v. 2.3.0.3., patient V.E.W.)

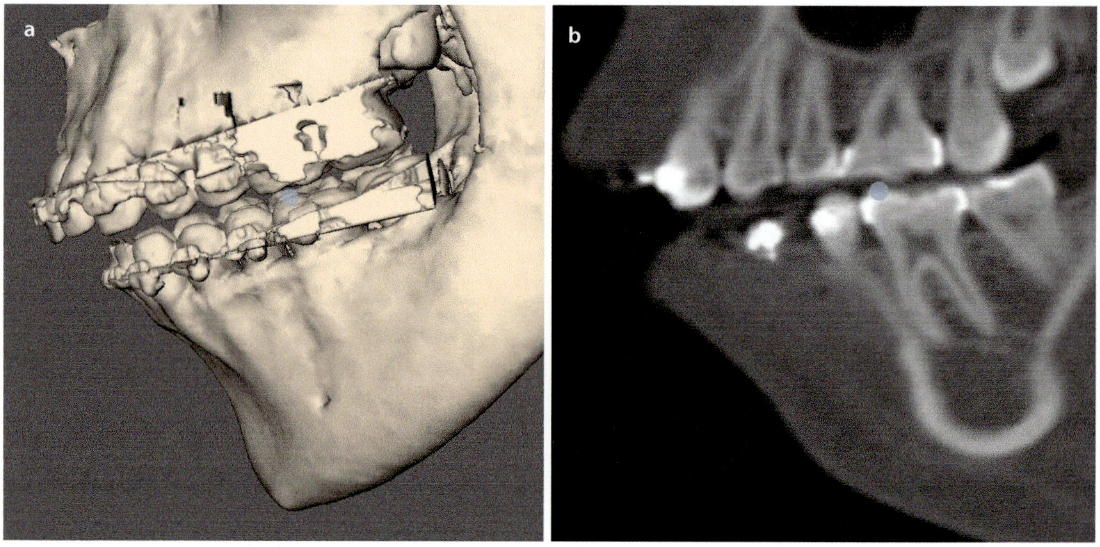

Fig. 2.118 *Lower Molar Cusp*$_l$. Profile view left (**a**) of the 3D "surface-rendered" hard tissue representation of the patient's head and sagittal reslice (**b**) (i-CAT, Imaging Sciences International Inc, Maxilim v. 2.3.0.3., patient V.E.W.)

Lower Molar Cusp (LMcusp$_r$-LM-cusp$_l$)

It can be helpful to hide the maxilla during 3D virtual definition of the *Lower Molar Cusp* Landmarks.

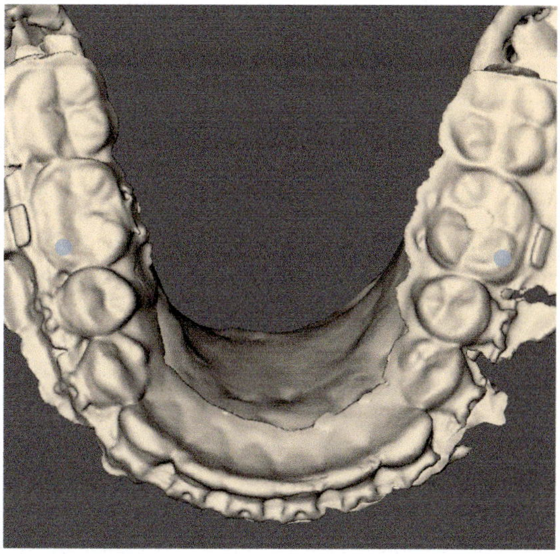

Fig. 2.119 *Lower Molar Cusp$_r$*. and *Lower Molar Cusp$_l$*. Base view left of the 3D "surface-rendered" hard tissue representation of the patient's head (i-CAT, Imaging Sciences International Inc, Maxilim v. 2.3.0.3., patient V.E.W.)

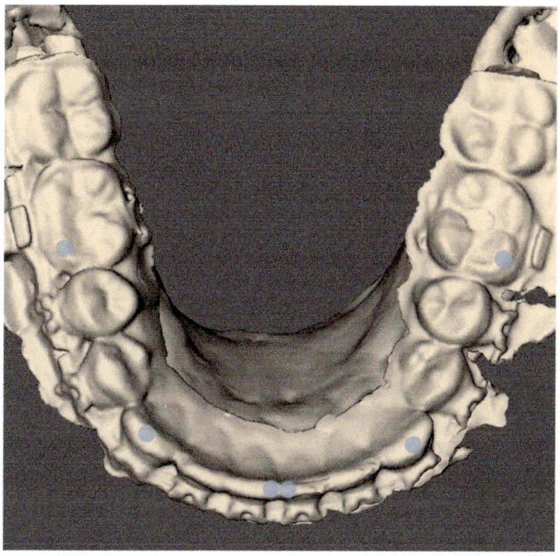

Fig. 2.120 *Lower Molar Cusp$_r$, Lower Canine$_r$, Lower Incisor$_r$*, Lower *Incisor$_l$, Lower Canine$_l$* and *Lower Molar Cusp$_l$*. Base view of the 3D "surface-rendered" hard tissue representation of the patient's head (i-CAT, Imaging Sciences International Inc, Maxilim v. 2.3.0.3., patient V.E.W.)

Menton - Men

Definition of the Menton (Men) landmark

"Menton (Men)" is the most inferior midpoint of the chin on the outline of the mandibular symphysis (Fig. 2.121).

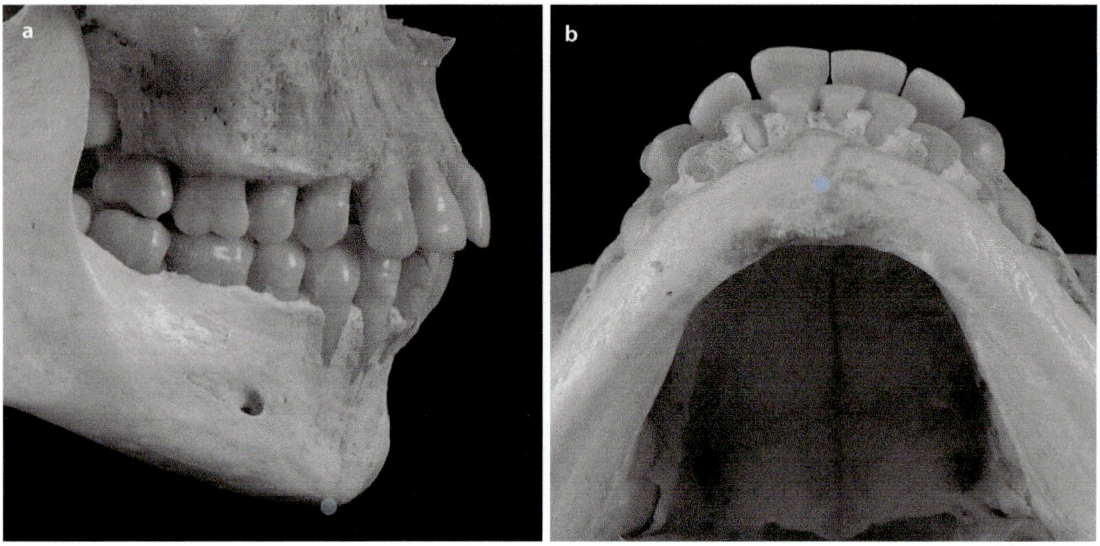

Fig. 2.121 *Menton*. Profile right (**a**) and base (**b**) views (cadaver skull)

Virtual definition of the *Menton* (Men) landmark

Step 1: Define *Menton* on the right profile view of the 3D hard tissue surface representation (Fig. 2.122a).

Step 2: Verify the midline position of the *Menton* landmark on the base view of the 3D hard tissue surface representation (Fig. 2.122b). Note that the *Menton* landmark is the skeletal midline point of the chin and can therefore be out of the facial midplane.

Step 3: Verify the midline position of the *Menton* landmark on the right and left (Fig. 2.123) profile views of the 3D hard tissue surface representation.

Menton (Men)

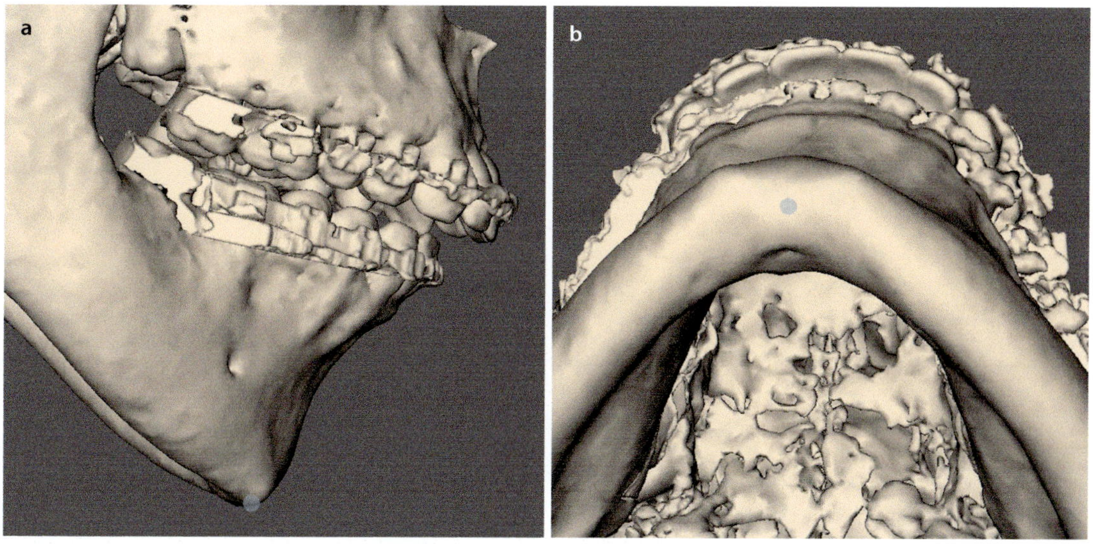

Fig. 2.122 *Menton*. Profile right (**a**) and base (**b**) views of the 3D "surface-rendered" hard tissue representation of the patient's head (i-CAT, Imaging Sciences International Inc, Maxilim v. 2.3.0.3., patient V.E.W.)

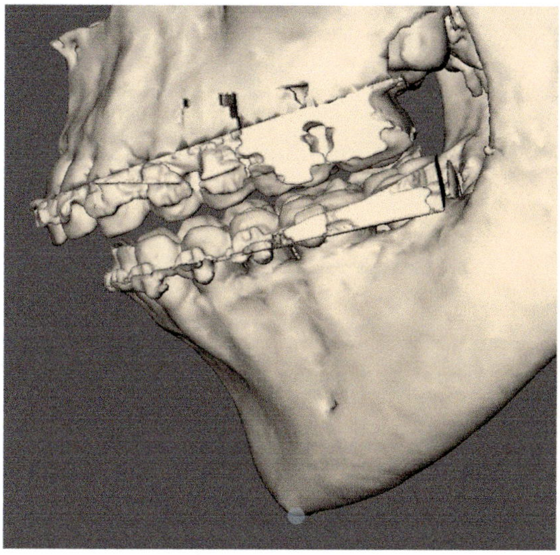

Fig. 2.123 *Menton*. Profile left view of the 3D "surface-rendered" hard tissue representation of the patient's head (i-CAT, Imaging Sciences International Inc, Maxilim v. 2.3.0.3., patient V.E.W.)

■ Gonion (Go_r-Go_l)

Definition of the *Gonion* (Go) landmark

Gonion (Go) is the point at the mandibular angle, defined by a perpendicular to the intersection point of the tangent lines to the posterior margin of the vertical ramus and to the inferior margin of the mandibular body (◘ Fig. 2.124).

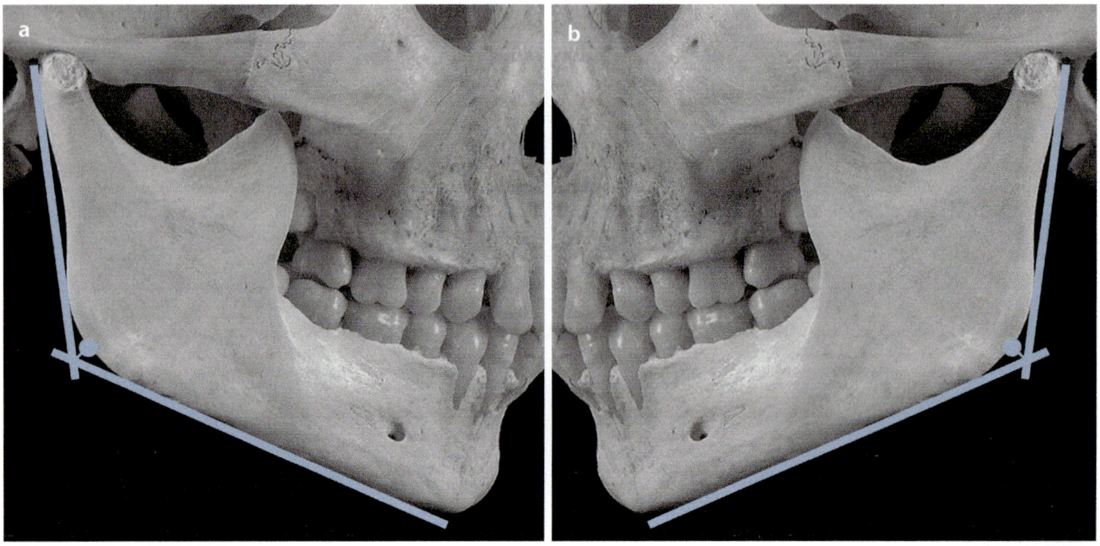

◘ **Fig. 2.124** *Gonion*$_r$ (**a**) and *Gonion*$_r$ (**b**) profile views (cadaver skull)

Virtual definition of the *Gonion* (Go) landmarks

Step 1: Define the *Gonion* landmarks on the right (◘ Fig. 2.125a) and left (◘ Fig. 2.125b) profile views of the 3D hard tissue surface representations.

Step 2: Verify the correct transversal position of the *Gonion* landmarks on the base view (◘ Fig. 2.126) of the 3D hard tissue surface representation.

Gonion (Go_r-Go_l)

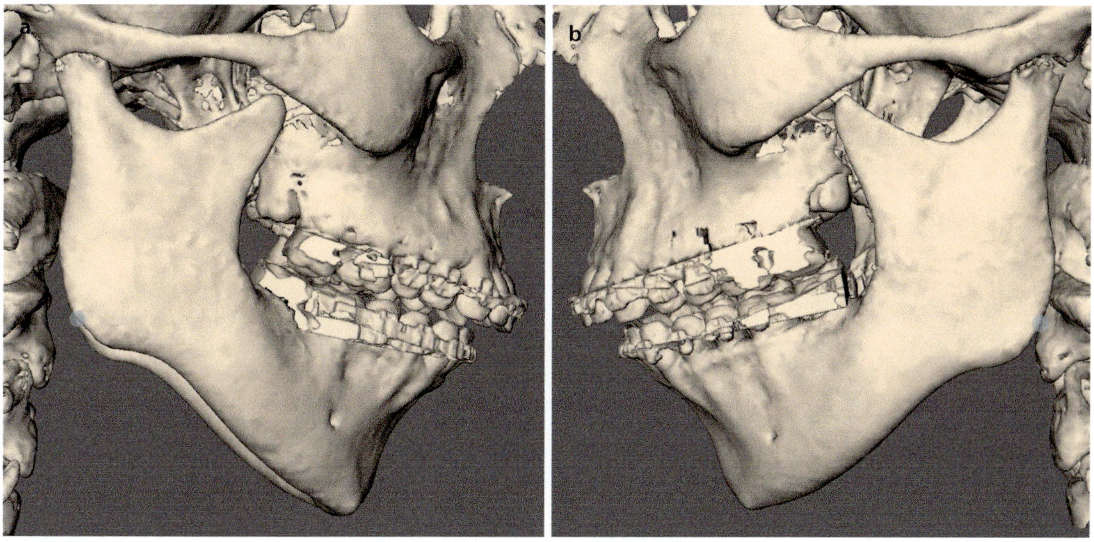

Fig. 2.125 *Gonion*$_r$ (**a**) *Gonion*$_l$ (**b**). Profile views of the 3D "surface-rendered" hard tissue representation of the patient's head (i-CAT, Imaging Sciences International Inc, Maxilim v. 2.3.0.3., patient V.E.W.)

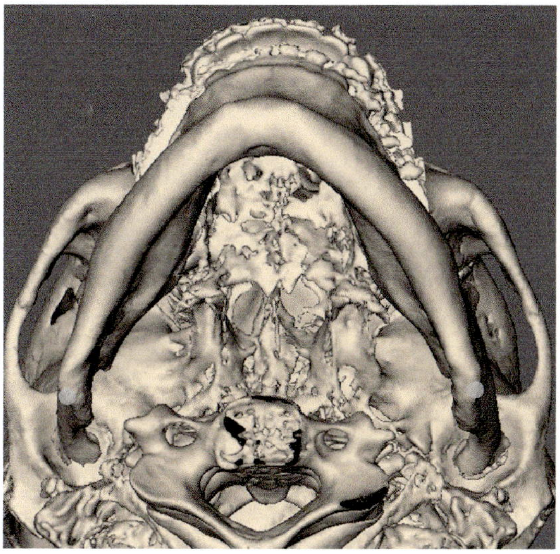

Fig. 2.126 *Gonion*$_r$ *Gonion*$_l$ Base view of the 3D "surface-rendered" hard tissue representation of the patient's head (i-CAT, Imaging Sciences International Inc, Maxilim v. 2.3.0.3., patient V.E.W.)

▪ Frontozygomatic Point (Fz_r-Fz_l)

Definition of the Frontozygomatic (Fz) landmark

"Frontozygomatic (Fz)" is the most medial and anterior point of the frontozygomatic suture at the level of the lateral orbital rim (▫ Fig. 2.127).

Virtual definition of the *Frontozygomatic* (Fz) landmark

Define *Frontozygomatic*$_r$ and *Frontozygomatic*$_l$ landmarks on the frontal view (▫ Fig. 2.128) of the 3D hard tissue surface representation.

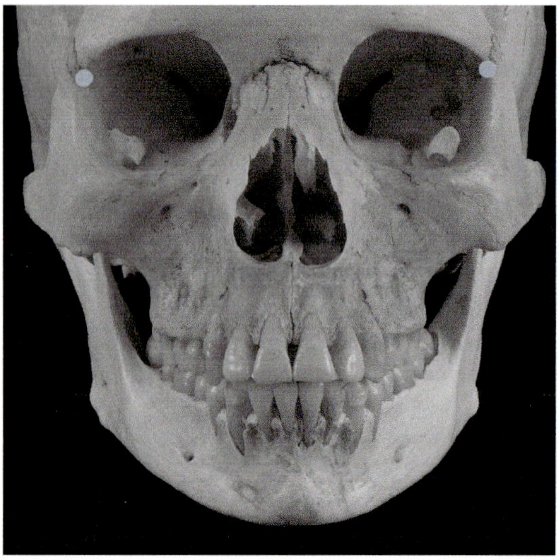

▫ **Fig. 2.127** *Frontozygomatic*$_r$ and *Frontozygomatic*$_l$. Frontal view (cadaver skull)

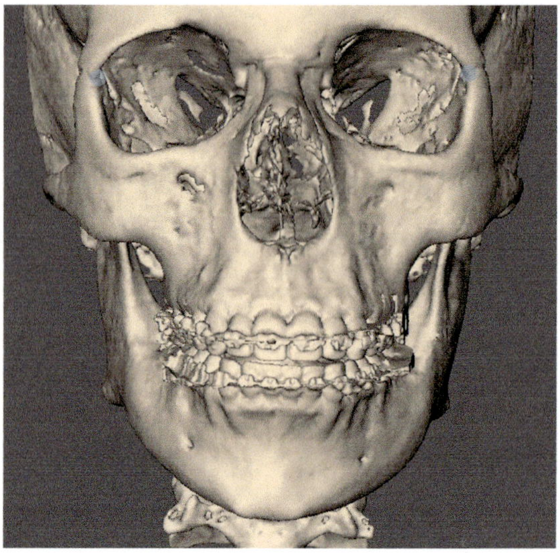

▫ **Fig. 2.128** *Frontozygomatic*$_r$ and *Frontozygomatic*$_l$. Frontal view of the 3D "surface-rendered" hard tissue representation of the patient's head (i-CAT, Imaging Sciences International Inc, Maxilim v. 2.3.0.3., patient V.E.W.)

Zygion (Zy(l)-Zy(r))

Definition of the *Zygion* (Zy) landmark

Zygion (Zy) is the most lateral point on the outline of the bony zygomatic arch (Fig. 2.129).

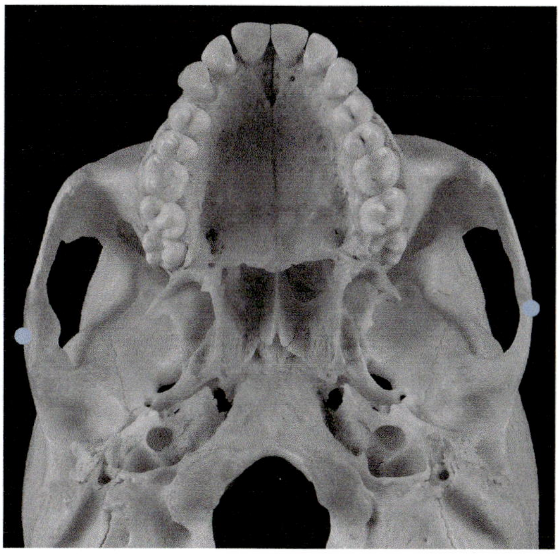

Fig. 2.129 *Zygion*$_r$ and *Zygion*$_l$. Base view (cadaver skull)

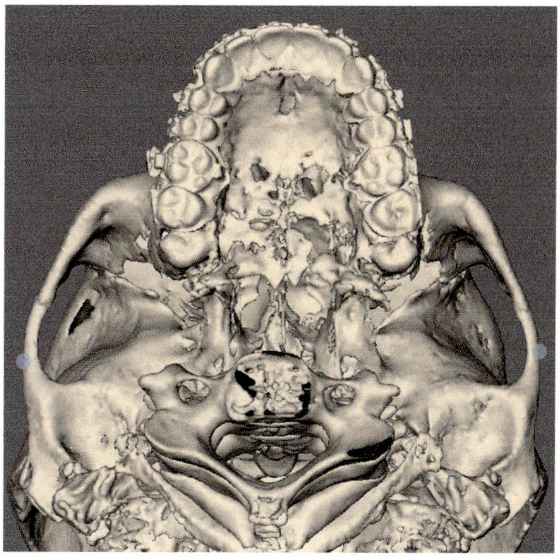

Fig. 2.130 *Zygion*$_r$ and *Zygion*$_l$. Base view of the 3D "surface-rendered" hard tissue representation of the patient's head (i-CAT, Imaging Sciences International Inc, Maxilim v. 2.3.0.3., patient V.E.)

Virtual definition of the *Zygion* (Zy) landmark

Step 1: Define *Zygion*$_r$ and Zygion$_l$ landmarks on the base view (Fig. 2.130) of the 3D hard tissue surface representation.

Step 2: Verify the vertical position of the *Zygion* landmarks on the profile (Fig. 2.131) and frontal (Fig. 2.132) views of the 3D hard tissue surface representations.

Zygion Point – Zy_r - Zy_l

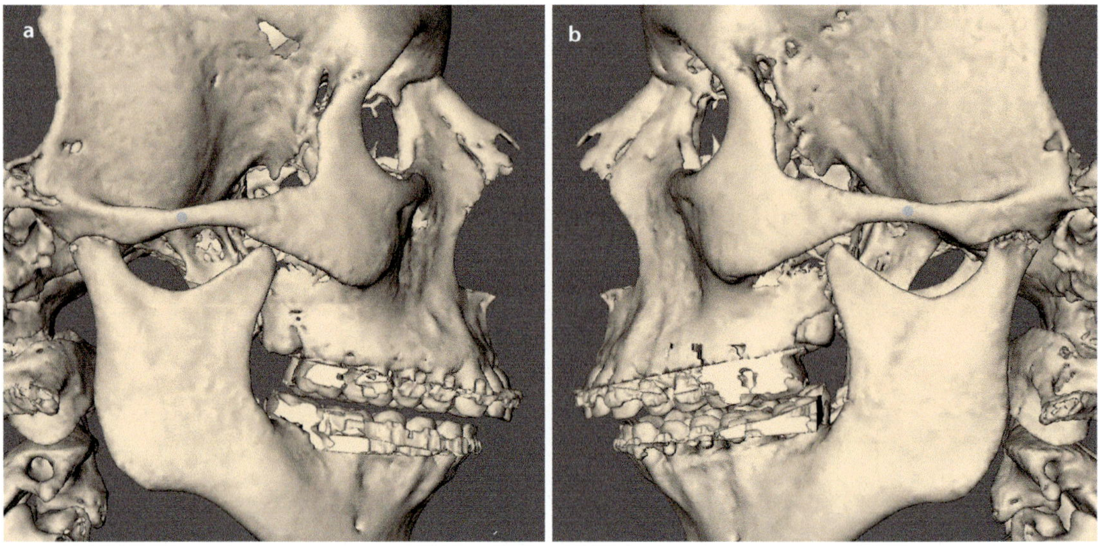

Fig. 2.131 *Zygion*$_r$ (**a**) and *Zygion*$_l$ (**b**). Profile views of the 3D "surface-rendered" hard tissue representation of the patient's head (i-CAT, Imaging Sciences International Inc, Maxilim v. 2.3.0.3., patient V.E.W.)

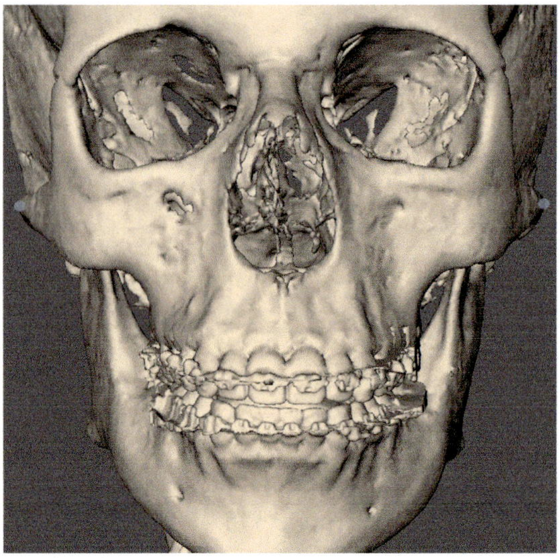

Fig. 2.132 *Zygion*$_r$ and *Zygion*$_l$. Frontal view of the 3D "surface-rendered" hard tissue representation of the patient's head (i-CAT, Imaging Sciences International Inc, Maxilim v. 2.3.0.3., patient V.E.W.)

A-Point

Definition of the A-Point (A) landmark

"A-Point (A)" is the point of maximum concavity in the midline of the dento-alveolar process of the maxilla (Fig. 2.133).

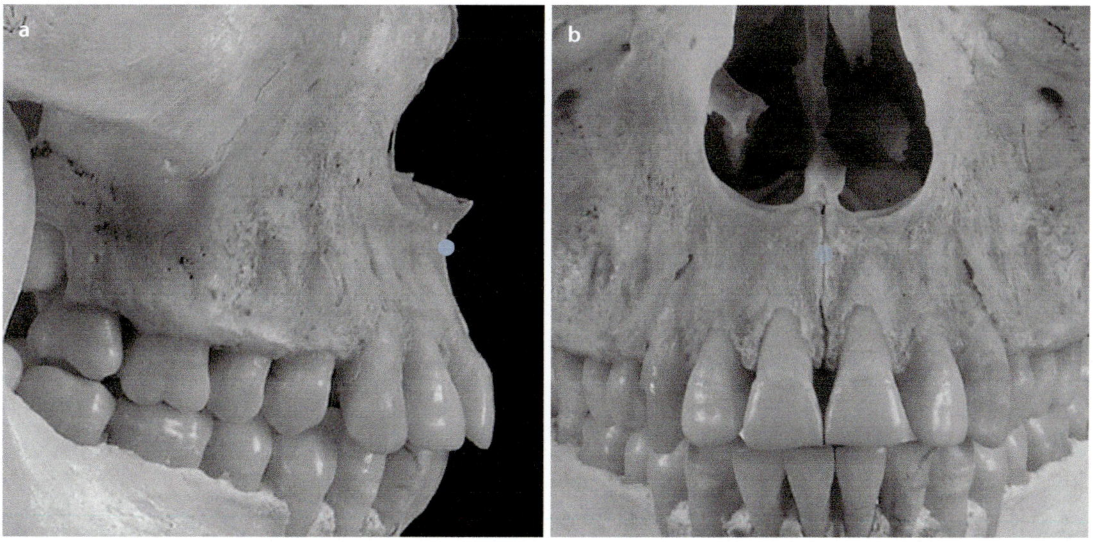

Fig. 2.133 *A-Point*. Profile right (**a**) and frontal (**b**) views (cadaver skull)

Virtual definition of the *A-Point* (A) landmark

Step 1: Define *A-Point* on the right profile view of the 3D hard tissue surface representation (Fig. 2.134a) and verify on the sagittal reslice (Fig. 2.134b)

Step 2: Verify and eventually correct the midline position of the *A-Point* landmark on the frontal view of the 3D hard tissue surface representation (Fig. 2.134c).

Step 3: The position of the *A-Point* landmark is verified on the right and left (Fig. 2.134d) profile views of the 3D hard tissue surface representations.

A- Point

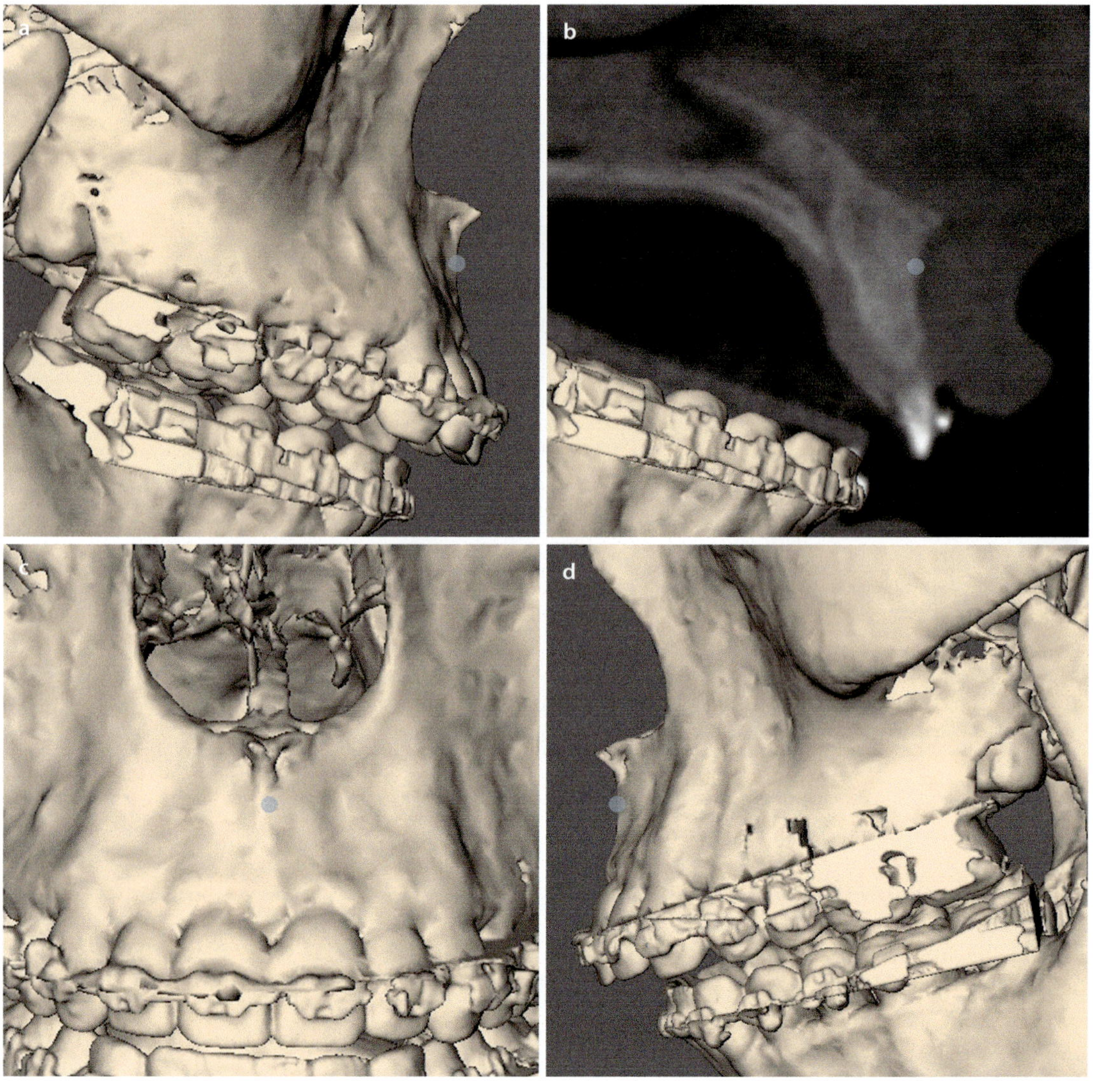

Fig. 2.134 *A-Point*. Profile right (**a**), sagittal reslice (**b**), frontal (**c**) and profile left (**d**) views of the 3D "surface-rendered" hard tissue representation of the patient's head (i-CAT, Imaging Sciences International Inc, Maxilim v. 2.3.0.3., patient V.E.W.)

B-Point

Definition of the B-Point (B) landmark

"B-Point (B)" is the point of maximum concavity in the midline of the dento-alveolar process of the mandible (Fig. 2.135).

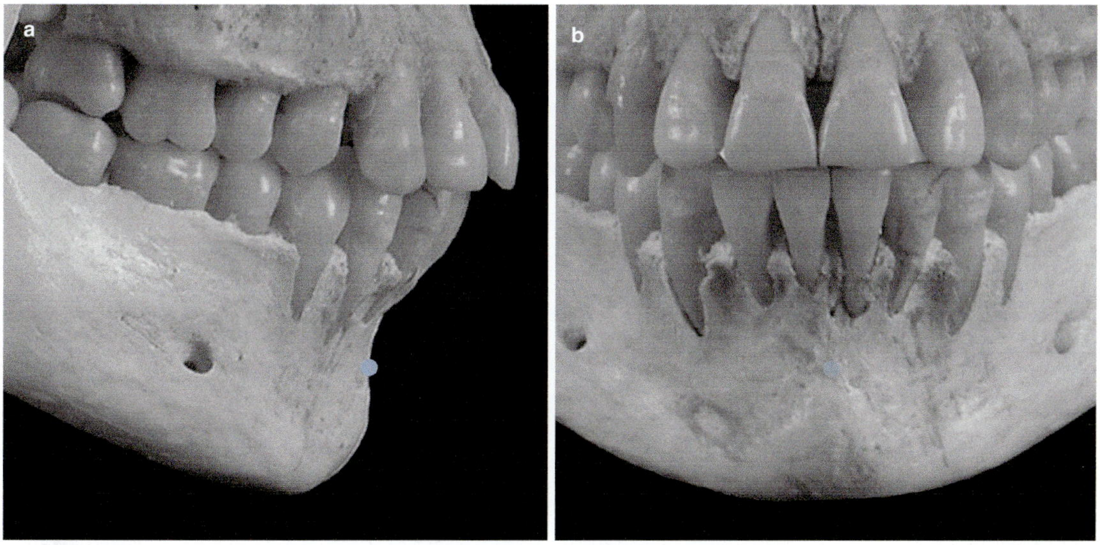

Fig. 2.135 *B-Point*. Profile right (**a**) and frontal (**b**) views (cadaver skull)

Virtual definition of the *B-Point (B)* landmark

Step 1: Define *B-Point* on the right profile view of the 3D hard tissue surface representation (Fig. 2.136a) and verify on the sagittal reslice (Fig. 2.136b)

Step 2: Verify and eventually correct the midline position of the *B-Point* landmark on the frontal view of the 3D hard tissue surface representation (Fig. 2.136c).

Step 3: The position of the *B-Point* landmark is verified on the right and left (Fig. 2.136d) profile views of the 3D hard tissue surface representations.

B- Point

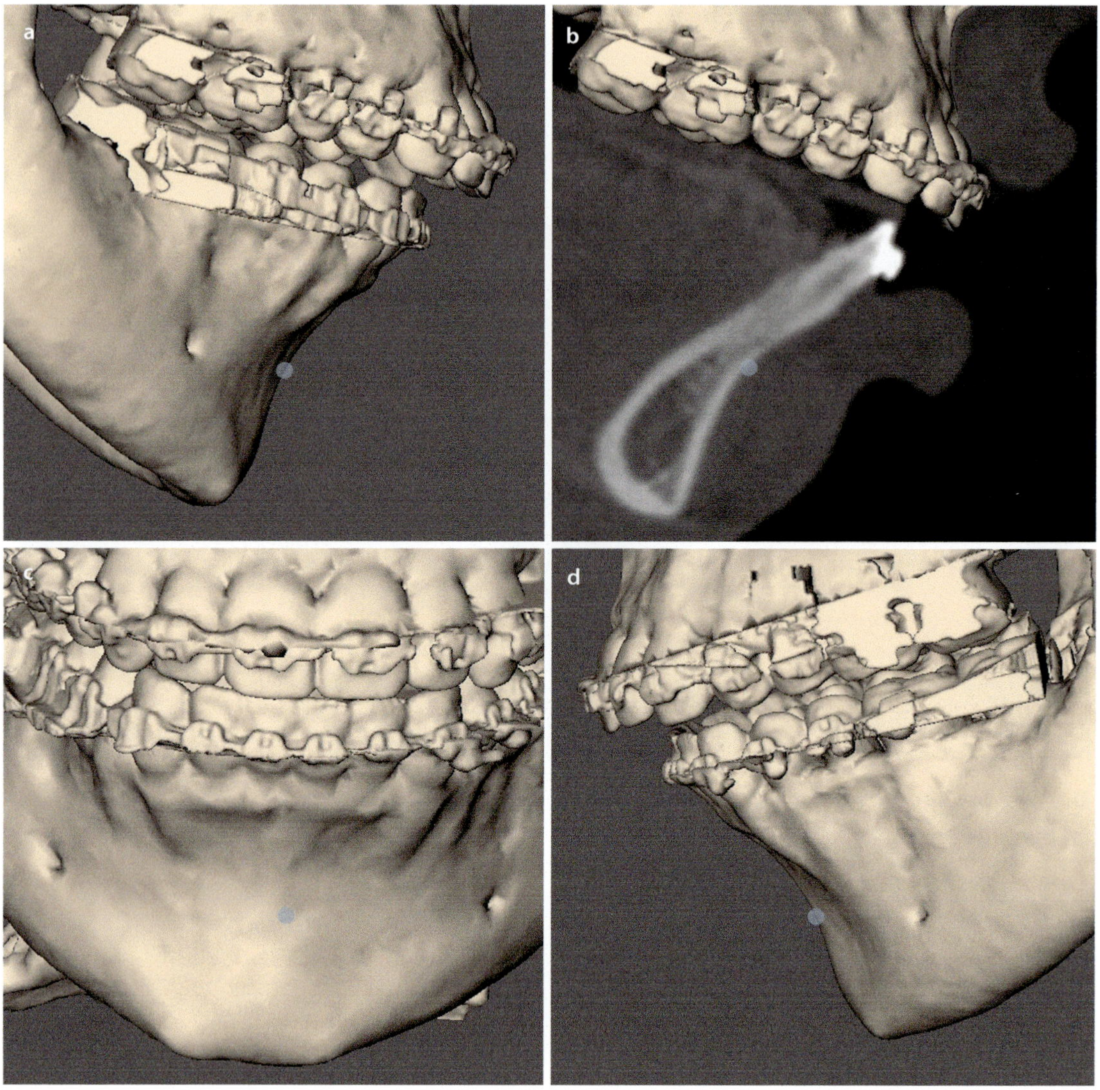

Fig. 2.136 *B-Point*. Profile right (**a**), sagittal reslice (**b**), frontal (**c**) and profile left (**d**) views of the 3D "surface-rendered" hard tissue representation of the patient's head (i-CAT, Imaging Sciences International Inc, Maxilim v. 2.3.0.3., patient V.E.W.)

Pogonion (Pog)

Definition of the Pogonion (Pog) landmark

"Pogonion (Pog)" is the most anterior midpoint of the chin on the outline of the mandibular symphysis (Fig. 2.137).

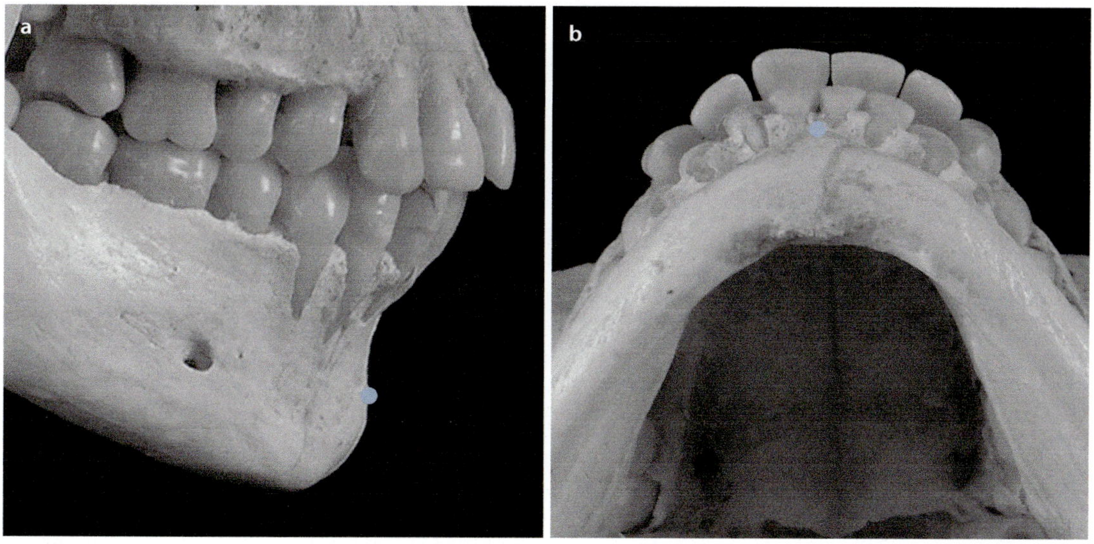

Fig. 2.137 *Pogonion.* Profile right (**a**) and base (**b**) views (cadaver skull)

Virtual definition of the *Pogonion* (Pog) landmark

Step 1: Define *Pogonion* on the right profile view of the 3D hard tissue surface representation (Fig. 2.138a).

Step 2: Verify and eventually correct the midline position of the *Pogonion* landmark on the base view of the 3D hard tissue surface representation (Fig. 2.138b). Note that the *Pogonion* landmark is the most anterior skeletal midline point of the chin and can therefore be out of the facial midplane.

Step 3: The position of the *Pogonion* landmark is verified on the right and left (Fig. 2.139) profile views of the 3D hard tissue surface representations.

Pogonion (Pog)

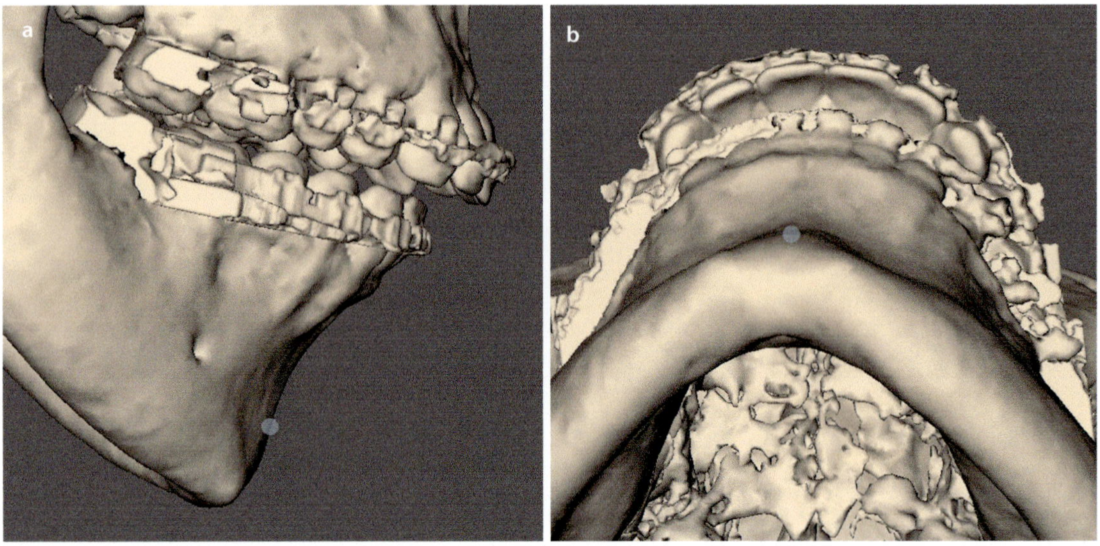

Fig. 2.138 *Pogonion*. Profile right (**a**) and base (**b**) views of the 3D "surface-rendered" hard tissue representation of the patient's head (i-CAT, Imaging Sciences International Inc, Maxilim v. 2.3.0.3., patient V.E.W.)

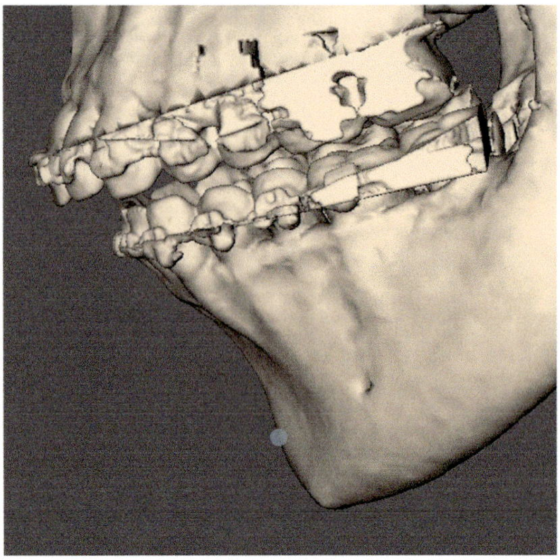

Fig. 2.139 *Pogonion*. Profile left view of the 3D "surface-rendered" hard tissue representation of the patient's head (i-CAT, Imaging Sciences International Inc, Maxilim v. 2.3.0.3., patient V.E.W.)

Basion (Ba)

Definition of the Basion (Ba) landmark

"Basion (Ba)" is the most anterior point of the great foramen (Foramen magnum) (Fig. 2.140).

Virtual definition of the *Basion* (Ba) landmark

Define *Basion* on the base view (Fig. 2.141.) of the 3D hard tissue surface representation.

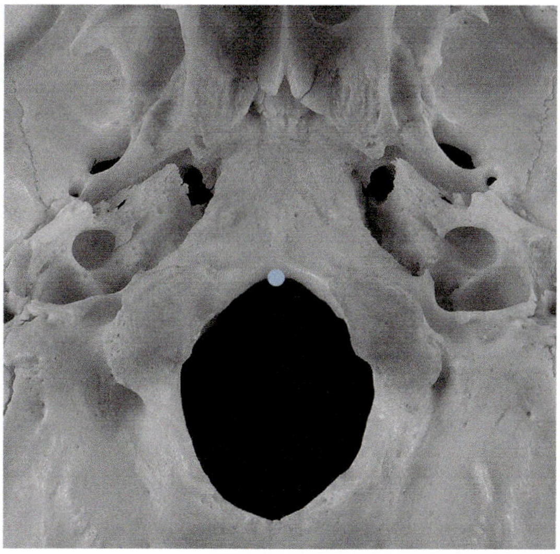

Fig. 2.140 *Basion*. Exocranial skullbase view (cadaver skull)

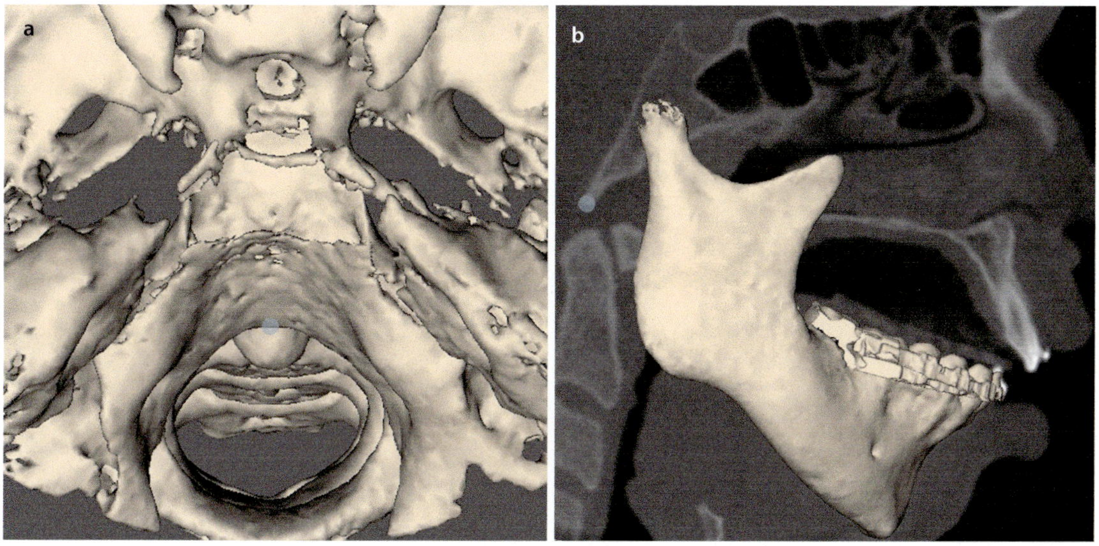

Fig. 2.141 *Basion*. Base view (**a**) and sagittal reslice (**b**) of the 3D "surface-rendered" hard tissue representation of the patient's head (i-CAT, Imaging Sciences International Inc, Maxilim v. 2.3.0.3., patient V.E.W.)

Condylion (Co_r-Co_l)

Definition of the Condylion (Co) landmark

"Condylion (Co)" is the most postero-superior point of the mandibular condyle in the sagittal plane (Figs. 2.142 and 2.145).

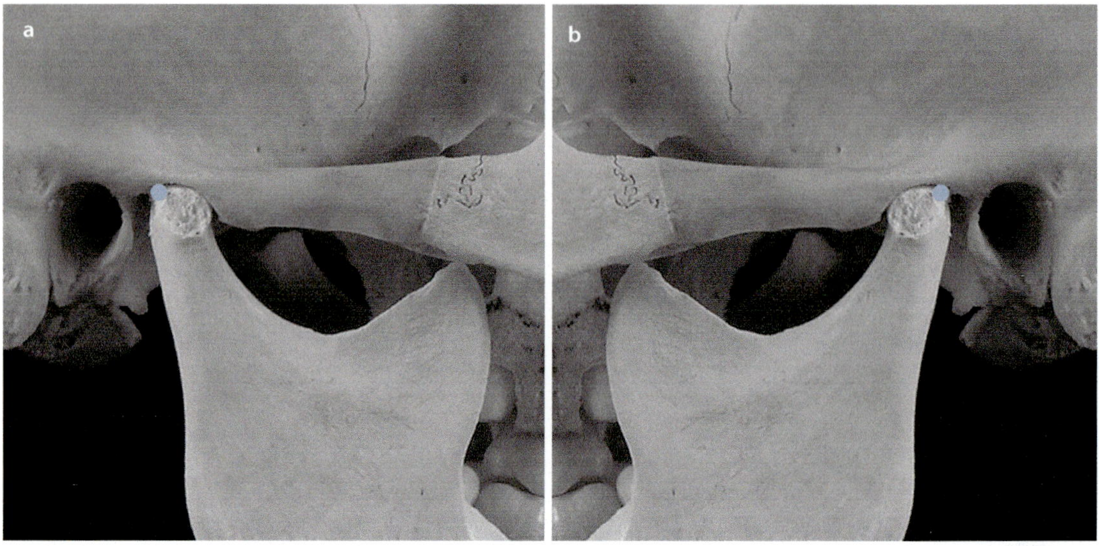

Fig. 2.142 *Condylion*$_r$ (**a**) and *Condylion*$_l$ (**b**). Profile views (cadaver skull)

Virtual definition of the *Condylion* (Co) landmark

Step 1: Define *Condylion*$_r$ and *Condylion*$_l$ on the right (Fig. 2.143a) and left (Fig. 2.144a) profile views of the 3D hard tissue surface representations.

Step 2: Verify and eventually correct the *Condylion*$_r$ and *Condylion*$_l$ landmarks on the sagittal reslices (Figs. 2.143b and 2.144b).

Condylion (Co_r-Co_l)

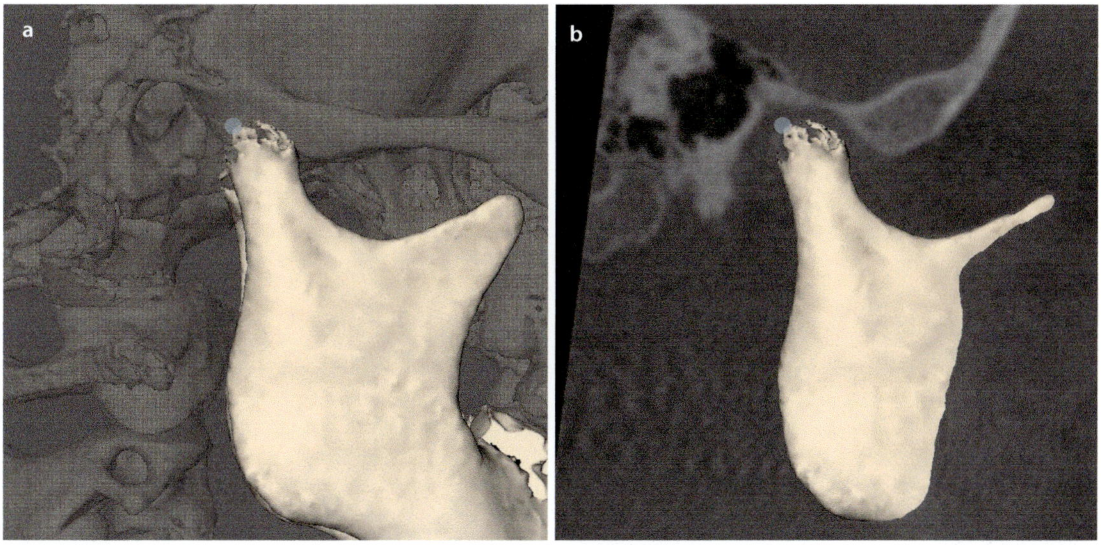

Fig. 2.143 *Condylion$_r$*. Profile view right (**a**) and superimposed sagittal reslice (**b**) of the 3D "surface-rendered" hard tissue representation of the patient's head (i-CAT, Imaging Sciences International Inc, Maxilim v. 2.3.0.3., patient V.E.W.)

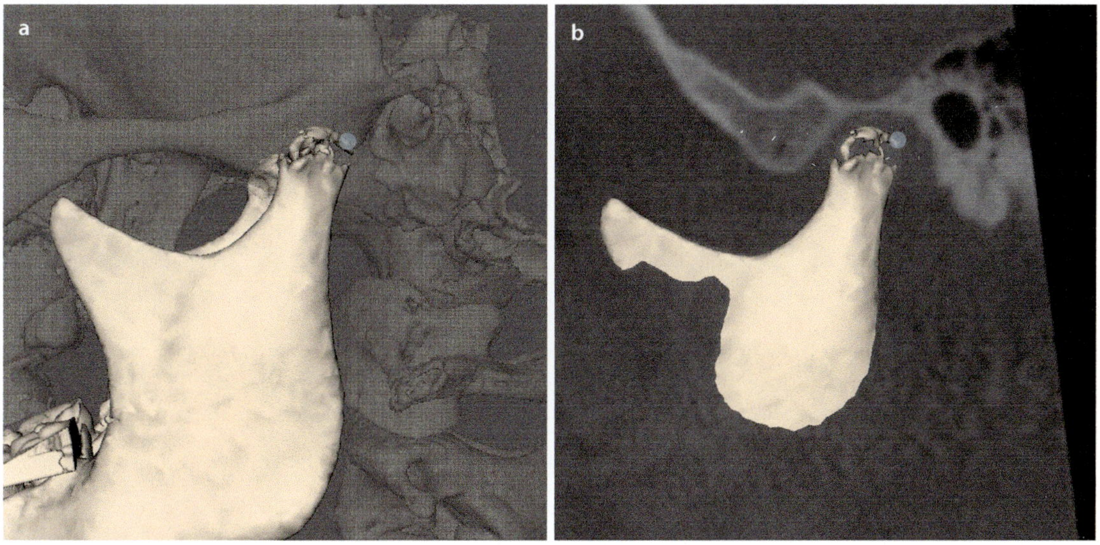

Fig. 2.144 *Condylion$_l$*. Profile view left (**a**) and superimposed sagittal reslice (**b**) of the 3D "surface-rendered" hard tissue representation of the patient's head (i-CAT, Imaging Sciences International Inc, Maxilim v. 2.3.0.3., patient V.E.W.)

Condylion (Co_r-Co_l)

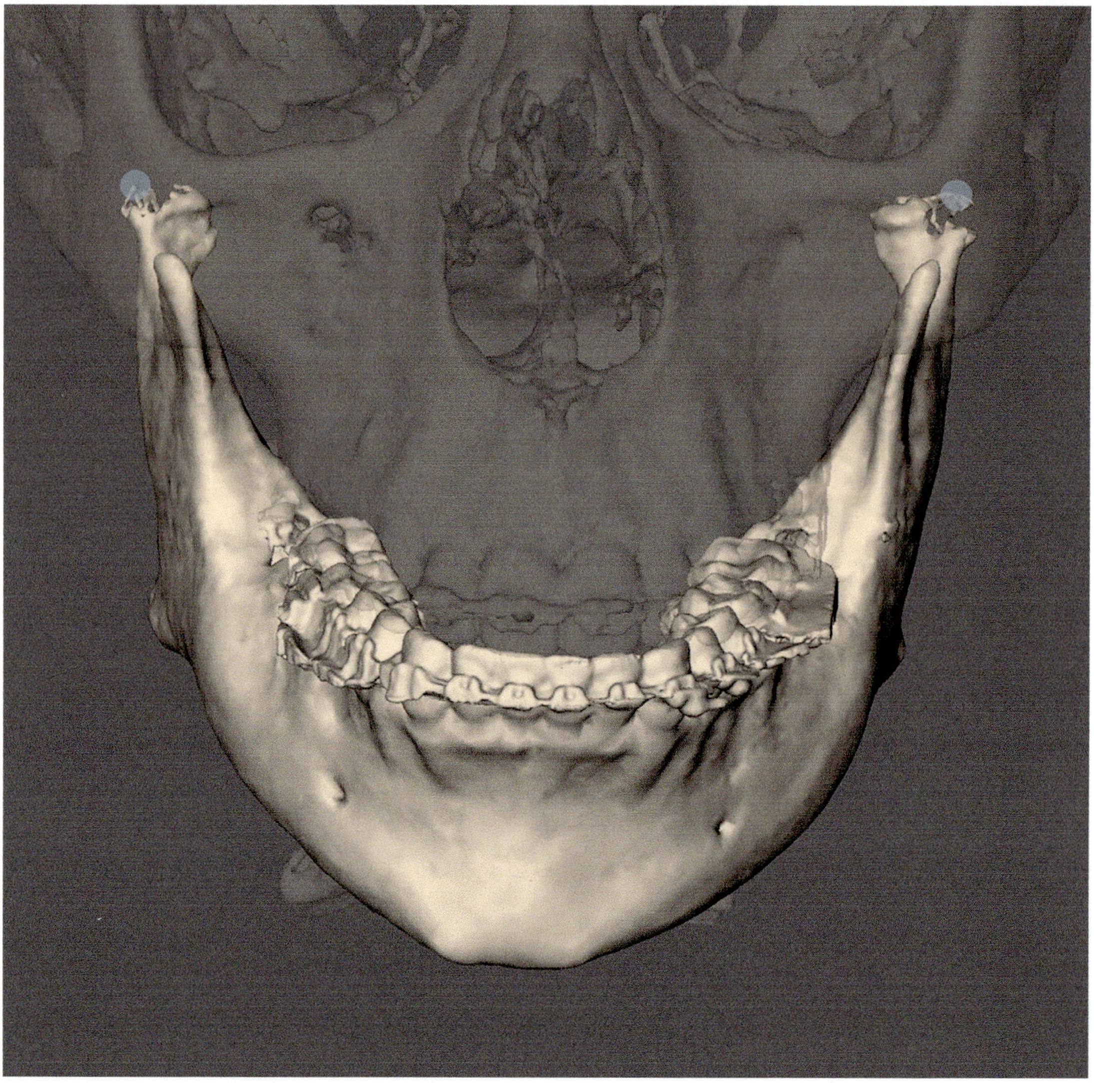

Fig. 2.145 *Condylion*$_r$ and *Condylion*$_l$. Frontal view of the 3D "surface-rendered" hard tissue representation of the patient's head (i-CAT, Imaging Sciences International Inc, Maxilim v. 2.3.0.3., patient V.E.W.)

Set-Up of 3D Cephalometric Hard Tissue and Teeth Landmarks

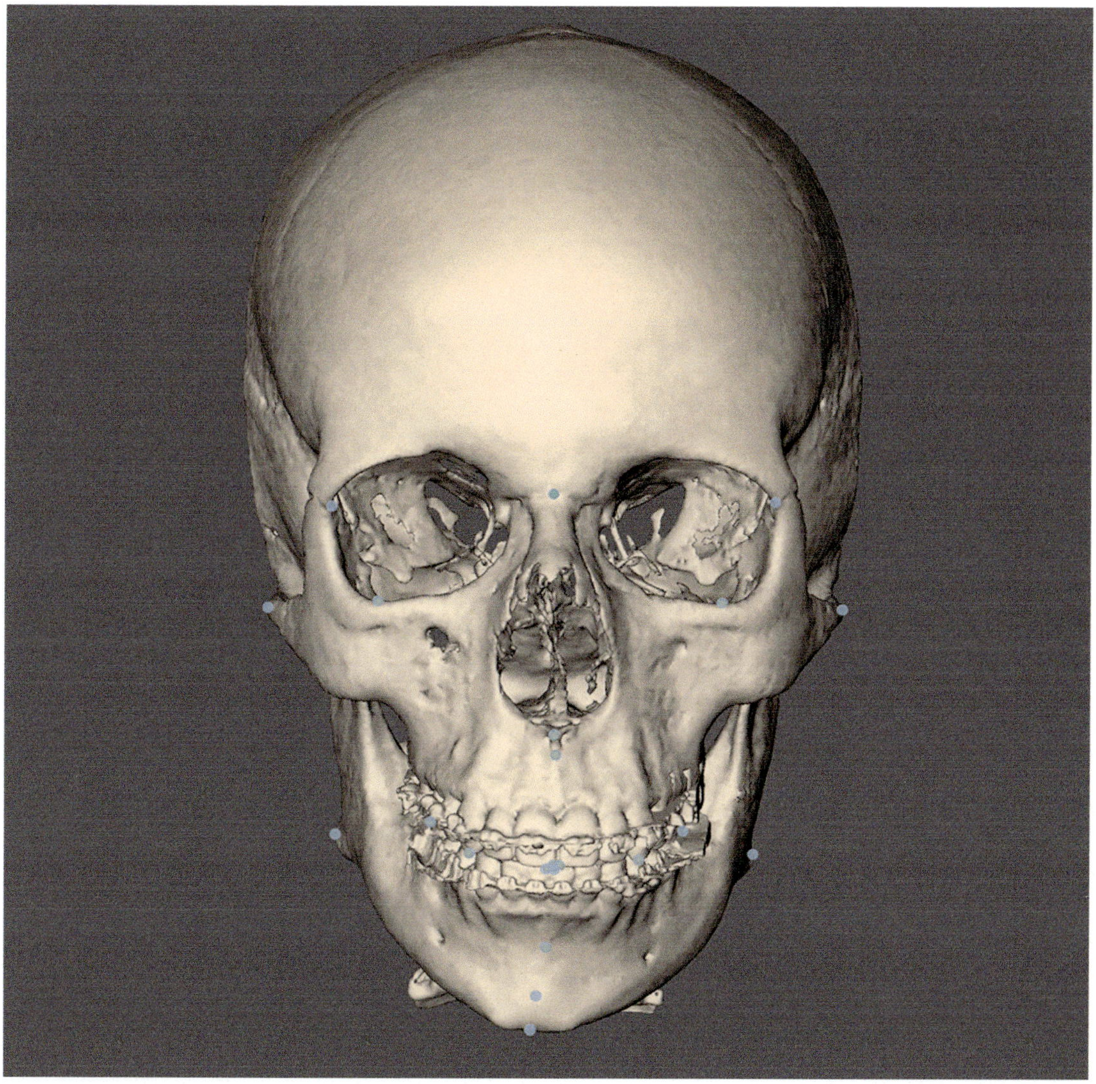

Fig. 2.146 Frontal view. Set-up of 3D cephalometric hard tissue and teeth landmarks. 3D "surface-rendered" hard tissue representation of the patient's head (i-CAT, Imaging Sciences International Inc, Maxilim v. 2.3.0.3., patient V.E.W.)

Set-Up of 3D Cephalometric Hard Tissue and Teeth Landmarks

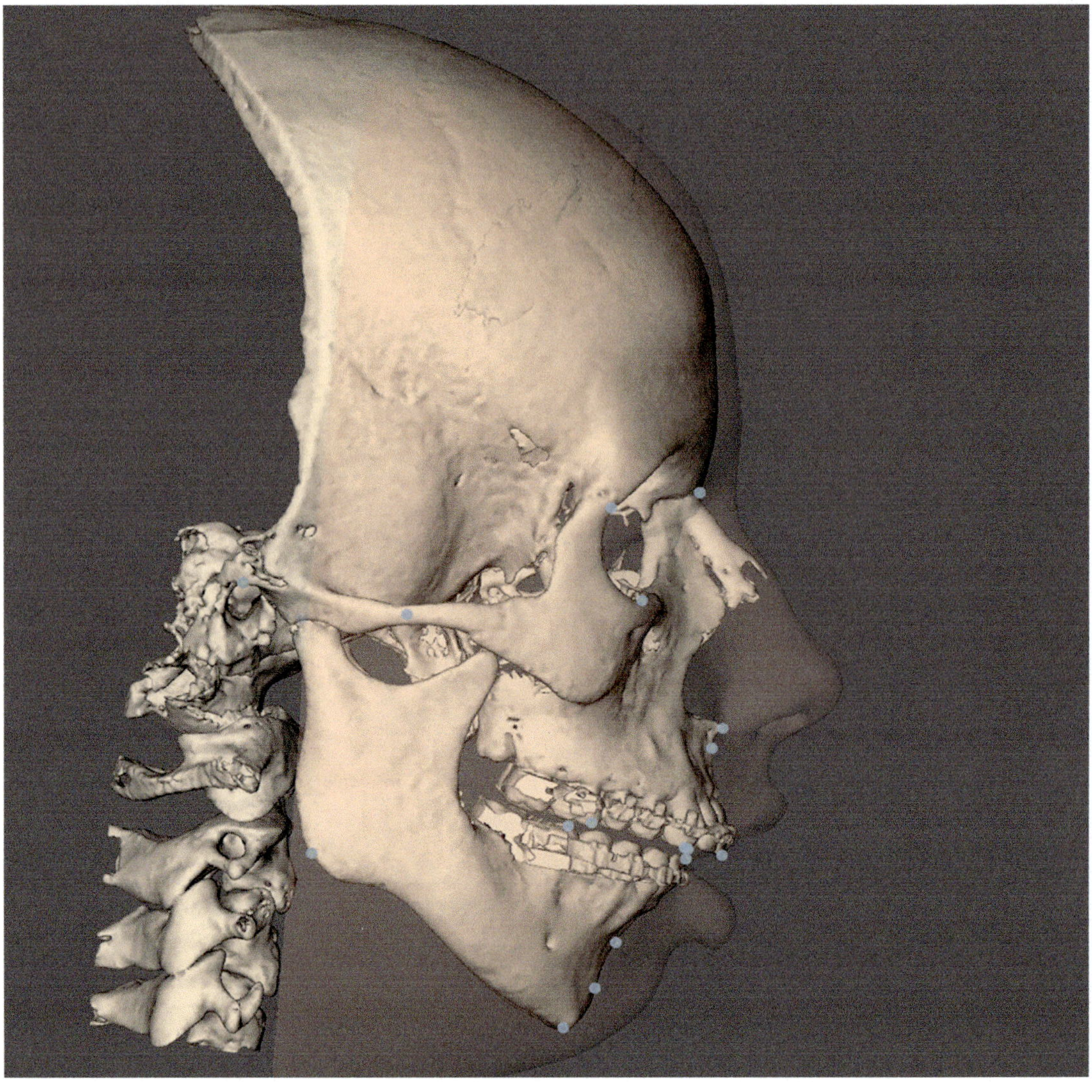

Fig. 2.147 Profile right view. Set-up of 3D cephalometric hard tissue and teeth landmarks. 3D "surface-rendered" hard tissue representation of the patient's head with transparent soft tissues (i-CAT, Imaging Sciences International Inc, Maxilim v. 2.3.0.3., patient V.E.W.)

Set-Up of 3D Cephalometric Hard Tissue and Teeth Landmarks

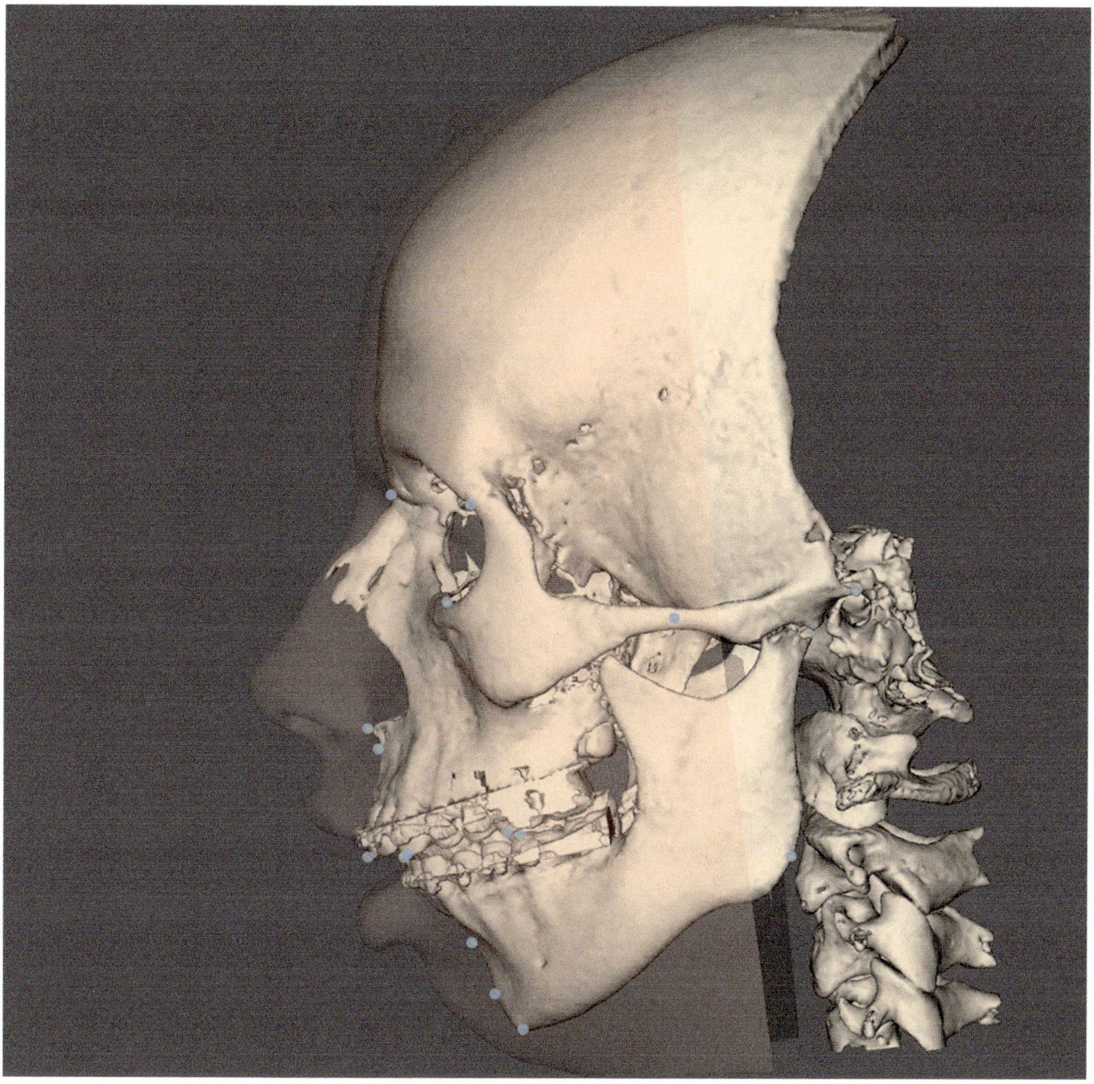

Fig. 2.148 Profile left view. Set-up of 3D cephalometric hard tissue and teeth landmarks. 3D "surface-rendered" hard tissue representation of the patient's head with transparent soft tissues (i-CAT, Imaging Sciences International Inc, Maxilim v. 2.3.0.3., patient V.E.W.)

Set-Up of 3D Cephalometric Hard Tissue and Teeth Landmarks

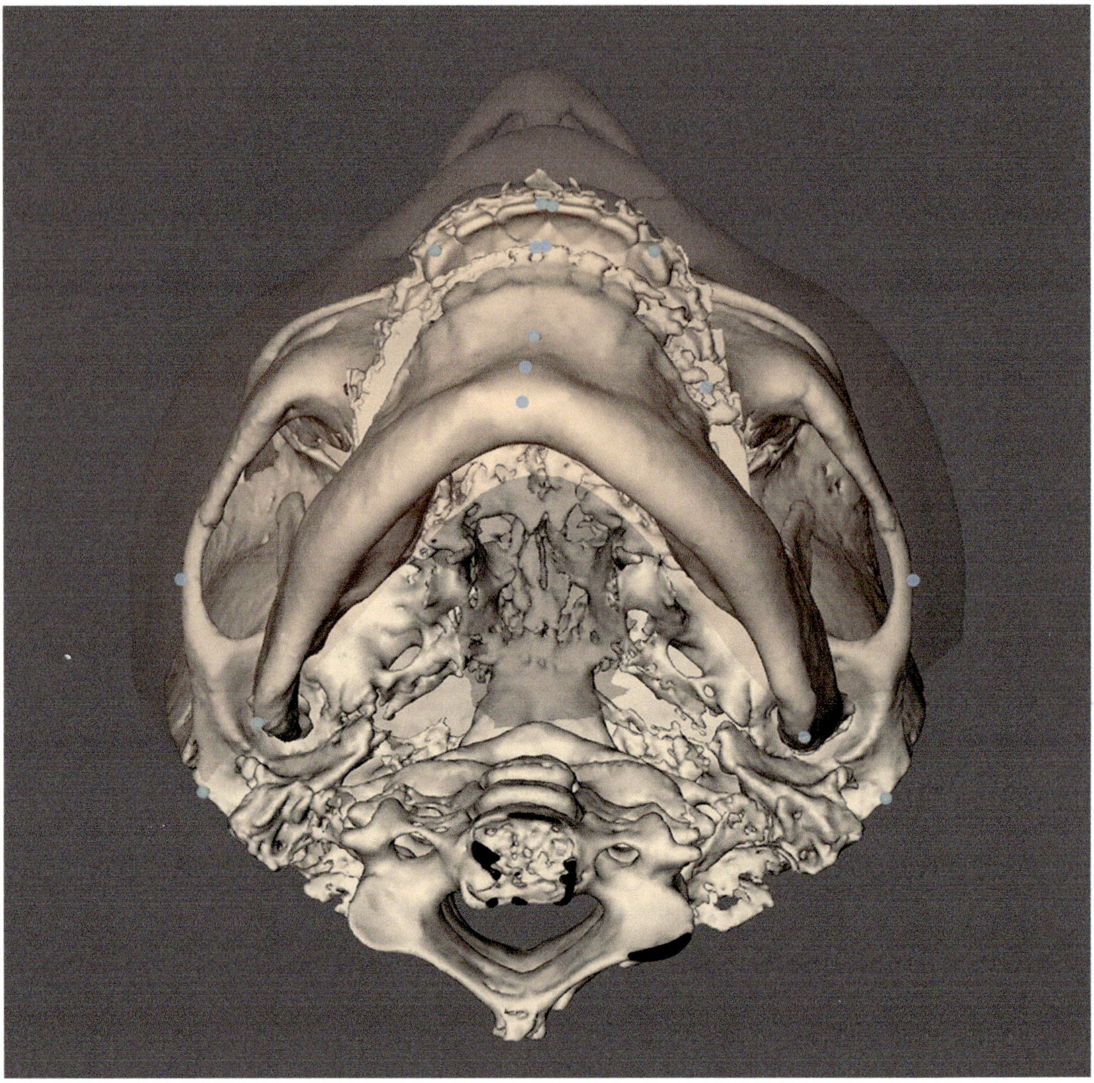

Fig. 2.149 Base view. Set-up of 3D cephalometric hard tissue and teeth landmarks. 3D "surface-rendered" hard tissue representation with transparent soft tissues of the patient's head (i-CAT, Imaging Sciences International Inc, Maxilim v. 2.3.0.3., patient V.E.W.)

Additional 3D Cephalometric Hard Tissue Landmarks

The following list provides other conventional cephalometric hard tissue landmarks described in the literature that could be implemented in 3D cephalometric analysis.

- *Antegonion.* The highest point of the notch or concavity of the lower border of the vertical mandibular ramus where it joins the body of the mandible
- *Articulare acc. to Bjork.* The intersection of the posterior border of the vertical mandibular ramus and the outer margin of the cranial base
- *Articulare acc. to Bolton.* The intersection of the posterior border of the condyle of the mandible with the Bolton plane (line joining the Bolton point and Nasion landmark on the lateral cephalogram)
- *Bolton point.* A point in space about the centre of the foramen magnum that is located on the lateral cephalogram by the highest point in the profile image of the postcondylare notches of the occipital bone
- *Bregma.* The crossing of the coronal and sagittal sutures on top of the skull
- *Coronoid Process.* The most superior point of the coronoid process
- *Dacryon.* Point on the inner wall of the orbit at the junction of the nasal process of the frontal bone, the frontal process of the maxilla and the lacrimal bone
- *Frontomaxillary Nasal Suture.* The junction of the frontal, maxillary and nasal bones

> The clinician (orthodontist or surgeon) can always modify, as shown in this chapter, his proper clinical routine 2D cephalometric landmarks towards 3D cephalometric landmarks or even create new 3D cephalometric landmarks.

Additional 3D Cephalometric Hard Tissue Landmarks

- *Frontotemporale.* Point near the root of the zygomatic process of the frontal bone at the most anterior point along the curvature of the temporal line
- *Glabella.* The most anterior point of the frontal bone
- *Gnathion.* The most anterior and inferior point on the contour of the mandibular symphysis
- *Infradentale.* The anterior superior point on the mandible at its labial contact between the mandibular central incisors
- *Inferior Zygoma.* The lowest point of the outline of each zygoma
- *O-Point.* The centre for convergence area of horizontal planes used in the Sassouni's analysis
- *Opisthion.* The posterior midsagittal point on the posterior margin of the foramen magnum
- *Prosthion.* The lowest, most anterior point on the alveolar portion of the premaxilla, in the median plane, between the upper central incisors
- *Sellion acc. to A.M. Schwarz.* The midpoint of the entrance of the sella turcica
- *Sphenoethmoidal Suture.* The most superior point of the sphenoethmoidal suture
- *Spheno-Occipital Synchondrosis.* The most superior point of the junction between the sphenoid and occipital bones
- *Staphylion.* Point in the medial line (interpalatal suture) of the posterior part of the hard palate where it is crossed by a line drawn tangent to the curves of the posterior margins of the palate
- *Supradentale.* The anterior inferior point on the maxilla at its labial contact between the lower central incisors
- *Supraorbitale.* The most superior point of the superior orbital rim
- *Temporale.* Point at the intersection of the shadows of the ethmoid and the anterior wall of the infratemporal fossa
- *Vertex.* The most superior point on the cranial vault

Set-Up of 3D Cephalometric Planes

After standardised 3D virtual definition of 3D cephalometric hard tissue and teeth landmarks, the "3D Virtual Scene Approach" allows to set-up different types of 3D cephalometric hard, soft tissue and teeth related planes in the "3D virtual scene" (Figs. 2.150, 2.151 and 2.152).

In 2005, Swennen described the generation of several types of 3D cephalometric planes that can automatically be computed based on one or several 3D cephalometric hard tissue, teeth and soft tissue (► see also Sect. 2.2.3) landmarks.

The following types of "3D cephalometric planes" can be set-up in the "3D virtual scene":

1. A 3D cephalometric plane computed from *one* 3D cephalometric landmark is defined by a plane that passes one landmark and that is parallel to one of the 3D cephalometric reference planes (*e.g. true vertical plane (TV-Pl),* ► see also Chap. 3).
2. A 3D cephalometric plane computed from *two* 3D cephalometric landmarks is defined by a plane that passes two landmarks and that is perpendicular to one of the 3D cephalometric reference planes (*e.g. ideal target lip profile plane (ITLP-Pl)*).
3. A 3D cephalometric plane computed from *three* 3D cephalometric landmarks is defined by a plane that passes three landmarks (*e.g. mandibular plane (Md-Pl)*).
4. A 3D cephalometric plane computed from *four* 3D cephalometric landmarks is defined by a plane that passes two landmarks and the mean of two other landmarks (*e.g. Frankfort horizontal plane (FH-Pl)*)
5. A 3D cephalometric plane computed from *more than four* 3D cephalometric landmarks is defined by a plane that passes the means of different pairs of landmarks (e.g. *upper occlusal plane (Uoccl-Pl) or maxillary occlusal plane (Mx-Occ-Pl)*)

The clinician (orthodontist or surgeon) can modify his proper clinical routine 2D cephalometric lines towards 3D cephalometric planes or create new 3D cephalometric planes.

Set-Up of 3D Cephalometric Planes

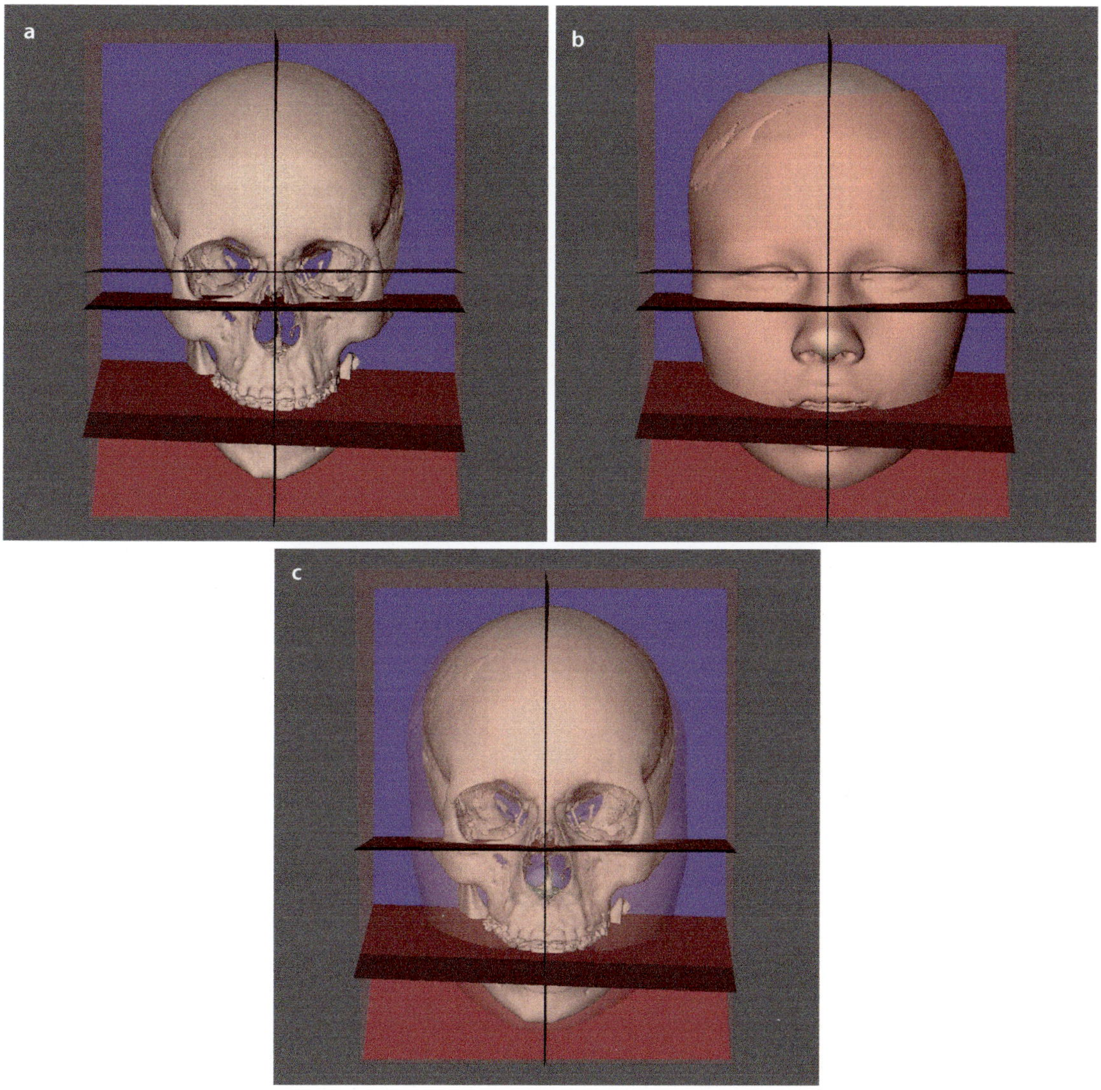

Fig. 2.150 Frontal views. Set-up of the true vertical plane (*TV-Pl*), ideal target lip profile plane (*ITLP-Pl*), mandibular plane (*Md-Pl*), Frankfort horizontal plane (*FH-Pl*) and upper occlusal plane (*Uoccl-Pl*) in conjunction with the "PHP 3D Cephalometric Reference Frame". 3D "surface-rendered" hard tissue representation (**a**) of the patient's head with soft tissues (**b**) and transparent soft tissues (**c**) (i-CAT, Imaging Sciences International Inc, Maxilim v. 2.3.0.3., patient V.E.W.)

Set-Up of 3D Cephalometric Planes

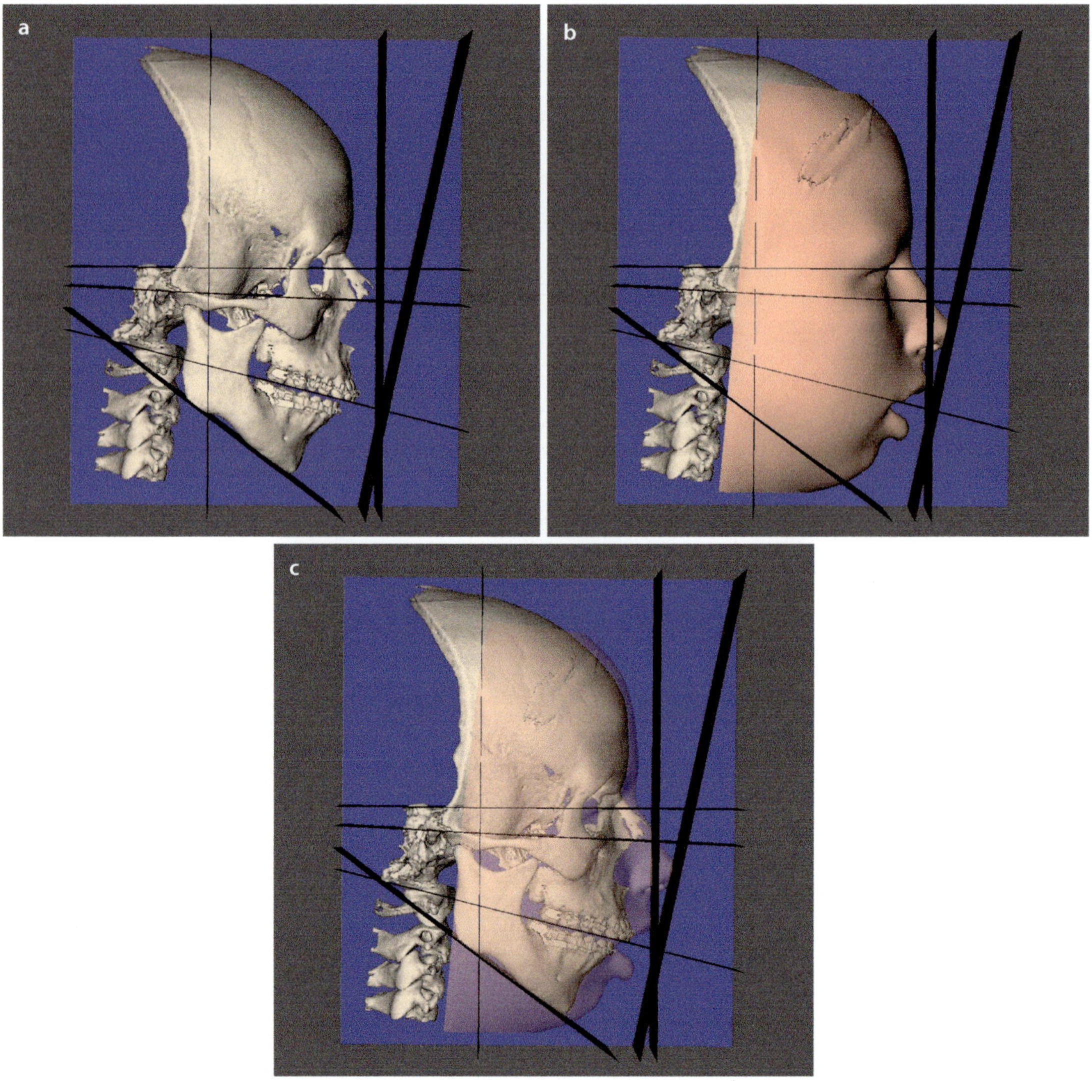

Fig. 2.151 Profile right views. Set-up of the true vertical plane (*TV-Pl*), ideal target lip profile plane (*ITLP-Pl*), mandibular plane (*Md-Pl*), Frankfort horizontal plane (*FH-Pl*) and upper occlusal plane (*Uoccl-Pl*) in conjunction with the "PHP 3D cephalometric reference frame". 3D "surface-rendered" hard tissue representation (**a**) of the patient's head with soft tissues (**b**) and transparent soft tissues (**c**) (i-CAT, Imaging Sciences International Inc, Maxilim v. 2.3.0.3., patient V.E.W.)

Set-Up of 3D Cephalometric Planes

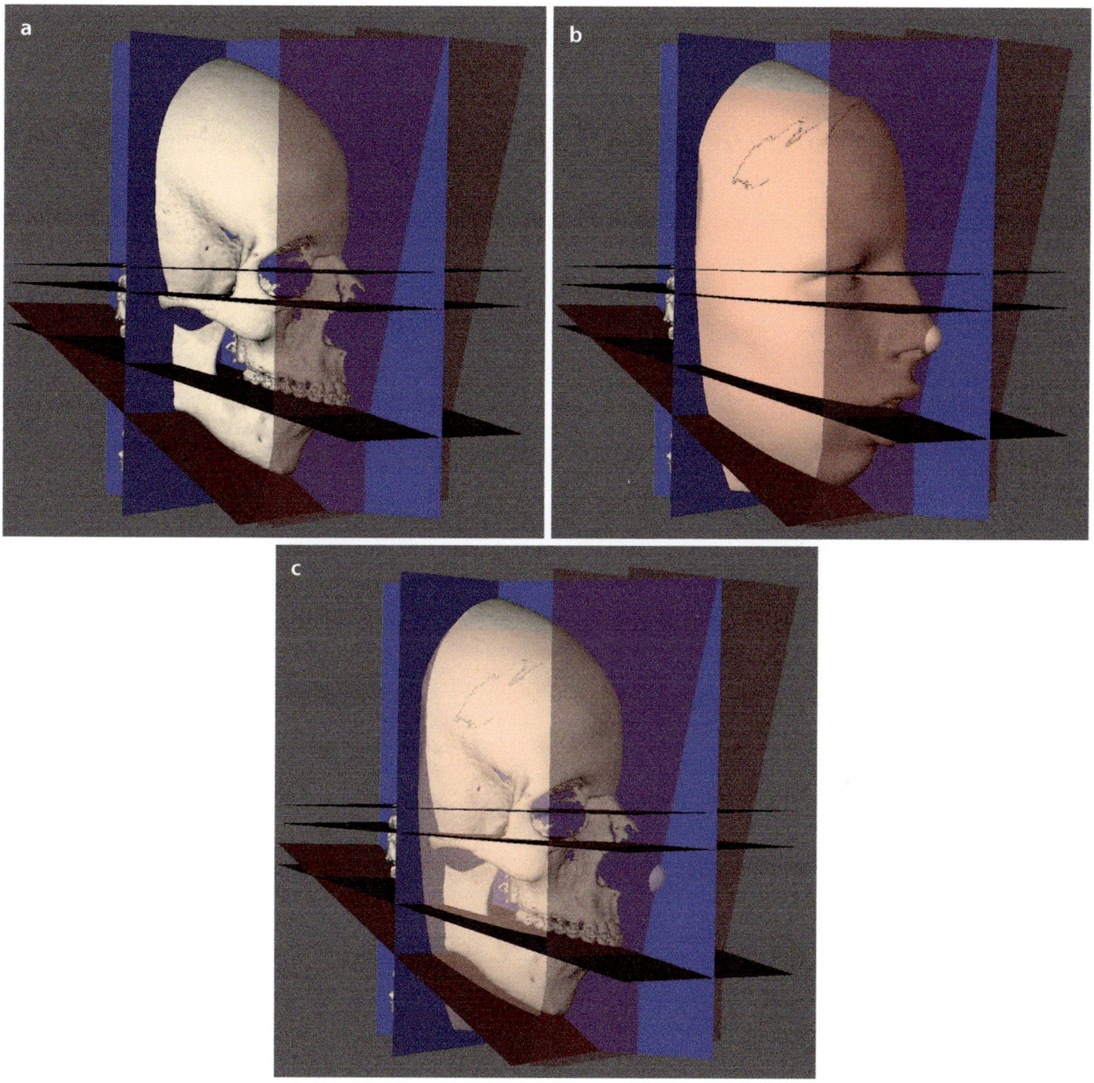

Fig. 2.152 2/3 Profile right views. Set-up of the true vertical plane (*TV-Pl*), ideal target lip profile plane (*ITLP-Pl*), mandibular plane (*Md-Pl*), Frankfort horizontal plane (*FH-Pl*) and upper occlusal plane (*Uoccl-Pl*) in conjunction with the "PHP 3D cephalometric reference frame". 3D "surface-rendered" hard tissue representation (**a**) of the patient's head with soft tissues (**b**) and transparent soft tissues (**c**) (i-CAT, Imaging Sciences International Inc, Maxilim v. 2.3.0.3., patient V.E.W.)

3D Cephalometric Analysis of the Patient

After generation of a 3D cephalometric reference frame, standardised 3D virtual definition of 3D cephalometric hard, soft tissue and teeth landmarks and set-up of 3D cephalometric planes, the following different types of "3D cephalometric hard, soft and teeth measurements" can be automatically computed in the "3D virtual scene":

1. Linear 3D measurements
2. Angular 3D measurements
3. Orthognonal 3D measurements
4. Proportional correlation 3D measurements

1. *Linear measurements*

- *Linear projective measurements* are measurements between two 3D cephalometric landmarks that are projected on one of the 3D cephalometric reference planes and are expressed in millimetres (mm):
  - *Linear projective width measurements* are horizontal measurements between two 3D cephalometric landmarks projected parallel to the median (z) and horizontal (x) plane on the vertical (y) plane.
  - *Linear projective height measurements* are vertical measurements between two 3D cephalometric landmarks projected parallel to the horizontal (x) and vertical (y) plane on the median (z) plane.
  - *Linear projective depth measurements* are sagittal projective measurements between two 3D cephalometric landmarks projected parallel to the horizontal (x) and vertical (y) plane on the median (z) plane.
- *3D distances* are direct linear measurements between two 3D cephalometric landmarks and are expressed in millimetres (mm).

2. *Angular measurements*
   - *Angular projective measurements (I)* are measurements between three or four 3D cephalometric landmarks that are projected on one of the 3D cephalometric reference planes and are expressed in degrees (°).
   - *Angular projective measurements (II)* are measurements between two 3D cephalometric landmarks and a 3D cephalometric reference plane projected on one of the 3D cephalometric reference planes and are expressed in degrees (°).
   - *Angular projective measurements (III)* are measurements between two 3D cephalometric planes projected on one of the 3D cephalometric reference planes and are expressed in degrees (°).
3. *Orthogonal measurements* are perpendicular measurements of the various 3D cephalometric landmarks to each of the 3D cephalometric reference planes and are expressed in millimetres (mm).
4. *Proportional correlation measurements* are ratio's between two 3D cephalometric measurements and are expressed in percentages (%).

The "Bruges Target Facial Mask" 3D cephalometric analysis is used in this section as an example to illustrate this transition ("making the bridge") of 2D cephalometric towards 3D cephalometric analysis.

"Bruges Target Facial Mask" 3D Cephalometric Analysis

The "Bruges Target Facial Mask" 3D cephalometric analysis is based on the conventional "Bruges Target Profile" 2D cephalometric analysis that has been clinically used in the department of OMF in Bruges for more than 25 years.

The "Bruges Target Facial Mask" 3D cephalometric analysis consists of:

1. Virtual definition of the "natural head position (NHP)" of the patient (► see also Sect. 3.1)
2. Generation of a "3D cephalometric reference frame" (► see also Sect. 2.2.1)
3. Virtual definition of 11 hard tissue, nine soft tissue and 12 dental 3D cephalometric landmarks
4. Automated calculation of six linear, ten angular, two proportional and 18 orthogonal 3D cephalometric hard and soft tissue measurements

A prospective ($n=350$) study in non-segmental cases (Swennen 2014) showed that the "Bruges Target Facial Mask" 3D cephalometric analysis (3D-VPS$_1$) could be performed in a more than acceptable time frame.

	Mean (min:s)	Range (min:s)
BSSO ($n=90$)	7:28	6:52 – 8:10
BSSO and chin ($n=18$)	7:23	6:48 – 8:04
Le Fort I and BSSO ($n=163$)	7:33	6:58 – 8:22
Le Fort I, BSSO and chin ($n=79$)	7:37	6:59 – 8:31

Case 1

(Patient V.E.W.) is used to demonstrate 3D-VPS$_1$ by means of the "Bruges Target Facial Mask" 3D cephalometric analysis (◘ Figs. 2.153 and 2.154).

"Bruges Target Facial Mask" 3D Cephalometric Analysis

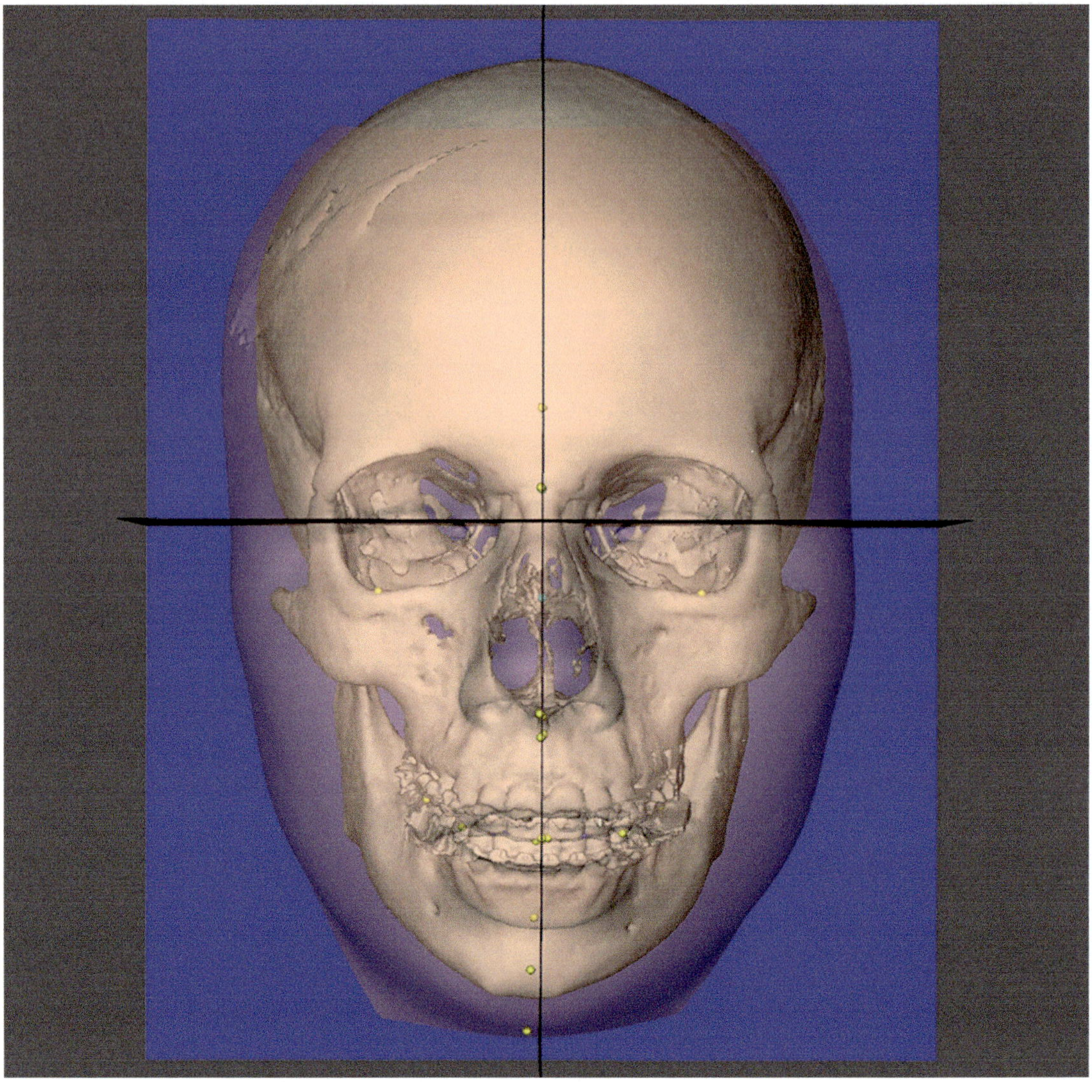

Fig. 2.153 Frontal view. Set-up of 3D cephalometric landmarks of the "Bruges Target Facial Mask" 3D cephalometric analysis. 3D "surface-rendered" hard tissue representation with transparent soft tissues of the patient's head (i-CAT, Imaging Sciences International Inc, Maxilim v. 2.3.0.3., patient V.E.W.)

"Bruges Target Facial Mask" 3D Cephalometric Analysis

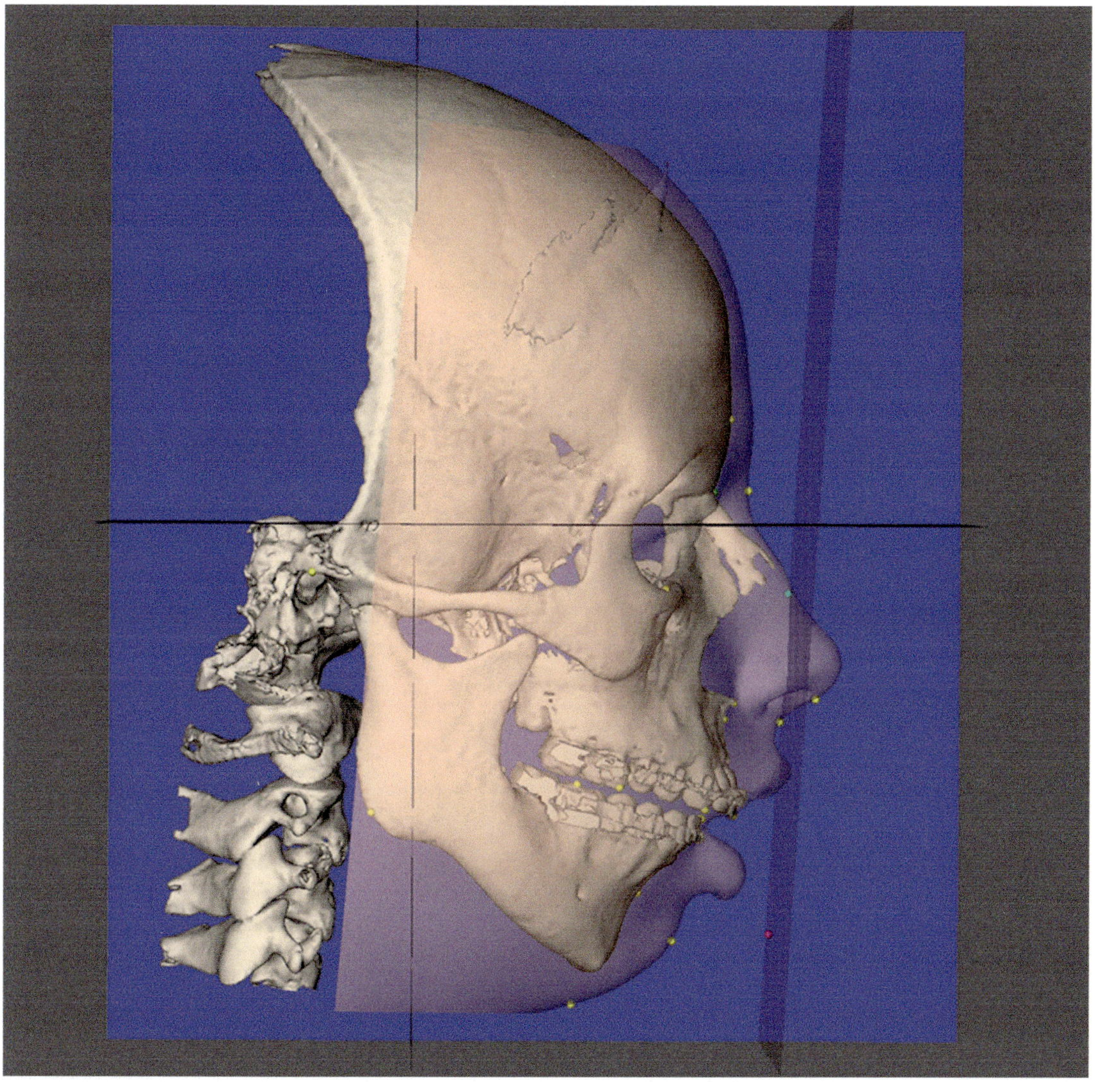

Fig. 2.154 Profile right view. Set-up of 3D cephalometric landmarks of the "Bruges Target Facial Mask" 3D cephalometric analysis. 3D "surface-rendered" hard tissue representation with transparent soft tissues of the patient's head (i-CAT, Imaging Sciences International Inc, Maxilim v. 2.3.0.3., patient V.E.W.)

"Bruges Target Facial Mask" 3D Cephalometric Analysis

3D cephalometry analysis (3D-VPS$_1$) report			
"Bruges Target Facial Mask" 3D cephalometric analysis			
Patient name: VEW			
Physician name: GS			
Linear measurement analysis (mm)			
Morphological height of the face (n-gn)	110.5		
Height of the face (gl-gn)	127.9		
Morphological height of the midface (n-sn)	53.7		
Height of the midface (gl-sn)	71.1		
Overjet	7.3		
Overbite	0.8		
Angular measurement analysis (deg)			
Upper incisor inclination (MxPl/Ulapex-UI)	119.3		
Lower incisor inclination (Md-Pl/Llapex-LI)	102.4		
Frontal inclination of the upper occlusal plane – x-Pl	2.1		
Frontal inclination of the lower occlusal plane – x-Pl	2.3		
Frontal inclination of the mandibular plane – x-Pl	1.5		
Lateral inclination of the upper occlusal plane – x-Pl	13.9		
Lateral inclination of the lower occlusal plane – x-Pl	15.6		
Lateral inclination of the mandibular plane – x-Pl	37.0		
Set- up of Bruges ideal target profile plane	88.0		
Set-up of Bruges ideal target lip profile plane	–		
Proportional measurement analysis (%)			
Morphological height of the midface/morphological height of the face (n-sn x 100/n-gn)	48.6		
Height of the midface/height of the face (gl-sn x 100/gl-gn)	55.6		
Orthogonal measurement analysis (mm)	x-Pl	y-Pl	z-Pl
UI_r	68.0	73.3	01.0
UI_l	68.0	73.3	-01.0
UC_r	65.9	66.1	16.8
UC_l	67.1	66.0	-17.3
$UMcusp_r$	60.5	46.6	24.6
$UMcusp_l$	61.8	44.6	-25.9

x-Pl horizontal plane, *y-Pl* vertical plane, *z-Pl* median plane

See Video 2.1.

2.2.3 3D Cephalometry of the Patient's Soft Tissues (3D-VPS_2)

"3D cephalometry of the patient's soft tissues (3D-VPS_2)" can be compared with direct anthropometric or indirect anthropometric (photogrammetric) assessment of the patient's face in conventional treatment planning.

Anthropometry of the head and face has been extensively developed and popularised by Farkas (1994). In 2005, Swennen introduced a "3D Virtual Scene Approach" towards "3D cephalometry of the soft tissues" based on the pioneering work of Farkas.

As for 3D cephalometry of the patient's hard tissues and teeth (3D-VPS_1) (► see also Sect. 2.2.2), the authors do not intend to promote a specific 3D cephalometric analysis of the patient's soft tissues (3D-VPS_2) but to provide:

1. "Step-by-step" 3D virtual definition of common 3D soft tissue cephalometric landmarks (◘ Figs. 2.211, 2.212 and 2.213)
2. The "Bruges Soft Tissue 3D Cephalometric Analysis" as an example

The principles of setting up 3D cephalometric soft tissue planes and creating 3D cephalometric measurements are the same as for (3D-VPS_1) and clearly outlined in Sect. 2.2.2.

This section will focus on "step-by-step" guidelines for precise and reliable definition of 3D cephalometric soft tissue landmarks and finally demonstrate 3D-VPS_2 by means of the "Bruges 3D Soft Tissue Cephalometric Analysis", illustrated on Case 1 (Patient V.E.W.), which is used throughout this book (► Chaps. 1, 3, 4, 5, and 6).

■ glabella (g)

Definition of glabella (g)

"*glabella* (*g*)" is the most anterior midpoint on the fronto-orbital soft tissue contour. In 3D cephalometry, this is a well-defined soft tissue landmark and is therefore not the same as the anthropometric "*Glabella* (*g*)" landmark acc. to *L.G. Farkas*, which is identical to the bony "*glabella*" landmark on the frontal bone.

3D virtual definition of the "glabella (g)" landmark

Step 1: Define *glabella (g)* on the right profile view of the 3D soft tissue surface representation (◘ Fig. 2.155a) and verify its position on the left profile view (◘ Figs. 2.155b and 2.156).

Step 2: Verify and eventually correct the midline position of the *glabella (g)* landmark on the frontal view of the 3D soft tissue surface representation (◘ Fig. 2.157).

glabella (g)

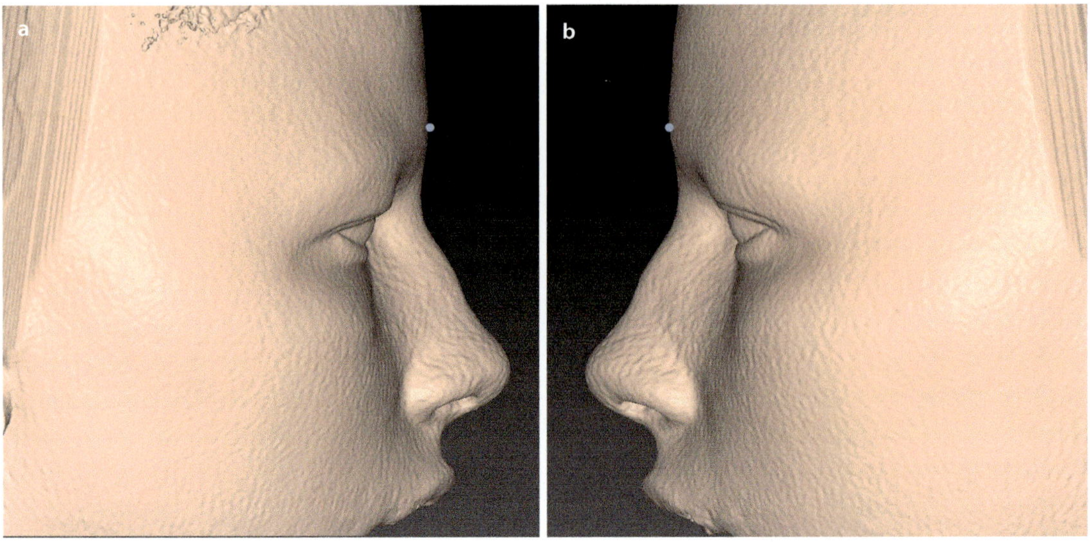

Fig. 2.155 *glabella*. Profile right (**a**) and left (**b**) views of the 3D "volume-rendered" representation of the patient's head (i-CAT, Imaging Sciences International Inc, IPS CaseDesigner ALPHA version, patient V.E.W.)

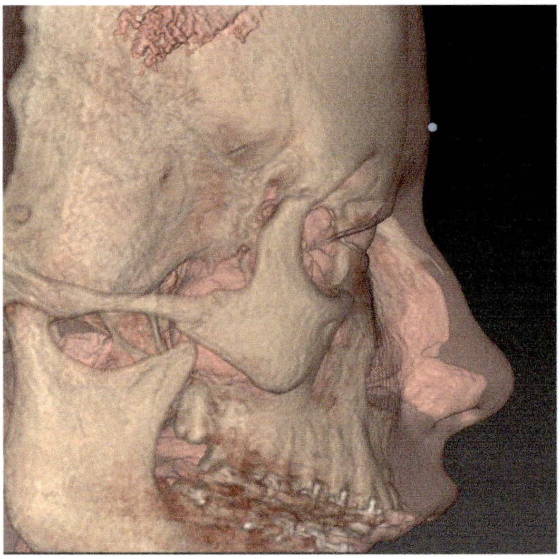

Fig. 2.156 *glabella*. Profile right view of the 3D "volume-rendered" hard and soft tissue (in transparency) representation of the patient's head (i-CAT, Imaging Sciences International Inc, IPS CaseDesigner ALPHA version, patient V.E.W.) Note that the 3D soft tissue cephalometric *glabella* landmark is located on the soft tissues and is therefore not identical to the anthropometric *glabella* landmark which is the same as the bony Glabella landmark

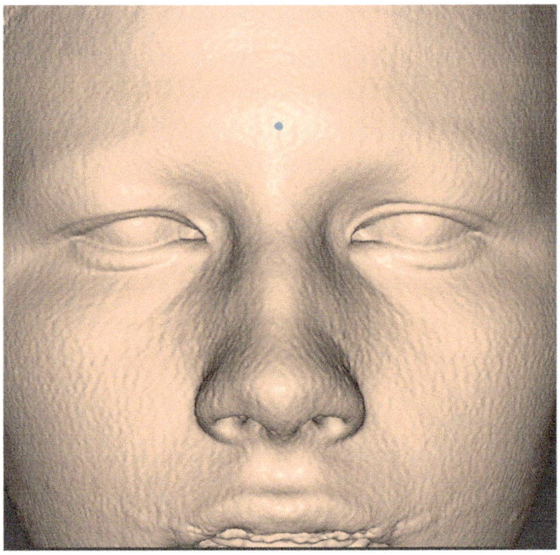

Fig. 2.157 *glabella*. Frontal view of the 3D "volume-rendered" representation of the patient's head (i-CAT, Imaging Sciences International Inc, IPS CaseDesigner ALPHA version, patient V.E.W.)

soft tissue nasion (n)

Definition of soft tissue nasion (n)

"*soft tissue nasion (n)*" is the midpoint on the soft tissue contour of the base of the nasal root, at the level of the frontonasal suture. In 3D cephalometry, this is a well-defined soft tissue landmark and is therefore not the same as the anthropometric soft nasion (n) landmark acc. to *L.G. Farkas*, which is identical to the bony "Nasion".

3D virtual definition of the "soft tissue nasion (n)" landmark

Step 1: Define *soft tissue nasion (n)* on the right profile view of the 3D transparent soft tissue surface representation (Fig. 2.158).

Step 2: Visualise the position of the *soft tissue nasion (n)* on the right (Fig. 2.159a) and left (Fig. 2.159b) profile view of the 3D soft tissue surface representation.

Step 3: Verify and eventually correct the midline position of the *soft tissue nasion (n)* landmark on the frontal view of the 3D soft tissue surface representation (Fig. 2.160).

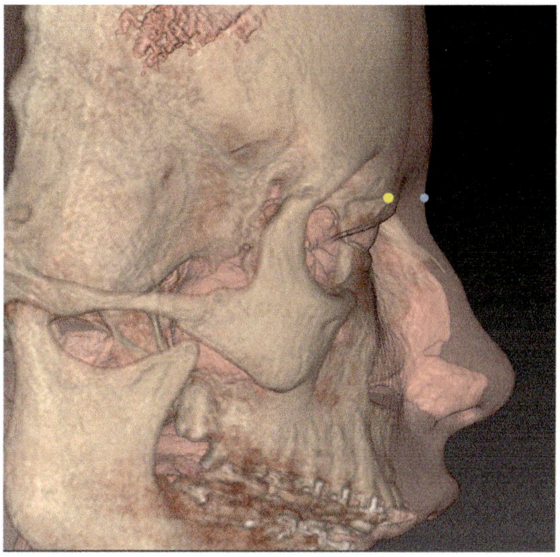

Fig. 2.158 *soft tissue nasion*. Profile right view of the 3D "volume-rendered" hard and soft tissue (in transparency) representation of the patient's head (i-CAT, Imaging Sciences International Inc, IPS CaseDesigner ALPHA version, patient V.E.W.). Note that the 3D cephalometric *soft tissue nasion* landmark is located on the soft tissues and is therefore not identical to the anthropometric *soft nasion* landmark which is the same as the bony Nasion (yellow dot) landmark

soft tissue nasion (n)

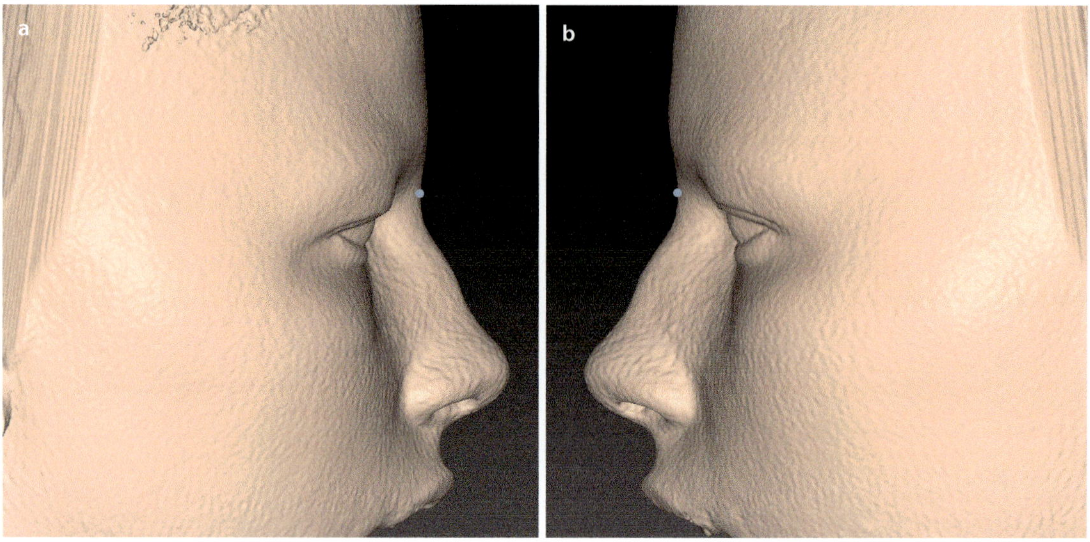

Fig. 2.159 *soft tissue nasion*. Profile right (**a**) and left (**b**) views of the 3D "volume-rendered" representation of the patient's head (i-CAT, Imaging Sciences International Inc, IPS CaseDesigner ALPHA version, patient V.E.W.)

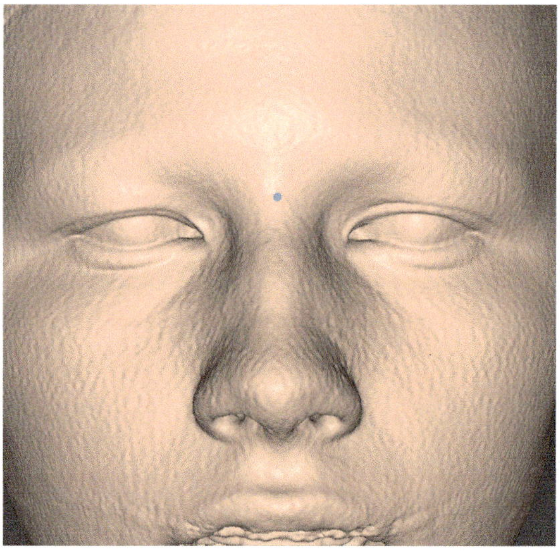

Fig. 2.160 *soft tissue nasion*. Frontal view of the 3D "volume-rendered" representation of the patient's head (i-CAT, Imaging Sciences International Inc, IPS CaseDesigner ALPHA version, patient V.E.W.)

■ sellion (se)

Definition of sellion (se)

"*sellion*" is the most posterior point of the fronto-nasal soft tissue contour in the midline of the base of the nasal root.

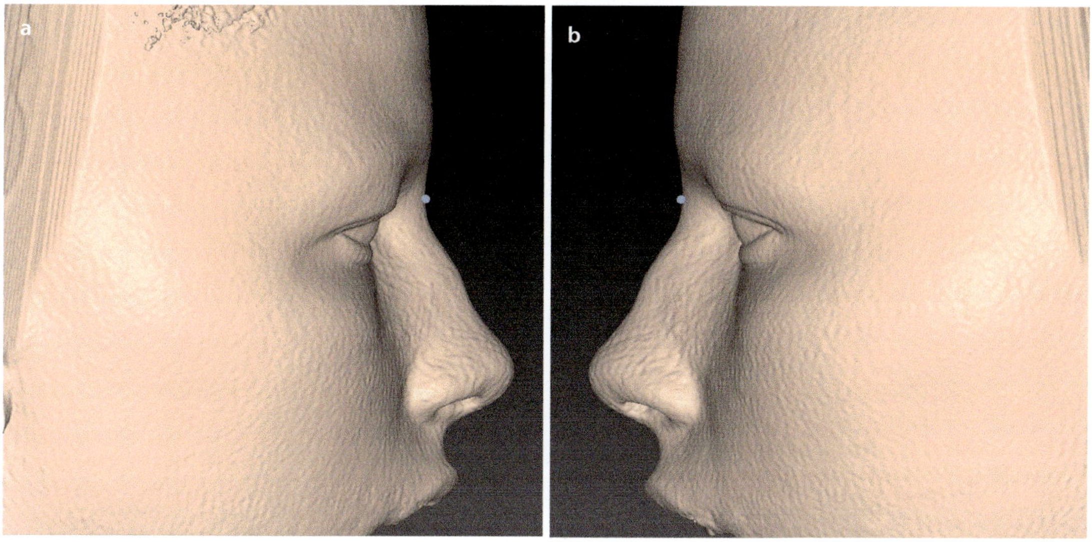

Fig. 2.161 *sellion*. Profile right (**a**) and left (**b**) views of the 3D "volume-rendered" representation of the patient's head (i-CAT, Imaging Sciences International Inc, IPS CaseDesigner ALPHA version, patient V.E.W.)

3D virtual definition of the sellion (se) landmark

Step 1: Define *sellion* (*se*) on the right profile view of the 3D soft tissue surface representation (Figs. 2.161a and 2.162) and verify its position on the left profile view (Fig. 2.161b).

Step 2: Verify and eventually correct the midline position of the *sellion* (*se*) landmark on the frontal view of the 3D soft tissue surface representation (Fig. 2.163). Note that *sellion* (*se*) is usually situated more inferiorly than *soft tissue nasion* (*n*).

sellion (se)

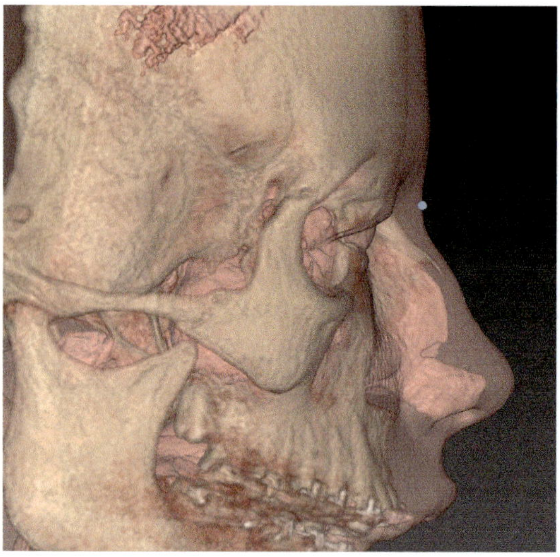

Fig. 2.162 *sellion*. Profile right view of the 3D "volume-rendered" hard and soft tissue (in transparency) representation of the patient's head (i-CAT, Imaging Sciences International Inc, IPS CaseDesigner ALPHA version, patient V.E.W.). Note that *sellion* is situated more inferiorly than *soft tissue nasion* (Fig. 2.158)

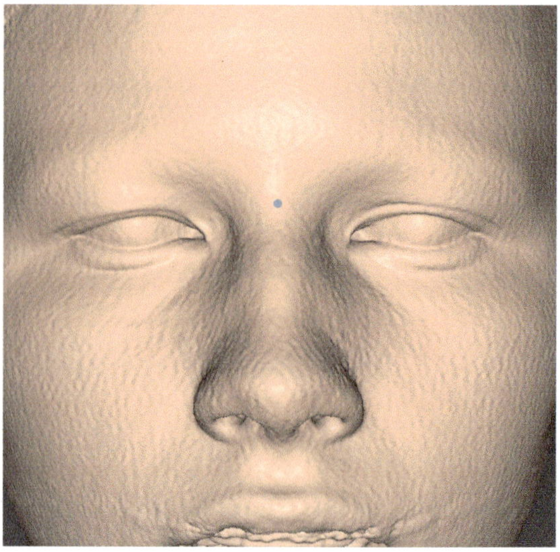

Fig. 2.163 *sellion*. Frontal view of the 3D "volume-rendered" representation of the patient's head (i-CAT, Imaging Sciences International Inc, IPS CaseDesigner ALPHA version, patient V.E.W.)

▪ endocanthion (en_r-en_l)

Definition of endocanthion (en)

"endocanthion (en)" is the soft tissue point located at the inner commissure of each eye fissure.

3D virtual definition of the endocanthion (en) landmarks

Define *endocanthion*$_r$ and *endocanthion*$_l$ on the frontal view of the 3D soft tissue surface representation (◘ Figs. 2.164 and 2.165).

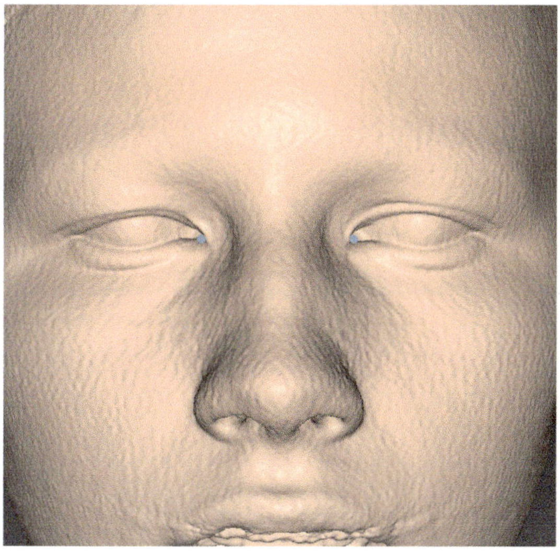

◘ **Fig. 2.164** *endocanthion*$_r$ and *endocanthion*$_l$. Frontal view of the 3D "volume-rendered" representation of the patient's head (i-CAT, Imaging Sciences International Inc, IPS CaseDesigner ALPHA version, patient V.E.W.)

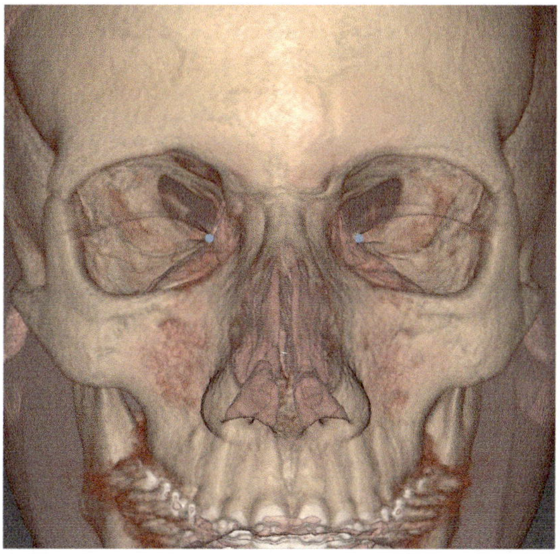

◘ **Fig. 2.165** *endocanthion*$_r$ and *endocanthion*$_l$. Frontal view of the 3D "volume-rendered" hard and soft tissue (in transparency) representation of the patient's head (i-CAT, Imaging Sciences International Inc, IPS CaseDesigner ALPHA version, patient V.E.W.). Note that the endocanthion landmarks are located laterally from the medial orbital wall

▪ exocanthion (ex_r-ex_l)

Definition of exocanthion (ex)

"exocanthion (ex)" is the soft tissue point located at the outer commissure of each eye fissure.

3D virtual definition of the exocanthion (ex) landmarks

Define *exocanthion*$_r$ and *exocanthion*$_r$ on the frontal view of the 3D soft tissue surface representation (▫ Figs. 2.166 and 2.167).

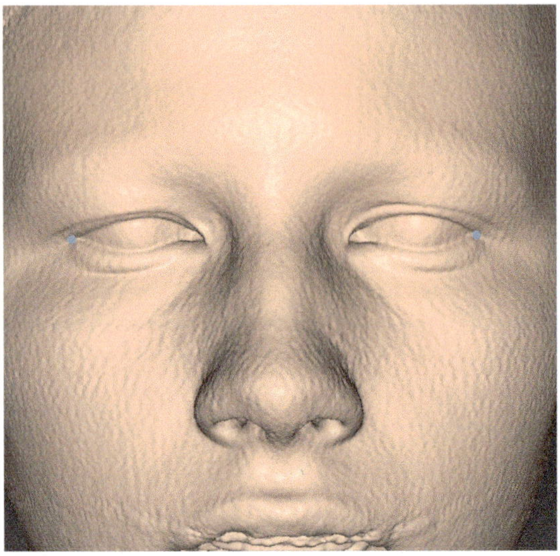

▫ **Fig. 2.166** *exocanthion*$_r$ and *exocanthion*$_r$. Frontal view of the 3D "volume-rendered" representation of the patient's head (i-CAT, Imaging Sciences International Inc, IPS CaseDesigner ALPHA version, patient V.E.W.)

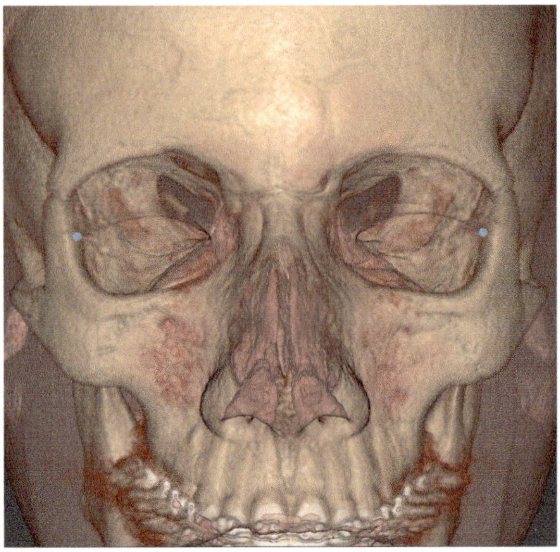

▫ **Fig. 2.167** *exocanthion*$_r$ and *exocanthion*$_r$. Frontal view of the 3D "volume-rendered" hard and soft tissue (in transparency) representation of the patient's head (i-CAT, Imaging Sciences International Inc, IPS CaseDesigner ALPHA version, patient V.E.W.). Note that although the exocanthion landmarks are most of the time located slightly medially from the lateral orbital rim, they can be projected directly on the lateral orbital rim, especially if CBCT scanning was done with closed eyes

▪ pupil (p_r-p_l)

Definition of pupil (p)

"pupil (p)" is the soft tissue point located at the centre of each bulbus.

3D virtual definition of the pupil (p) landmarks

Define *pupil$_r$* and *pupil$_l$* on the frontal view of the 3D soft tissue surface representation (Figs. 2.168 and 2.169).

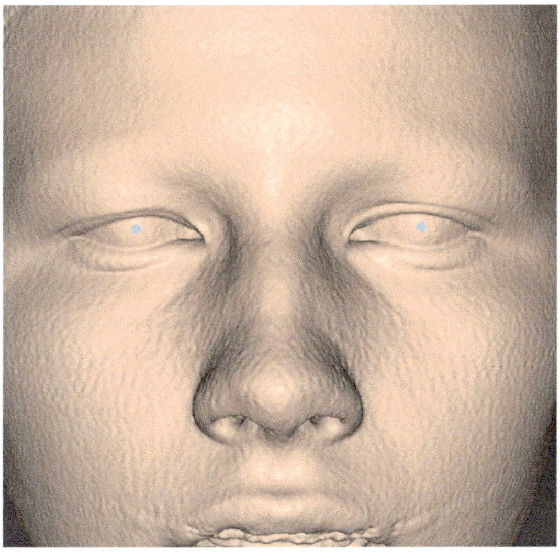

Fig. 2.168 *pupil$_r$* and *pupil$_l$*. Frontal view of the 3D "volume-rendered" representation of the patient's head (i-CAT, Imaging Sciences International Inc, IPS CaseDesigner ALPHA version, patient V.E.W.). Note that it is crucial that the patient is scanned with the eyes open to define the pupil landmarks. Additional mapping of 2D or 3D facial photographs in order to define the pupil landmarks does not lead to increased accuracy neither reliability

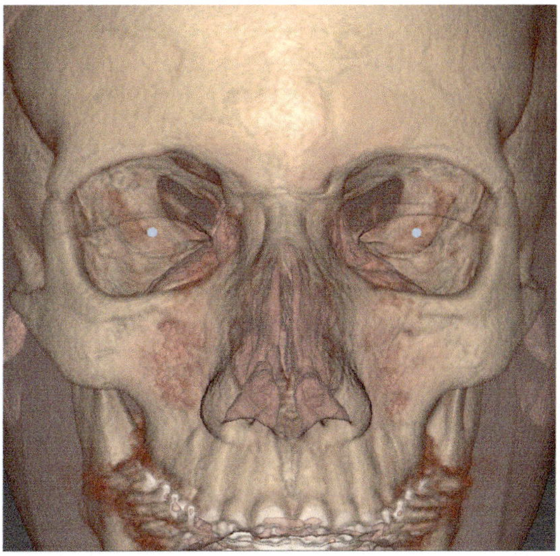

Fig. 2.169 *pupil$_r$* and *pupil$_l$*. Frontal view of the 3D "volume-rendered" hard and soft tissue (in transparency) representation of the patient's head (i-CAT, Imaging Sciences International Inc, IPS CaseDesigner ALPHA version, patient V.E.W.)

soft tissue orbitale (or_r-or_l)

Definition of soft tissue orbitale (or)

"*soft tissue orbitale* (or)" is the soft tissue point located at the most inferior level of each infraorbital rim and located at the level of the 3D hard tissue cephalometric "orbitale" landmark. In 3D cephalometry, this is a well-defined soft tissue landmark and is therefore not the same as the anthropometric orbitale (or) landmark acc. to *L.G. Farkas*, which is identical to the bony "Orbitale".

3D virtual definition of the soft tissue orbitale (or) landmarks

Step 1: Define *soft tissue orbitale$_r$* and *soft tissue orbitale$_l$* on the frontal view of the 3D transparent soft tissue surface representation (Fig. 2.170).

Step 2: Visualise both *soft tissue orbitale* landmarks on the frontal view of the 3D soft tissue surface representation (Fig. 2.171).

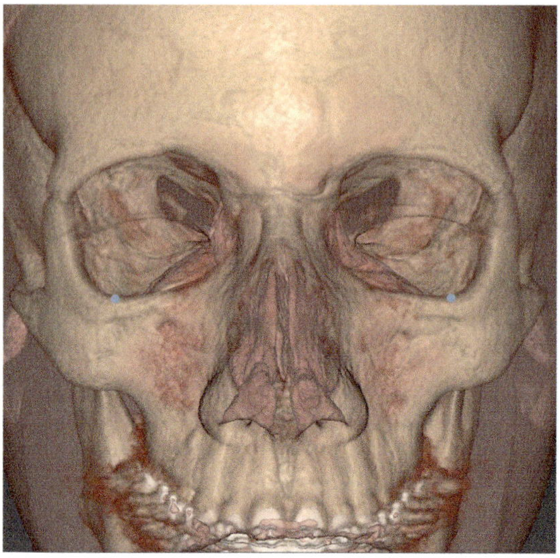

Fig. 2.170 *soft tissue orbitale$_r$* and *soft tissue orbitale$_l$*. Frontal view of the 3D "volume-rendered" hard and soft tissue (in transparency) representation of the patient's head (i-CAT, Imaging Sciences International Inc, IPS CaseDesigner ALPHA version, patient V.E.W.). Note that the transparent soft tissue representation shows the underlying bony structures and allows accurate definition of the *soft tissue orbitale* landmarks

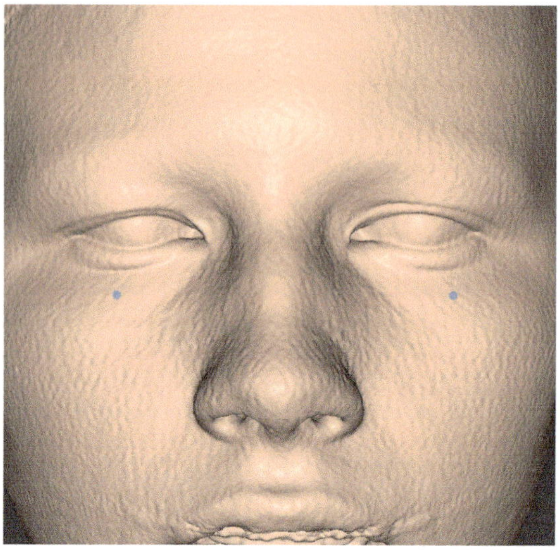

Fig. 2.171 *soft tissue orbitale$_r$* and *soft tissue orbitale$_l$*. Frontal view of the 3D "volume-rendered" representation of the patient's head (i-CAT, Imaging Sciences International Inc, IPS CaseDesigner ALPHA version, patient V.E.W.)

▪ orbitale superius (os_r-os_l)

Definition of orbitale superius (os)

"*orbitale superius* (os)" is the soft tissue point located at the most superior level of each supraorbital rim. This landmark is close to the anthropometric orbitale (os) landmark acc. to *L.G. Farkas*, which is defined as the highest point on the lower border of the eyebrow.

3D virtual definition of the orbitale superius (os) landmarks

Step 1: Define *orbitale superius*$_r$ and *orbitale superius*$_l$ on the frontal view of the 3D transparent soft tissue surface representation (▪ Fig. 2.172).

Step 2: Visualise both *orbitale superius* landmarks on the frontal view of the 3D soft tissue surface representation (▪ Fig. 2.173).

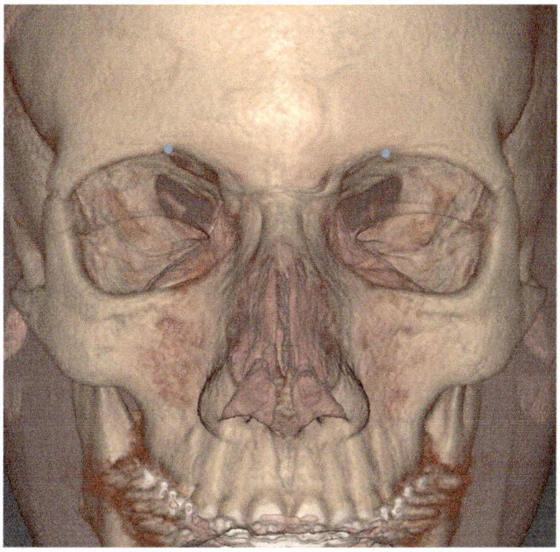

▪ **Fig. 2.172** *orbitale superius*$_r$ and *orbitale superius*$_l$. Frontal view of the 3D "volume-rendered" hard and soft tissue (in transparency) representation of the patient's head (i-CAT, Imaging Sciences International Inc, IPS CaseDesigner ALPHA version, patient V.E.W.). Note that the transparent soft tissue representation shows the underlying bony structures and allows accurate definition of the *orbitale superius* landmarks

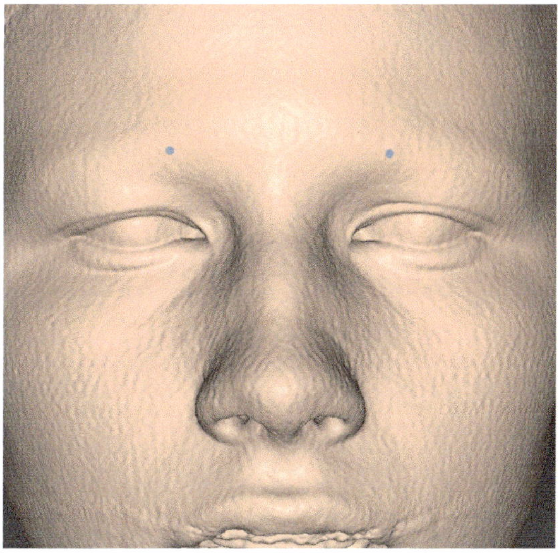

▪ **Fig. 2.173** *orbitale superius*$_r$ and *orbitale superius*$_l$. Frontal view of the 3D "volume-rendered" representation of the patient's head (i-CAT, Imaging Sciences International Inc, IPS CaseDesigner ALPHA version, patient V.E.W.)

zygion (zy_l-zy_r)

Definition of zygion (zy)

"*zygion* (zy)" is the most lateral point on the soft tissue contour of each zygomatic arch, located at the level of the 3D hard tissue cephalometric "zygion" landmark. In 3D cephalometry, *zygion* (*zy*) is a well-defined soft tissue landmark and is therefore not the same as the anthropometric *zygion* (*zy*) landmark acc. to *L.G. Farkas*, which is identical to the bony "Zygion".

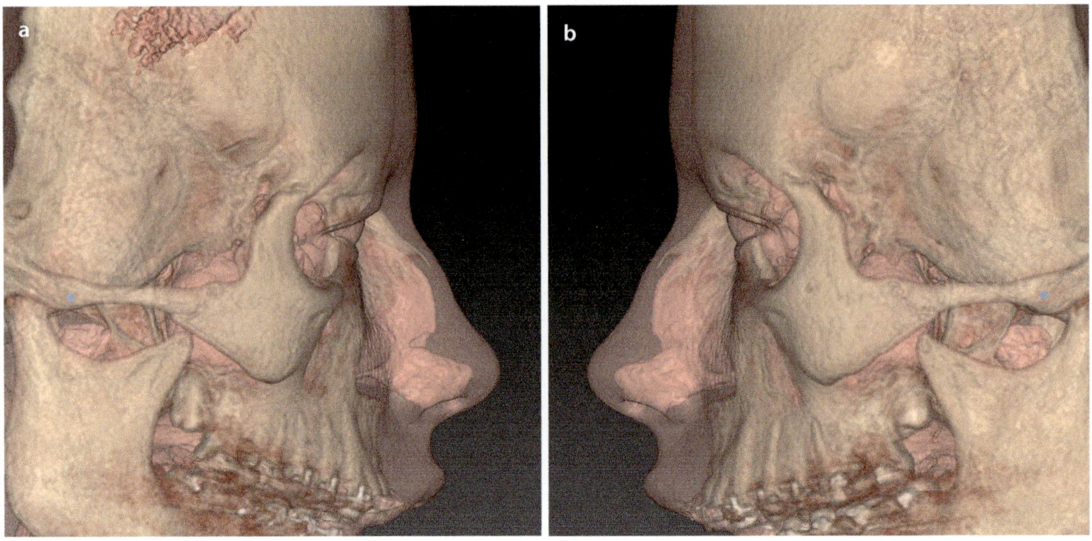

Fig. 2.174 *zygion*$_r$ and *zygion*$_l$. Profile view right (**a**) and left (**b**) of the 3D "volume-rendered" hard and soft tissue (in transparency) representation of the patient's head (i-CAT, Imaging Sciences International Inc, IPS CaseDesigner ALPHA version, patient V.E.W.). Note that the transparent soft tissue representation shows the underlying bony structures and allows accurate definition of the *zygion* landmarks

3D virtual definition of the zygion (zy) landmarks

Step 1: Define *zygion*$_r$ and *zygion*$_l$ on the right (Fig. 2.174a) and left (Fig. 2.174b) profile views of the 3D transparent soft tissue surface representation at the level of the 3D hard tissue cephalometric Zygion landmarks.

Step 2: Verify and eventually correct the position of both *zygion* landmarks on the frontal view of the 3D soft tissue surface representation (Figs. 2.175 and 2.176).

zygion (zy_l-zy_r)

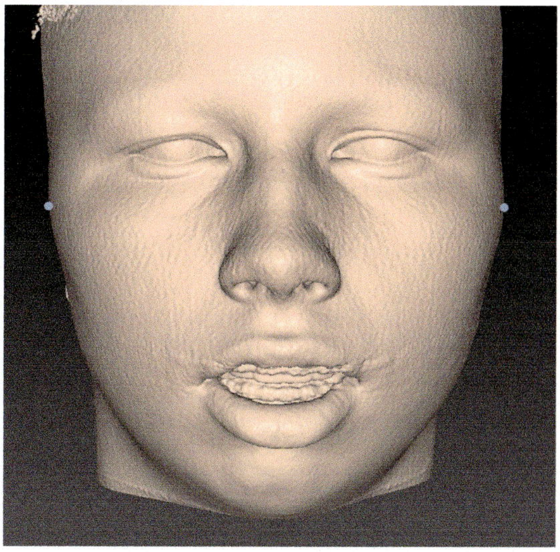

Fig. 2.175 *zygion*$_r$ and *zygion*$_l$. Frontal view of the 3D "volume-rendered" representation of the patient's head (i-CAT, Imaging Sciences International Inc, IPS CaseDesigner ALPHA version, patient V.E.W.)

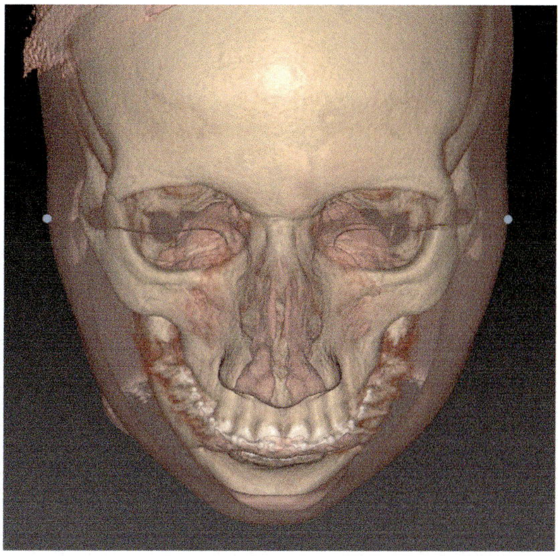

Fig. 2.176 *zygion*$_r$ and *zygion*$_l$. Inferior inclined frontal view of the 3D "volume-rendered" hard and soft tissue (in transparency) representation of the patient's head (i-CAT, Imaging Sciences International Inc, IPS CaseDesigner ALPHA version, patient V.E.W.)

pronasale (prn)

Definition of pronasale (prn)

"*pronasale* (prn)" is the most anterior midpoint of the nasal tip. In case a bifid nose is present, the more protruding tip is chosen to determine *pronasale* as proposed by *L.G. Farkas*.

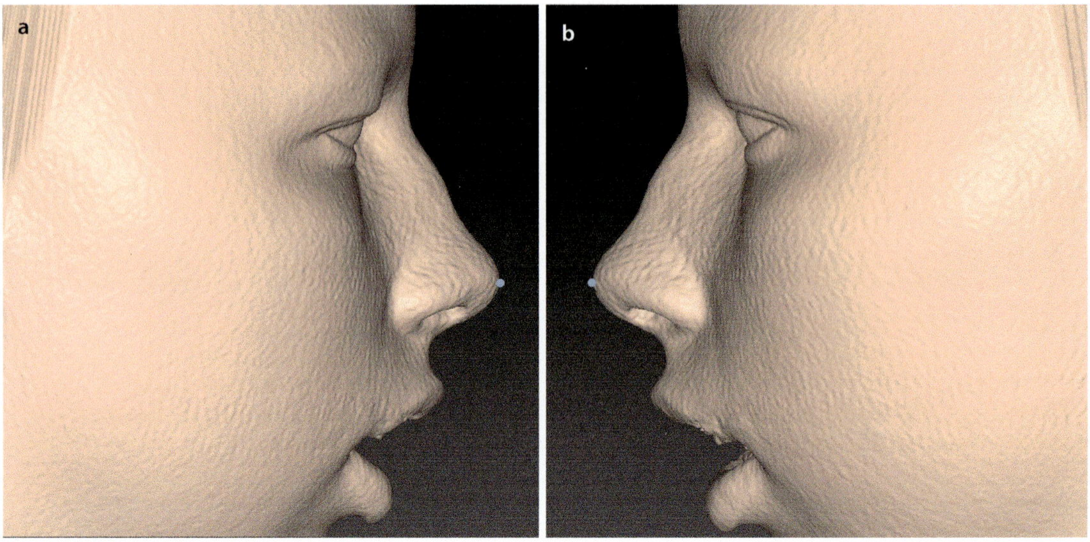

Fig. 2.177 *pronasale*. Profile right (**a**) and left (**b**) views of the 3D "volume-rendered" representation of the patient's head (i-CAT, Imaging Sciences International Inc, IPS CaseDesigner ALPHA version, patient V.E.W.)

3D virtual definition of the pronasale (prn) landmark

Step 1: Define *pronasale (prn)* on the right profile view of the 3D soft tissue surface representation (Fig. 2.177a) and verify its position on the left profile view (Fig. 2.177b).

Step 2: Verify and eventually correct the midline position of the *pronasale (prn)* landmark on the base view of the 3D soft tissue surface representation (Fig. 2.178).

pronasale (prn)

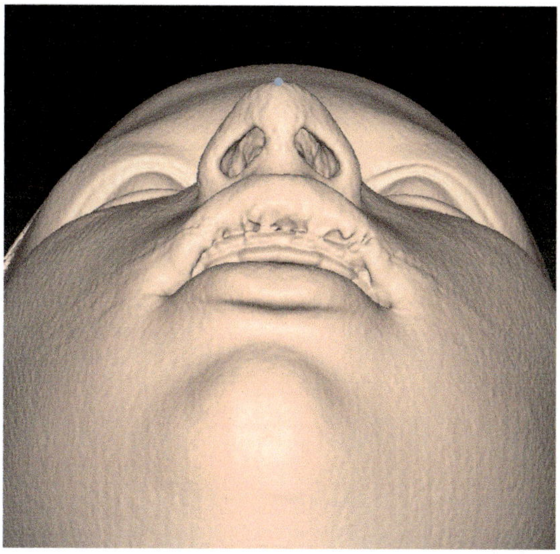

Fig. 2.178 *pronasale*. Base view of the 3D "volume-rendered" representation of the patient's head (i-CAT, Imaging Sciences International Inc, IPS CaseDesigner ALPHA version, patient V.E.W.)

▪ subnasale (sn)

Definition of subnasale (sn)

"*subnasale* (sn)" is the midpoint on the nasolabial soft tissue contour between the columella crest and the upper lip.

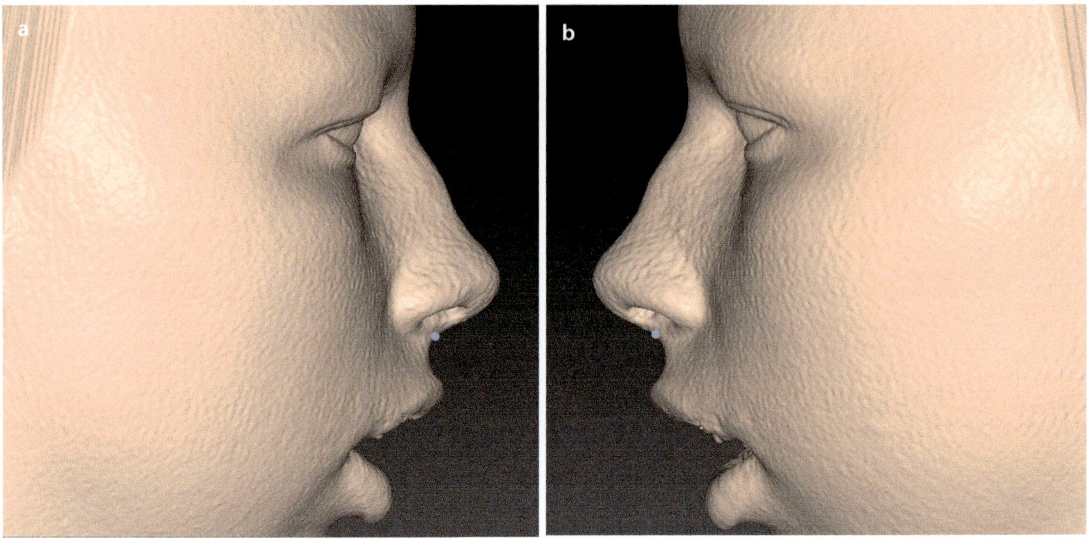

Fig. 2.179 *subnasale*. Profile right (**a**) and left (**b**) views of the 3D "volume-rendered" representation of the patient's head (i-CAT, Imaging Sciences International Inc, IPS CaseDesigner ALPHA version, patient V.E.W.)

3D virtual definition of the subnasale (sn) landmark

Step 1: Define *subnasale* (*sn*) on the right profile view of the 3D soft tissue surface representation (Fig. 2.179a) and verify its position on the left profile view (Fig. 2.179b).

Step 2: Verify and eventually correct the midline position of the *subnasale* (*sn*) landmark on the base view of the 3D soft tissue surface representation (Fig. 2.180).

subnasale (sn)

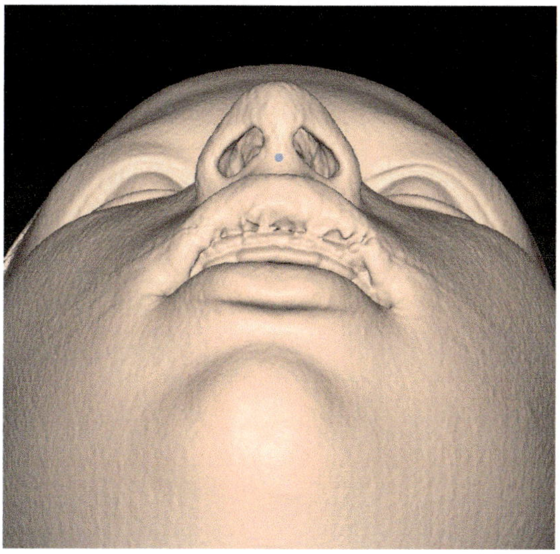

Fig. 2.180 *subnasale*. Base view of the 3D "volume-rendered" representation of the patient's head (i-CAT, Imaging Sciences International Inc, IPS CaseDesigner ALPHA version, patient V.E.W.)

▪ alare (al_r-al_l)

Definition of alare (al)

"*alare* (al)" is the most lateral point on each alar contour.

3D virtual definition of the alare (al) landmarks

Define *alare*$_r$ and *alare*$_l$ on the base view of the 3D soft tissue surface representation (▣ Fig. 2.181).

▪ alar curvature point (ac_r-ac_l)

Definition of alar curvature point (ac)

"*alar curvature point* (ac)" is the point located at the facial insertion of each alar base.

3D Virtual definition of the alar curvature point (ac) landmarks

Define *alar curvature point*$_r$ and *alar curvature point*$_l$ on the submental view of the 3D soft tissue surface representation (▣ Fig. 2.182).

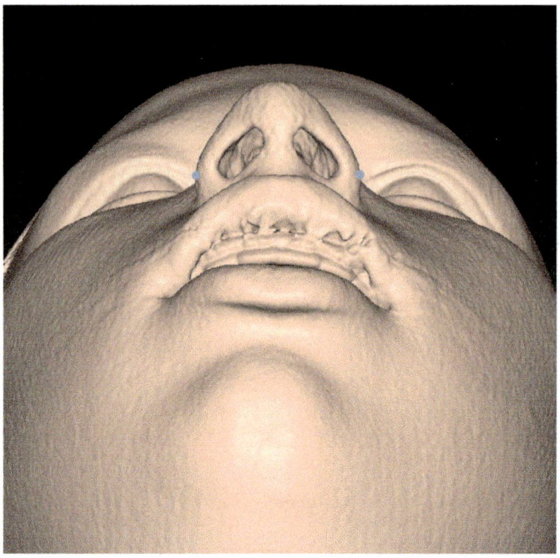

▣ **Fig. 2.181** *alare*$_r$ and *alare*$_l$. Base view of the 3D "volume-rendered" representation of the patient's head (i-CAT, Imaging Sciences International Inc, IPS CaseDesigner ALPHA version, patient V.E.W.)

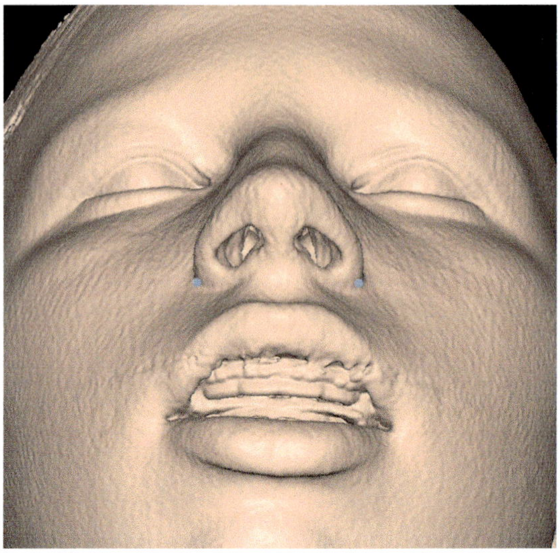

▣ **Fig. 2.182** *alar curvature point*$_r$ and *alar curvature point*$_l$. Submental view of the 3D "volume-rendered" representation of the patient's head (i-CAT, Imaging Sciences International Inc, IPS CaseDesigner ALPHA version, patient V.E.W.)

▪ nostril top point (nt_r-nt_l)

Definition of nostril top point (nt)

"*nostril top point* (*nt*)" is the highest point of each nostril or the superior terminal point of each nostril axis.

3D virtual definition of the nostril top point (nt) landmarks

Define *nostril top point$_r$* and *nostril top point$_l$* on the base view of the 3D soft tissue surface representation (▪ Fig. 2.183).

▪ columella constructed point (c´´)

Definition of columella constructed point (c´´)

"*columella constructed point* (c´´)" is the midpoint of the columella crest at the level of the "nostril top points". This 3D cephalometric soft tissue landmark is a constructed landmark in order to define the nasolabial angle in the "3D virtual scene".

3D Virtual definition of the columella constructed (c´´) landmark

Define *columella constructed point* (*c´´*) on the base view of the 3D soft tissue surface representation (▪ Fig. 2.184).

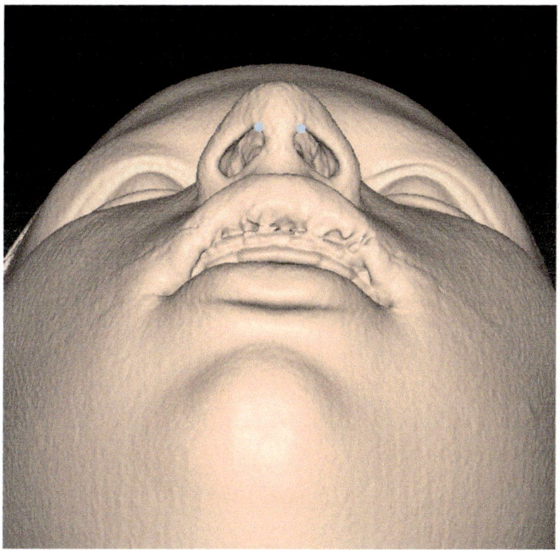

▪ **Fig. 2.183** *nostril top point$_r$* and *nostril top point$_l$*. Base view of the 3D "volume-rendered" representation of the patient's head (i-CAT, Imaging Sciences International Inc, IPS CaseDesigner ALPHA version, patient V.E.W.)

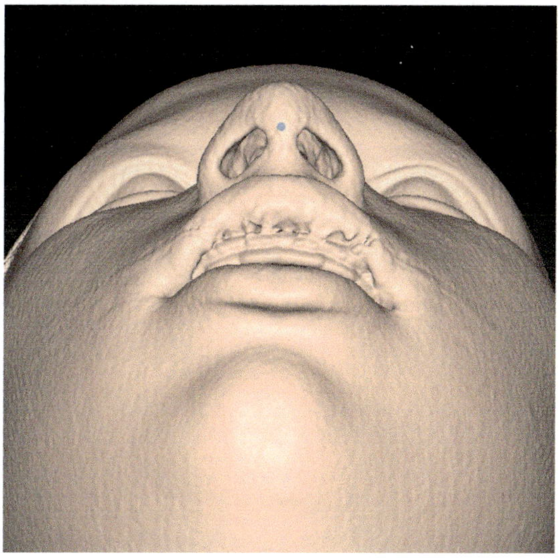

▪ **Fig. 2.184** *columella constructed point*. Base view of the 3D "volume-rendered" representation of the patient's head (i-CAT, Imaging Sciences International Inc, IPS CaseDesigner ALPHA version, patient V.E.W.)

▪ nostril base point (nb_r-nb_l)

Definition of nostril base point (nb)

"*nostril base point* (*nb*)" is the lowest point of each nostril or the inferior terminal point of each nostril axis.

3D virtual definition of the nostril base point (nb) landmarks

Define *nostril base point*$_r$ and *nostril base point*$_l$ on the base view of the 3D soft tissue surface representation (◘ Fig. 2.185).

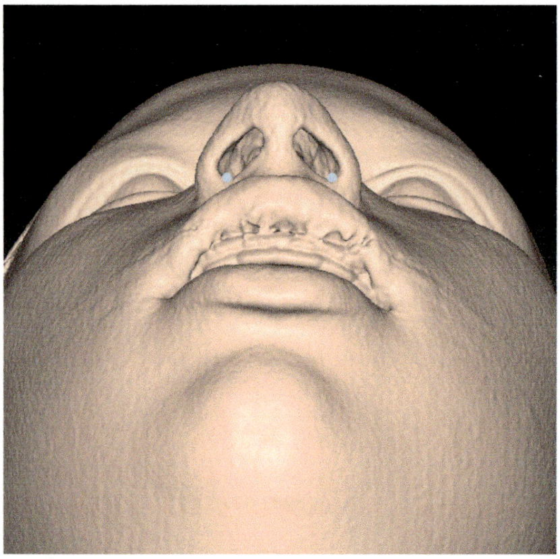

◘ **Fig. 2.185** *nostril base point*$_r$ and *nostril base point*$_l$. Base view of the 3D "volume-rendered" representation of the patient's head (i-CAT, Imaging Sciences International Inc, IPS CaseDesigner ALPHA version, patient V.E.W.)

▪ subspinale (ss)

Definition of subspinale (ss)

"*subspinale* (ss)" is the most posterior midpoint of the philtrum.

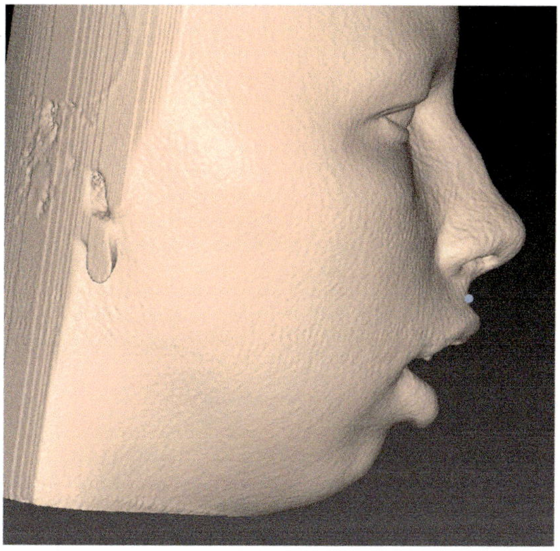

▪ **Fig. 2.186** *subspinale*. Profile view right of the 3D "volume-rendered" representation of the patient's head (i-CAT, Imaging Sciences International Inc, IPS CaseDesigner ALPHA version, patient V.E.W.)

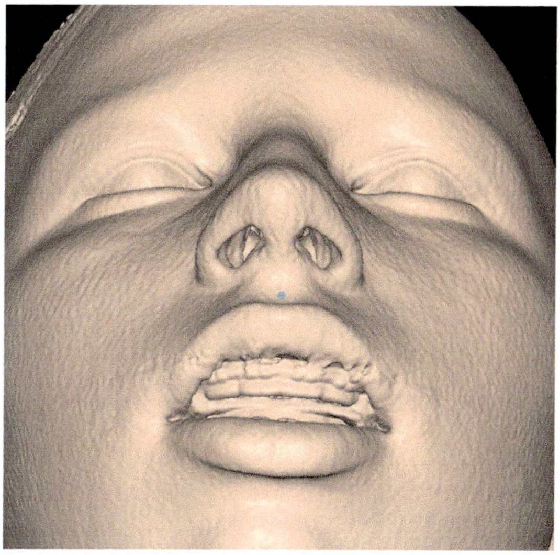

▪ **Fig. 2.187** *subspinale*. Submental view of the 3D "volume-rendered" representation of the patient's head (i-CAT, Imaging Sciences International Inc, IPS CaseDesigner ALPHA version, patient V.E.W.)

3D virtual definition of the subspinale (ss) landmark

Step 1: Define *subspinale* (*ss*) on the right or left profile view of the 3D soft tissue surface representation (▪ Fig. 2.186).

Step 2: Correct the midline position of the *subspinale* (*ss*) landmark on the submental view of the 3D soft tissue surface representation (▪ Fig. 2.187). In most cases the landmark will not be visible anymore on the right and left profile views of the 3D soft tissue surface representation, because of the philtral column (▪ Fig. 2.188). However, it is still visible on the profile 3D transparent soft tissue surface representation (▪ Fig. 2.189).

Step 3: Verify the position of the *subspinale* (*ss*) landmark on the right (▪ Fig. 2.190a) and left (▪ Fig. 2.190b) 2/3 profile views of the 3D soft tissue surface representation.

subspinale (ss)

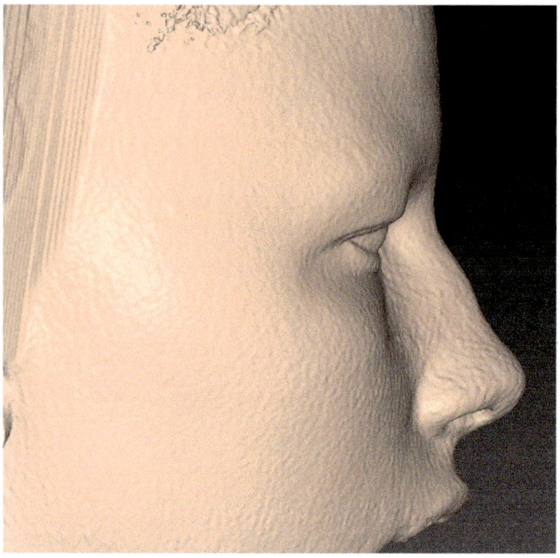

Fig. 2.188 *subspinale*. Profile view right of the 3D "volume-rendered" representation of the patient's head (i-CAT, Imaging Sciences International Inc, IPS CaseDesigner ALPHA version, patient V.E.W.). Note that the landmark is not visible anymore because of the philtral column

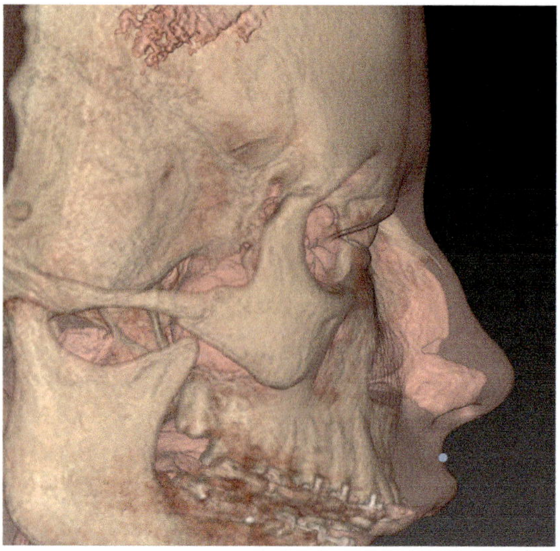

Fig. 2.189 *subspinale*. Profile view right with transparent soft tissue of the 3D "volume-rendered" representation of the patient's head (i-CAT, Imaging Sciences International Inc, IPS CaseDesigner ALPHA version, patient V.E.W.). Note that the transparent soft tissue representation allows the visualisation of the *subspinale* landmark

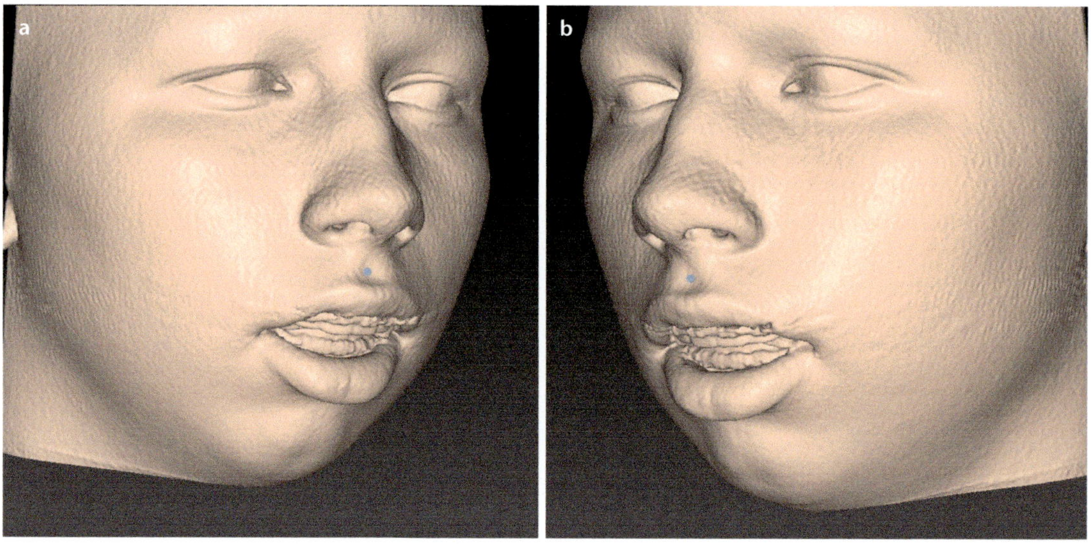

Fig. 2.190 *subspinale*. 2/3 profile view right (**a**) and left (**b**) of the 3D "volume-rendered" representation of the patient's head (i-CAT, Imaging Sciences International Inc, IPS CaseDesigner ALPHA version, patient V.E.W.)

labiale (or labrale) superius (ls)

Definition of labiale superius (ls)

"*labiale superius* (ls)" is the midpoint of the vermilion line of the upper lip.

3D virtual definition of the labiale superius (ls) landmark

Step 1: Define *labiale superius* (*ls*) on the submental view of the 3D soft tissue surface representation (Fig. 2.191).

Step 2: Verify and eventually correct the position of the *labiale superius* (*ls*) landmark on the right (Fig. 2.192a) and left (Fig. 2.192b) 2/3 profile views of the 3D soft tissue surface representation.

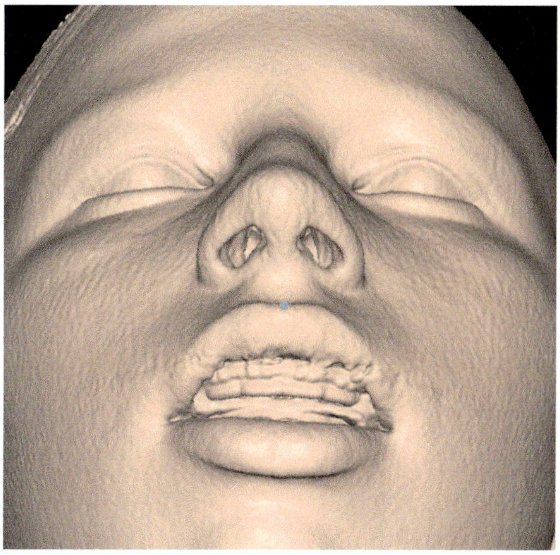

Fig. 2.191 *labiale superius*. Submental view of the 3D "volume-rendered" representation of the patient's head (i-CAT, Imaging Sciences International Inc, IPS CaseDesigner ALPHA version, patient V.E.W.)

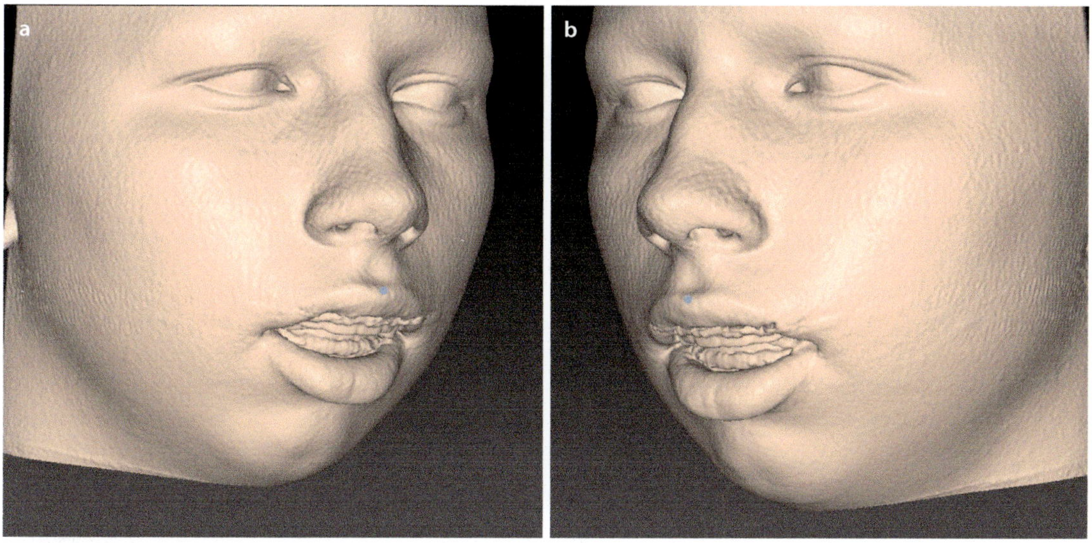

Fig. 2.192 *labiale superius*. 2/3 profile view right (**a**) and left (**b**) of the 3D "volume-rendered" representation of the patient's head (i-CAT, Imaging Sciences International Inc, IPS CaseDesigner ALPHA version, patient V.E.W.)

stomion superius (st_s)

Definition of stomion superius (st_s)

"*stomion superius* (st_s)" is the most inferior point of the upper lip, in the midsagittal plane.

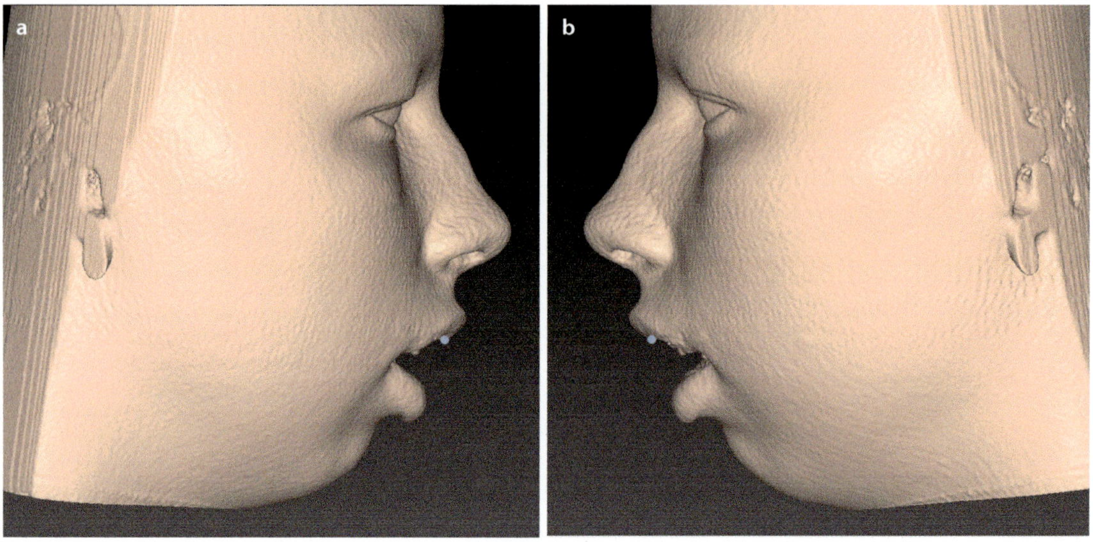

Fig. 2.193 *stomion superius*. Profile right (**a**) and left (**b**) views of the 3D "volume-rendered" representation of the patient's head (i-CAT, Imaging Sciences International Inc, IPS CaseDesigner ALPHA version, patient V.E.W.)

3D virtual definition of the stomion superius (st_s) landmark

Step 1: Define *stomion superius* (st_s) on the right profile view of the 3D soft tissue surface representation (Fig. 2.193a) and verify its position on the left profile view (Fig. 2.193b).

Step 2: Verify and eventually correct the midline position of the *stomion superius* (st_s) landmark on the frontal view of the 3D soft tissue surface representation (Fig. 2.194).

stomion superius – st_s

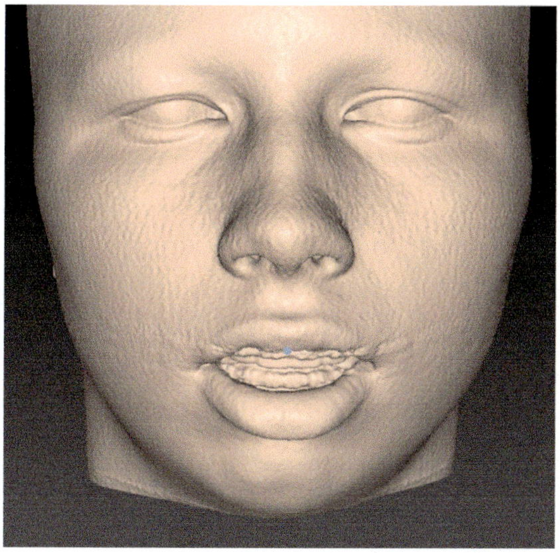

Fig. 2.194 *stomion superius*. Frontal view of the 3D "volume-rendered" representation of the patient's head (i-CAT, Imaging Sciences International Inc, IPS CaseDesigner ALPHA version, patient V.E.W.)

stomion Inferius (st_i)

Definition of stomion inferius (st_i)

"*stomion inferius* (st_i)" is the most inferior point of the lower lip, in the midsagittal plane.

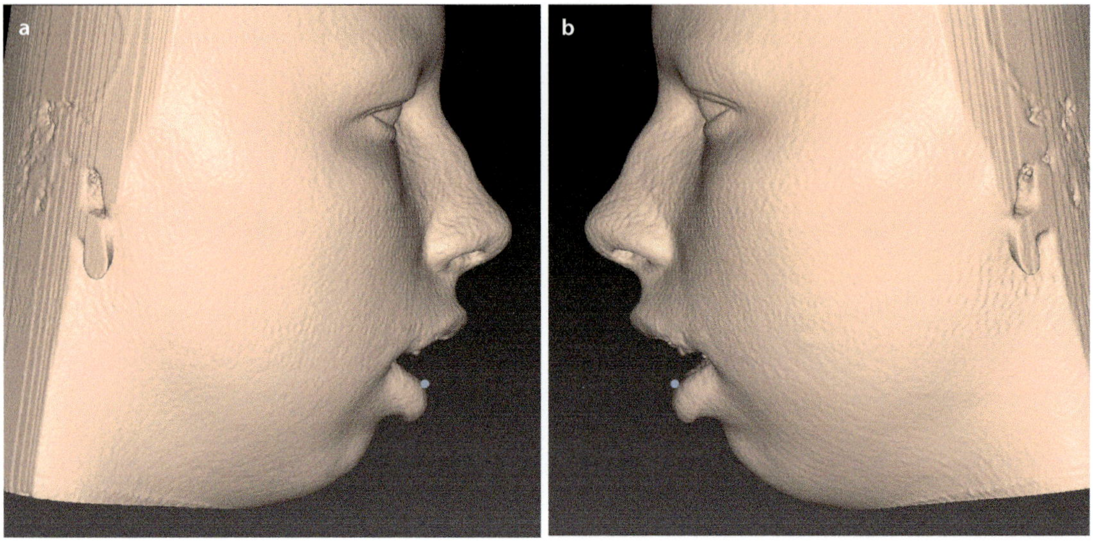

Fig. 2.195 *stomion inferius*. Profile right (**a**) and left (**b**) views of the 3D "volume-rendered" representation of the patient's head (i-CAT, Imaging Sciences International Inc, IPS CaseDesigner ALPHA version, patient V.E.W.)

3D definition of the stomion inferius (st_i) landmark

Step 1: Define *stomion inferius* (st_i) on the right profile view of the 3D soft tissue surface representation (Fig. 2.195a), and verify its position on the left profile view (Fig. 2.195b).

Step 2: Verify and eventually correct the midline position of the *stomion inferius* (st_i) landmark on the frontal view of the 3D soft tissue surface representation (Fig. 2.196).

stomion inferius (st_i)

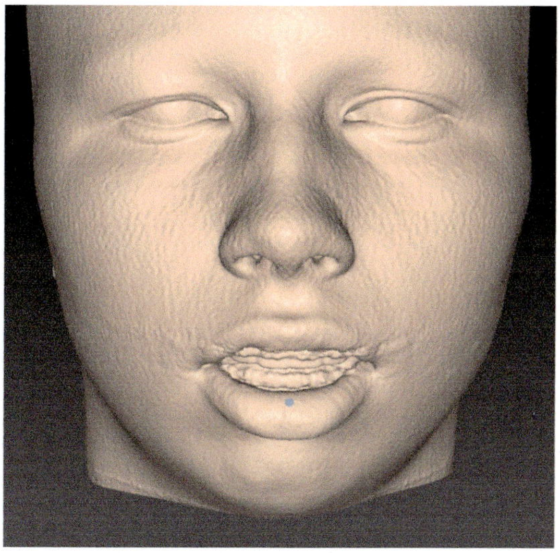

Fig. 2.196 *stomion inferius*. Frontal view of the 3D "volume-rendered" representation of the patient's head (i-CAT, Imaging Sciences International Inc, IPS CaseDesigner ALPHA version, patient V.E.W.)

cheilion (ch_r-ch_l)

Definition of cheilion (ch)

"*cheilion* (ch)" is the point located at each labial commissure.

3D virtual definition of the cheilion (ch) landmarks

Step 1: Define $cheilion_r$ and $cheilion_l$ on the frontal view of the 3D soft tissue surface representation (Fig. 2.197).

Step 2: Verify and eventually correct the position of the $cheilion_r$ and $cheilion_l$ on the right (Fig. 2.198a) and left (Fig. 2.198b) 2/3 profile views of the 3D soft tissue surface representation.

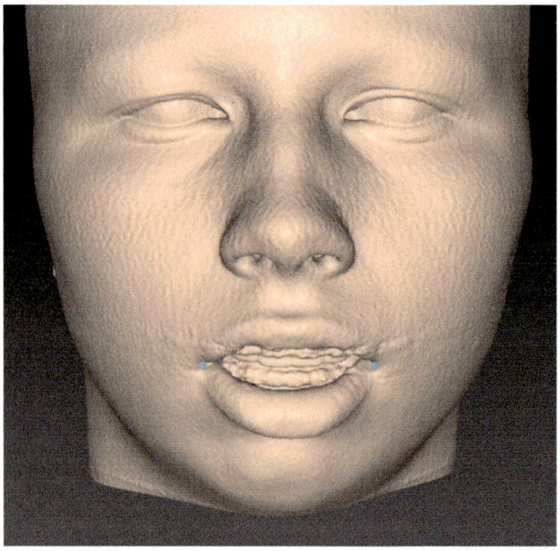

Fig. 2.197 $cheilion_r$ and $cheilion_l$. Frontal view of the 3D "volume-rendered" representation of the patient's head (i-CAT, Imaging Sciences International Inc, IPS CaseDesigner ALPHA version, patient V.E.W.)

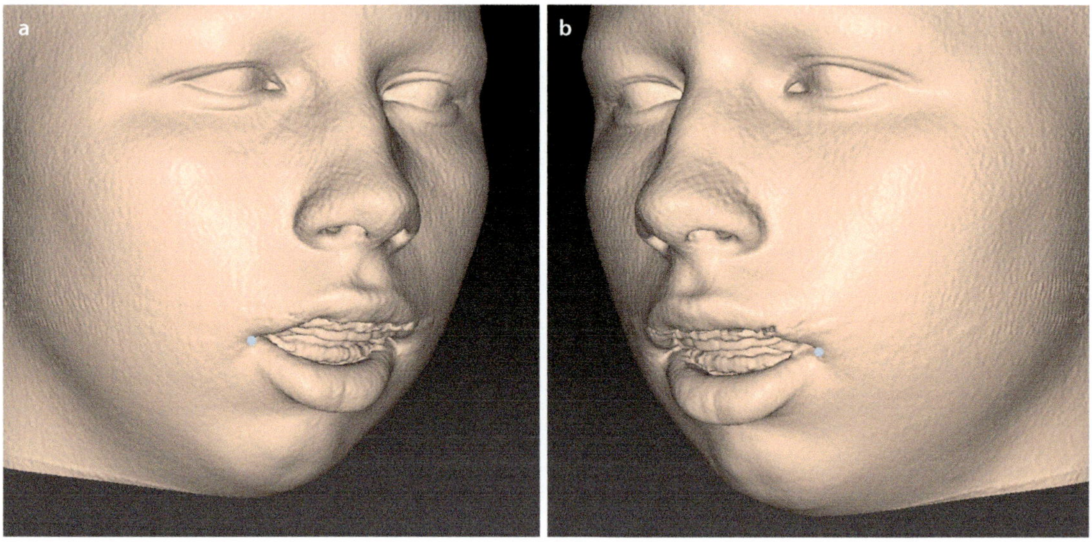

Fig. 2.198 $cheilion_r$ and $cheilion_l$. 2/3 profile view right (**a**) and left (**b**) of the 3D "volume-rendered" representation of the patient's head (i-CAT, Imaging Sciences International Inc, IPS CaseDesigner ALPHA version, patient V.E.W.)

labiale (or labrale) inferius (li)

Definition of labiale inferius (li)

"*labiale inferius* (li)" is the midpoint of the vermilion line of the lower lip.

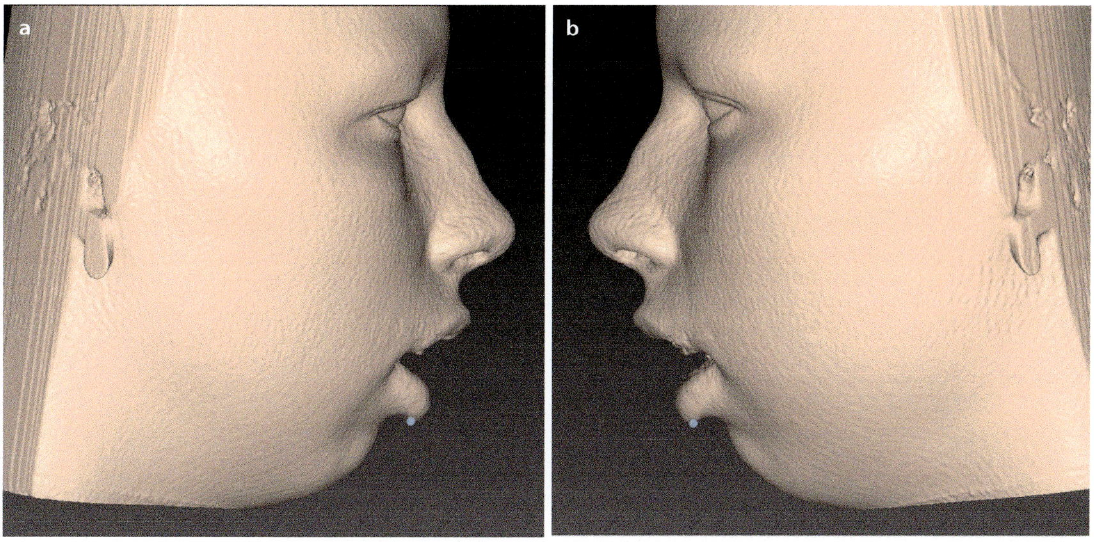

Fig. 2.199 *labiale inferius*. Profile right (**a**) and left (**b**) views of the 3D "volume-rendered" representation of the patient's head (i-CAT, Imaging Sciences International Inc, IPS CaseDesigner ALPHA version, patient V.E.W.)

3D virtual definition of the labiale inferius (li) landmark

Step 1: Define *labiale inferius* (*li*) on the right profile view of the 3D soft tissue surface representation (Fig. 2.199a), and verify its position on the left profile view (Fig. 2.199b).

Step 2: Verify and eventually correct the midline position of the *labiale inferius* (*li*) landmark on the submental view of the 3D soft tissue surface representation (Fig. 2.200).

labiale (or labrale) inferius (li)

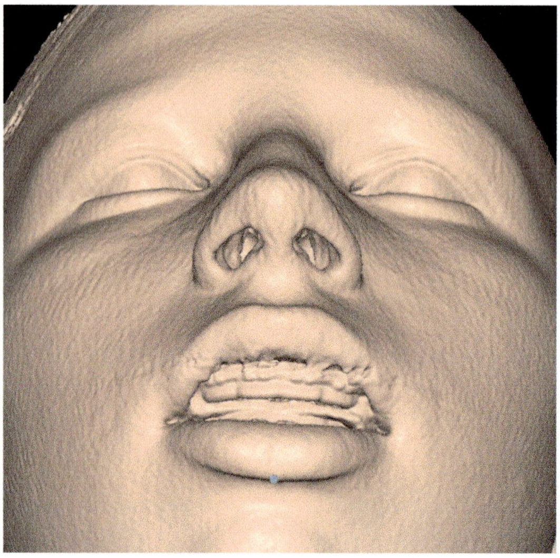

Fig. 2.200 *labiale inferius*. Submental view of the 3D "volume-rendered" representation of the patient's head (i-CAT, Imaging Sciences International Inc, IPS CaseDesigner ALPHA version, patient V.E.W.)

soft tissue gonion (go_r-go_l)

Definition of soft tissue gonion (go)

"*soft tissue gonion* (go)" is the most lateral point on the soft tissue contour of each mandibular angle, located at the same level as the 3D hard tissue cephalometric "Gonion" landmark (► see also Sect. 2.2.2).

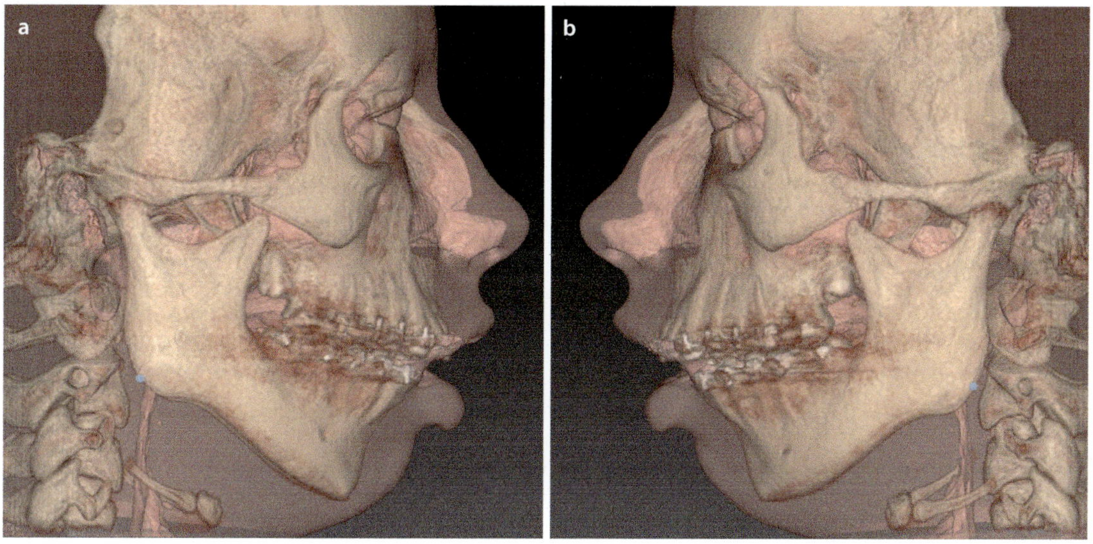

Fig. 2.201 *soft tissue gonion*$_r$ and *soft tissue gonion*$_l$. Profile right (**a**) and left (**b**) views with transparent soft tissue of the 3D "volume-rendered" representation of the patient's head (i-CAT, Imaging Sciences International Inc, IPS CaseDesigner ALPHA version, patient V.E.W.)

3D virtual definition of the soft tissue gonion (go) landmarks

Step 1: Define *soft tissue gonion*$_r$ and *soft tissue gonion*$_l$ on the right (Fig. 2.201a) and left profile (Fig. 2.201b) views of the 3D transparent soft tissue surface representation.

Step 2: Verify and eventually correct the position of both *soft tissue gonion* landmarks on the frontal view of the 3D transparent soft tissue surface representation (Fig. 2.202).

Step 3: Visualise both *soft tissue gonion* landmarks on the frontal view of the 3D soft tissue surface representation (Fig. 2.203).

2

soft tissue gonion (go_r-go_l)

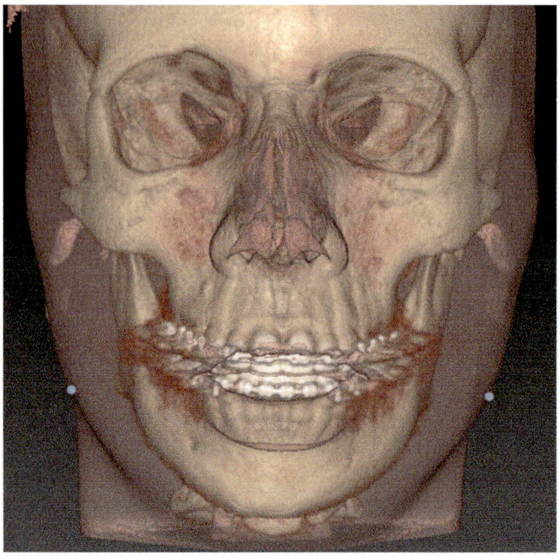

Fig. 2.202 *soft tissue gonion$_r$* and *soft tissue gonion$_l$*. Frontal view with transparent soft tissues of the 3D "volume-rendered" representation of the patient's head (i-CAT, Imaging Sciences International Inc, IPS CaseDesigner ALPHA version, patient V.E.W.). Note that the transparent soft tissue representation shows the underlying bony structures and allows accurate definition of the *soft tissue gonion* landmarks

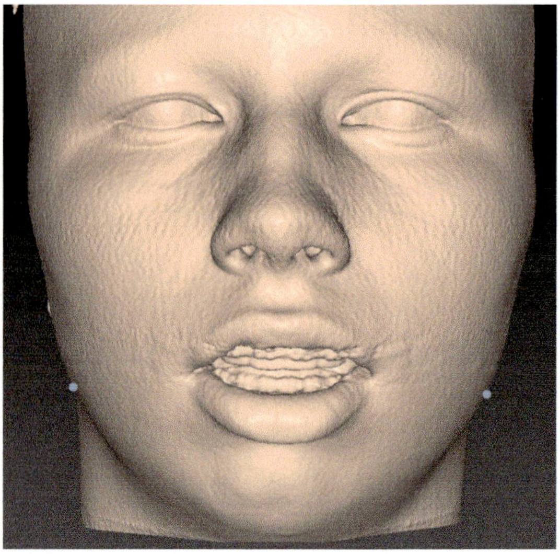

Fig. 2.203 *soft tissue gonion$_r$* and *soft tissue gonion$_l$*. Frontal view of the 3D "volume-rendered" representation of the patient's head (i-CAT, Imaging Sciences International Inc, IPS CaseDesigner ALPHA version, patient V.E.W.)

▪ sublabiale (sl)

Definition of sublabiale (sl)

"*sublabiale* (sl)" is the most posterior midpoint on the labiomental soft tissue contour that defines the border between the lower lip and the chin.

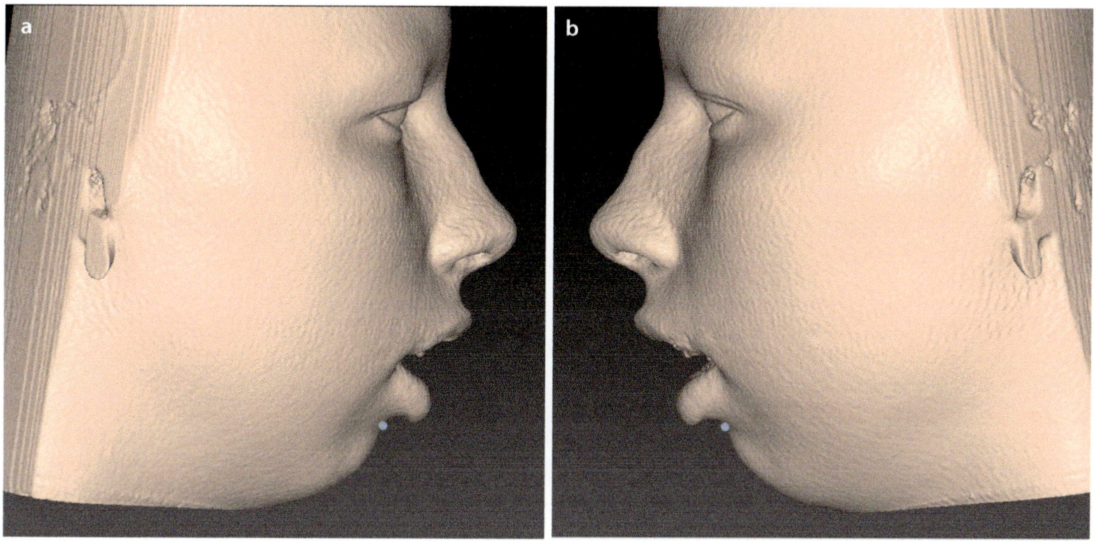

Fig. 2.204 *sublabiale*. Profile right (**a**) and left (**b**) views of the 3D "volume-rendered" representation of the patient's head (i-CAT, Imaging Sciences International Inc, IPS CaseDesigner ALPHA version, patient V.E.W.)

3D virtual definition of the sublabiale (sl) landmark

Step 1: Define *sublabiale* (*sl*) on the right profile view of the 3D soft tissue surface representation (Fig. 2.204a) and verify its position on the left profile view (Fig. 2.204b).

Step 2: Verify and eventually correct the midline position of the *sublabiale* (*sl*) landmark on the submental view of the 3D soft tissue surface representation (Fig. 2.205).

sublabiale (sl)

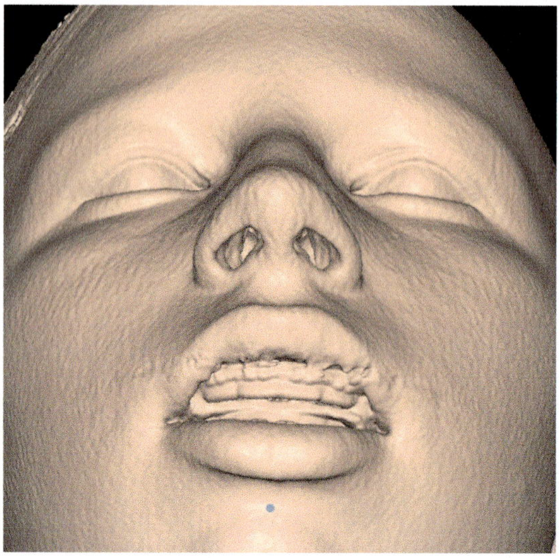

Fig. 2.205 *sublabiale*. Submental view of the 3D "volume-rendered" representation of the patient's head (i-CAT, Imaging Sciences International Inc, IPS CaseDesigner ALPHA version, patient V.E.W.)

▪ soft tissue pogonion (pg)

Definition of soft tissue pogonion (pg)

"*soft tissue pogonion* (pg)" is the most anterior midpoint of the chin.

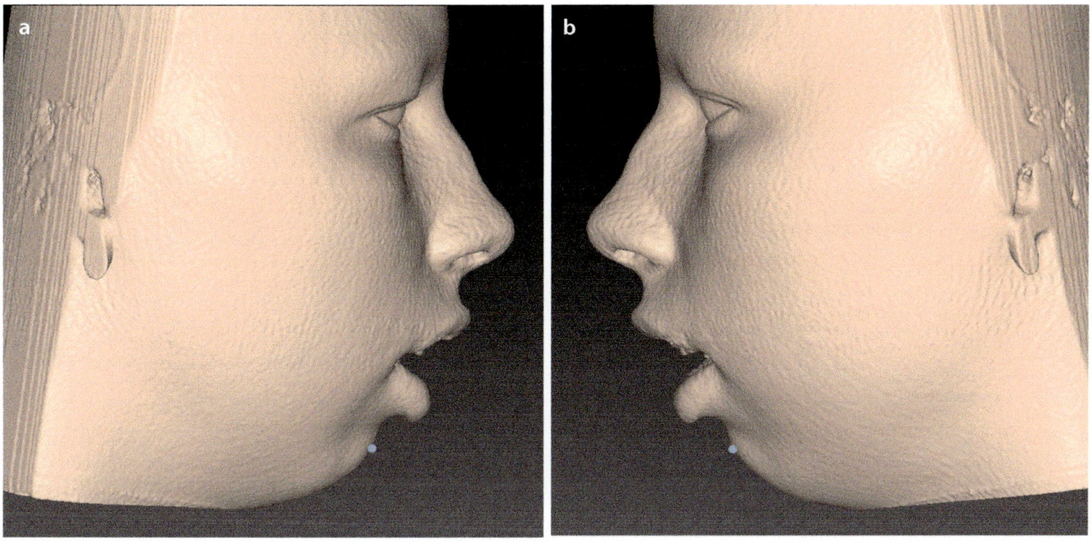

◘ **Fig. 2.206** *soft tissue pogonion.* Profile right (**a**) and left (**b**) views of the 3D "volume-rendered" representation of the patient's head (i-CAT, Imaging Sciences International Inc, IPS CaseDesigner ALPHA version, patient V.E.W.)

3D virtual definition of the soft tissue pogonion (pg) landmark

Step 1: Define *soft tissue pogonion (pg)* on the right profile view of the 3D soft tissue surface representation (◘ Figs. 2.206a and 2.208), and verify its position on the left profile view (◘ Fig. 2.206b).

Step 2: Verify and eventually correct the midline position of the *soft tissue pogonion (pg)* landmark on the submental view of the 3D soft tissue surface representation (◘ Fig. 2.207).

soft tissue pogonion (pg)

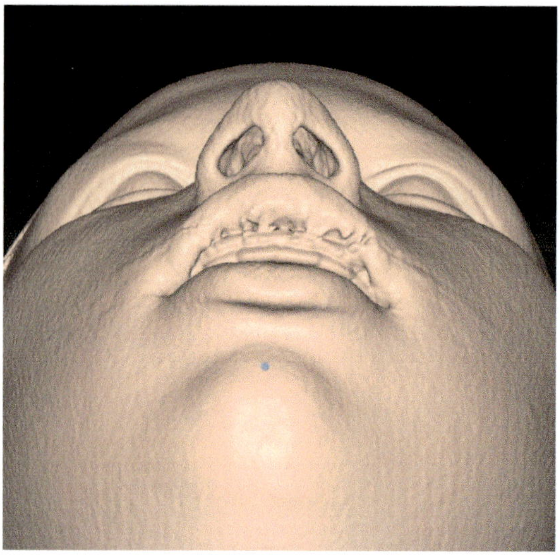

Fig. 2.207 *soft tissue pogonion*. Submental view of the 3D "volume-rendered" representation of the patient's head (i-CAT, Imaging Sciences International Inc, IPS CaseDesigner ALPHA version, patient V.E.W.)

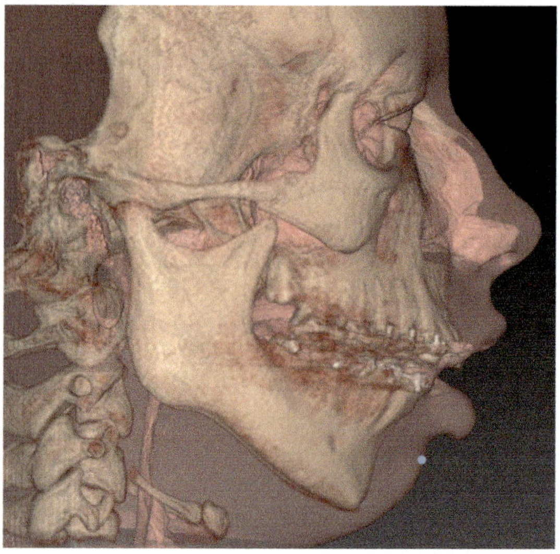

Fig. 2.208 *soft tissue pogonion*. Profile view right with transparent soft tissues of the 3D "volume-rendered" representation of the patient's head (i-CAT, Imaging Sciences International Inc, IPS CaseDesigner ALPHA version, patient V.E.W.). Note that the *soft tissue pogonion* landmark is located in a more superior position compared to the bony Pogonion landmark

■ soft tissue gnathion (or menton) (gn)

Definition of soft tissue gnathion (gn)

"*soft tissue gnathion* (gn)" is the most inferior midpoint on the soft tissue contour of the chin located at the level of the 3D cephalometric hard tissue "menton" landmark (► see also Sect. 2.2.2). In 3D cephalometry, "*soft tissue gnathion* (*gn*)" is a well-defined soft tissue landmark and is therefore not the same as the anthropometric *gnathion* (*gn*) landmark acc. to *L.G. Farkas*, which is identical to the bony "Gnathion".

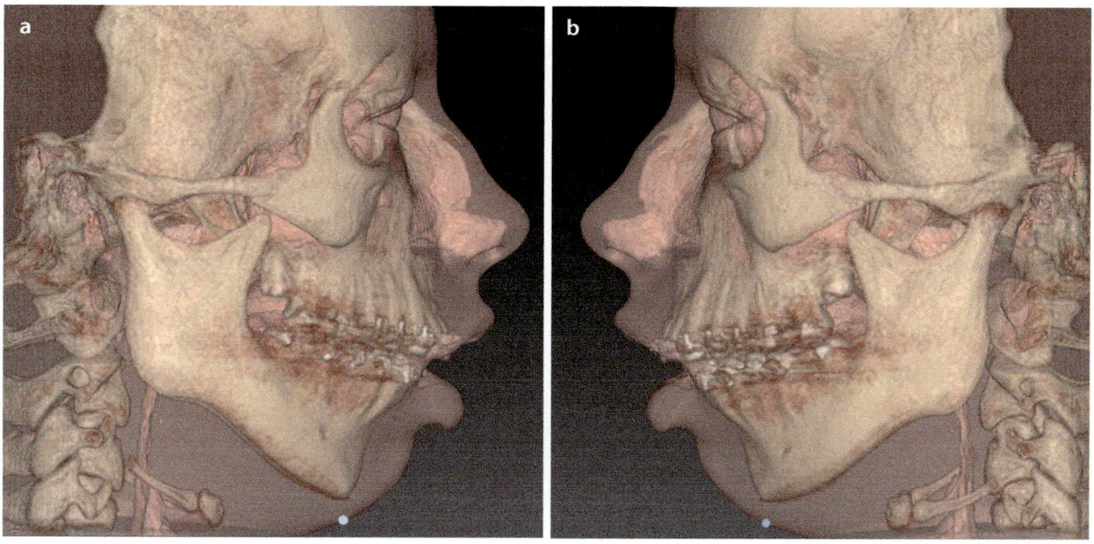

■ **Fig. 2.209** *soft tissue gnathion*. Profile right (**a**) and left (**b**) views with transparent soft tissues of the 3D "volume-rendered" representation of the patient's head (i-CAT, Imaging Sciences International Inc, IPS CaseDesigner ALPHA version, patient V.E.W.)

3D virtual definition of the soft tissue gnathion (gn) landmark

Step 1: Define *soft tissue gnathion (gn)* on the right profile view of the transparent 3D soft tissue surface representation (■ Fig. 2.209a), and verify its position on the left profile view of the transparent 3D soft tissue surface representation (■ Fig. 2.209b).

Step 2: Verify and eventually correct the midline position of the *soft tissue gnathion (gn)* landmark on the base view of the 3D soft tissue surface representation (■ Fig. 2.210).

soft tissue gnathion (or menton) (gn)

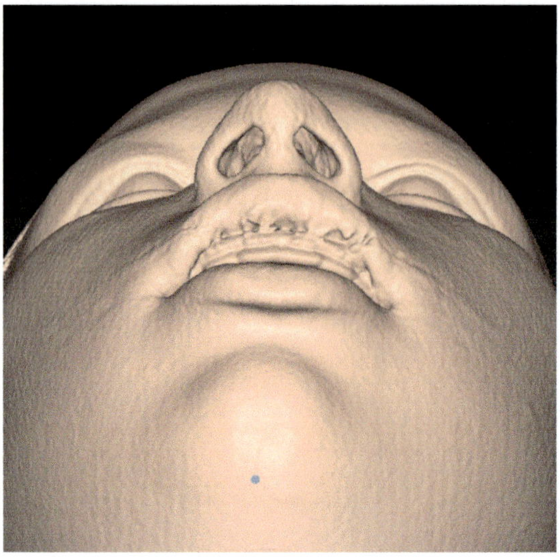

Fig. 2.210 *soft tissue gnathion*. Base view left of the 3D "volume-rendered" representation of the patient's head (i-CAT, Imaging Sciences International Inc, IPS CaseDesigner ALPHA version, patient V.E.W.). Note that this landmark is positioned in the centre of the chin aesthetic unit and could therefore be out of the true facial midline

Set-Up of 3D Cephalometric Soft Tissue Landmarks

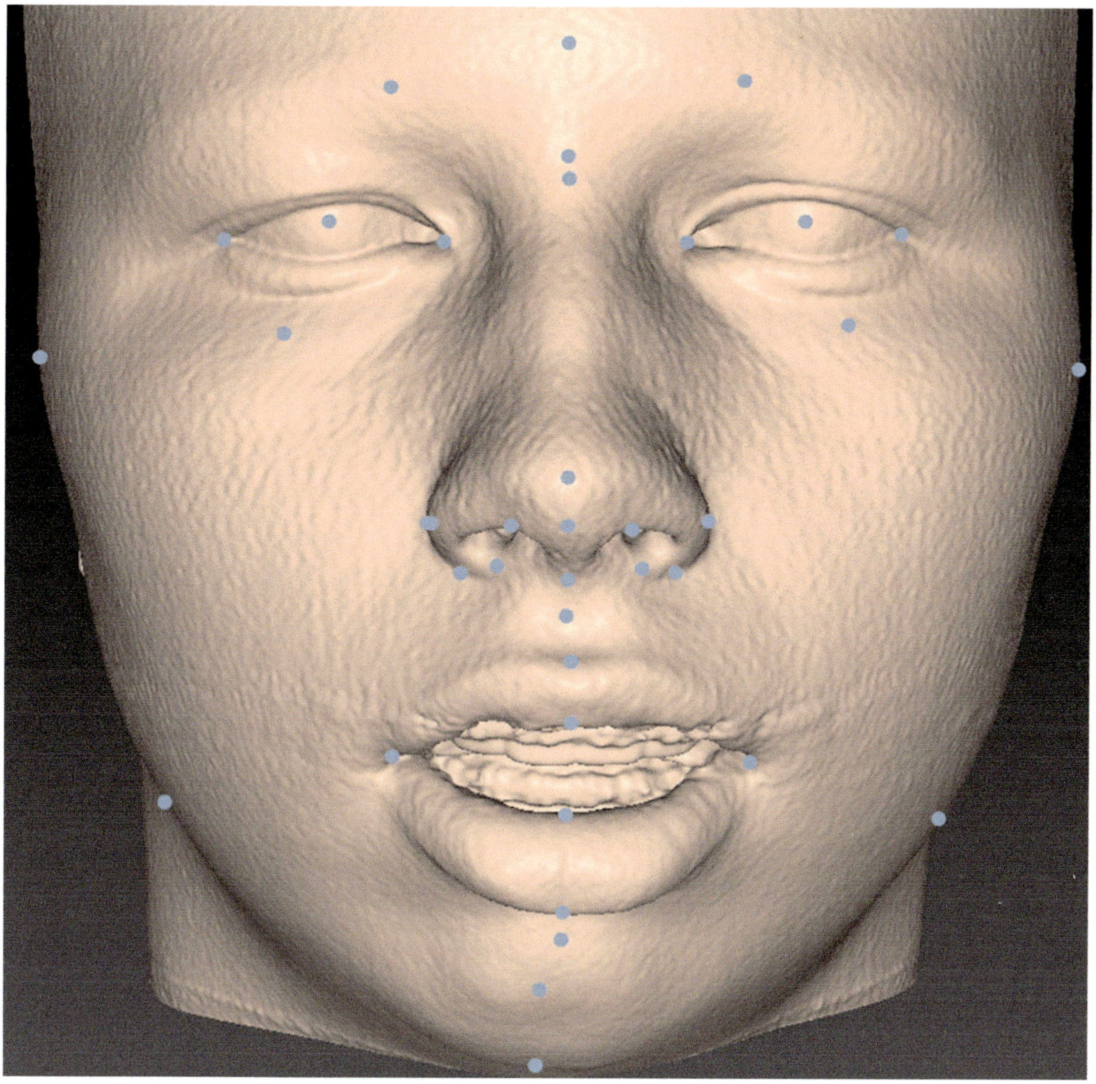

Fig. 2.211 Frontal view. Set-up of 3D cephalometric soft tissue landmarks. 3D "volume-rendered" representation of the patient's head (i-CAT, Imaging Sciences International Inc, IPS CaseDesigner ALPHA version, patient V.E.W.). Note that midpoint landmarks are positioned in the centre of each aesthetic unit and could therefore be out of the true facial midline

Set-Up of 3D Cephalometric Soft Tissue Landmarks

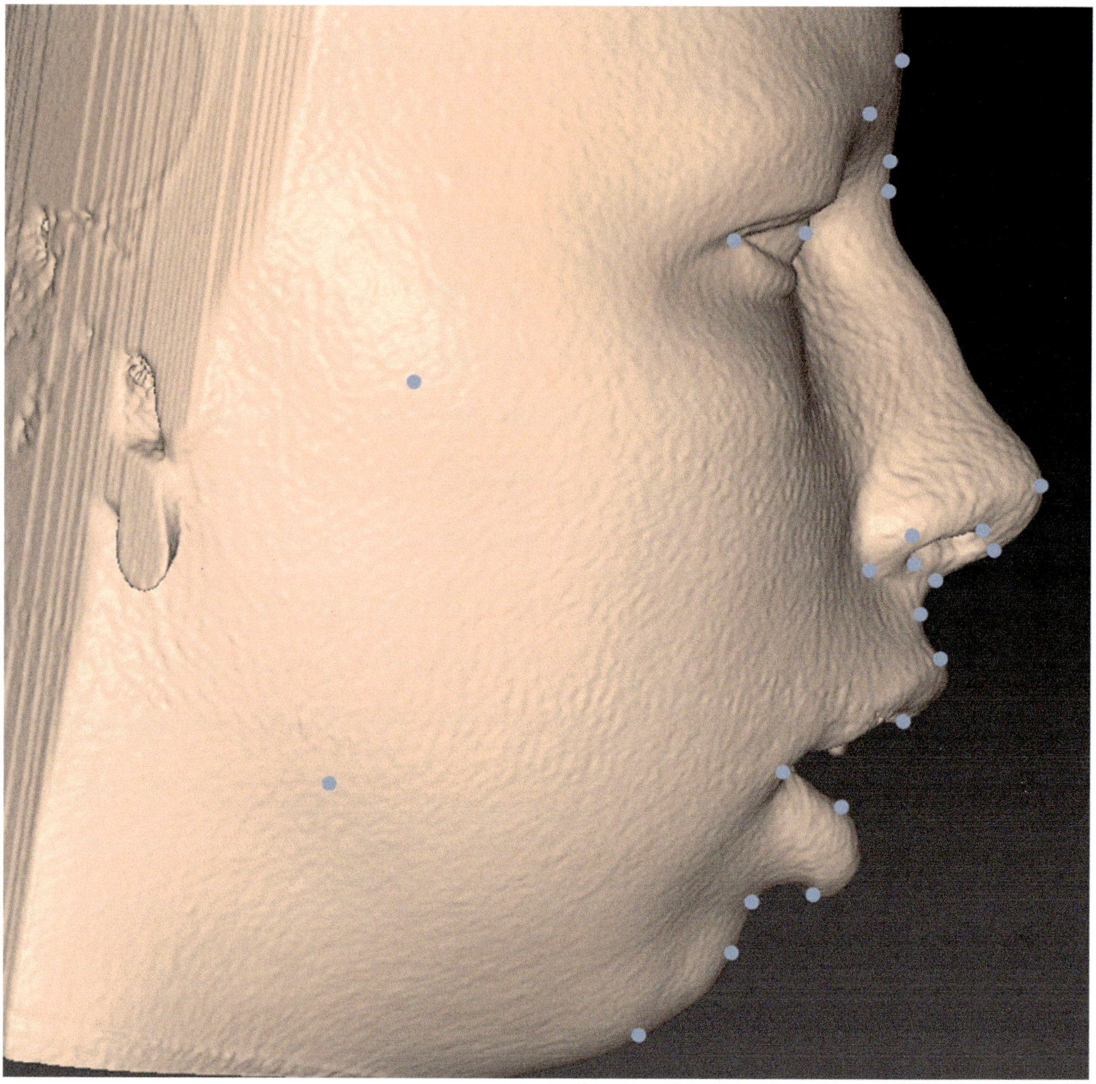

Fig. 2.212 Profile right view. Set-up of 3D cephalometric soft tissue landmarks. 3D "volume-rendered" representation of the patient's head (i-CAT, Imaging Sciences International Inc, IPS CaseDesigner ALPHA version, patient V.E.W.)

Set-Up of 3D Cephalometric Soft Tissue Landmarks

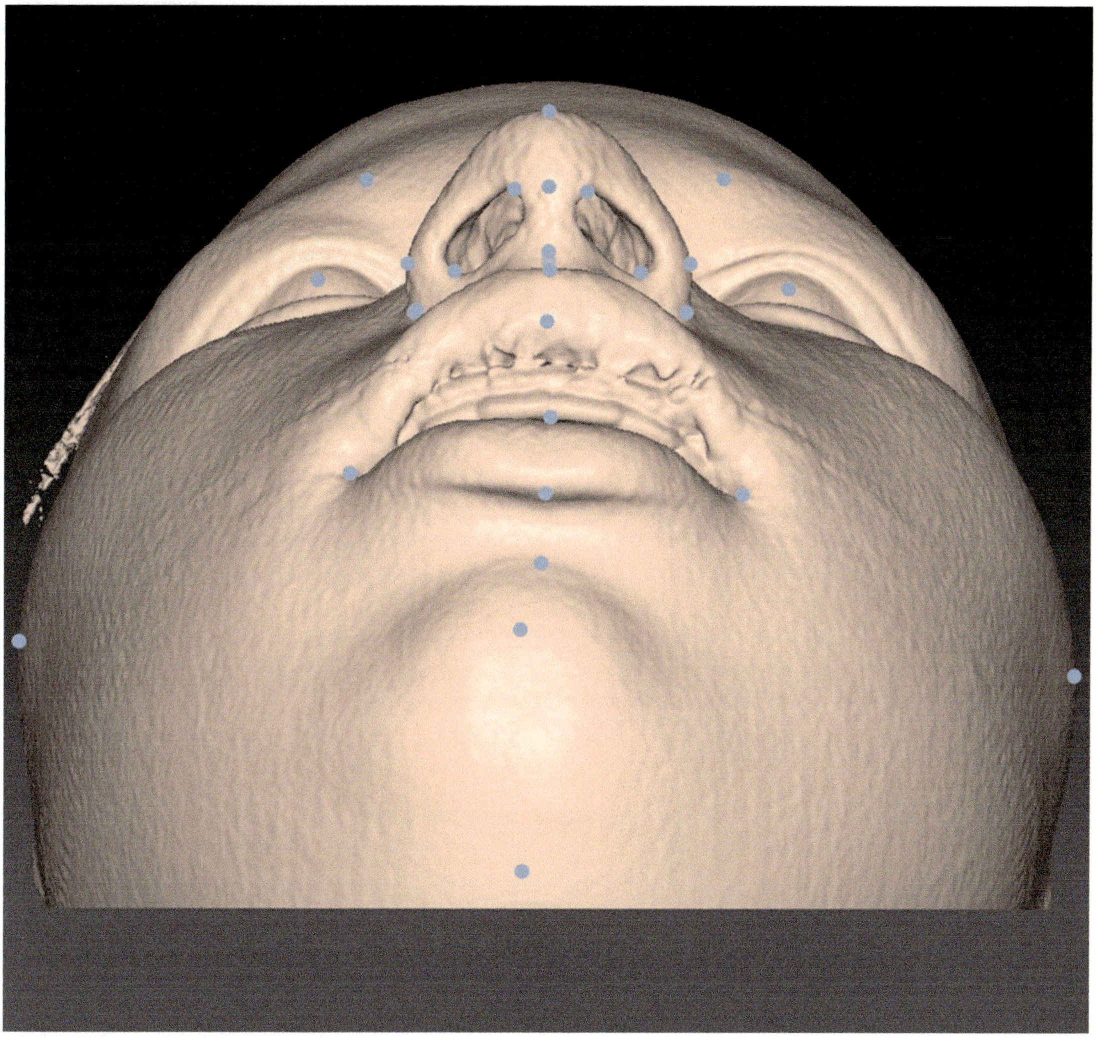

Fig. 2.213 Profile left view. Set-up of 3D cephalometric soft tissue landmarks. 3D "volume-rendered" representation of the patient's head (i-CAT, Imaging Sciences International Inc, IPS CaseDesigner ALPHA version, patient V.E.W.). Note that midpoint landmarks are positioned in the centre of each aesthetic unit and could therefore be out of the true facial midline

2

Additional 3D Cephalometric Soft Tissue Landmarks

The following list provides other anthropometric landmarks described by Farkas (1994) that could be implemented in 3D cephalometric soft tissue analysis.

> The clinician (orthodontist or surgeon) can modify his proper direct or indirect anthropometric landmarks towards 3D cephalometric soft tissue landmarks or even create new 3D cephalometric soft tissue landmarks.

- *maxillofrontale (mf).* The soft tissue point located at each lateral margin of the base of the nasal root at the level of the endocanthion *(en).*
- *eurion (eu).* Landmark defined as the most lateral point of the parieto-temporal region of the skull.
- *opisthocranion (op).* Landmark defined as the most posterior point of the occipital region of the head and the most distant from *glabella (g).*
- *otobasion inferius (obi).* Landmark defined as the point of attachment of the ear lobe to the cheek, which determines the lower border of the ear insertion.
- *otobasion superius (obs).* Landmark defined as the point of attachment of the helix in the temporal region, which determines the upper border of the ear insertion.
- *porion (soft) (po).* Landmark defined as the highest point on the upper margin of the cutaneous auditory meatus.
- *postaurale (pa).* Landmark defined as the most posterior point on the free margin of the ear.
- *preaurale (pra).* Landmark defined as the most anterior point of the ear, located at the level of the helix attachment to the head.
- *subaurale (sba).* Landmark defined as the lowest point on the free margin of the ear lobe.
- *superaurale (sa).* Landmark defined as the highest point on the free margin of the auricle.
- *tragion (t).* The point located at the upper margin of each tragus.
- *vertex (v).* Landmark defined as the highest point of the head when the head is orientated to the FH.

"Bruges 3D Soft Tissue Cephalometric Analysis"

The "Bruges Soft Tissue 3D Cephalometric Analysis" is based on the direct anthropometric measurements that have been used in the department of OMF in Bruges for more than 25 years (Fig. 2.214, 2.215 and 2.216).

The "Bruges 3D Soft Tissue Cephalometric Analysis" consists of:

1. Virtual definition of the natural head position (NHP) of the patient (▶ see also Sect. 3.1)
2. Generation of a 3D cephalometric reference frame (▶ see also Sect. 2.2.1)
3. Virtual definition of 18 soft tissue 3D cephalometric landmarks
4. Automated calculation of 11 linear, two angular and five proportional 3D cephalometric soft tissue measurements

A prospective ($n = 350$) study in (Swennen 2014) showed that the "Bruges 3D Soft Tissue Cephalometric Analysis" 3D-VPS_2 could be performed in a more than acceptable time frame.

	Mean (min:s)	Range (min:s)
BSSO ($n = 90$)	2:41	2:31 – 2:45
BSSO and chin ($n = 18$)	2:43	2:34 – 2:48
Le Fort I and BSSO ($n = 163$)	2:38	2:27 – 2:41
Le Fort I, BSSO and chin ($n = 79$)	2:40	2:33 – 2:47

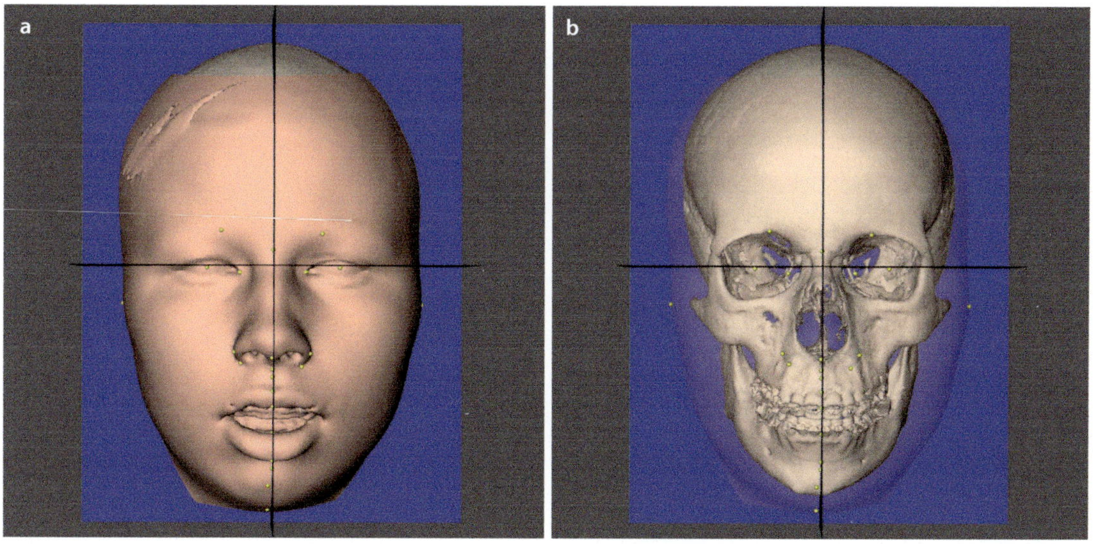

Fig. 2.214 Frontal view. Set-up of 3D soft tissue cephalometric landmarks of the "Bruges 3D Soft Tissue Cephalometric Analysis". 3D "surface-rendered" soft tissue representation of the patient's head (**a**), with transparent soft tissues (**b**) (i-CAT, Imaging Sciences International Inc, Maxilim v. 2.3.0.3., patient V.E.W.)

"Bruges 3D Soft Tissue Cephalometric Analysis"

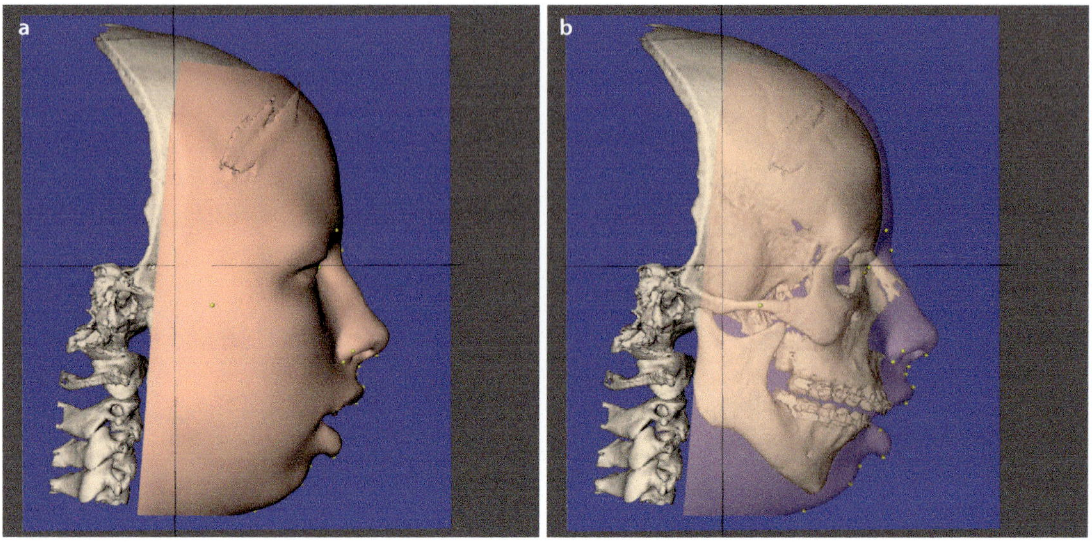

Fig. 2.215 Profile right view. Set-up of 3D soft tissue cephalometric landmarks of the "Bruges 3D Soft Tissue Cephalometric Analysis". 3D "surface-rendered" soft tissue representation of the patient's head (**a**), with transparent soft tissues (**b**) (i-CAT, Imaging Sciences International Inc, Maxilim v. 2.3.0.3., patient V.E.W.)

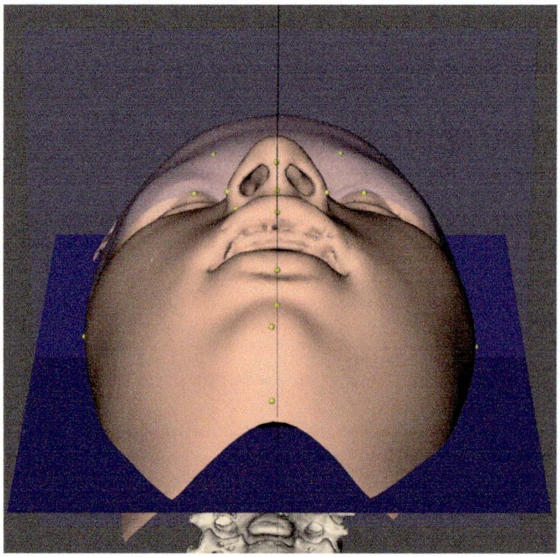

Fig. 2.216 Base view. Set-up of 3D soft tissue cephalometric landmarks of the "Bruges 3D Soft Tissue Cephalometric Analysis". 3D "surface-rendered" soft tissue representation of the patient's head (i-CAT, Imaging Sciences International Inc, Maxilim v. 2.3.0.3., patient V.E.W.)

Bruges 3D Soft Tissue Cephalometric Analysis

3D Cephalometry Analysis (3D-VPS$_2$) Report	
"Bruges 3D soft tissue cephalometric analysis"	
Patient name: VEW	
Physician Name: GS	
Linear measurement analysis (mm)	
Height of the lower face (sn-gn)	65.7
Height of the face according to da Vinci (right) (os_r-gn)	127.8
Height of the face according to da Vinci (left) (os_l-gn)	126.3
Height of the skin portion of the upper lip (philtrum) (sn-ls)	9.6
Height of the upper lip (sn-sto_u)	16.7
Interlabial gap (ILG) (sto_u-sto_l)	12.3
Height of the mandible (sto_l-gn)	36.7
Interpupillary distance (IPD) (p_r-p_l)	59.7
Intercanthal width (en_r-en_l)	29.7
Upper face width (zy_r-zy_l)	138.2
Morphological width of the nose according to Farkas (al_r-al_l)	33.6
Angular measurement analysis (deg)	
Nasolabial angle (c″-sn/ss-ls)	116.8
Mentolabial angle (li-sl-pg)	137.5
Proportional measurement analysis (%)	
Facial index (zy_r-zy_l) x 100/(sn-gn)	116.2
Bruges index(r) (p_r-p_l) x 100/(os_r-gn)	23.2
Bruges index(l) (p_r-p_l) x 100/(os_l-gn)	23.5
Height of the mandible/height of the lower face (sto_l-gn) x 100/(sn-gn)	55.9
Philtrum/height of the upper lip (sn-ls) x 100/(sn-sto_u)	57.6

See Video 2.1.

2.3 The Potential of 3D Mirroring and Colour Distance Maps in Enhanced Patient Diagnostics

After systematic virtual diagnosis of the patient's deformity, anatomy and pathology (▶ see Sect. 2.1) and subsequent 3D cephalometric analysis (▶ see Sect. 2.2), the "3D Virtual Visualisation Paradigm" (▶ see also Sect. 1.1.1), offers the clinician (both orthodontists and surgeons) some additional virtual tools for more enhanced patient diagnostics:

1. 3D virtual mirroring
2. Colour distance maps

■ Case 1

Patient (V.E.W.) is used to demonstrate these more enhanced features, while other patient's specific applications are demonstrated on other clinical cases (▶ see also Chaps. 4 and 6).

2.3.1 3D Virtual Mirroring

To assess overall facial symmetry or asymmetry of the patient's head, "3D virtual mirroring" can be used as an enhanced tool in the "3D virtual scene" to mirror both the patient's soft and hard tissues.

The most crucial issue in "3D virtual mirroring" is the virtual definition of the "3D virtual mirror plane", which needs to be defined by the clinician and is independent of cranial reference planes.

For overall assessment of facial symmetry or asymmetry, the "3D virtual mirror plane" is set up on the 3D soft tissues of the patient's head in its PHP position (▶ see also Sect. 3.1). It is therefore defined by the median ("z") plane of the "3D PHP cephalometric reference frame" (◘ Fig. 2.217–2.227). (▶ see also Sect. 2.2.1).

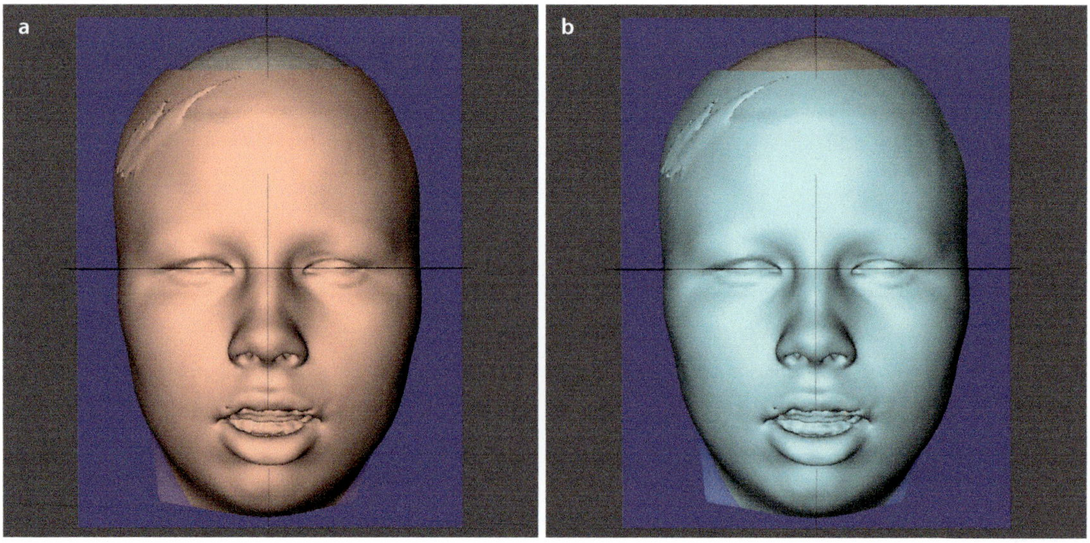

◘ **Fig. 2.217** Frontal view. The patient's head is positioned in the "3D virtual scene" towards its individual PHP with visualisation of the "3D PHP cephalometric reference frame" (**a**). The 3D "surface-rendered" soft tissue representation of the patient's head is virtually marked in blue (**b**) prior to "3D virtual mirroring" (i-CAT, Imaging Sciences International Inc, Maxilim v. 2.3.0.3., patient V.E.W.)

▪ 3D Virtual Mirroring of the Soft Tissues of the Patient's Head

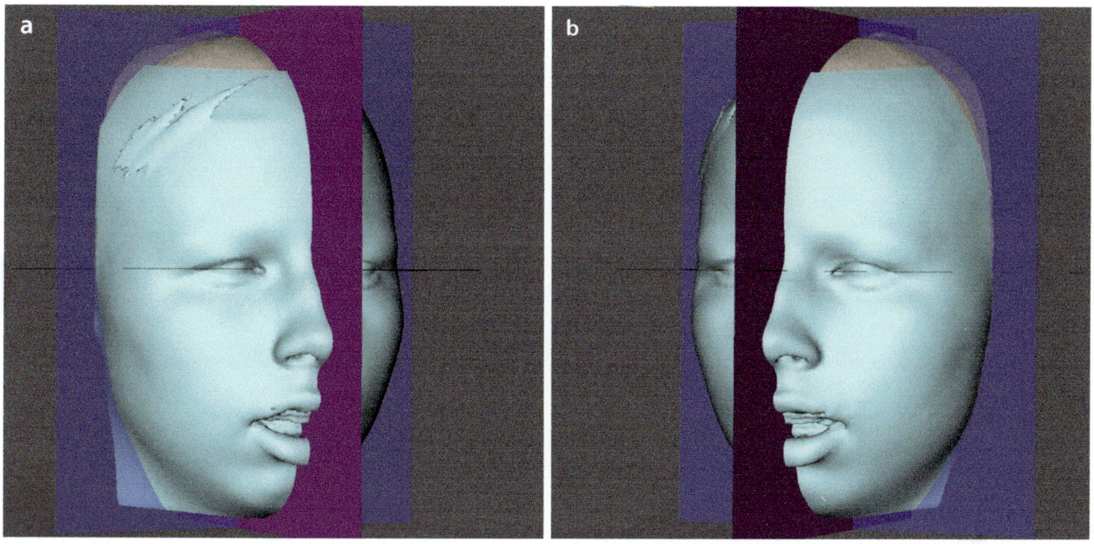

Fig. 2.218 Profile 2/3 right (**a**) and left (**b**) views. The patient's head is positioned in the "3D virtual scene" towards its individual PHP with visualisation of the "3D PHP cephalometric reference frame" and "3D virtual mirror plane (purple)". 3D "surface-rendered" soft tissue representations of the patient's head (i-CAT, Imaging Sciences International Inc, Maxilim v. 2.3.0.3., patient V.E.W.)

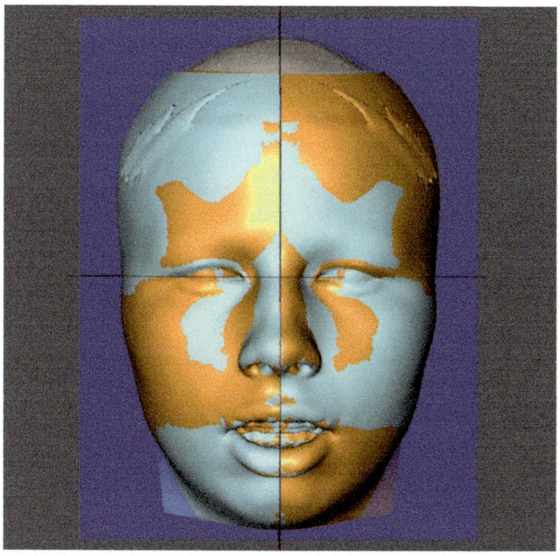

Fig. 2.219 Frontal view. 3D virtual mirroring of the soft tissues of the patient's head along the median (z) plane of the "3D PHP cephalometric reference frame" in the "3D virtual scene" (i-CAT, Imaging Sciences International Inc, Maxilim v. 2.3.0.3., patient V.E.W.)

3D Virtual Mirroring of the Soft Tissues of the Patient's Head

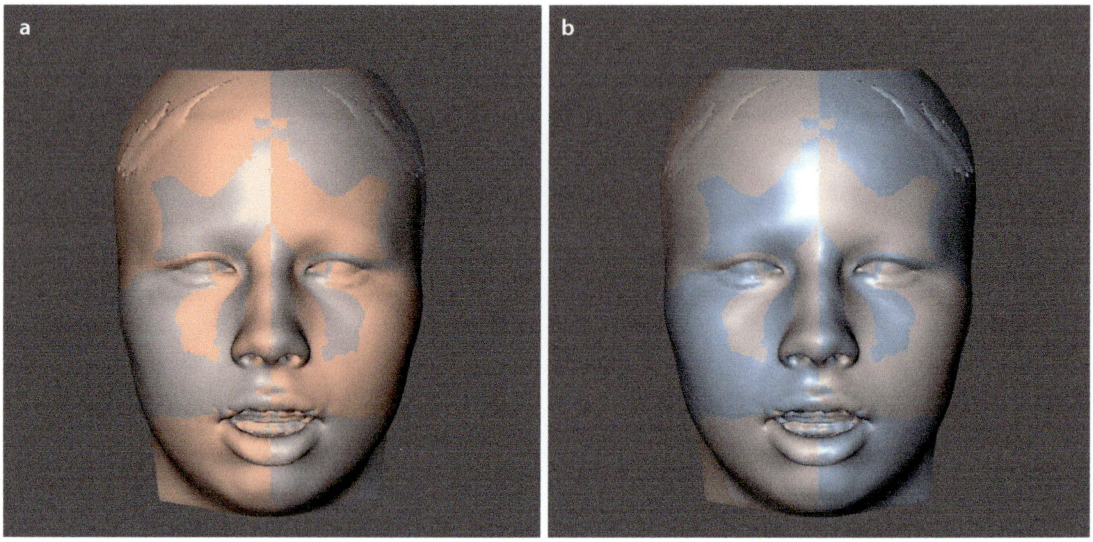

Fig. 2.220 Frontal view. "Transparent 3D virtual mirrored soft tissues" superimposed on the actual soft tissues (**a**) and 3D virtual mirrored soft tissues superimposed on "the actual soft tissues in transparency" (**b**) of the patient's head. (i-CAT, Imaging Sciences International Inc, Maxilim v. 2.3.0.3., patient V.E.W.). Note that 3D virtual mirroring does not identify obvious facial asymmetries

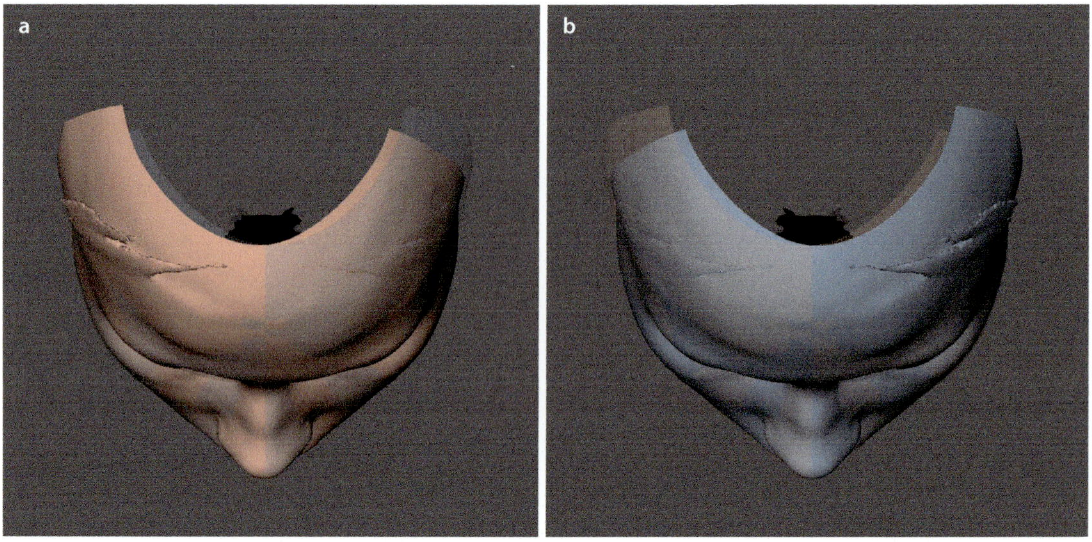

Fig. 2.221 Frontal downward inclined view. "Transparent 3D virtual mirrored soft tissues" superimposed on the actual soft tissues (**a**) and 3D virtual mirrored soft tissues superimposed on "the actual soft tissues in transparency" (**b**) of the patient's head. (i-CAT, Imaging Sciences International Inc, Maxilim v. 2.3.0.3., patient V.E.W.). Note that 3D virtual mirroring does not identify obvious facial asymmetries

3D Virtual Mirroring of the Soft and Hard Tissues of the Patient's Head

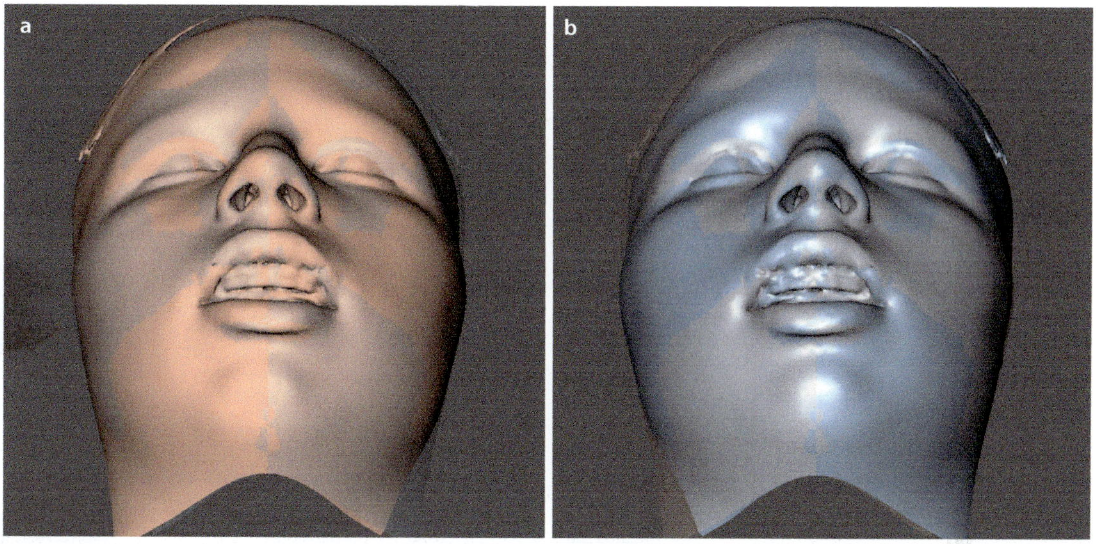

Fig. 2.222 Base view. "Transparent 3D virtual mirrored soft tissues" superimposed on the actual soft tissues (**a**) and 3D virtual mirrored soft tissues superimposed on "the actual soft tissues in transparency" (**b**) of the patient's head. (i-CAT, Imaging Sciences International Inc, Maxilim v. 2.3.0.3., patient V.E.W.). Note that 3D virtual mirroring does not identify obvious facial asymmetries

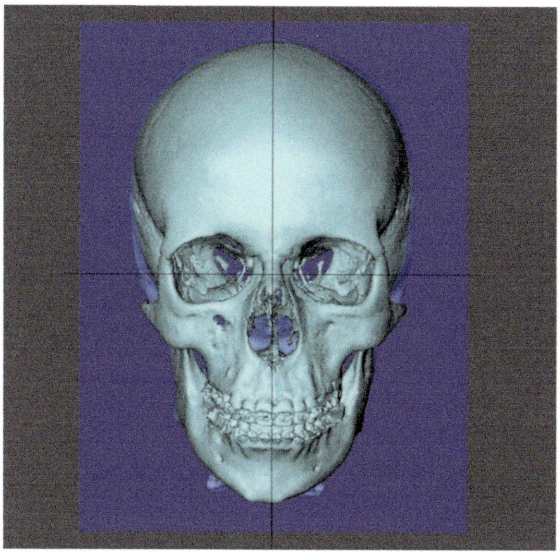

Fig. 2.223 Frontal view. The patient's head is positioned in the "3D virtual scene" towards its individual PHP with visualisation of the "3D PHP cephalometric reference frame". The 3D "surface-rendered" hard tissue representation of the patient's head is virtually marked in blue prior to "3D virtual mirroring" (i-CAT, Imaging Sciences International Inc, Maxilim v. 2.3.0.3., patient V.E.W.)

3D Virtual Mirroring of the Hard Tissues of the Patient's Head

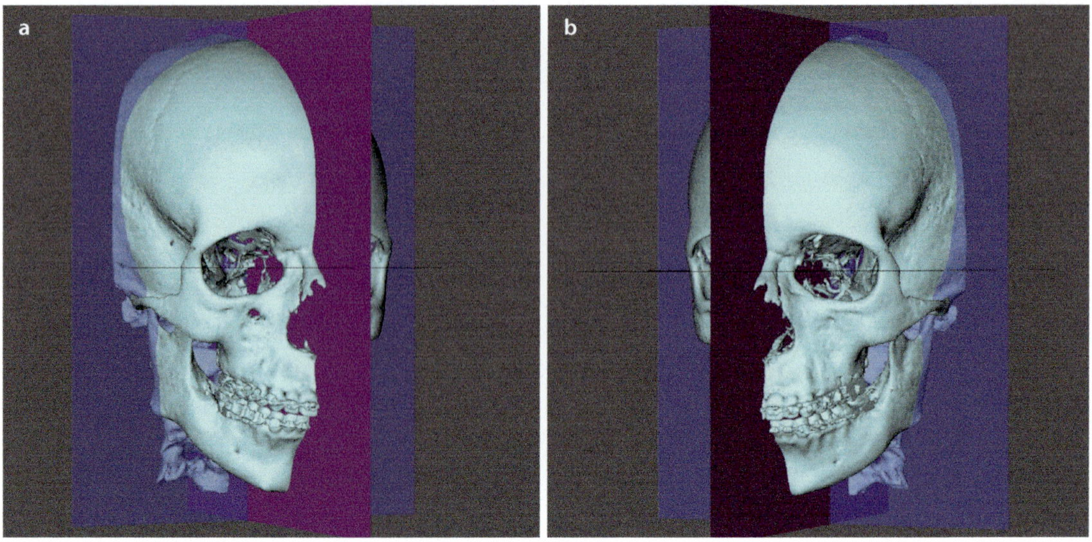

Fig. 2.224 Profile 2/3 right (**a**) and left (**b**) views. The patient's head is positioned in the "3D Virtual Scene" towards its individual PHP with visualisation of the "3D PHP Cephalometric Reference Frame" and "3D Virtual Mirror Plane (*purple*)". 3D "surface-rendered" hard tissue representations of the patient's head (i-CAT, Imaging Sciences International Inc, Maxilim v. 2.3.0.3., patient V.E.W.)

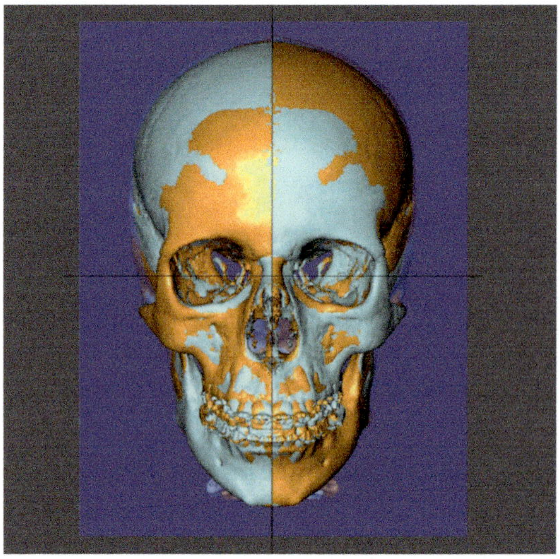

Fig. 2.225 Frontal view. 3D virtual mirroring of the hard tissues of the patient's head along the median (z) plane of the "3D PHP Cephalometric Reference Frame" in the "3D Virtual Scene" (i-CAT, Imaging Sciences International Inc, Maxilim v. 2.3.0.3., patient V.E.W.)

3D Virtual Mirroring of the Hard Tissues of the Patient's Head

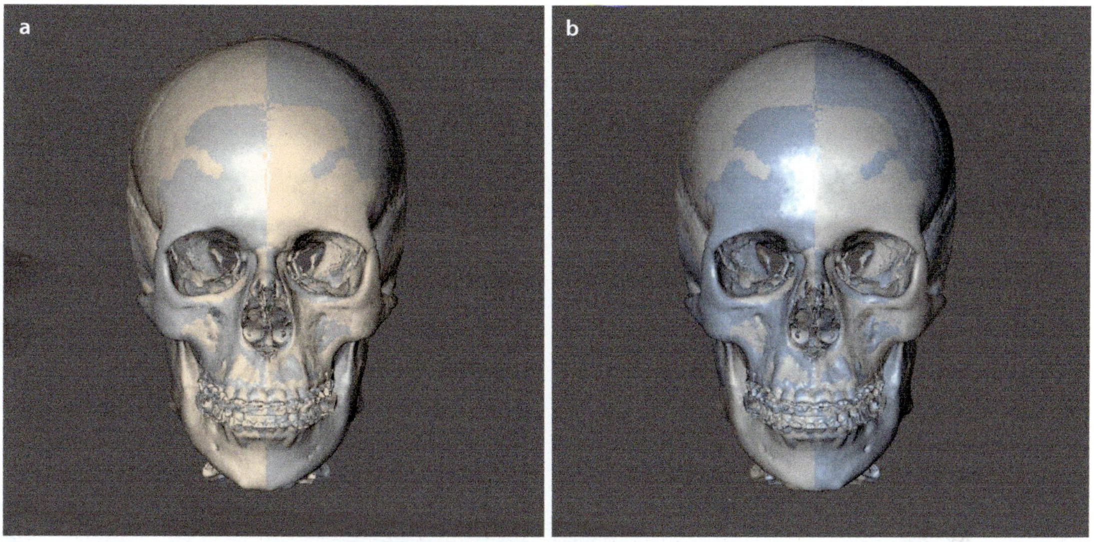

Fig. 2.226 Frontal view. "Transparent 3D virtual mirrored hard tissues" superimposed on the actual hard tissues (**a**) and 3D virtual mirrored hard tissues superimposed on "the actual hard tissues in transparency" (**b**) of the patient's head. (i-CAT, Imaging Sciences International Inc, Maxilim v. 2.3.0.3., patient V.E.W.). Note that 3D virtual mirroring identifies a skeletal mandibular asymmetry at the gonial angles and chin

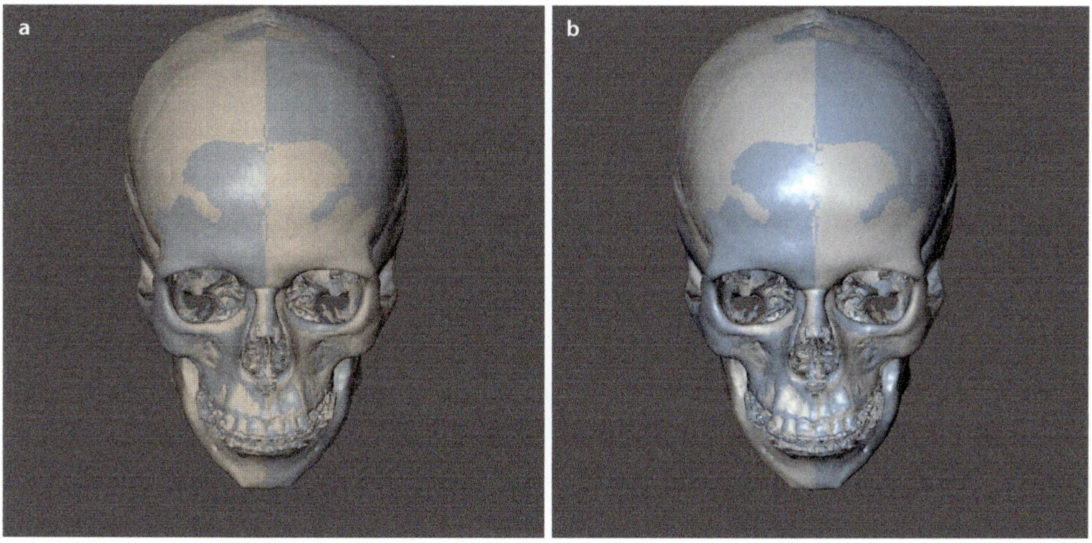

Fig. 2.227 Frontal downward inclined view. "Transparent 3D virtual mirrored hard tissues" superimposed on the actual hard tissues (**a**) and 3D virtual mirrored hard tissues superimposed on "the actual hard tissues in transparency" (**b**) of the patient's head. (i-CAT, Imaging Sciences International Inc, Maxilim v. 2.3.0.3., patient V.E.W.). Note that 3D virtual mirroring identifies a skeletal mandibular asymmetry at the gonial angles, mandibular border and chin

2.3.2 Colour Distance Maps

After "3D virtual mirroring", the "3D Virtual Visualisation Paradigm" allows (1) to calculate the inter-surface distance between the "original" and "3D mirrored" surface representations of the patient's head and (2) to visualise this inter-surface distance by "colour distance maps" (Fig. 2.228).

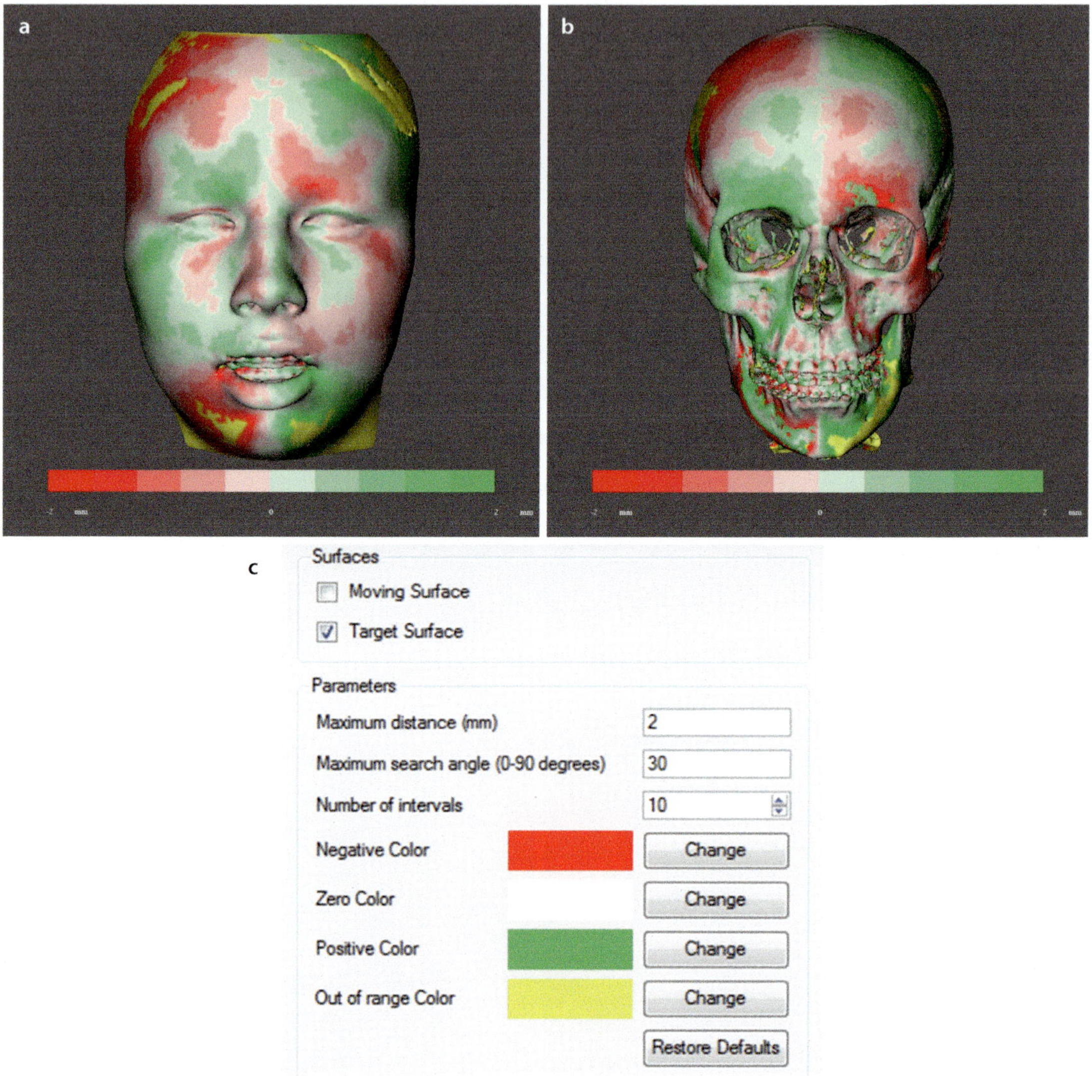

Fig. 2.228 Colour surface distance maps visualising the inter-surface distance between the "original" and "3D mirrored" soft (**a**) and hard (**b**) surface representations of the patient's head. (**c**) 3D virtual mirror parameters (i-CAT, Imaging Sciences International Inc, Maxilim v. 2.3.0.3., patient V.E.W.)

Additional Recommended Reading

Farkas LG (1994) Anthropometry of the head and face. Raven, New York

Gateno J, Xia JJ, Teichgraeber JF (2011) New 3-dimensional cephalometric analysis for orthognathic surgery. J Oral Maxillofac Surg 69:606–622

Guijarro-Martínez R, Swennen GR (2011) Cone-beam computerized tomography imaging and analysis of the upper airway: a systematic review of the literature. Int J Oral Maxillofac Surg 40:1227–1237

Guijarro-Martínez R, Swennen GR (2013) Three-dimensional cone beam computed tomography definition of the anatomical subregions of the upper airway: a validation study. Int J Oral Maxillofac Surg 42:1140–1149

Olszewski R, Frison L, Wisniewski M, Denis JM, Vynckier S, Cosnard G, Zech F, Reychler H (2013) Reproducibility of three-dimensional cephalometric landmarks in cone-beam and low-dose computed tomography. Clin Oral Investig 17:285–292

Proffit WR, Phillips C, Dann C, Turvey TA (1991) Stability after surgical-orthodontic correction of skeletal class III malocclusion I mandibular setback. Int J Adult Orthodon Orthognath Surg 6:7–18

Swennen GRJ (2005a) 3-D cephalometric reference system. In: Swennen GRJ, Schutyser F, Hausamen JE (eds) Three-dimensional cephalometry, vol 3. Springer, Heidelberg, pp 91–112

Swennen GRJ (2005b) 3-D cephalometric hard tissue landmarks. In: Swennen GRJ, Schutyser F, Hausamen JE (eds) Three-dimensional cephalometry, vol 4. Springer, Heidelberg, pp 113–181

Swennen GRJ (2005c) 3-D cephalometric soft tissue landmarks. In: Swennen GRJ, Schutyser F, Hausamen JE (eds) Three-dimensional cephalometry, vol 5. Springer, Heidelberg, pp 183–226

Swennen GRJ (2005d) 3-D cephalometric planes. In: Swennen GRJ, Schutyser F, Hausamen JE (eds) Three-dimensional cephalometry, vol 6. Springer, Heidelberg, pp 227–240

Swennen GRJ (2005e) 3-D cephalometric analysis. In: Swennen GRJ, Schutyser F, Hausamen JE (eds) Three-dimensional cephalometry, vol 7. Springer, Heidelberg, pp 241–288

Swennen GRJ (2014) Timing of three-dimensional virtual treatment planning of orthognathic surgery: a prospective single-surgeon evaluation on 350 consecutive cases. Oral Maxillofac Surg Clin North Am 26:475–485

Swennen GRJ, Schutyser F (2006) Three-dimensional cephalometry. Spiral multi-slice versus cone-beam CT. Am J Orthod Dentofac Orthop 130:410–416

Swennen GRJ, Schutyser F (2007) Three-dimensional virtual approach to diagnosis and treatment planning of maxillo-facial deformity. In: Bell WH, Guerrero CA (eds) Distraction osteogenesis of the facial skeleton, vol 6. Decker Inc, Hamilton, pp 55–79

Swennen GRJ, Schutyser F, Barth EL, De Groeve P, De Mey A (2006) A new method of 3-D cephalometry. Part I. The anatomic cartesian 3-D reference system. J Craniofac Surg 17:314–325

Xi T, van Loon B, Fudalej P, Bergé S, Swennen G, Maal T (2013) Validation of a novel semi-automated method for three-dimensional surface rendering of condyles using cone beam computed tomography data. Int J Oral Maxillofac Surg 42:1023–1029

3D Virtual Treatment Planning of Orthognathic Surgery

Gwen R.J. Swennen

Electronic supplementary material The online version of this chapter (doi:10.1007/978-3-662-47389-4_3) contains supplementary material, which is available to authorized users.

G.R.J. Swennen (ed.), *3D Virtual Treatment Planning of Orthognathic Surgery*,
DOI 10.1007/978-3-662-47389-4_3

3.1 The Virtual Natural Head Position (*v*-NHP) and Planning Head Position (PHP)

Treatment planning of orthognathic and orthofacial surgery needs to be based on the individual natural head position (NHP) of the patient, which is independent of intracranial reference planes and determined by the clinician.

The concept of NHP has been introduced in orthodontics approximately in the late 1950s by Downs (1956), Bjerin (1957) and Moorrees and Kean (1958). A standardised technique for registration of the patient's NHP was developed by Solow and Tallgren (1971), and the reproducibility of NHP was confirmed by Cooke and colleagues (1988, 1990, 1999). In order to incorporate NHP into cephalometrics, Lundström (1992, 1995) defined NHP as "the head orientation of the patient in a standing position with relaxed body and head posture looking at a distant point at eye level, perceived by the clinician based on general experience". Finally, Arnett and McLaughlin (2004) further maximised the contribution of NHP towards facial and dental planning in orthognathic surgery.

A new concept of "*c*-NHP", "*v*-NHP" and "PHP" towards 3D virtual treatment planning of orthognathic and orthofacial surgery in the clinical routine is introduced and outlined "step by step" in this chapter.

1. "**c-NHP**": For proper 3D virtual treatment planning of orthognathic and orthofacial surgery, the patient needs to be scanned in its "clinical natural head position (*c*-NHP)", in "centric relation (CR)" and without deformation of the facial soft tissue mask (▶ Chap. 1). The patient's head position and orientation during CBCT image acquisition unfortunately never correspond to its true *c*-NHP according to the author's experience. Xia and colleagues (2009) introduced a digital orientation device to record NHP in 3D. This apparatus consists of a digital orientation sensor attached to the patient through a facebow and bite jig. A limit of this technique is that the bite jig will invariably disturb lip morphology and posture. The use of lasers on the other hand (Damstra et al. 2010) can certainly help to record the patient's *c*-NHP.
2. "**v-NHP**": Virtual modification of the scanned head position of the patient is therefore necessary towards its *c*-NHP, which needs to be defined by the clinician, and will ultimately result in the "virtual modified natural head position (*v*-NHP)".
3. "**PHP**": The *v*-NHP finally corresponds to the individual "planning head position (PHP)" of the patient. A correct determination of the patient's individual PHP at the onset of 3D virtual treatment planning is of major clinical importance, since it defines the 3D PHP coordinate reference frame, which directly relates to:

- 3D cephalometric measurements of soft, hard tissues and teeth
- "Roll", "Yaw", "Pitch" and translational movements of the maxilla, mandible and chin

A "step-by-step" approach is described to virtually modify the patient's head position towards its *c*-NHP, which results in the *v*-NHP, or individual patient's PHP.

Attention
It is essential that the virtual modified natural head position (*v*-NHP) is determined by the clinician.

Case 1: Class II/1 Long-Face (Patient V.E.W.), Video

To illustrate the concept towards "step-by-step" integrated "individualised 3D virtual treatment planning" of orthognathic surgery, patient V.E.W. is used throughout the book (▶ Chaps. 1, 2, 4, 5 and 6) (◘ Figs. 3.1 and 3.2).

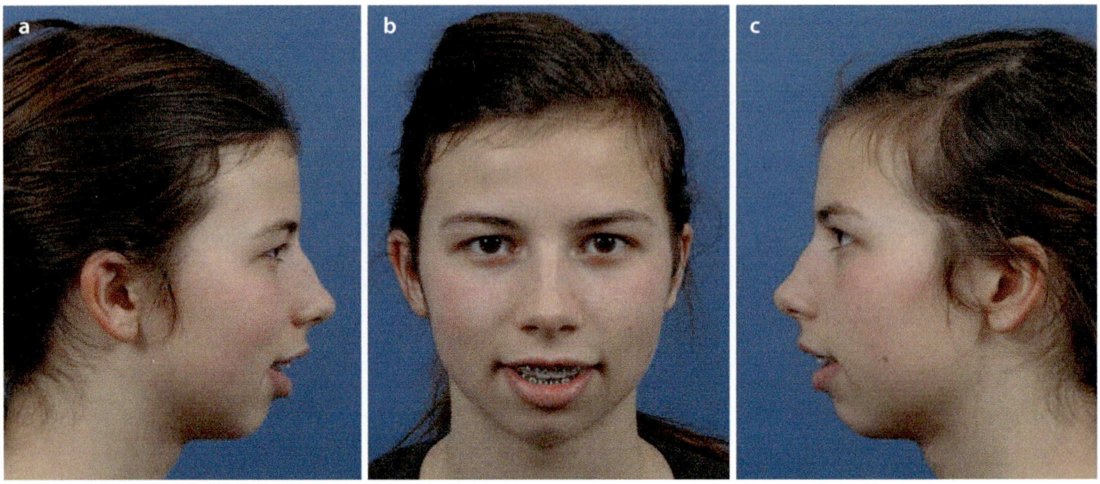

◘ **Fig. 3.1** Pre-surgical clinical right profile (**a**), frontal (**b**) and left profile (**c**) views in rest of a 16-year-old girl with Class II/1, long-face (> maxillary vertical excess) maxillofacial deformity, at the time of the workup (patient V.E.W.)

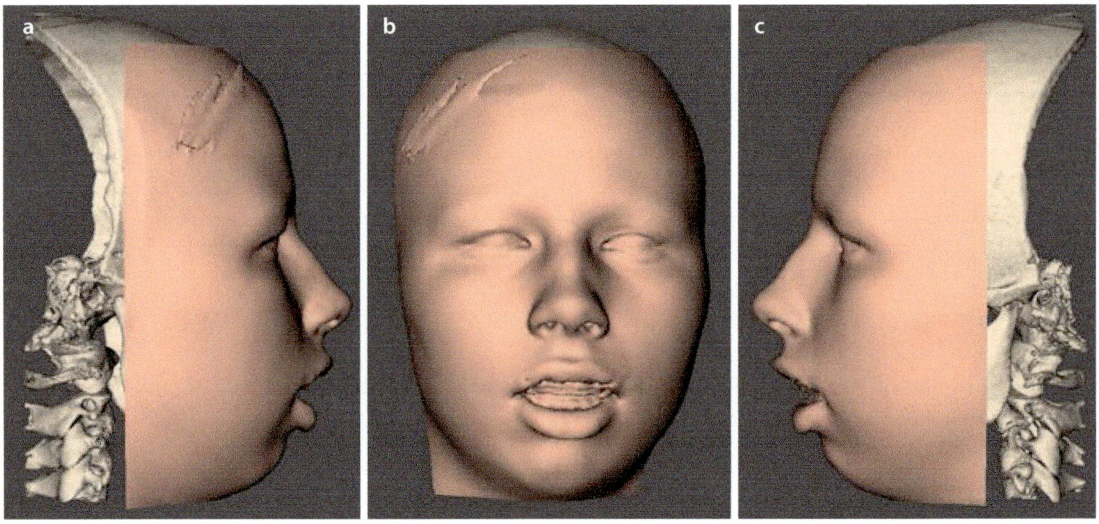

◘ **Fig. 3.2** Pre-surgical 3D "surface-rendered" soft and hard tissue representations of the patient's head, as generated during CBCT image acquisition, at the time of the workup. Right profile (**a**), frontal (**b**) and left profile (**c**) views (patient V.E.W., Maxilim v. 2.3.0.3). Note the incorrect position and orientation of the patient's head compared to the clinical pictures of the patient (◘ Fig. 3.1), although it was attempted to scan the patient in its correct NHP

▪ Virtual Modification of the Patient's Head Position Towards its Individual "*v*-NHP" or "PHP"

Step 1: Position and orientate the patient's skull in the frontal plane using paired "non-pathological" anatomical structures (e.g. the fronto-temporo-parietal bones, the bony orbits, the frontal process of the maxilla, the zygomatic arch, the zygomatic bone, the mastoid process, etc.) (▣ Figs. 3.3 and 3.4).

This step is essential since setting up the patient's *v*-NHP only based on its 3D soft tissues (▣ Fig. 3.5) could include a potential "Yaw" error in the individual patient's PHP. On clinical examination and during standardised clinical photography, correct symmetric positioning of the patient's ears in the frontal view allows to avoid incorrect "Yaw" rotations of the patient's head. Unfortunately, the ears are seldom incorporated in the 3D virtual model of the patient due to the limited FOV during CBCT image acquisition.

Step 2: Position and orientate the patient's 3D facial soft tissue mask in the frontal plane towards its *c*-NHP (▣ Figs. 3.5, 3.6 and 3.7). This "crucial" planning step should be based on precise evaluation of standardised clinical frontal photographs in rest and by clinical examination of the patient in both a vertical seated and standing position, ideally at different time intervals. In many patients, the horizontal *c*-NHP reference plane corresponds with the bi-pupillary plane.

- The clinician should especially be aware of patients with an habitual frontal modified *c*-NHP, compensating for an underlying facial asymmetry.
- Especially in patients with facial asymmetry, the horizontal *c*-NHP reference plane can be totally different than the bi-pupillary plane. In these cases, it can be helpful to additionally visualise the endocranial view and reorientate the patient's skull towards the crista galli and foramen magnum (▣ Fig. 3.8). This can be of particular interest in patients with orbital dystopia, cranial base asymmetry and torticollis, but also in patients with a habitual modified *c*-NHP.

Step 3: Position and orientate the patient's 3D facial soft tissue mask in the profile planes towards the vertical c-NHP reference plane which corresponds to the "True Vertical Plane (TVP)" (► see Chap. 2). This planning step should be based on evaluation of standardised clinical right and left photographs and by clinical examination of the patient in both a vertical seated and standing position (▣ Figs. 3.9–3.13).

Attention
The (*v*-NHP) corresponds to the individual patient's planning head position (PHP) which is crucial at the onset of 3D virtual treatment planning.

Step 1: Virtual Modification of the Patient's Head Position Towards its Individual "*v*-NHP" or "PHP"

Position and orientate the patient's skull in the frontal plane using paired "non-pathological" anatomical structures. "Step 1" is essentially performed by a combination of "Roll" and "Yaw" movements (► see also Sect. 3.4) of the skull of the patient.

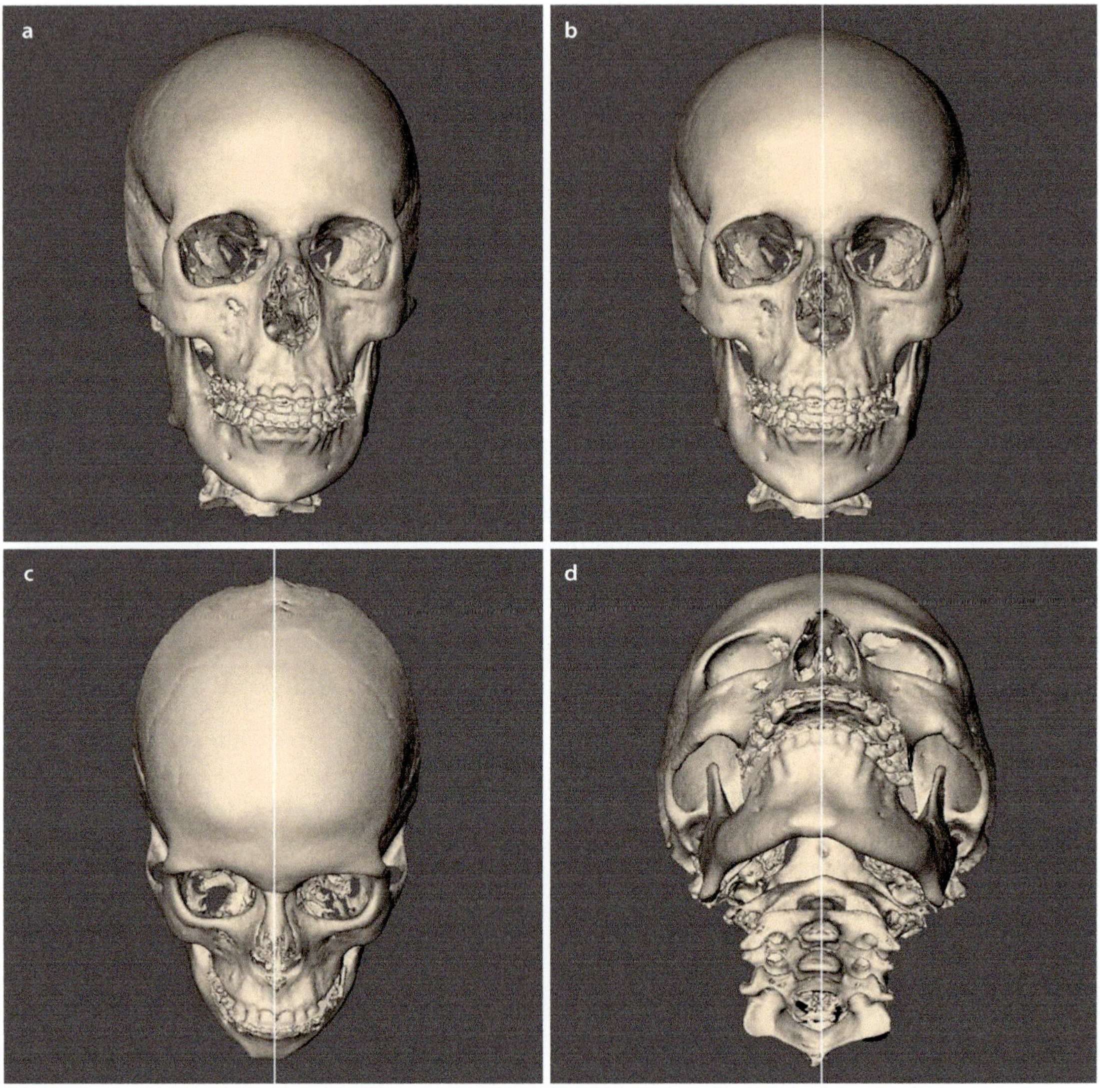

Fig. 3.3 The patient's skull (**a**) is orientated in the frontal plane using paired non-pathological anatomic structures: the temporal bones and bony orbits (**b**), the zygomatic arches (**c**) and the zygomatic bones (**d**) (3D "surface-rendered" representations, patient V.E.W., Maxilim v. 2.3.0.3)

Step 1: Virtual Modification of the Patient's Head Position Towards its Individual "*v*-NHP" or "PHP"

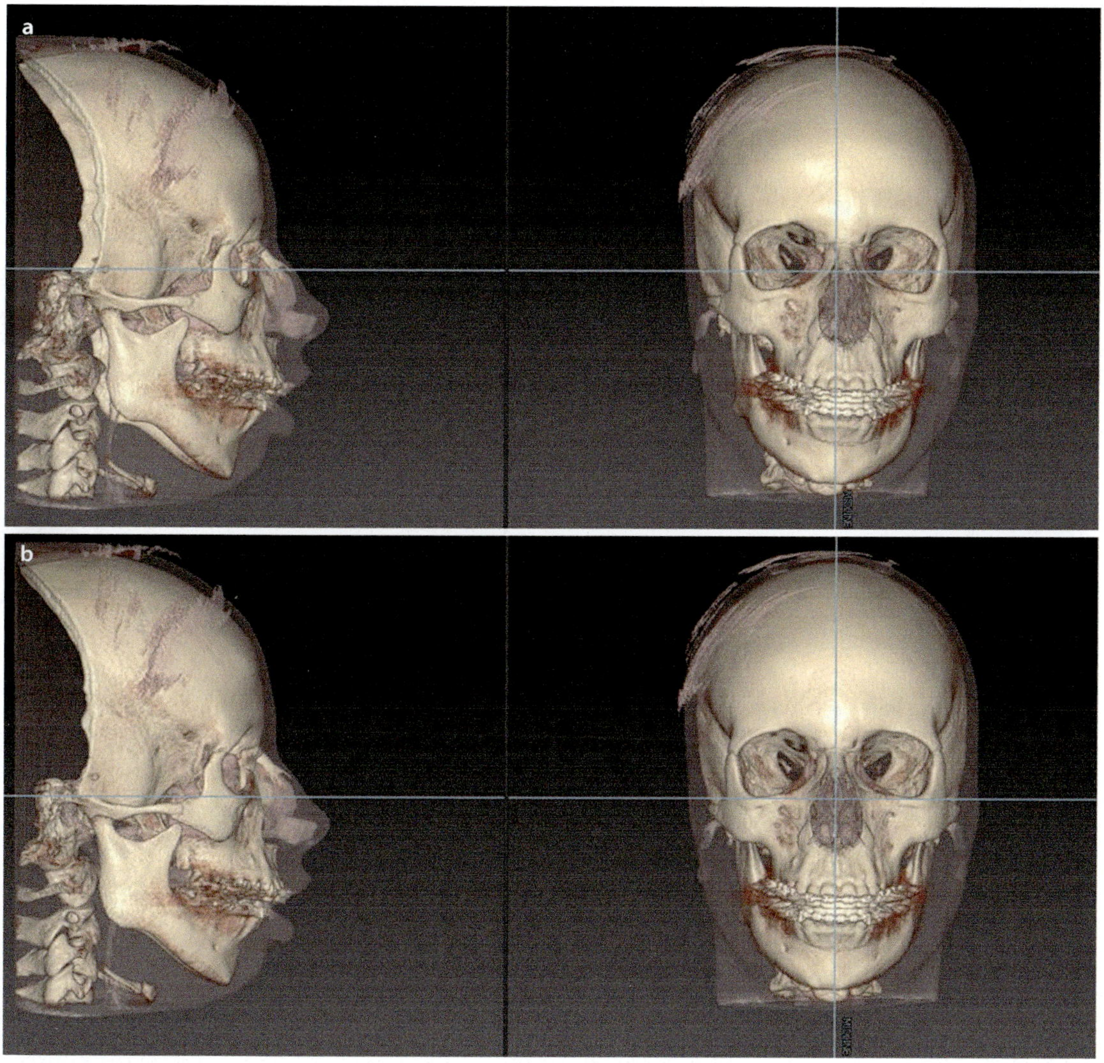

Fig. 3.4 The patient's skull (**a**) is semiautomatically oriented in the frontal plane (**b**) (3D "volume-rendered" representations, patient V.E.W, IPS CaseDesigner ALPHA version)

Step 2: Virtual Modification of the Patient's Head Position Towards its Individual "*v*-NHP" or "PHP"

Position and orientate the patient's 3D facial soft tissue mask in the frontal plane towards its *c*-NHP. "Step 2" is essentially performed by a "Roll" movement (▶ see also Sect. 3.4) of the patient's head.

Attention
As in conventional treatment planning of orthognathic surgery, the clinical NHP (*c*-NHP) of the patient is determined by the clinician.

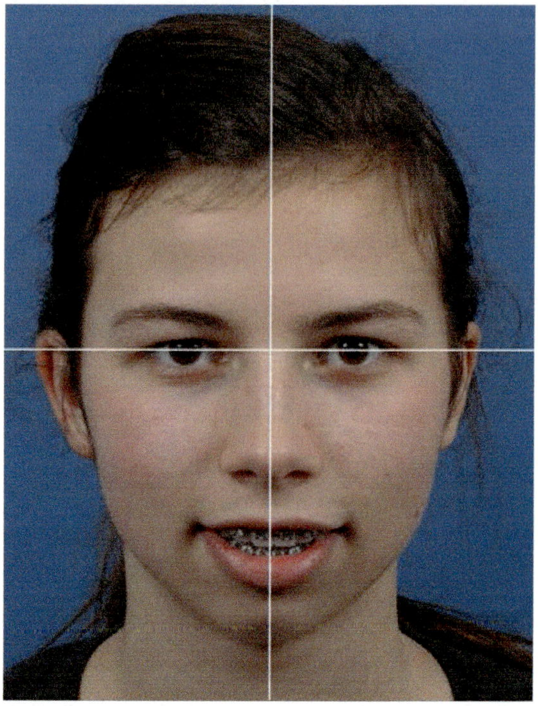

Fig. 3.5 Pre-surgical frontal view of the patient in its *c*-NHP in rest, at the time of the workup (patient V.E.W.)

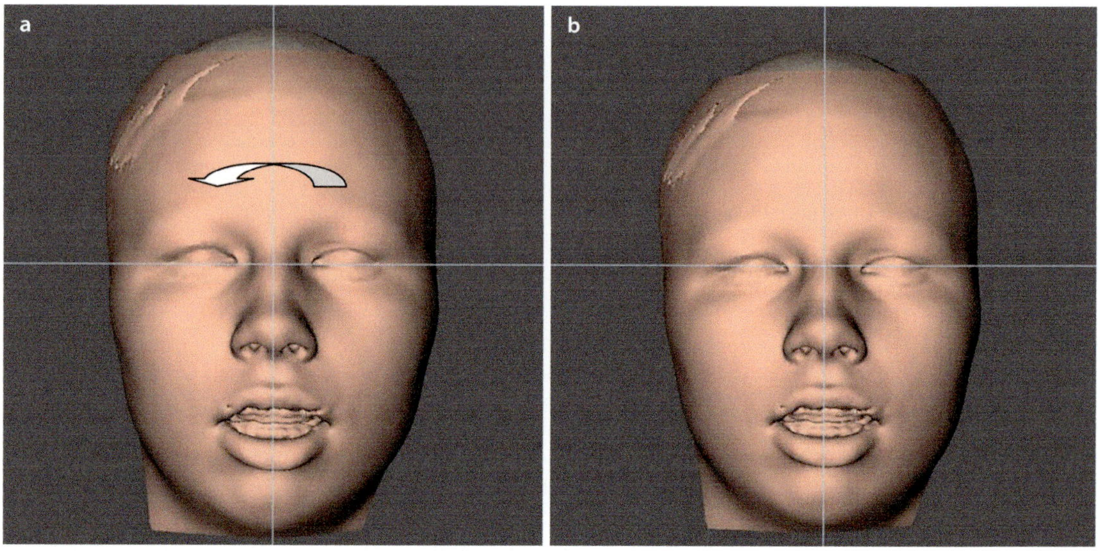

Fig. 3.6 The 3D facial soft tissue mask of the patient (**a**) is orientated in the frontal plane by a slight "Roll" of the patient's head towards its *c*-NHP (**b**) (3D "surface-rendered" representations, patient V.E.W., Maxilim v. 2.3.0.3)

Step 2: Virtual Modification of the Patient's Head Position Towards its Individual "v-NHP" or "PHP"

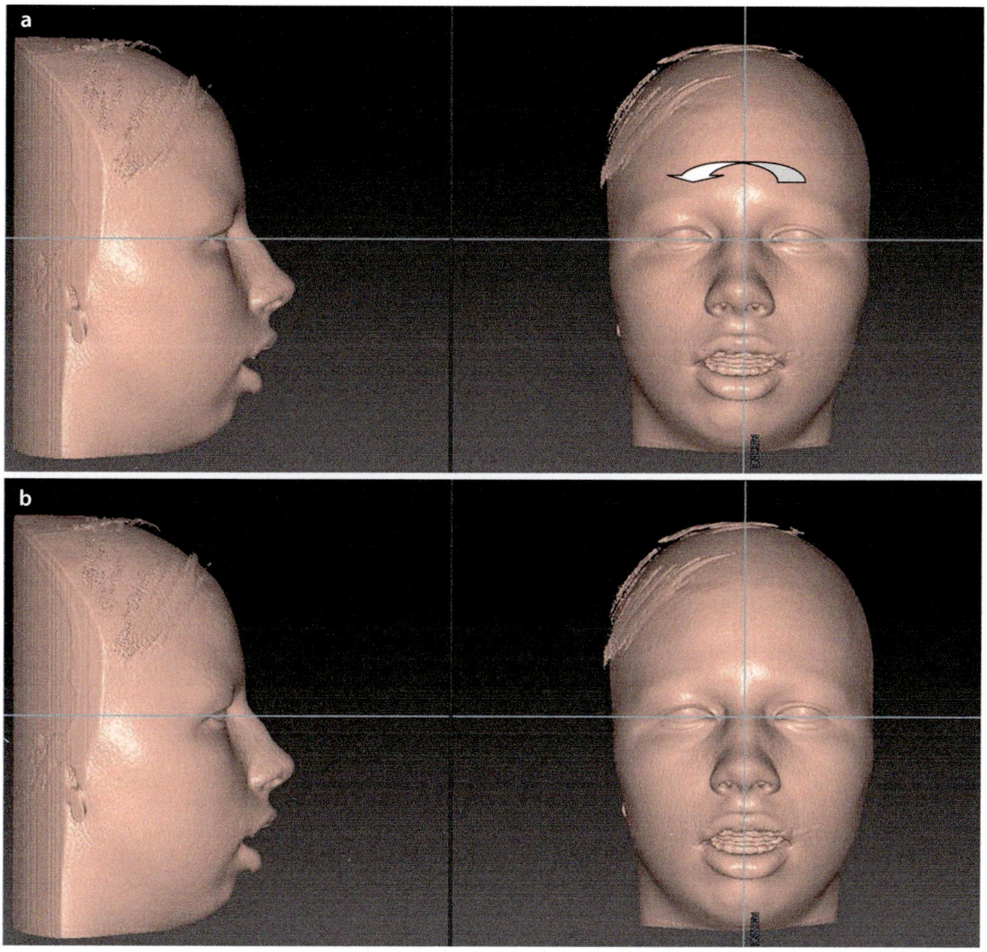

Fig. 3.7 The 3D facial soft tissue mask of the patient (**a**) is semiautomatically orientated in the frontal plane by a slight "Roll" of the patient's head towards its *c*-NHP (**b**) (3D "volume-rendered" representations, patient V.E.W., IPS CaseDesigner ALPHA version)

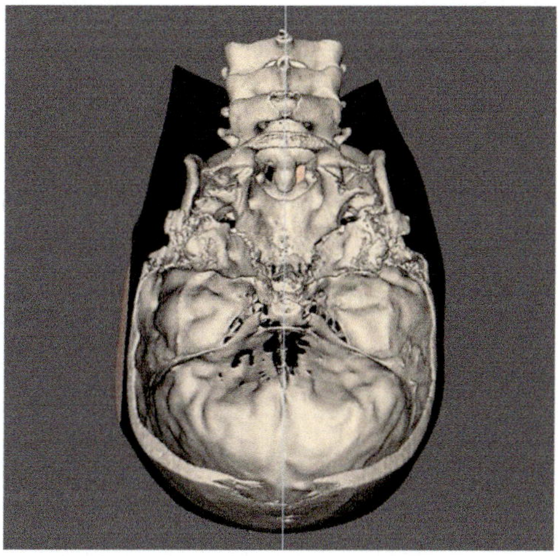

Fig. 3.8 The patient's head is rotated to the endocranial view to visualise the crista galli and the foramen magnum. Note that there is no significant cranial base asymmetry (3D "surface-rendered" representations, patient V.E.W., Maxilim v. 2.3.0.3)

Step 3: Virtual Modification of the Patient's Head Position Towards its Individual "*v*-NHP" or "PHP"

Position and orientate the patient's 3D facial soft tissue mask in the profile planes towards its *c*-NHP. "Step 3" is essentially performed by a "Pitch" movement (▶ see also Sect. 3.4).

Attention

The TVL (True Vertical Line) in conventional treatment planning becomes the TVP (True Vertical Plane) in 3D virtual treatment planning.

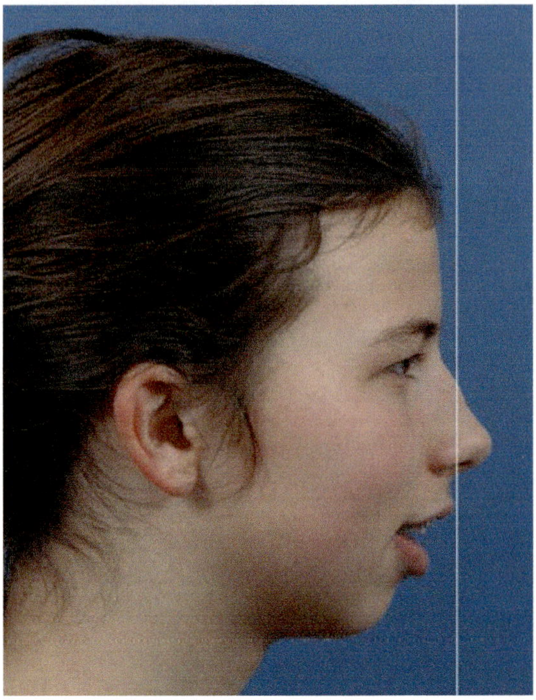

Fig. 3.9 Pre-surgical profile right view of the patient in its *c*-NHP in rest, at the time of the workup, with the TVL (True Vertical Line) visualised (patient V.E.W.)

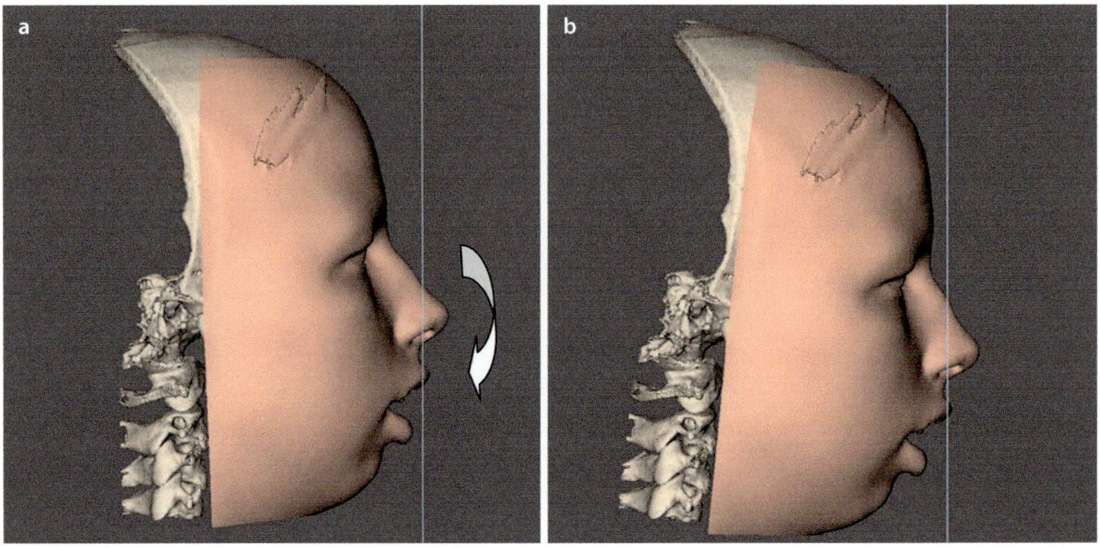

Fig. 3.10 The 3D facial soft tissue mask of the patient is orientated in the right profile plane (**a**) by a "Pitch" movement towards the TVP (True Vertical Plane) (**b**) (3D "surface-rendered" representations, patient V.E.W., Maxilim v. 2.3.0.3)

Step 3: Virtual Modification of the Patient's Head Position Towards Its Individual "v-NHP" or "PHP"

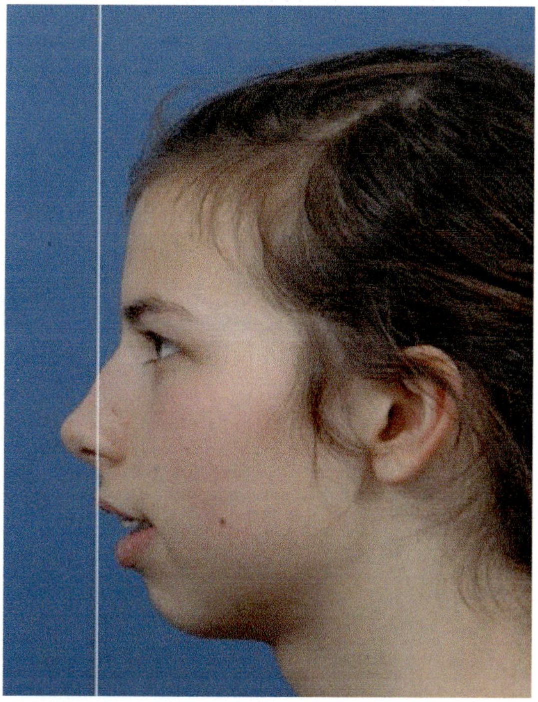

Fig. 3.11 Pre-surgical profile left view of the patient in its *c*-NHP, at the time of the workup, with the TVL (True Vertical Line) visualised (patient V.E.W.)

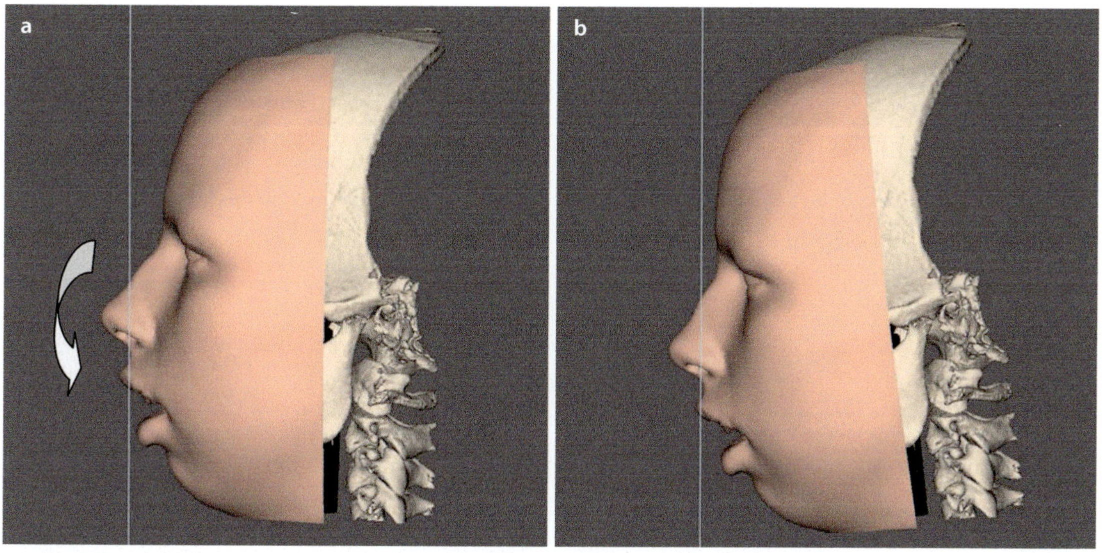

Fig. 3.12 The 3D facial soft tissue mask of the patient is orientated in the left profile plane (**a**) by a "Pitch" movement towards the TVP (True Vertical Plane) (**b**) (3D "surface-rendered" representations, patient V.E.W., Maxilim v. 2.3.0.3)

Step 3: Virtual Modification of the Patient's Head Position Towards Its Individual "v-NHP" or "PHP"

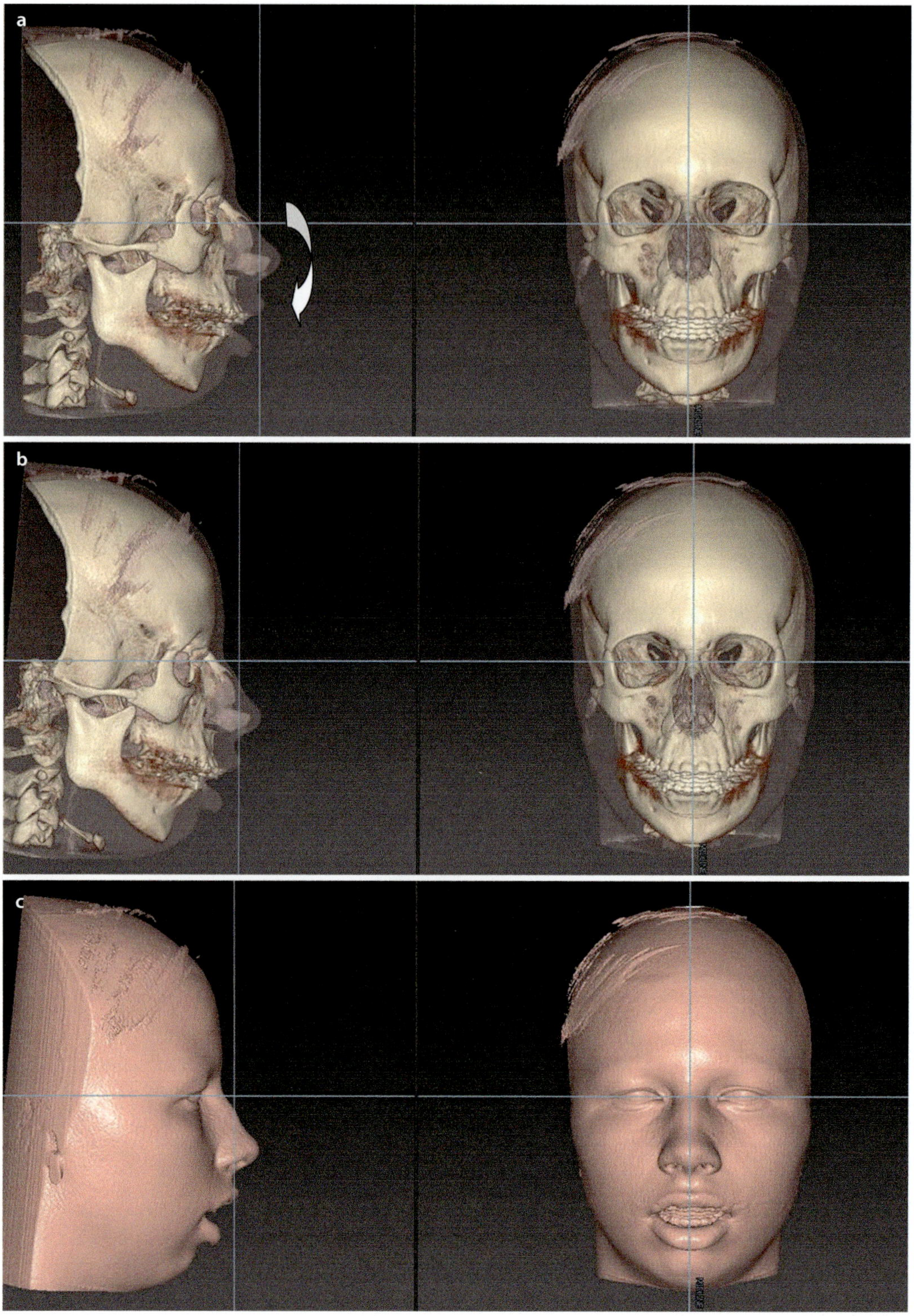

Fig. 3.13 The 3D facial soft tissue mask of the patient (**a**) is semiautomatically orientated in the left and right profile planes by a "Pitch" movement of the patient's head towards the TVP (True Vertical Plane) (**b, c**) (3D "volume-rendered" representations, patient V.E.W, IPS CaseDesigner ALPHA version)

3.2 3D Virtual Osteotomies ($3D\text{-}VPS_3$)

Compared to conventional treatment planning, the 3D virtual approach offers a major advantage. It allows the clinician to individually design the 3D virtual osteotomy planes in regard to the patient's specific (1) dento-maxillo-facial deformity and bite, (2) anatomy and (3) pathology.

A prospective ($n = 350$) study (Swennen 2014) showed that $3D\text{-}VPS_3$ (one-piece Le Fort I, bilateral sagittal split and chin osteotomy) could be virtually performed in a clinical acceptable time frame (overall mean, 3:46 min; range, 3:44–3:48 min).

The 3D virtual approach allows to individually customise all type of osteotomies (▶ see also Sect. 3.2.4). It is crucial that during the entire 3D virtual planning process, the 3D virtual osteotomy planes of the patient can be modified at each step if necessary (◘ Figs. 3.14 to 3.26).

3.2.1 Le Fort I Osteotomy: Video

Attention

It is crucial that all 3D virtual osteotomy planes can be modified at each stage of the "10 step-by-step" protocol.

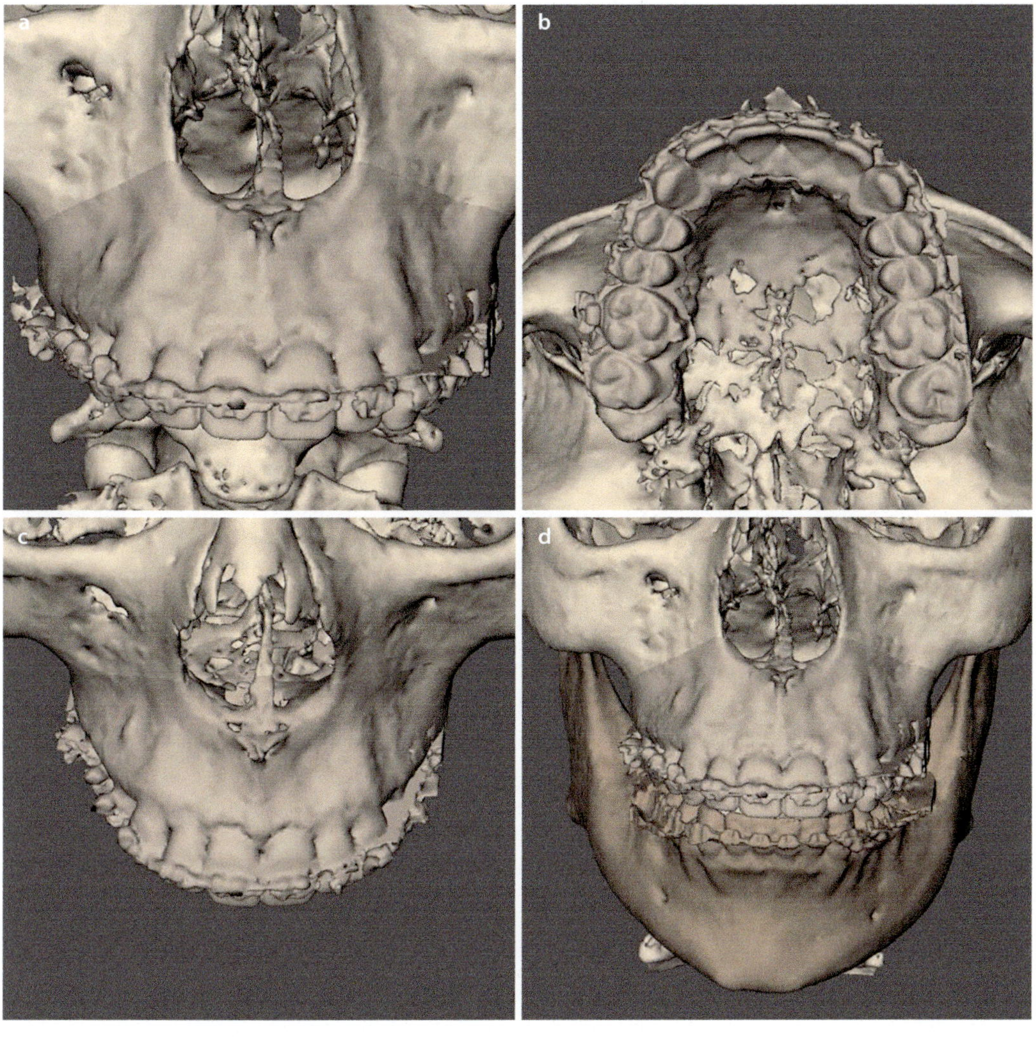

◘ **Fig. 3.14** 3D virtual one-piece Le Fort I osteotomy as it has virtually been planned (3D "volume-rendered" representations, patient V.E.W., Maxilim v. 2.3.0.3). (**a**) Frontal view (**b**) base view (**c**) 2/3 downward inclined view (**d**) full frontal view with mandible visualised

3.2.2 Bilateral Sagittal Split Osteotomy: Video

Advantage
The 3D virtual approach allows to individually customise the 3D virtual osteotomy planes.

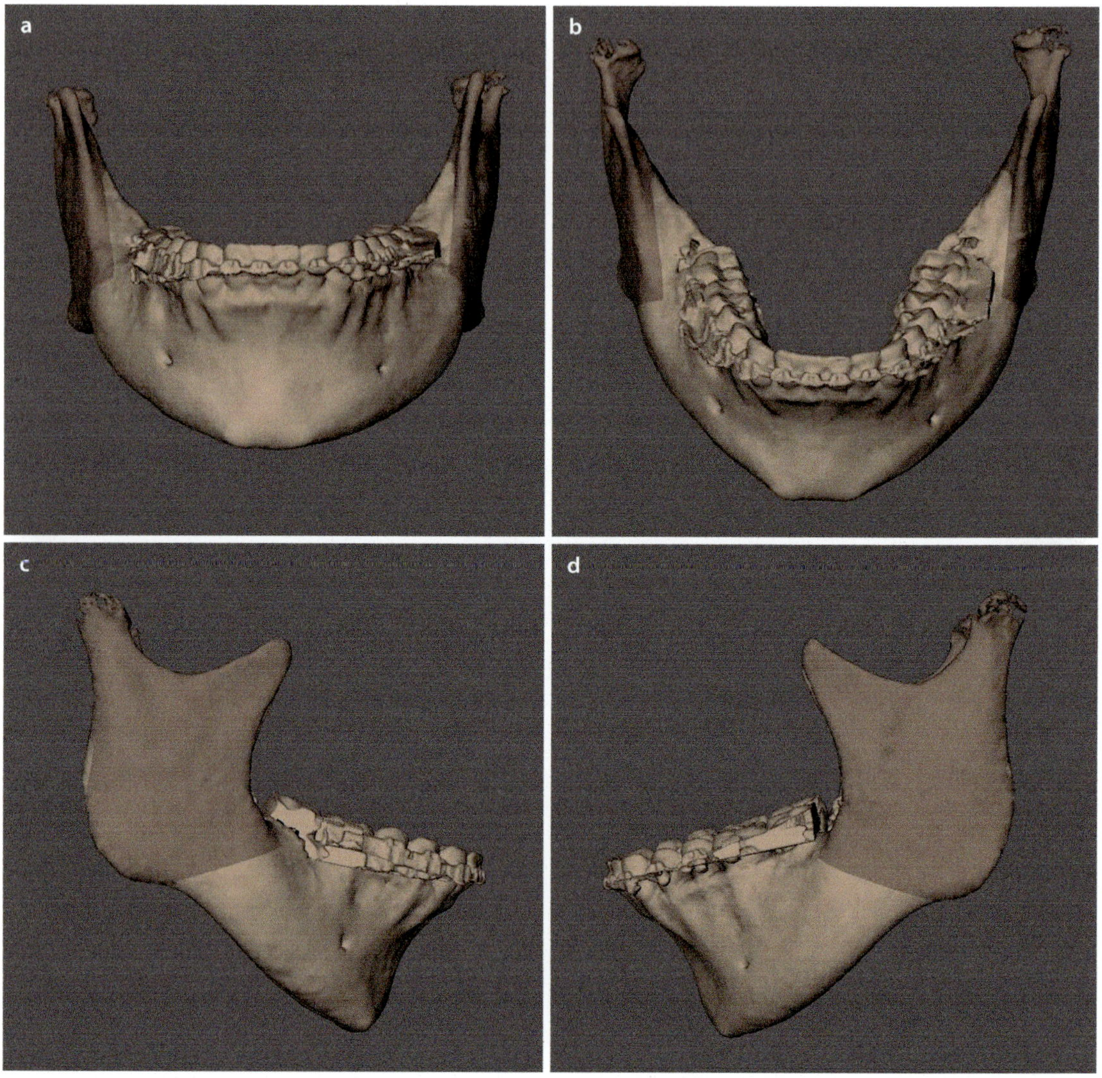

Fig. 3.15 3D virtual bilateral sagittal split osteotomy (BSSO) as it has virtually been planned. Note that the buccal corticotomy is inclined towards the ante-gonial notch (3D "surface-rendered" representations, patient V.E.W., Maxilim v. 2.3.0.3). (**a**) Frontal view (**b**) 2/3 downward inclined view (**c**) profile right view (**d**) profile left view

3.2.3 Chin Osteotomy: Video

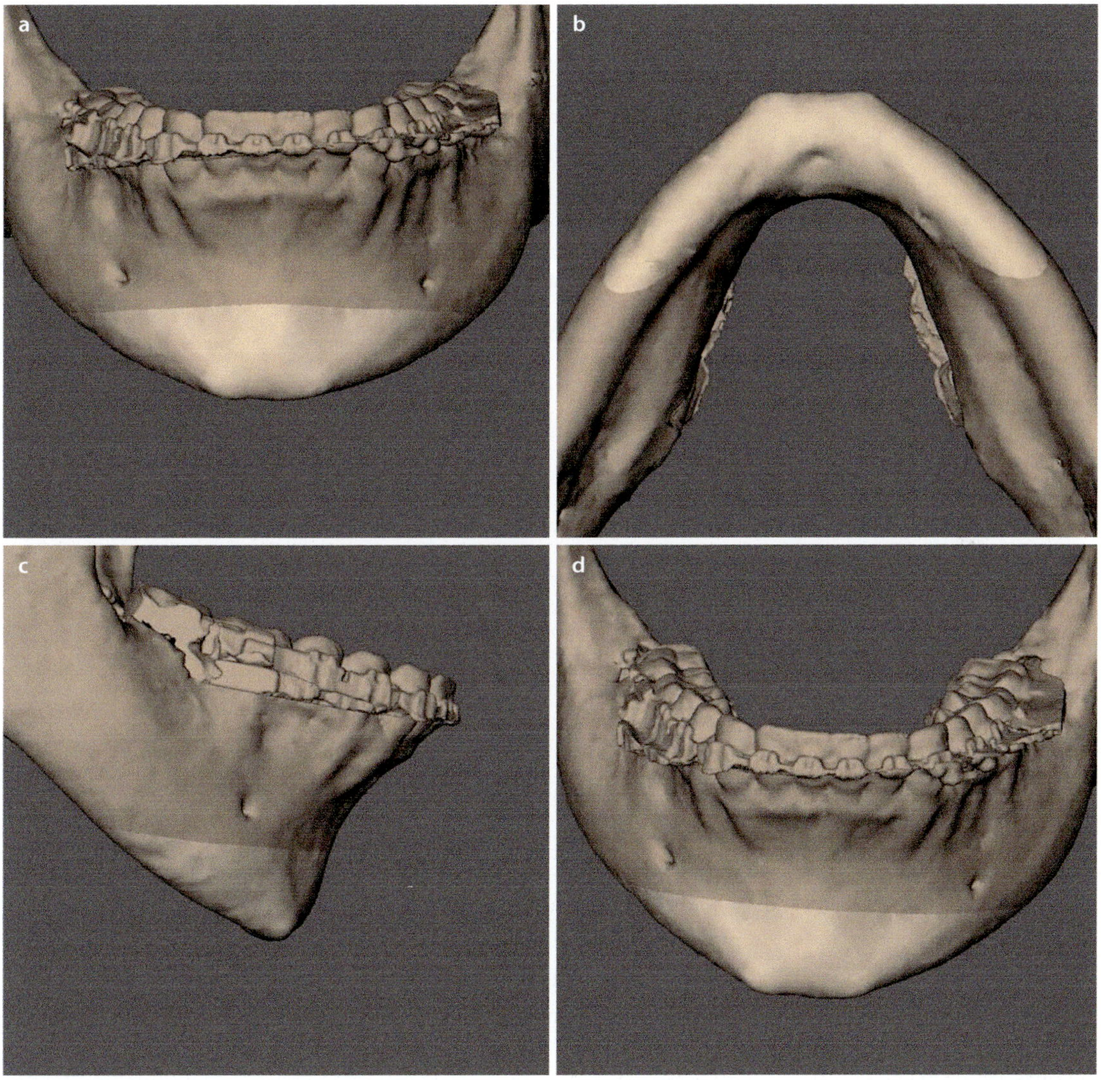

Fig. 3.16 3D virtual chin osteotomy as it has virtually been planned. Note that the foramen mentale are not on the same vertical level (3D "surface-rendered" representations, patient V.E.W., Maxilim v. 2.3.0.3). (**a**) Frontal view (**b**) base view (**c**) profile right view (**d**) frontal view in PHP

3.2.4 Additional Facial Osteotomies

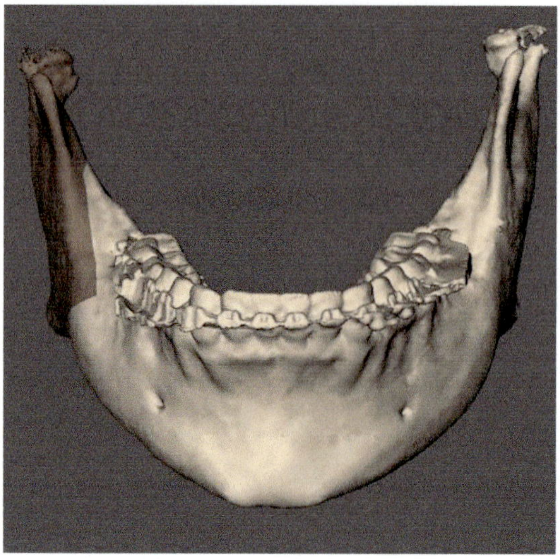

Fig. 3.17 Right unilateral sagittal split osteotomy (USSO) to illustrate additional osteotomies, which was clinically not performed on the patient (3D "surface-rendered" representations, patient V.E.W., Maxilim v. 2.3.0.3)

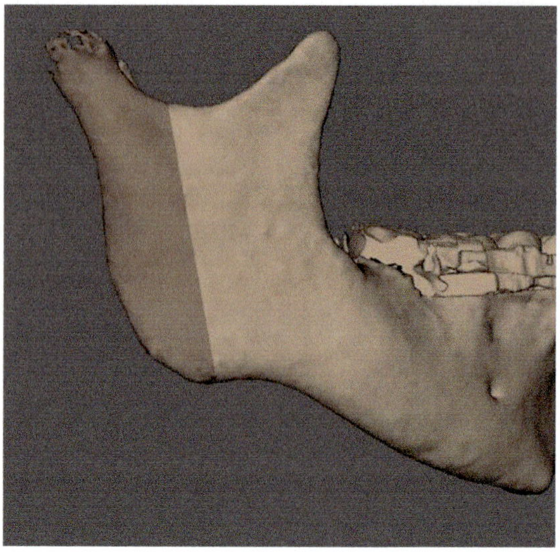

Fig. 3.18 Right vertical ramus osteotomy (VRO) to illustrate additional osteotomies, which was clinically not performed on the patient (3D "surface-rendered" representations, patient V.E.W., Maxilim v. 2.3.0.3)

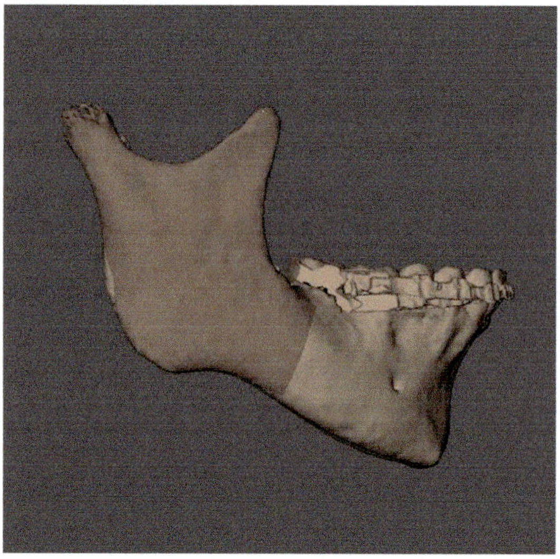

Fig. 3.19 Right SSO with vertical corticotomy according to Dal Pont to illustrate additional osteotomies, which was clinically not performed on the patient (3D "surface-rendered" representations, patient V.E.W., Maxilim v. 2.3.0.3)

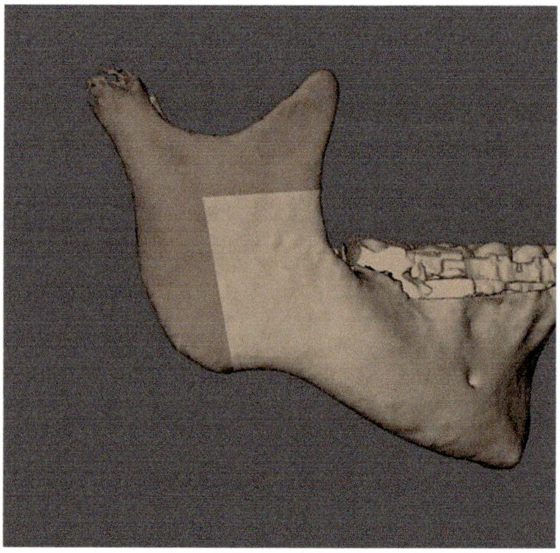

Fig. 3.20 Right inverted L-osteotomy to illustrate additional osteotomies, which was clinically not performed on the patient (3D "surface-rendered" representations, patient V.E.W., Maxilim v. 2.3.0.3)

Additional Facial Osteotomies

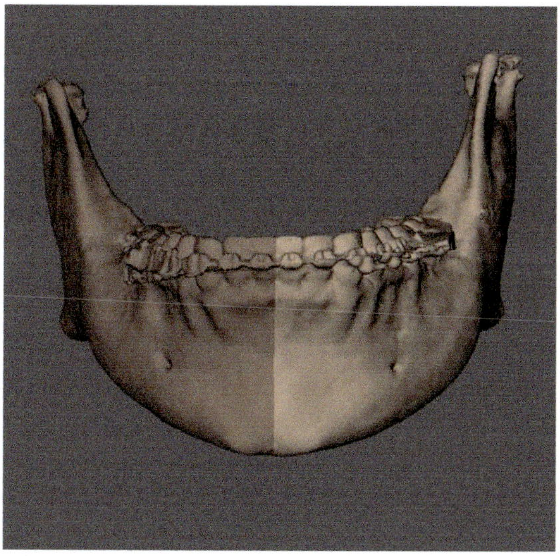

Fig. 3.21 Two-piece mandible midline osteotomy to illustrate additional osteotomies, which was clinically not performed on the patient (3D "surface-rendered" representations, patient V.E.W., Maxilim v. 2.3.0.3)

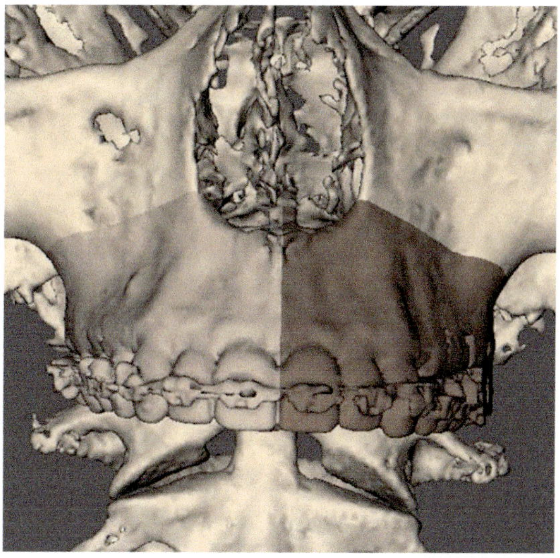

Fig. 3.22 Two-piece Le Fort I midline osteotomy to illustrate additional osteotomies, which was clinically not performed on the patient (3D "surface-rendered" representations, patient V.E.W., Maxilim v. 2.3.0.3)

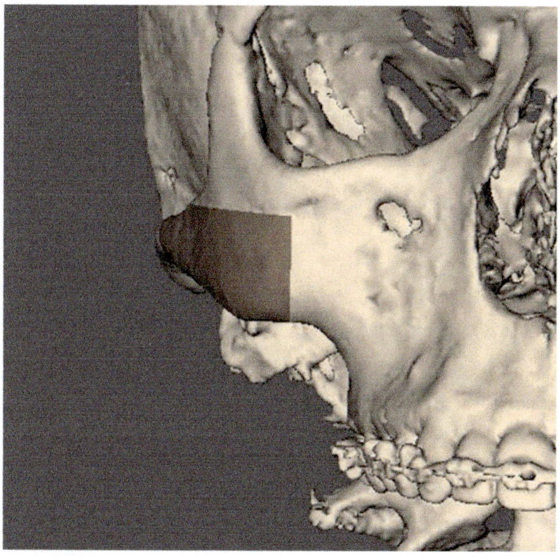

Fig. 3.23 3D virtual unilateral "zygoma" osteotomy according to Prof. M. Mommaerts to illustrate additional osteotomies, which was clinically not performed on the patient (3D "surface-rendered" representations, patient V.E.W., Maxilim v. 2.3.0.3)

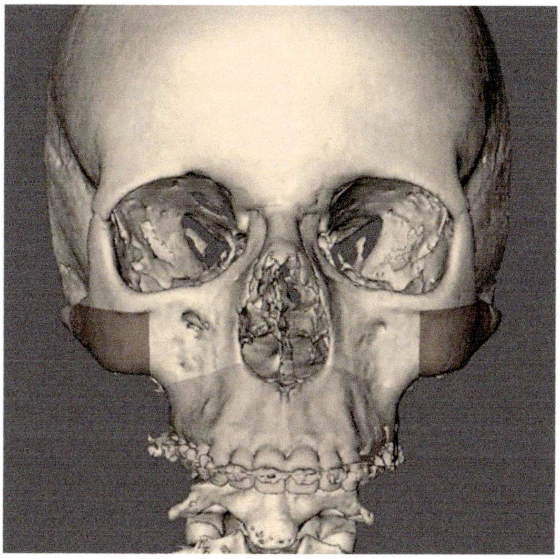

Fig. 3.24 3D virtual bilateral "zygoma" osteotomies according to Prof. M. Mommaerts, in combination with a one-piece Le Fort I osteotomy to illustrate additional osteotomies, which were not performed clinically on the patient (3D "surface-rendered" representations, patient V.E.W., Maxilim v. 2.3.0.3). Note that the foramen infraorbitale are not at the same level

Additional Facial Osteotomies

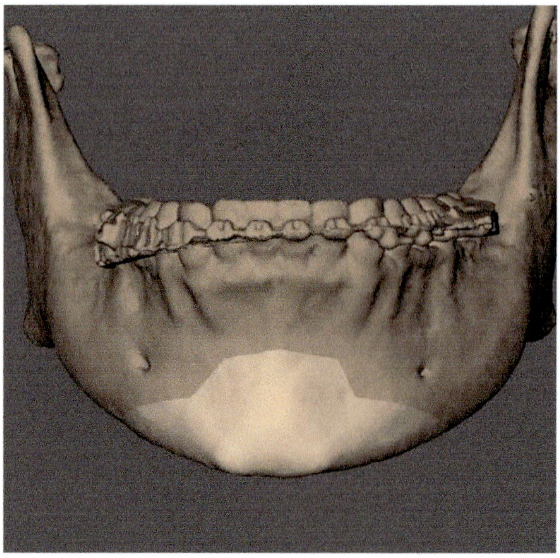

Fig. 3.25 3D virtual "chin shield" osteotomy to illustrate additional osteotomies, which was clinically not performed on the patient (3D "surface-rendered" representations, patient V.E.W., Maxilim v. 2.3.0.3)

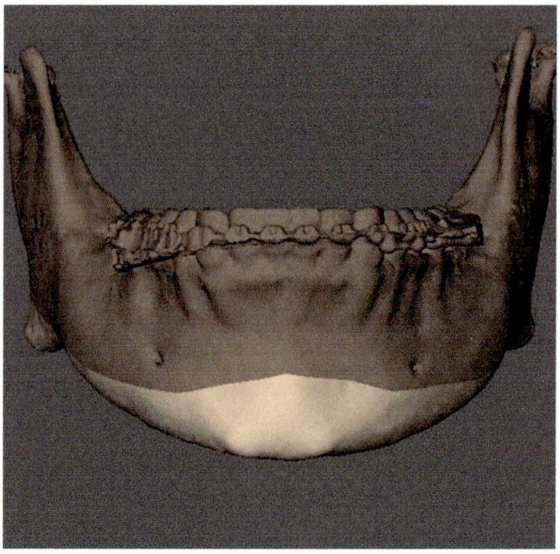

Fig. 3.26 3D virtual "chin wing" osteotomy according to Prof. A. Triaca to illustrate additional osteotomies, which was clinically not performed on the patient (3D "surface-rendered" representations, patient V.E.W., Maxilim v. 2.3.0.3)

3.3 3D Virtual Occlusal Definition ($3D\text{-}VPS_4$)

Compared to conventional treatment planning, "3D virtual occlusal definition" corresponds to conventional occlusal definition on plaster dental models" in non-segmental and segmental cases.

3.3.1 Non-segmental Occlusal Definition

Non-segmental occlusal definition can be performed either (1) virtually (without the use of plaster dental models) based on 3D upper and lower dentition models generated from scanning of impressions or intra-oral scanning (▶ see also Sect. 1.2) or (2) semi-virtually (with the use of plaster dental models).

▪ "Virtual" Non-segmental Occlusal Definition: Video

Virtual non-segmental occlusal definition is performed without the use of plaster dental models and has the inherent advantages: (1) to be faster in the clinical workflow compared to semi-virtual occlusal definition which still requires the manufacturing of plaster dental models and (2) does not necessitates an additional registration process of plaster dental models in occlusion which always implements a potential additional error in the virtual workflow. On the other hand, virtual occlusal definition in non-segmental cases is still highly demanding to the clinician, mostly because of its lack of tactile sense. In order to virtually define the final occlusion, "best fit" and "collision detecting" algorithms, visualised to the clinician by colour distance maps, are integrated (◘ Figs. 3.27, 3.28, 3.29 and 3.30).

A prospective ($n = 350$) study in non-segmental cases (Swennen 2014) showed that $3D\text{-}VPS_4$ was currently still time consuming (overall mean, 8:26 min; range, 7:40–9:13 min) compared to conventional treatment planning.

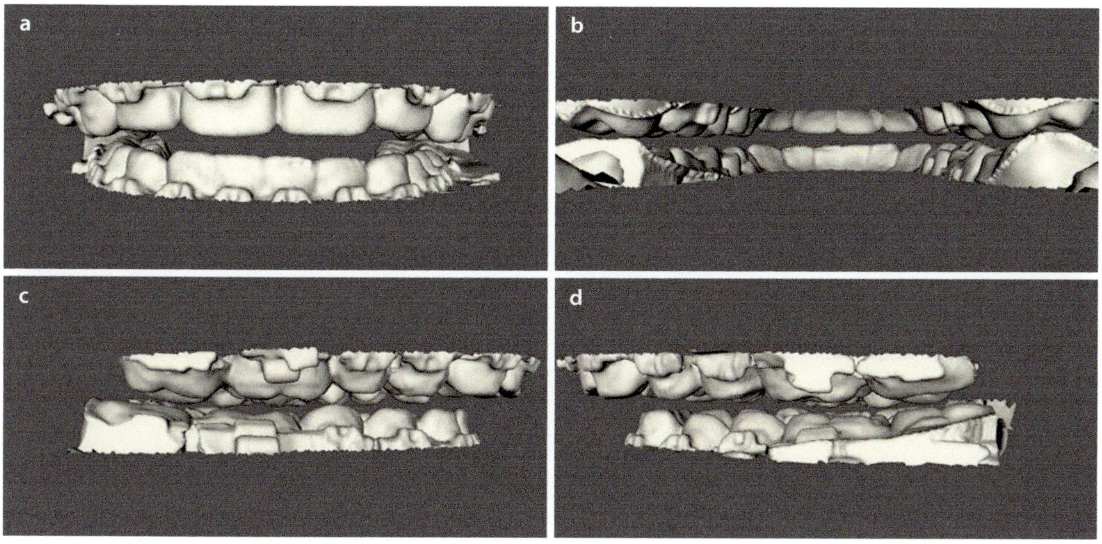

◘ **Fig. 3.27** 3D upper and lower dentition models, in "centric relation (CR)", as scanned during CBCT image acquisition (▶ see also Chap. 1) (3D "surface-rendered" representations, Triple Scan Protocol, patient V.E.W., Maxilim v. 2.3.0.3). (**a**) Frontal view (**b**) posterior view (**c**) profile right view (**d**) profile left view

"Virtual" Non-segmental Occlusal Definition

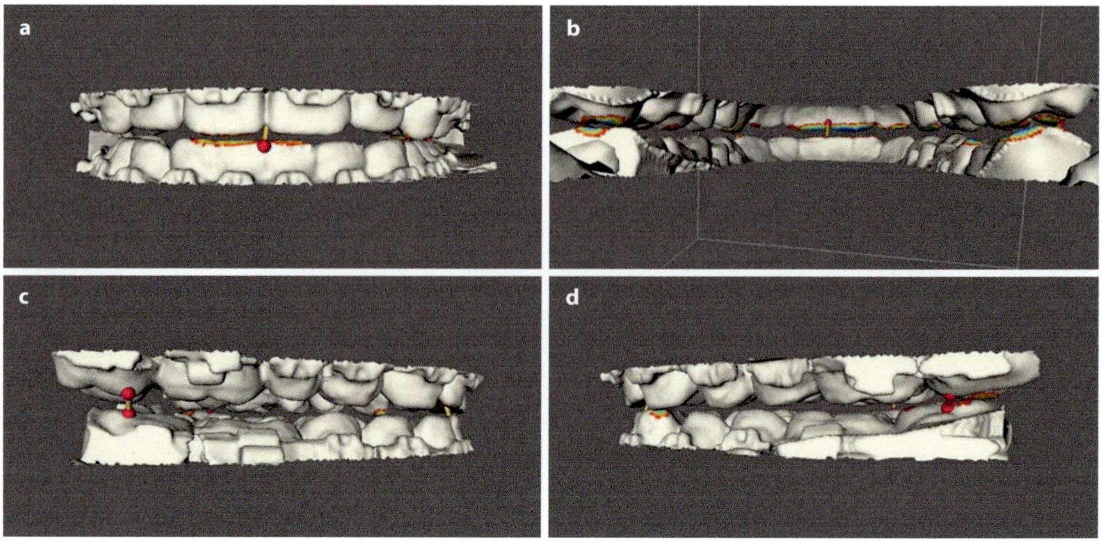

Fig. 3.28 After initial manual alignment, the 3D upper and lower dentition models are guided into final virtual occlusion by use of virtual springs and "best fit" and "collision detecting" algorithms. Selective virtual tooth grinding may be necessary to achieve ideal final virtual occlusion (3D "surface-rendered" representations, Triple Scan Protocol, patient V.E.W., Maxilim v. 2.3.0.3). (**a**) Frontal view (**b**) posterior view (**c**) profile right view (**d**) profile left view

"Virtual" Non-segmental Occlusal Definition

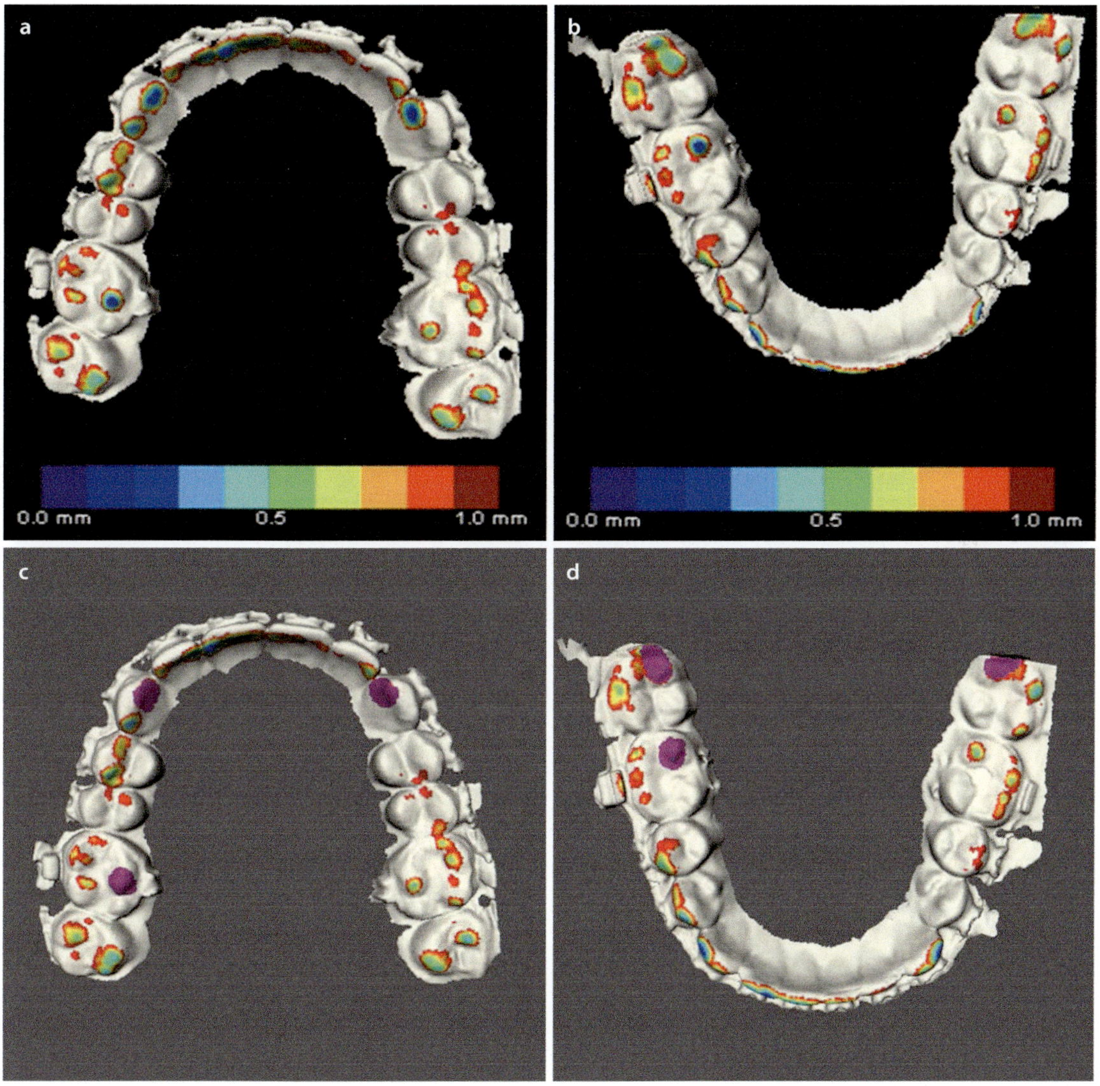

Fig. 3.29 After the final occlusion has been virtually defined by the clinician, an occlusogram tool allows visualisation of the inter-arch dental contacts. A colour distance map provides additional quantification of the degree of the latter occlusal contacts (**a, b**). In some cases, selective virtual tooth grinding may be necessary to achieve ideal final virtual occlusion (**c, d**). Note that neither virtual nor clinical tooth grinding was performed on the patient (3D "surface-rendered" representations, Triple Scan Protocol, patient V.E.W., Maxilim v. 2.3.0.3)

"Virtual" Non-segmental Occlusal Definition

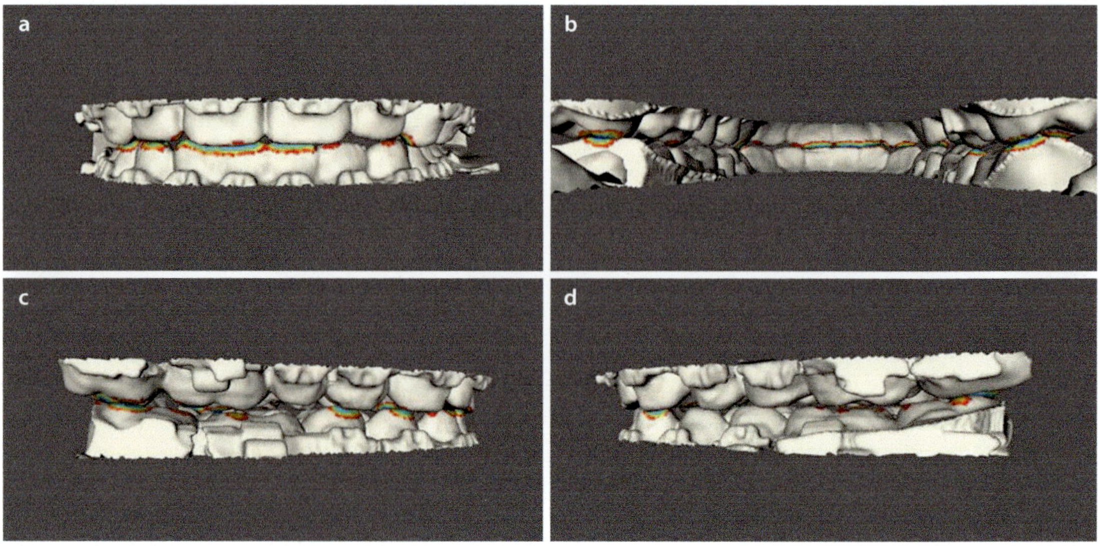

Fig. 3.30 Final virtual occlusal definition with good canine and first molar Angle Class I relationship. Note that neither virtual nor clinical tooth grinding was performed on the patient (3D "surface-rendered" representations, Triple Scan Protocol, patient V.E.W., Maxilim v. 2.3.0.3). (**a**) Frontal view (**b**) posterior view (**c**) profile right view (**d**) profile left view

"Semi-virtual" Non-segmental Occlusal Definition

Semi-virtual non-segmental occlusal definition is performed based on image acquisition of plaster dental models:

1. "**Dental model CBCT1**": CBCT image acquisition of upper and lower dental plaster models separated from each other (Fig. 3.31).
2. "**Dental model CBCT2**": CBCT image acquisition of upper and lower plaster dental models that were placed manually into final occlusion by the clinician (Fig. 3.32).

Based on "rigid registration" (► see also Sect. 1.2.1), "Dental model CBCT2" is superimposed (registered) to "Dental model CBCT1". To evaluate the accuracy of the registration process, multiplanar reslices along the dental arches are essential to verify the final occlusion (Fig. 3.32). Compared to "virtual occlusal definition", "semi-virtual occlusal definition" has the following disadvantages: (1) Slower in the clinical workflow since it requires the manufacturing of plaster dental models and (2) necessitates an additional registration process. On the other hand, it is certainly less demanding in the 3D virtual workflow.

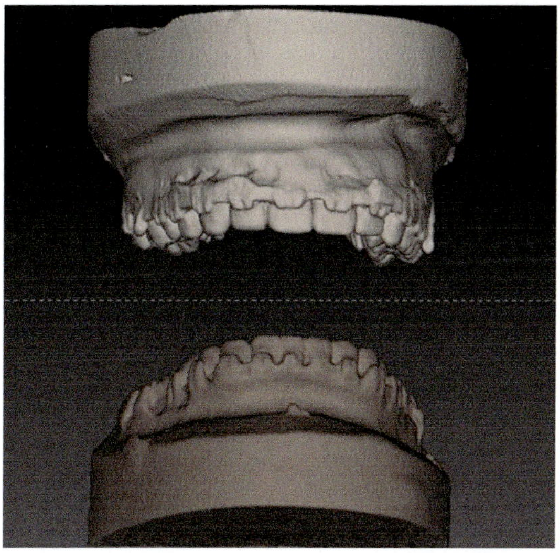

Fig. 3.31 3D upper and lower dentitions models, based on CBCT scanning of the plaster dental models made from the "all-in-one" impression of the upper and lower dental arches (► see also Sect. 1.2.2). "Dental model CBCT 1" is acquired with the plaster dental models separated from each other by a sponge (3D "volume-rendered" representations, patient V.E.W, IPS CaseDesigner ALPHA version)

"Semi-virtual" Non-segmental Occlusal Definition

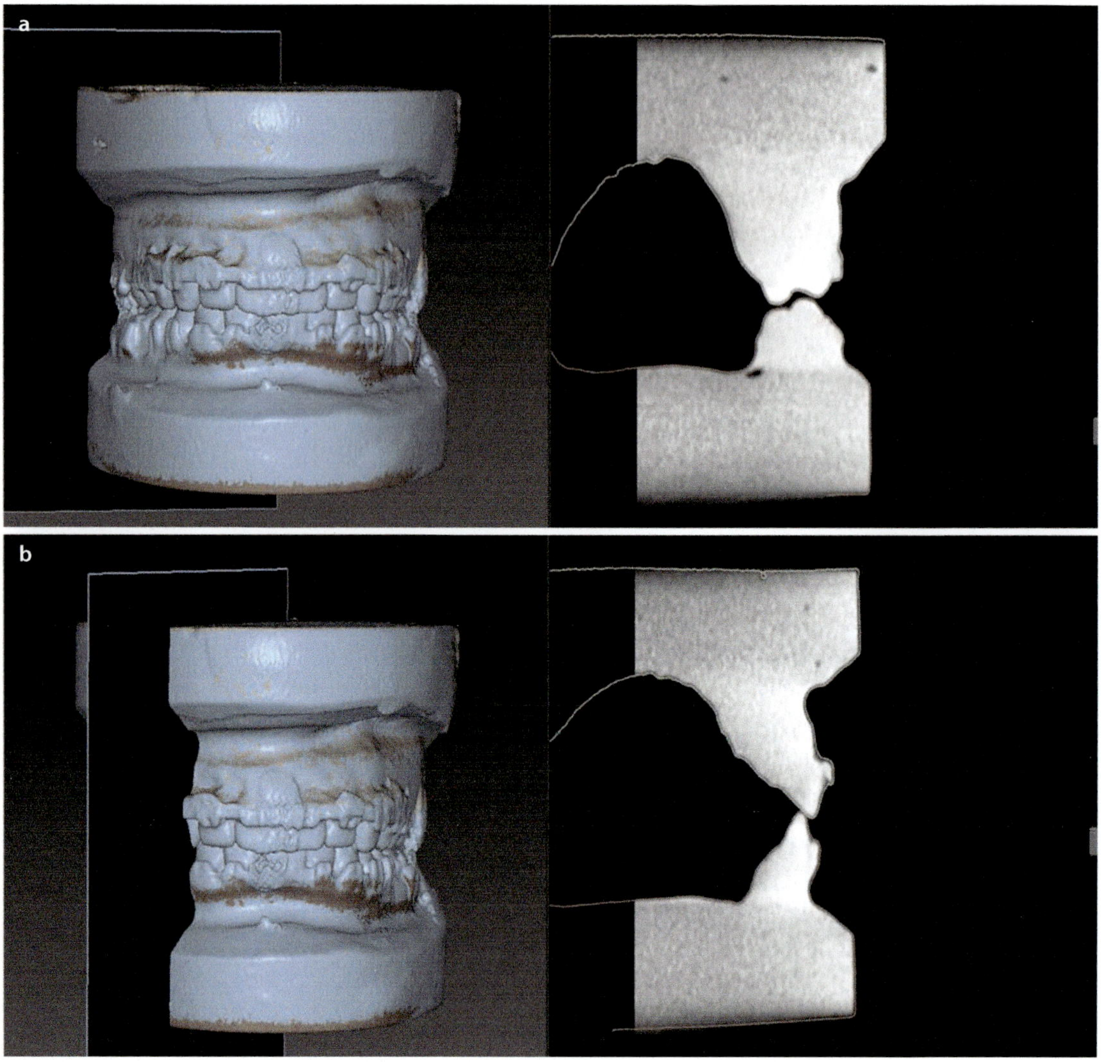

Fig. 3.32 3D upper and lower dentition models, based on CBCT scanning of the plaster dental models made from the "all-in-one" impression of the upper and lower dental arches (► see also Chap. 1) in virtual final occlusion. The plaster dental models were manually placed into final occlusion by the clinician before image acquisition (Dental model CBCT2). The 3D upper and lower dentition models in virtual occlusion from "Dental model CBCT2" were then superimposed (registered) to "Dental model CBCT1". Multiplanar reslices along the dental arches are provided to evaluate the accuracy of the registration process. Multiplanar reslices at the canine (**b**, **c**) and first molar level (**a**, **d**) (3D "volume-rendered" representations, patient V.E.W, IPS CaseDesigner ALPHA version)

"Semi-virtual" Non-segmental Occlusal Definition

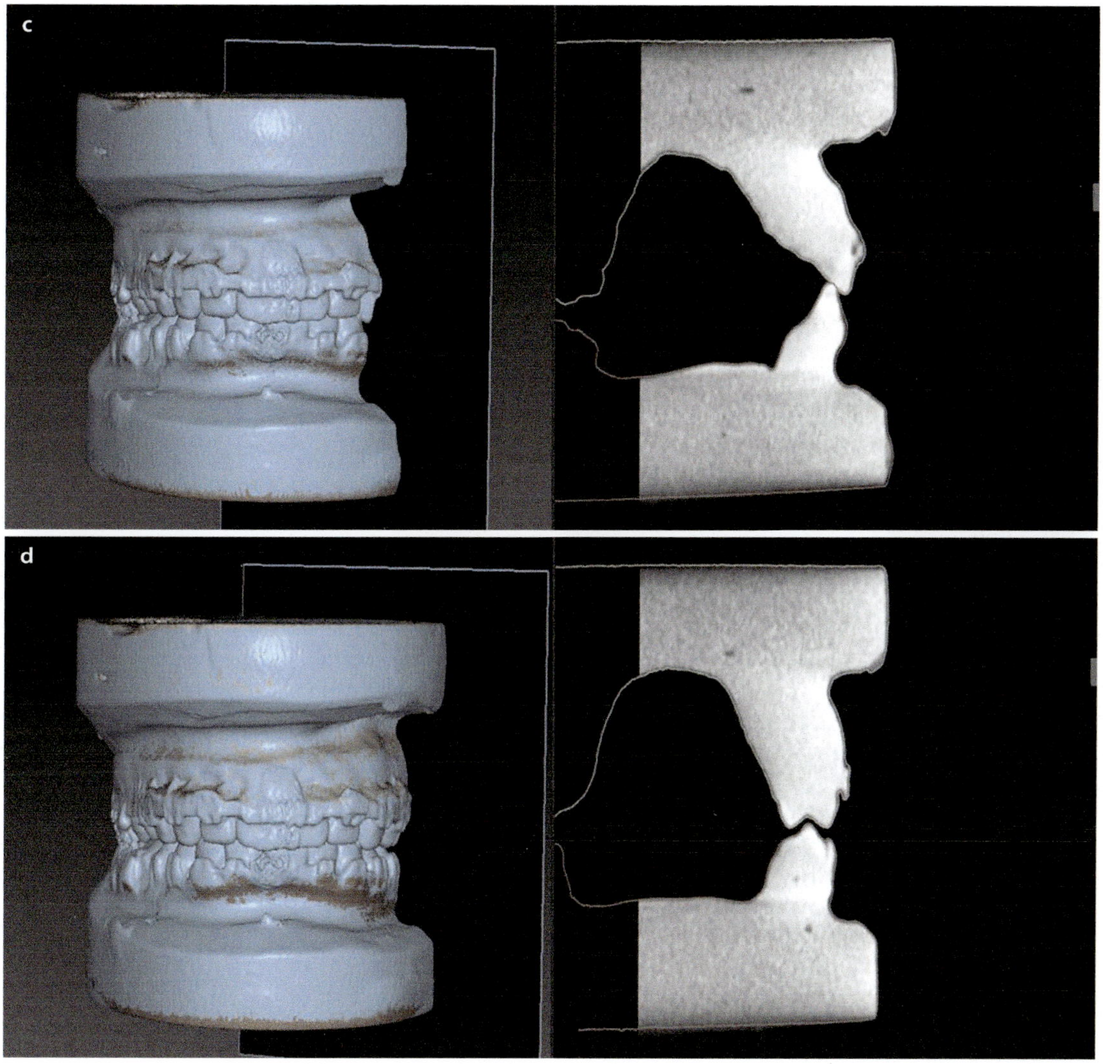

Fig. 3.32 (continued)

3.3.2 Segmental Occlusal Definition

Currently, segmental occlusal definition is still performed semi-virtually based on image acquisition of plaster dental models since virtual (without the use of plaster dental models) occlusal definition in segmental cases is still prone to errors:

1. **"Dental model CBCT1"**. CBCT image acquisition of upper and lower dental plaster models separated from each other (◘ Fig. 3.33).
2. "**Dental model CBCT2**". CBCT image acquisition of upper and lower plaster dental models that were manually segmented and placed into final occlusion by the clinician (◘ Fig. 3.34).

Based on "rigid registration" (► see also Sect. 1.2.1), "Dental model CBCT2" is superimposed (registered) to "Dental model CBCT1". To evaluate the accuracy of the rigid registration process, multiplanar reslices along the dental arches are essential to verify the final occlusion (◘ Fig. 3.34).

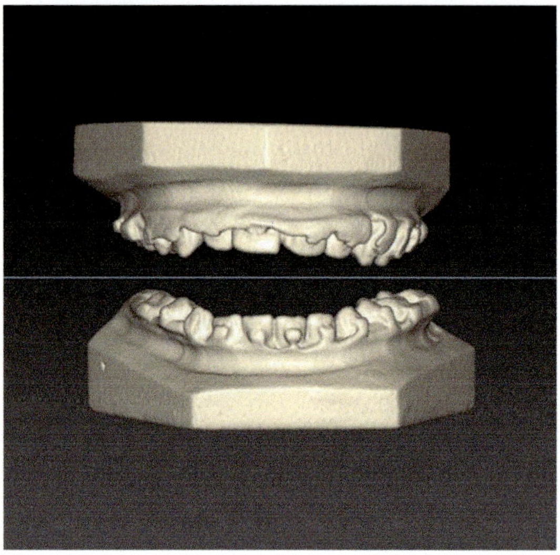

◘ **Fig. 3.33** 3D upper and lower dentitions models, based on CBCT scanning of the plaster dental models made from the "all-in-one" impression of the upper and lower dental arches (► see also Chap. 1). "Dental model CBCT 1" is acquired with the plaster dental models separated from each other by a sponge (3D "volume-rendered" representations, patient L.A., IPS CaseDesigner ALPHA version)

"Semi-virtual" Segmental Occlusal Definition

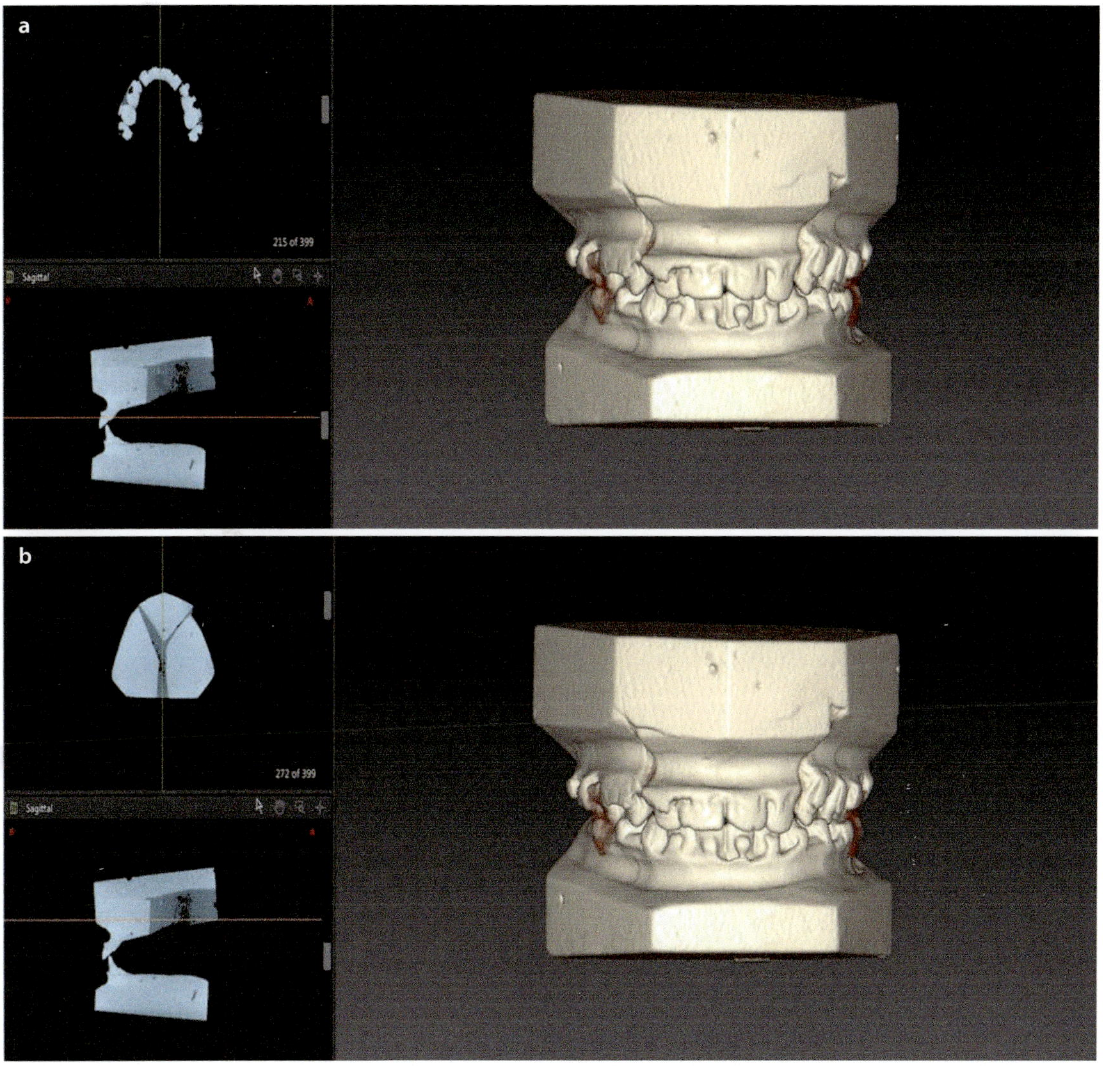

Fig. 3.34 3D upper and lower dentition models, based on CBCT scanning of the plaster dental models made from the "all-in-one" impression of the upper and lower dental arches (▶ see also Chap. 1) in virtual final occlusion. The plaster dental models were manually placed into final occlusion by the clinician before image acquisition (Dental model CBCT2). The 3D upper and lower dentition models in virtual occlusion from "Dental model CBCT2" were then superimposed (registered) to "Dental model CBCT1". Multiplanar reslices along the dental arches are provided to evaluate the accuracy of the registration process. Multiplanar reslices at the upper midline (**a**, **b**) and canine level (**c**, **d**) (3D "volume-rendered" representations, patient L.A., IPS CaseDesigner ALPHA version)

"Semi-virtual" Segmental Occlusal Definition

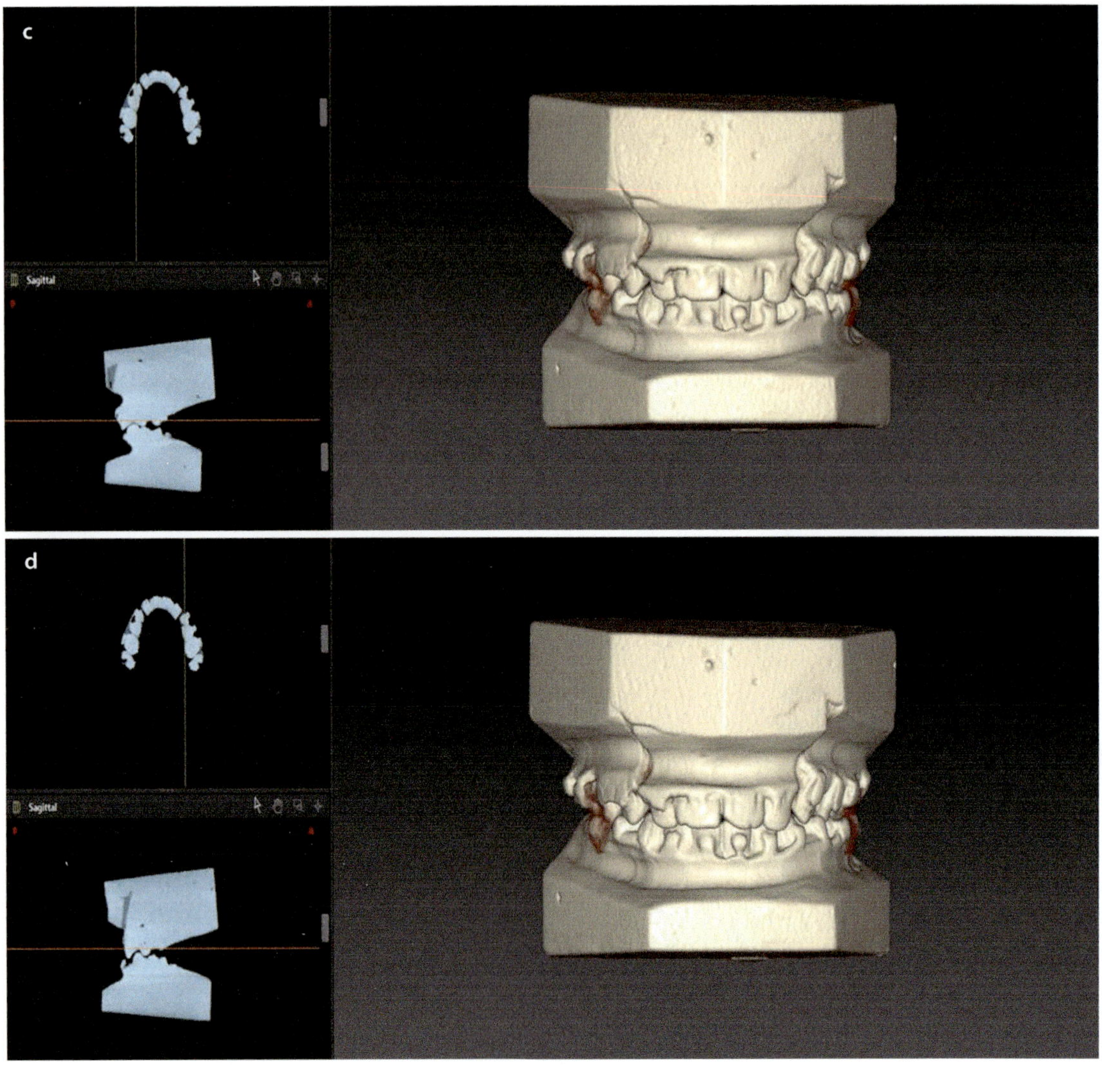

■ **Fig. 3.34** (continued)

3.4 Principles of "Roll", "Yaw" and "Pitch" in the 3D Virtual Scene

From conventional treatment planning of orthognathic surgery, it is well known that "rotational movements of the maxillo-mandibular complex" are a very powerful tool in both functional and aesthetic management of maxillofacial deformity.

In the 3D virtual scene, rotational movements ("Roll", "Yaw" and "Pitch") can be performed in all 3D planes, in a clockwise (CW) or counterclockwise (CCW) manner, or, more simply, to the right or left (◘ Figs. 3.35 to 3.51).

1. "**Roll**": Rotational movement around the "*z*-axis" in the frontal plane that can be performed CW or CCW
2. "**Yaw**": Rotational movement around the "*y*-axis" in the base or frontal plane that can be performed CW or CCW, but sometimes more simply described to the right or to the left
3. "**Pitch**": Rotational movement around the "*x*-axis" in the profile plane that can be performed CW or CCW

"Roll", "Yaw" and "Pitch" rotational movements are used in the 3D virtual approach towards:

1. Virtual modification of the scanned head position of the patient towards its "clinical natural head position (*c*-NHP)", resulting in the "virtual modified natural head position (*v*-NHP) or individual "planning head position (PHP)" of the patient (▶ see also Sect. 3.1).
2. Virtual surgical rotational movements of the maxilla, mandible, chin, proximal fragments of the mandible or maxillo-mandibular complex in final occlusion (▶ see also Sect. 3.5).

▪ "Roll", "Yaw" and "Pitch" Rotational Movements for Virtual Modification of the Head Position

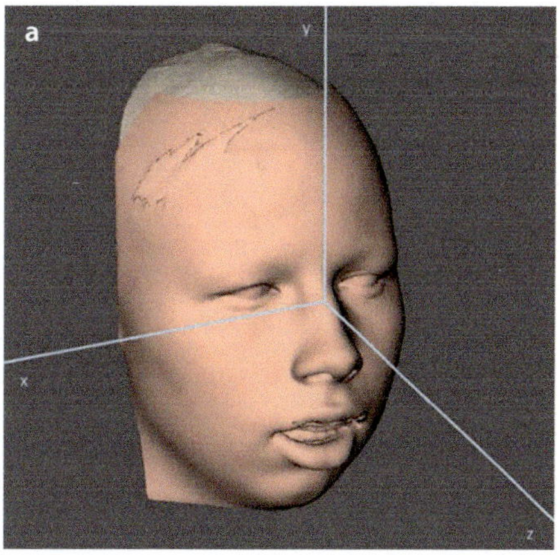

◘ **Fig. 3.35** After setting the *v*-NHP, a new 3D coordinate reference frame is generated, as a basis for the individual PHP of the patient (**a**). 3D cephalometric measurements and surgical movements of the maxilla, mandible and chin are both related to the 3D PHP coordinate reference frame. The "Roll" movement is performed around the "z"-axis, while the "Pitch" movement is around the "x"-axis and the "Yaw" movement around the "y"-axis (**b**, **c**) (3D "surface-rendered" representations, patient V.E.W., Maxilim v. 2.3.0.3)

"Roll", "Yaw" and "Pitch" Rotational Movements for Virtual Modification of the Head Position

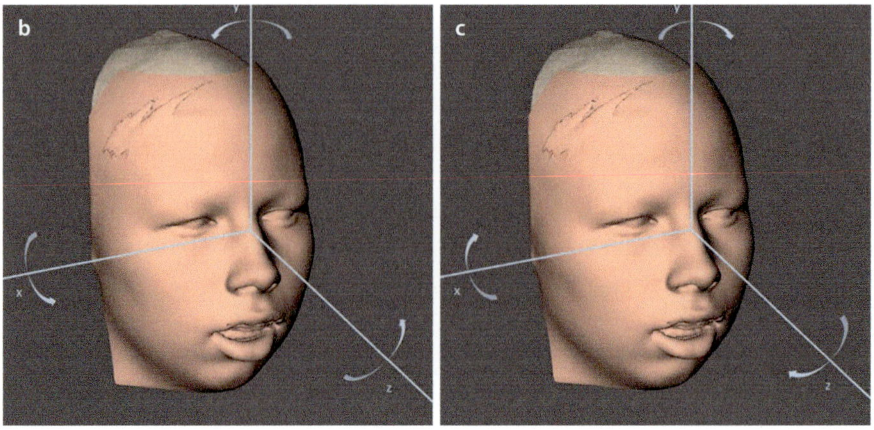

■ **Fig. 3.35** (continued)

▪ "Roll", "Yaw" and "Pitch" Rotational Movements for Virtual Surgery

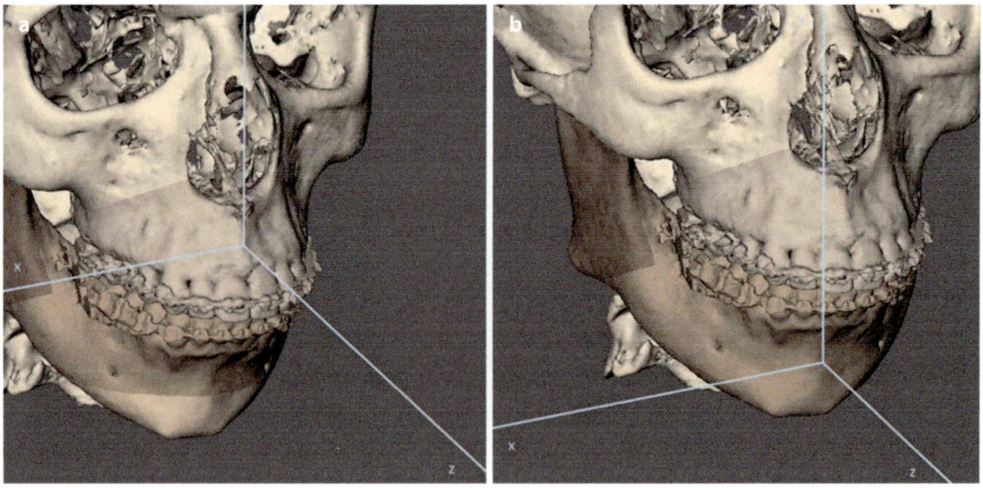

■ **Fig. 3.36** The principles of "Roll", "Yaw" and "Pitch" can be individually related to the maxilla (**a**), the distal fragment of the mandible (**b**), the chin (**c**), the proximal segments of the mandible (**d**) and finally the maxillo-mandibular complex (**e**) (3D "surface-rendered" representations, patient V.E.W., Maxilim v. 2.3.0.3)

"Roll", "Yaw" and "Pitch" Rotational Movements for Virtual Surgery

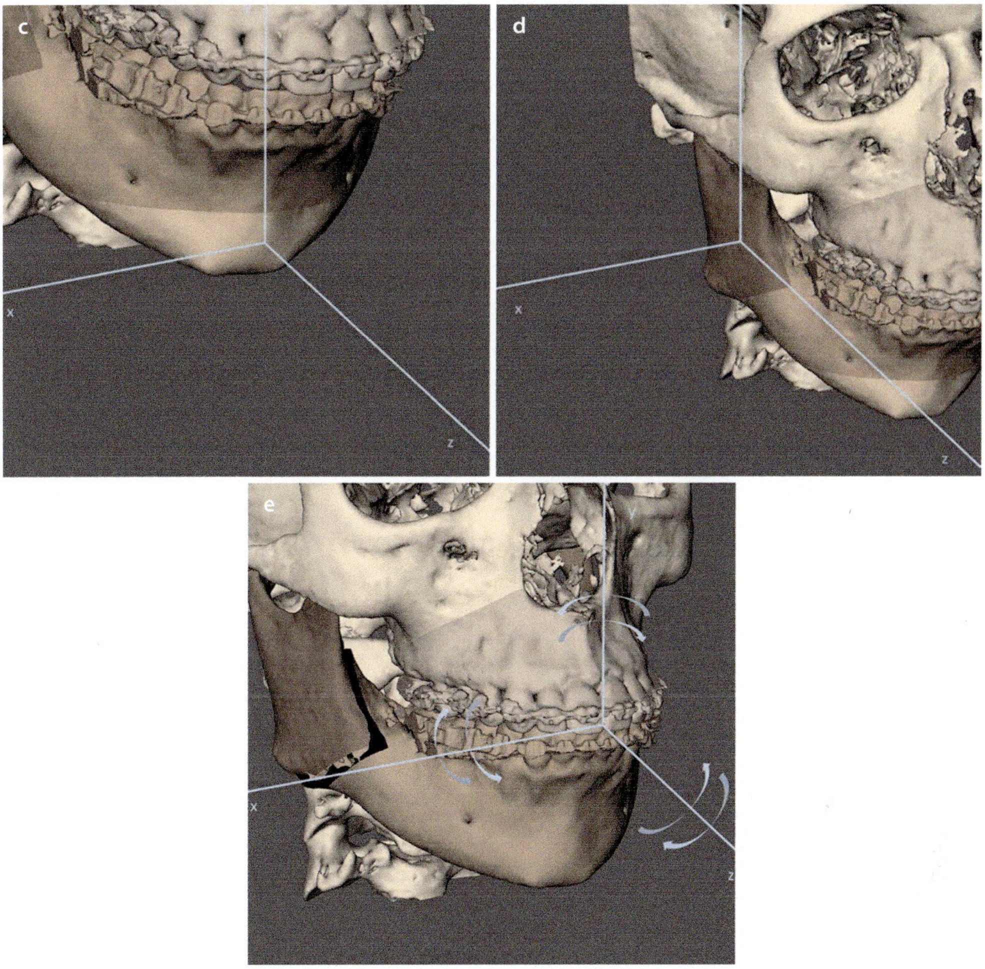

Fig. 3.36 (continued)

■ "Roll": Rotational Movement Around the *Z*-Axis in the Frontal Plane (CW or CCW)

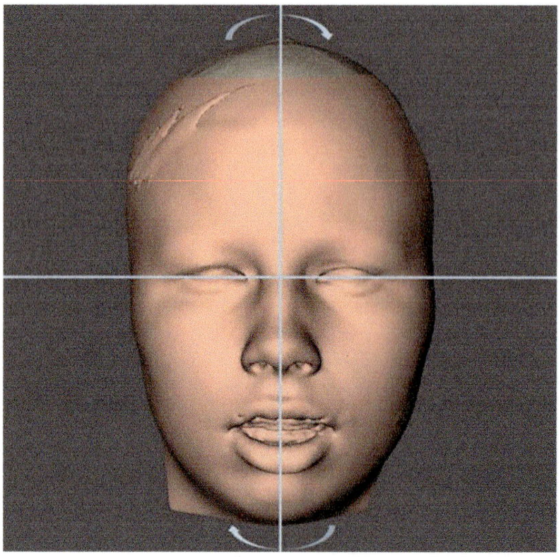

Fig. 3.37 The principle of "Roll" is related to a rotational movement around the "z"-axis. In the frontal plane, it can be conceptually correlated to the direction of a clock's hands. CW refers to a circular rotation to the right, while CCW refers to a circular rotation to the left (3D "surface-rendered" representations, patient V.E.W., Maxilim v. 2.3.0.3)

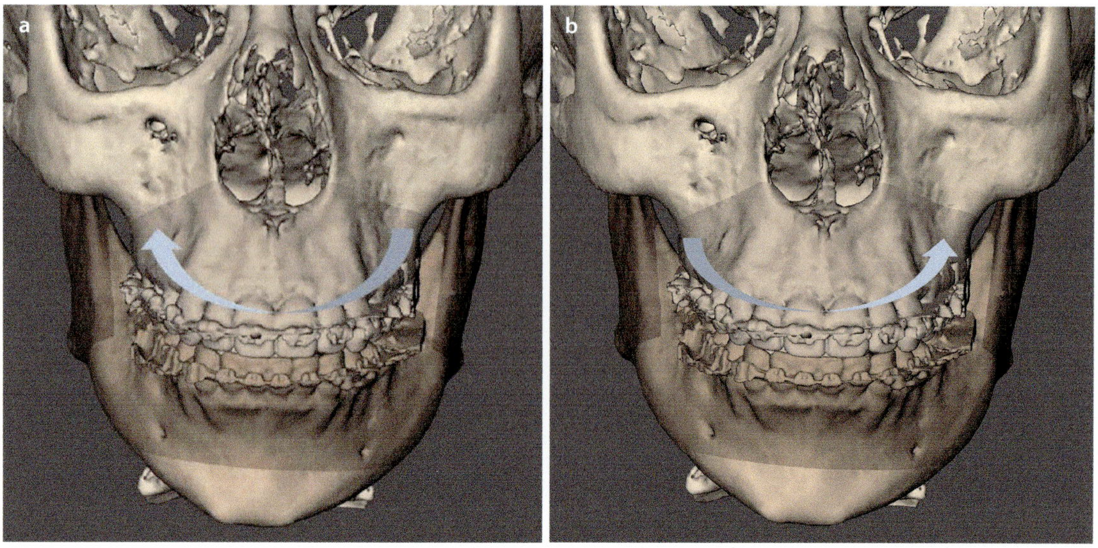

Fig. 3.38 In maxillary surgery, the "Roll" concept is related to "Cant" correction, and the maxilla can therefore be rotated in a CW or CCW manner (3D "surface-rendered" representations, patient V.E.W., Maxilim v. 2.3.0.3). (**a**) CW (**b**) CCW

"Roll": Rotational Movement Around the *Z*-Axis in the Frontal Plane (CW or CCW)

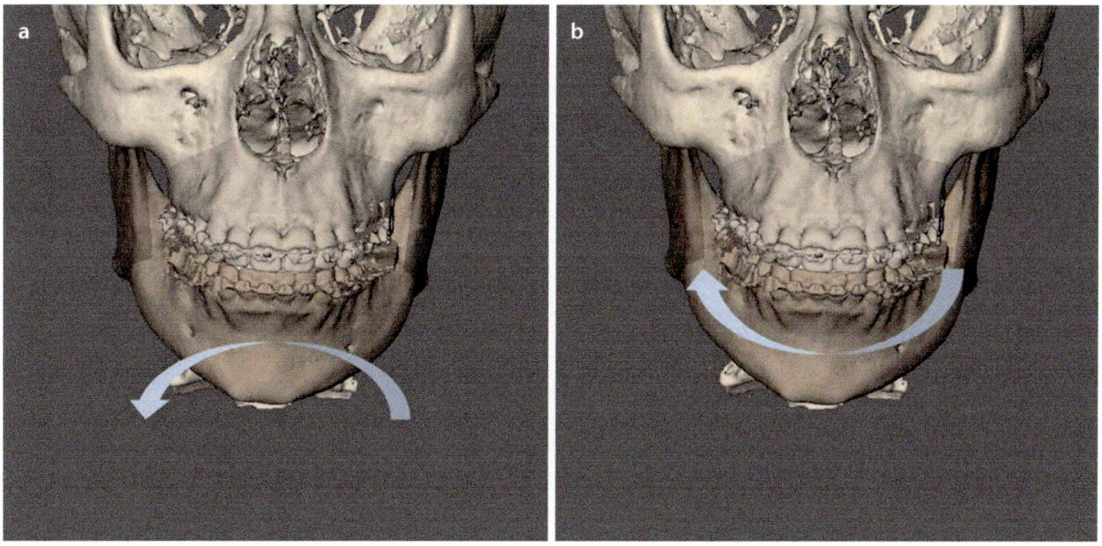

Fig. 3.39 In mandibular surgery, the "Roll" concept is related to "Cant" correction, and the distal segment of the mandible can therefore be rotated in a CW or CCW manner. The mandible can be individually evaluated for the presence of a "Cant", but will most often be assessed as part of the maxillo-mandibular complex, after final virtual occlusal definition (3D "surface-rendered" representations, patient V.E.W., Maxilim v. 2.3.0.3). (**a**) CCW (**b**) CW

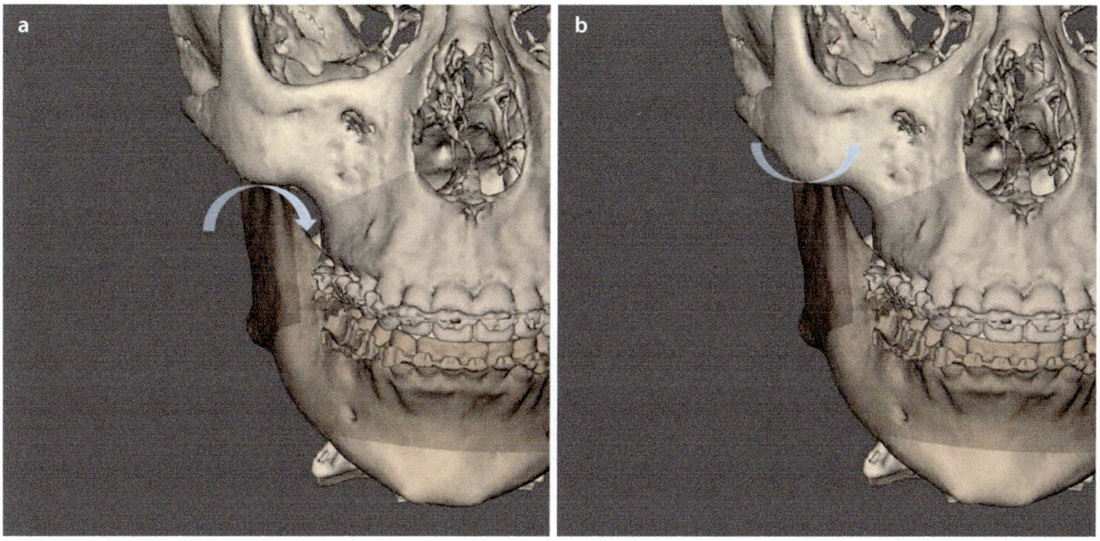

Fig. 3.40 In mandibular surgery, the "Roll" concept can also be related to the management of the proximal segment during USSO or BSSO. The condylar-ramus unit can therefore rotate laterally (**a**) or medially (**b**), around a centre of rotation based at the condylar head. Movement of the proximal segments should be minimised during surgery to prevent any deleterious effect on the condyle (3D "surface-rendered" representations, patient V.E.W., Maxilim v. 2.3.0.3)

"Roll": Rotational Movement Around the *Z*-Axis in the Frontal Plane (CW or CCW)

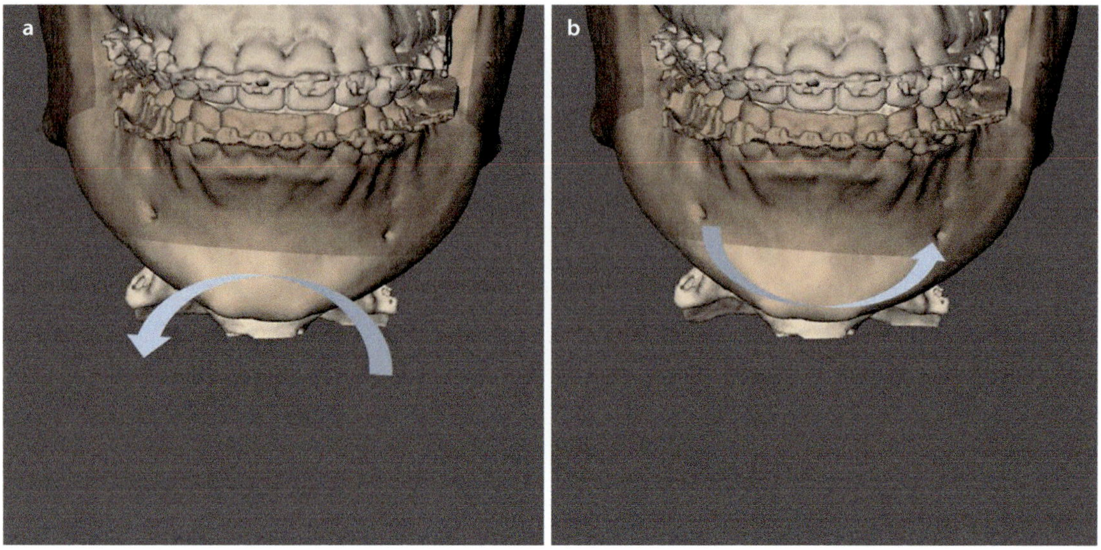

Fig. 3.41 In genioplasty, the "Roll" concept is related to "Cant" correction, and the mandibular symphysis can therefore be rotated in a CW or CCW manner (3D "surface-rendered" representations, patient V.E.W., Maxilim v. 2.3.0.3). (**a**) CCW rotation for cant correction with extrusion at the right, (**b**) CCW rotation for cant correction with intrusion at the left

"Yaw": Rotational Movement Around the *Y*-Axis in the Base or Frontal Plane

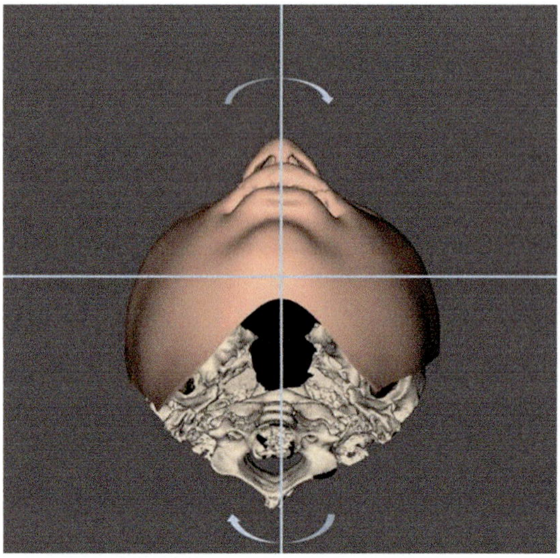

Fig. 3.42 The principle of "Yaw" is related to a rotational movement around the "y"-axis. In the base plane, it can be conceptually correlated to the direction of a clock's hands. CW refers to a circular rotation to the right, while CCW refers to a circular rotation to the left (3D "surface-rendered" representations, patient V.E.W., Maxilim v. 2.3.0.3)

"Yaw": Rotational Movement Around the *Y*-Axis in the Base or Frontal Plane

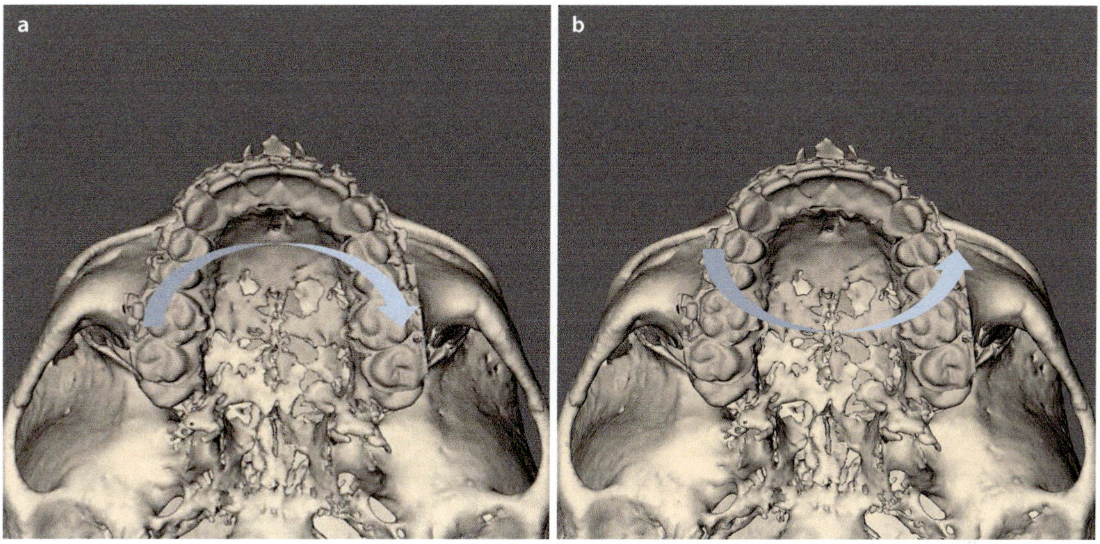

Fig. 3.43 The principle of "Yaw" is related to a rotational movement around the "y" axis. In maxillary surgery, the maxilla can therefore be rotated in a CW or CCW manner, depending on the clinical situation (3D "surface-rendered" representations, patient V.E.W., Maxilim v. 2.3.0.3). (**a**) CW (**b**) CCW

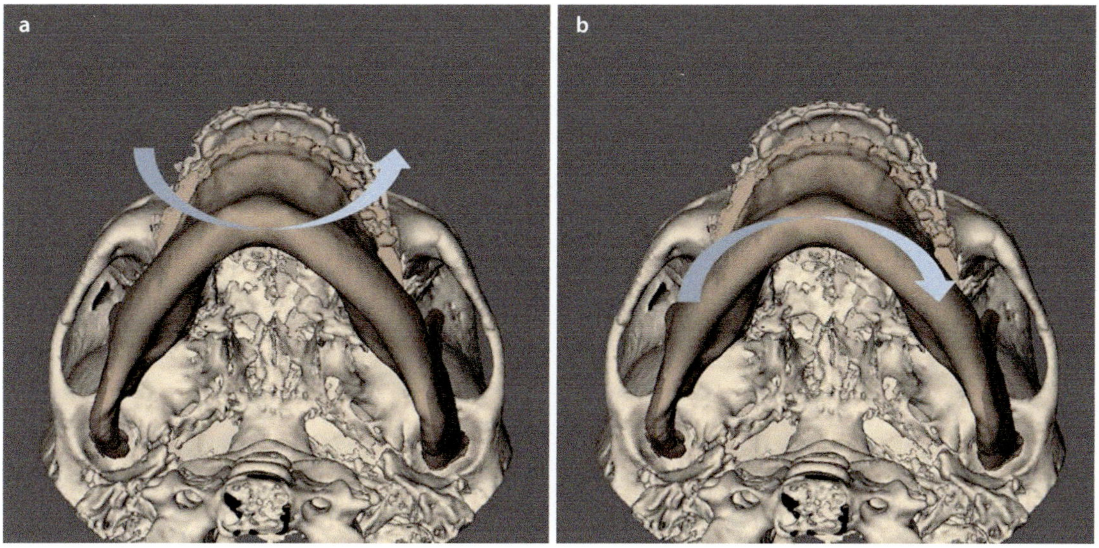

Fig. 3.44 In mandibular surgery, the "Yaw" concept is related to asymmetry correction and inter-fragmentary bony adaptation between the proximal and distal segment. In BSSO, the distal segment can therefore be rotated in a CW or CCW manner, depending on the clinical situation (3D "surface-rendered" representations, patient V.E.W., Maxilim v. 2.3.0.3). (**a**) CCW (**b**) CW

"Yaw": Rotational Movement Around the *Y*-Axis in the Base or Frontal Plane

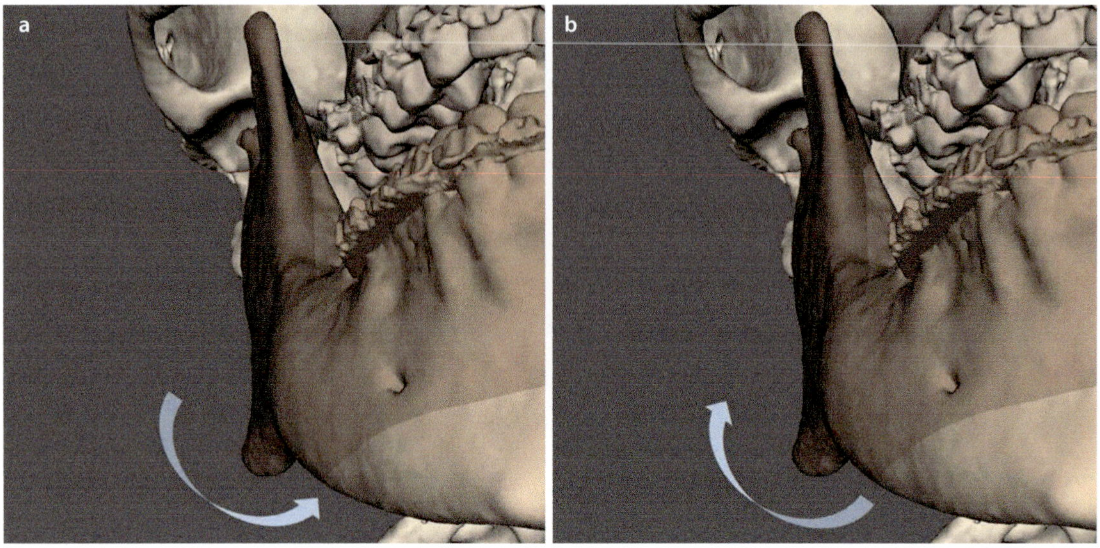

Fig. 3.45 In mandibular surgery, the "Yaw" concept can also be related to the management of the proximal segment during BSSO. The condylar-ramus unit can therefore be rotated in the base plane to the right or to the left. Movement of the proximal segments should be minimised during surgery to prevent any deleterious effect on the condyle (3D "surface-rendered" representations, patient V.E.W., Maxilim v. 2.3.0.3). (**a**) CCW (left) (**b**) CW (right)

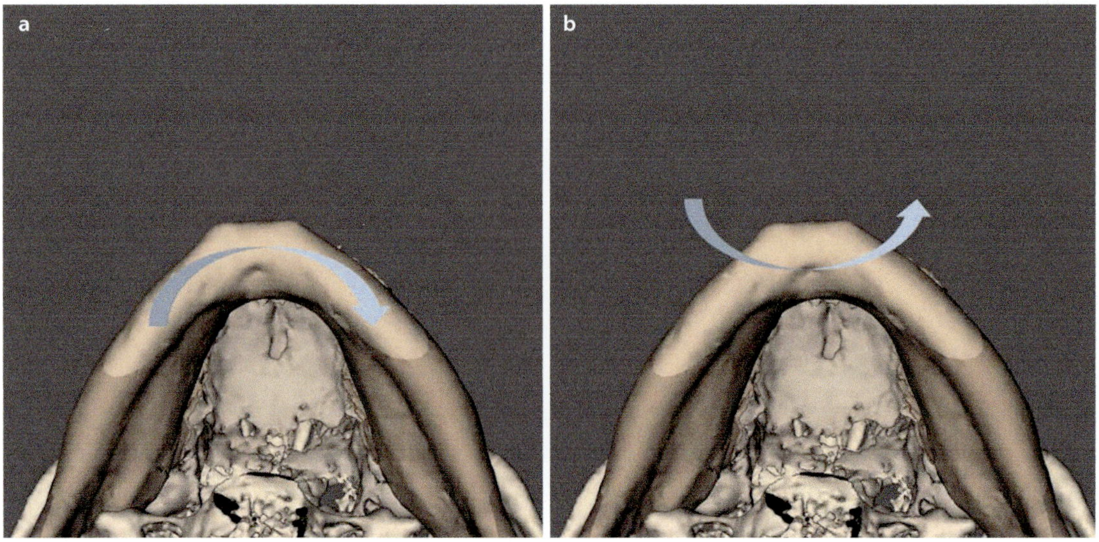

Fig. 3.46 In genioplasty, the "Yaw" concept is related to asymmetry correction. The mandibular symphysis can therefore be rotated in a CW or CCW manner, depending on the clinical situation (3D "surface-rendered" representations, patient V.E.W., Maxilim v. 2.3.0.3). (**a**) CW (**b**) CCW

■ "Pitch": Rotational Movement Around the *X*-Axis in the Profile Plane (CW or CCW)

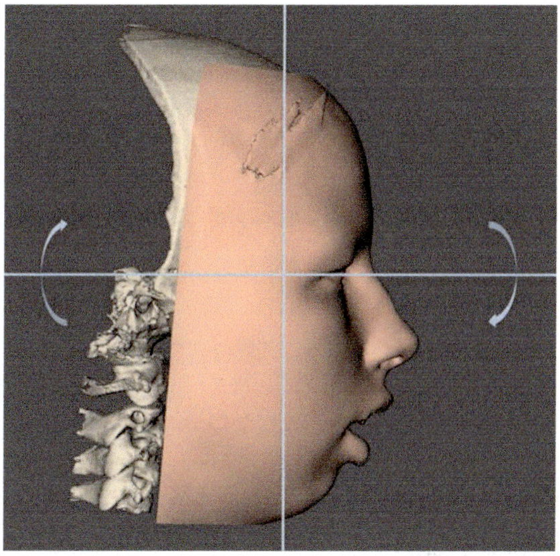

Fig. 3.47 The principle of "Pitch" is related to a rotational movement around the "x"-axis. In the profile plane, it can be conceptually correlated to the direction of a clock's hands. CW refers to a circular rotation to the right, while CCW refers to a circular rotation to the left (3D "surface-rendered" representations, patient V.E.W., Maxilim v. 2.3.0.3)

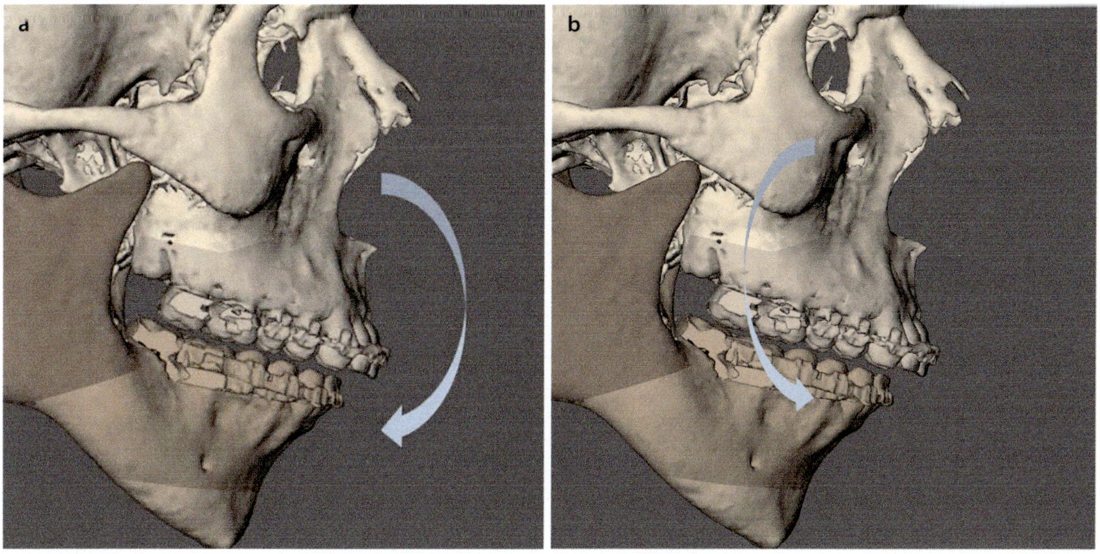

Fig. 3.48 In orthognathic surgery, the "Pitch" concept is related to occlusal plane modification, therefore, in maxillary surgery, the maxilla can be rotated in a CW or CCW manner, depending on the clinical situation (3D "surface-rendered" representations, patient V.E.W., Maxilim v. 2.3.0.3). (**a**) CW (**b**) CCW

"Pitch": Rotational Movement Around the *X*-Axis in the Profile Plane (CW or CCW)

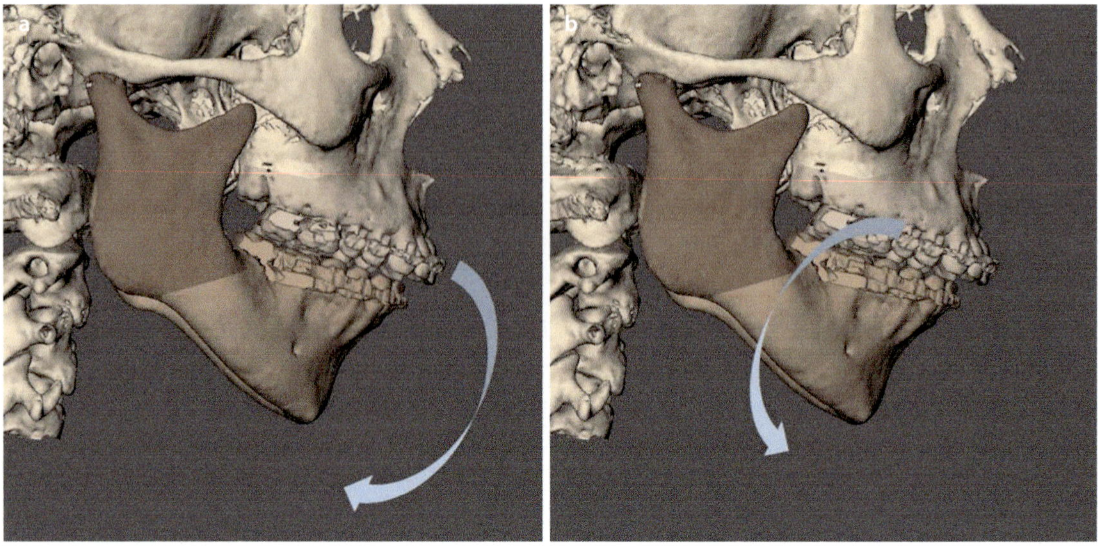

Fig. 3.49 The mandible can be individually evaluated according to the "Pitch" concept for occlusal plane modification. Most often the mandible will be assessed as a part of the maxillo-mandibular complex, after final virtual occlusal definition and can be rotated in a CW or CCW manner (3D "surface-rendered" representations, patient V.E.W., Maxilim v. 2.3.0.3). (**a**) CW (**b**) CCW

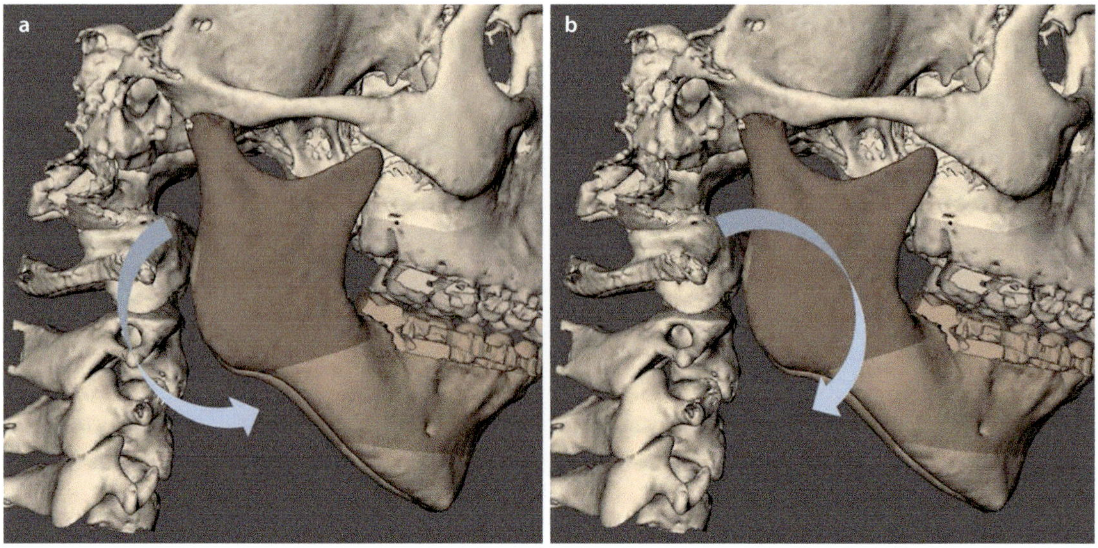

Fig. 3.50 In mandibular surgery, the "Pitch" concept can also be related to the management of the proximal segment during USSO or BSSO. The condylar-ramus unit can therefore be rotated in a CW or CCW manner. Movement of the proximal segments should be minimised to prevent any deleterious effect on the condyle (3D "surface-rendered" representations, patient V.E.W., Maxilim v. 2.3.0.3). (**a**) CCW (**b**) CW

"Pitch": Rotational Movement Around the *X*-Axis in the Profile Plane (CW or CCW)

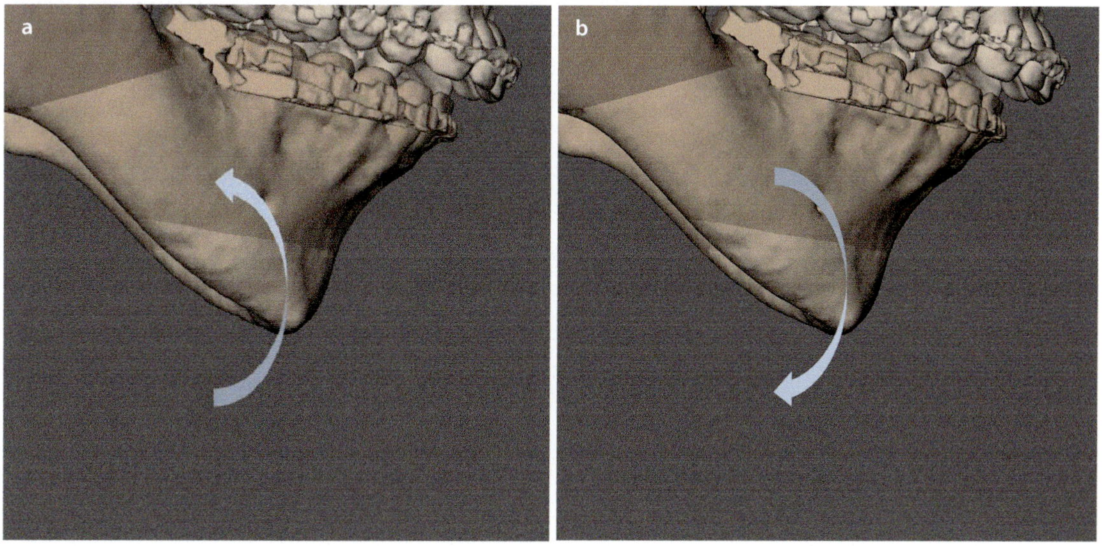

Fig. 3.51 In genioplasty, the "Pitch" concept is related to chin prominence and mandibular border contour. The mandibular symphysis can therefore be rotated in a CW or CCW manner, depending on the clinical situation (3D "surface-rendered" representations, patient V.E.W., Maxilim v. 2.3.0.3). (**a**) CW (**b**) CCW

3

3.5 "Step-by-Step" Individualised 3D Virtual Treatment Planning (3D-VPS$_5$)

The "10 step-by-step" integrated "individualised 3D virtual treatment planning" approach outlined in this chapter aims to provide a standardised and systematic way of using "3D virtual treatment planning" in the daily clinical routine planning of orthognathic surgery.

The backbone of the described approach is "individualised treatment planning" in order to:

1. Offer an "individualised treatment plan" towards each patient, depending on his particular functional needs, aesthetic concerns or as in most cases, a combination of both.
2. Provide the clinician (orthodontist, surgeon or most ideal the ortho-surgical team) a manner of "individualising 3D virtual treatment planning", based on his personal educational background (e.g. cephalometric analysis, etc.) and treatment planning philosophies (e.g. maxilla first/mandible first/surgery first, clockwise (CW)/counterclockwise (CCW) rotation, non-segmental/segmental surgery, one-stage/two-stage surgery, etc).

Step 1 – Maxillary occlusal cant evaluation/correction ("Roll")
Step 2 – Upper dental midline evaluation/correction
Step 3 – Overall evaluation of facial asymmetry after virtual occlusal definition
Step 4 – Evaluation/correction of flaring ("Yaw")
Step 5 – Upper vertical incisal position evaluation/correction
Step 6 – Upper sagittal incisal position evaluation/correction
Step 7 – Profile evaluation/occlusal plane correction ("Pitch")
Step 8 – 3D chin position evaluation/correction ("Roll", "Yaw" and "Pitch")
Step 9 – Patient communication of the "individualised 3D virtual treatment plan"
Step 10 – Final adjustments of the "individualised 3D virtual treatment plan"

Although the "10 step-by-step" integrated virtual planning approach necessitates 3D virtual definition of some cephalometric landmarks (▶ see also Chap. 2), it is not based on any particular cephalometric analysis described in the literature. The planning approach is based on "clinical decision-making", starting from the individual patient's "planning head position (PHP)" (▶ see Sect. 3.1).

The clinician is nevertheless able to incorporate any specific 2D or 3D cephalometric measurements in each of the ten planning steps to individualise his treatment planning approach.

A prospective ($n = 350$) study in non-segmental cases (Swennen 2014) showed that 3D-VPS$_5$ could be performed in an acceptable time frame compared to conventional treatment planning.

	Mean (min:s)	Range (min:s)
BSSO ($n = 90$)	7:45	6:32–8:12
BSSO and chin ($n = 18$)	8:05	7:48–10:03
Le Fort I and BSSO ($n = 163$)	16:23	11:12–19:43
Le Fort I, BSSO and chin ($n = 79$)	17:59	12:58–21:24

Attention
3D-VPS$_5$ starts from the virtual modified natural head position (v-NHP) which correspondents to the individual patient's planning head position (PHP) determined by the clinician (▶ see Sect. 3.1).

(3D-VPS$_5$) "10 step-by-step" integrated "individualised 3D virtual treatment planning" is illustrated on several clinical cases with different types of maxillofacial deformity in Chap. 6.

■ **Case 1: Class II/1 Long-Face (Patient V.E.W.): Video**

3.5.1 "Step 1": Maxillary Occlusal Cant Evaluation/Correction ("Roll")

The maxillary occlusal plane is evaluated in the frontal plane as in conventional treatment planning, by clinical examination of the patient in rest and during smiling and by evaluation of clinical photographs (ideally with a cheek retractor) (▸ see also Chap. 1) (◘ Fig. 3.52).

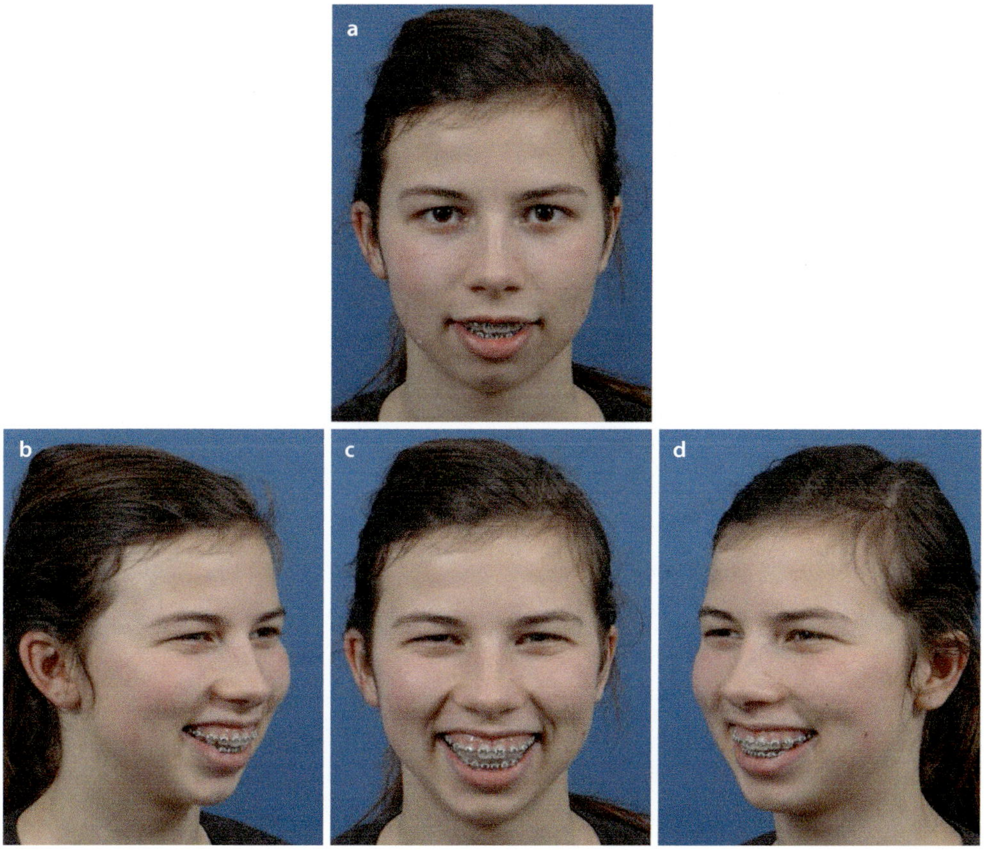

◘ **Fig. 3.52** Pre-surgical clinical frontal views in rest (**a**), smiling 2/3 right profile (**b**), smiling frontal (**c**) and smiling 2/3 profile left (**d**). Note that clinically, there is no obvious cant of the maxilla neither of the mandible (patient V.E.W.)

"Step 1": Maxillary Occlusal Cant Evaluation/Correction ("Roll")

In the 3D virtual approach, a potential maxillary occlusal cant is evaluated in "Step 1" in the frontal individual PHP of the patient that has been defined by the clinician (► see also Sect. 3.1) (▣ Fig. 3.53).

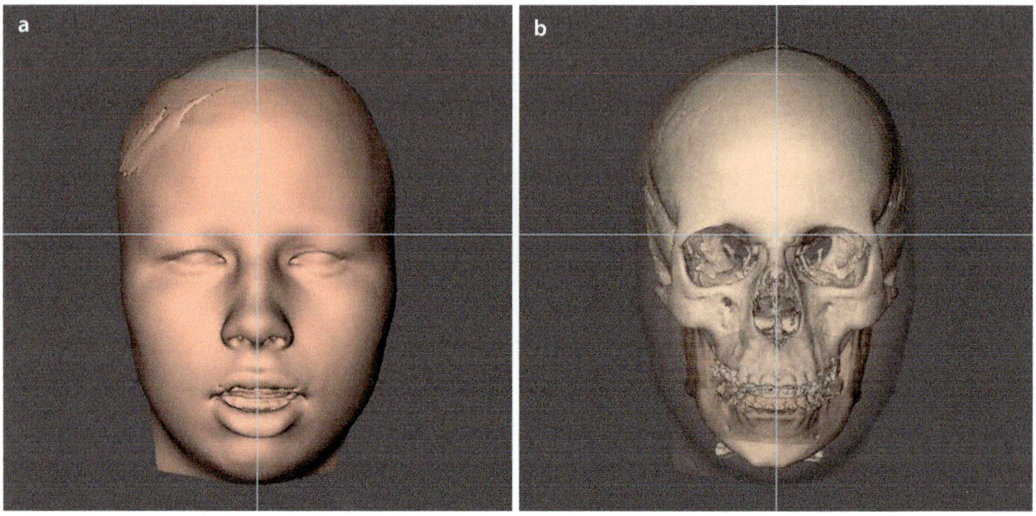

▣ **Fig. 3.53** Frontal PHP views at the start of the "10 step-by-step" integrated 3D virtual planning approach. Note that the 3D virtual patient model does not clearly show a maxillary occlusal cant. On the other hand, compared to the clinical photographs, a clear cant of the mandible with chin deviation to the right becomes noticeable (3D "surface-rendered" representations, patient V.E.W., Maxilim v. 2.3.0.3). (**a**) Frontal view (**b**) frontal view with soft tissues in transparency.

The maxillary occlusal plane (Mx-Occ-Pl) is additionally visualised and evaluated. As described in Chap. 2, the Mx-Occ-Pl is theoretically defined by a plane that connects (1) the mean of *upper incisor*$_r$, *upper incisor*$_l$, (2) *upper molar cusp*$_r$ and (3) *upper molar cusp*$_l$ 3D cephalometric dental landmarks (▣ Fig. 3.54).

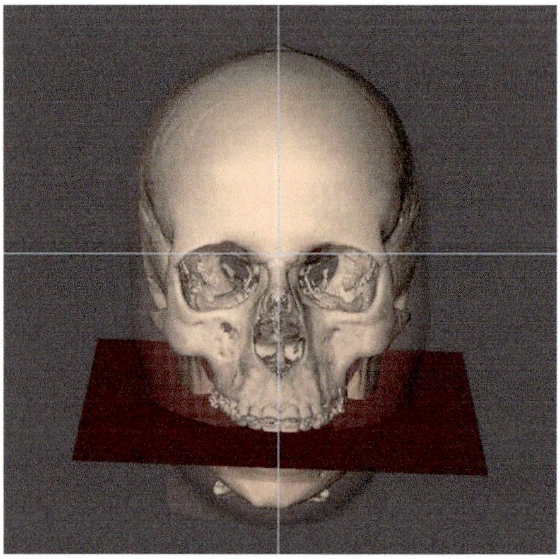

▣ **Fig. 3.54** Visualisation of the Mx-Occ-Pl shows a maxillary cant that was clinically not evident (3D "surface-rendered" representations, patient V.E.W., Maxilim v. 2.3.0.3)

Pitfall
Always check that the 3D cephalometric dental landmarks correctly determine the maxillary occlusal plane (Mx-Occ-Pl).

"Step 1": Maxillary Occlusal Cant Evaluation/Correction ("Roll")

The above-mentioned 3D cephalometric definition of the Mx-Occ-Pl is true in non-segmental cases where the upper dental arch is orthodontically well aligned and levelled. Since this is not always the case in daily clinical routine, the clinician needs to verify if the above-mentioned 3D cephalometric dental landmarks truly define the "maxillary occlusal plane" and if not modify them. In segmental cases (e.g. two-pieces and three-pieces Le Fort I with stepwise orthodontic pre-surgical preparation), the "maxillary occlusal plane" needs to be defined by the clinician by at least four 3D cephalometric dental landmarks.

In case a cant of the "maxillary occlusal plane" is present, it is corrected by a "Roll" movement (CW or CCW) towards the horizontal 3D PHP reference plane, in the frontal view (◻ Figs. 3.55 and 3.56).

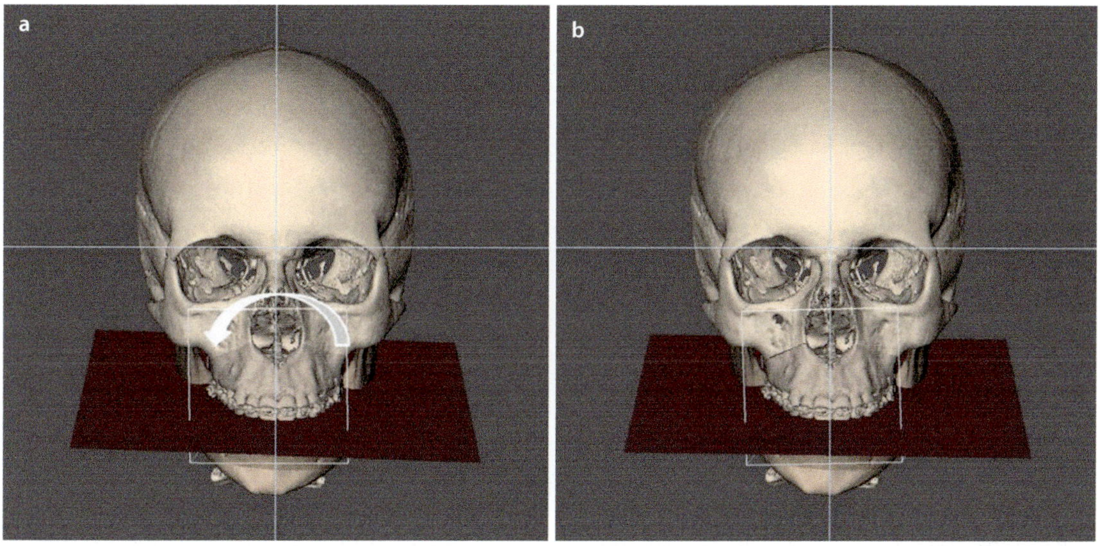

◻ **Fig. 3.55** The maxillary cant is corrected towards the horizontal 3D PHP reference plane by a CCW "Roll" rotational movement (3D "surface-rendered" representations, patient V.E.W., Maxilim v. 2.3.0.3). (**a**) Before correction (**b**) after correction

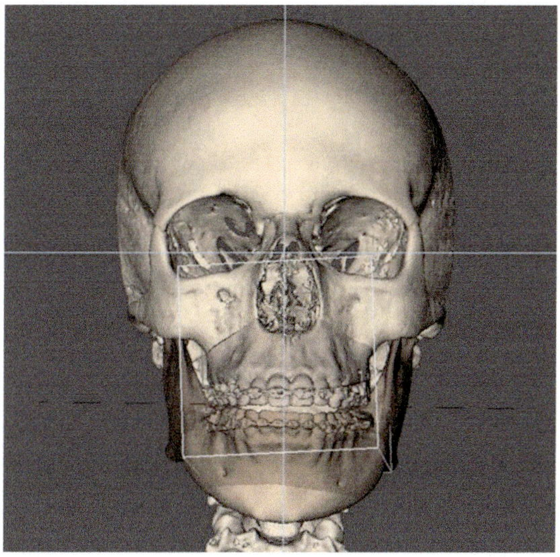

◻ **Fig. 3.56** Slight virtual rotation of the patient's skull to the back more clearly shows that the maxillary cant is corrected towards the horizontal 3D PHP reference plane (3D "surface-rendered" representations, patient V.E.W., Maxilim v. 2.3.0.3)

3.5.2 "Step 2": Upper Dental Midline Evaluation/Correction

The upper dental midline is evaluated in the frontal plane towards the nasophiltrum and the facial midline, as in conventional treatment planning, by clinical examination of the patient in rest and by evaluation of the clinical standardised photographs (Fig. 3.57).

In the daily clinical routine, discrepancies often occur in the assessment of the upper dental midline towards the nasophiltrum versus the facial midline. This can be of myofunctional origin but mostly caused by positional changes of the nasolabial aesthetic unit of the face by (1) a septal deviation, (2) a deviation of the anterior nasal spine (ANS), (3) an asymmetric nasal base, (4) a maxillary asymmetry, (5) a nasal asymmetry, (6) a mandibular asymmetry or (7) a combination. Systematic virtual diagnosis of the patient's individual anatomy and pathology (▶ see also Chap. 2) can help to identify the underlying cause. In the 3D virtual approach, the upper dental midline is evaluated in "Step 2" towards the vertical 3D PHP reference plane (▶ see also Sect. 3.1).

Attention

Clinical discrepancies of the upper dental midline often occur towards the nasophiltrum versus the facial midline.

Systematic virtual diagnosis of the patient's individual anatomy and pathology (▶ see also Sect. 2.1.2) can help to identify the underlying cause.

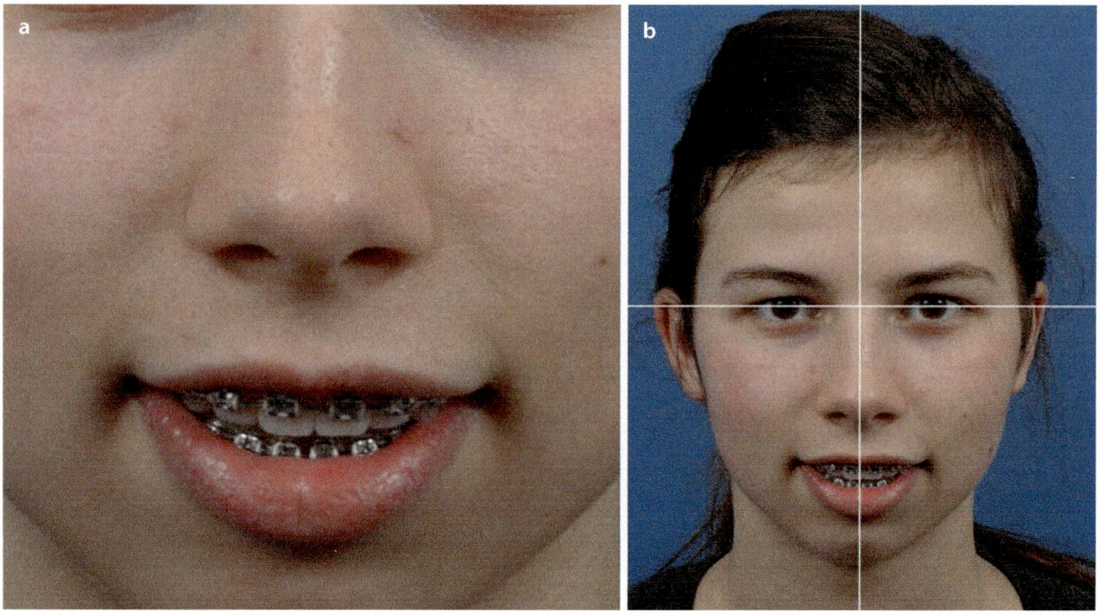

Fig. 3.57 Pre-surgical clinical frontal views in rest, with details of the nasolabial aesthetic unit (**a**) and full frontal view in *c*-NHP (**b**). Note that clinically, there is no deviation of the upper dental midline towards the nasophiltrum, although there is a slight but obvious deviation to the left towards the facial midline (patient V.E.W.)

"Step 2": Upper Dental Midline Evaluation/Correction

An upper dental midline deviation can be corrected virtually by (1) a translation to the right or left, (2) by a rotation in the base plane ("Yaw"), (3) by a combined translation and rotation, (4) by a cant correction of the maxilla ("Roll") or (5) by a combination of all these movements.

Since in "Step 1", an eventual cant of the maxillary occlusal plane has already been corrected by a "Roll", the upper dental midline in "Step 2" is only modified by a translation, a rotation in the base plane ("Yaw") or a combination of both (◘ Fig. 3.58).

In "Step 2", it is important and of clinical benefit to also virtually hide the mandible in order to

Advantage
The 3D virtual approach helps the clinician in the assessment of the upper dental midline.

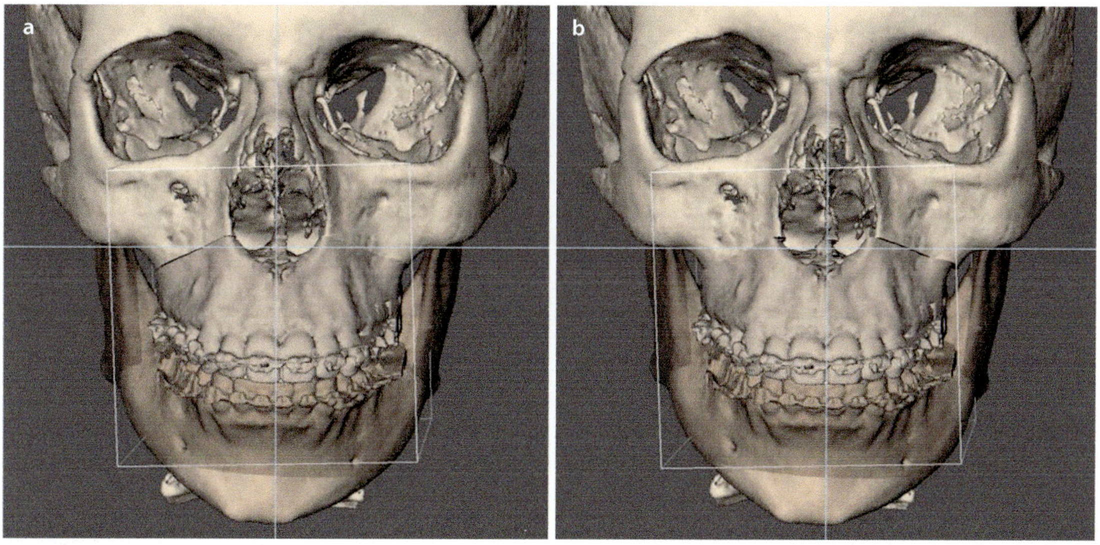

◘ **Fig. 3.58** The deviation of the upper dental midline to the left (**a**) is corrected towards the facial midline 3D PHP reference plane, by a pure translation movement to the right (**b**) (3D "surface-rendered" representations, patient V.E.W., Maxilim v. 2.3.0.3)

"Step 2": Upper Dental Midline Evaluation/Correction

assess the position of the maxillary dental arch towards the midface (e.g. zygomatic prominence and zygomatic arches) in the base view (◘ Fig. 3.59).

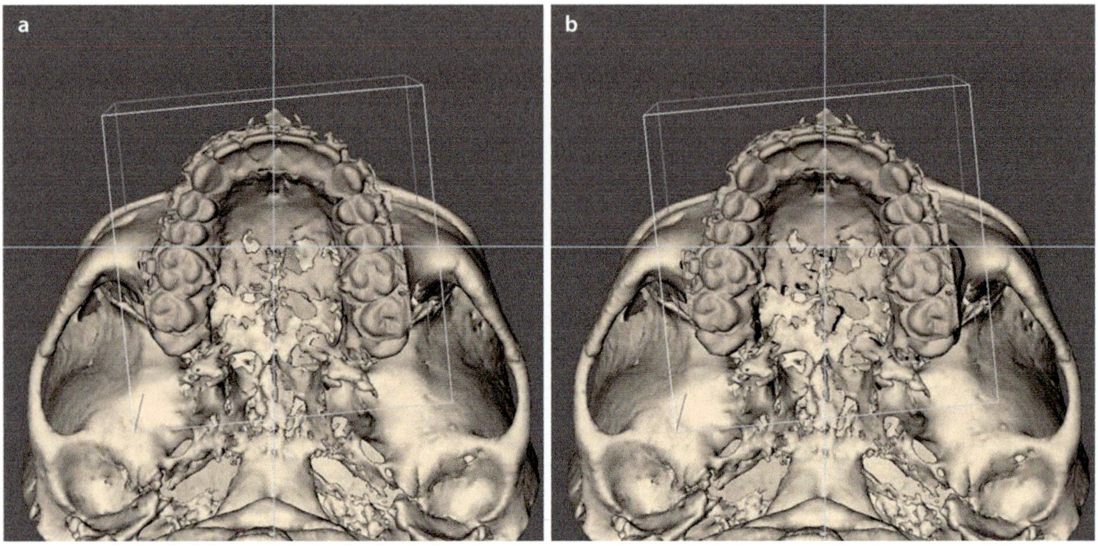

◘ **Fig. 3.59** The base views illustrate a slight correction of the upper dental midline to the right by a pure translation of the maxilla to the right towards the facial midline 3D PHP reference plane (3D "surface-rendered" representations, patient V.E.W., Maxilim v. 2.3.0.3). (**a**) Before correction (**b**) after correction

3.5.3 "Step 3": Overall Evaluation of Facial Asymmetry After Virtual Occlusal Definition

In "Step 3" overall facial symmetry/asymmetry is evaluated after "virtual occlusal definition" (3D-VPS_4) (► see also Sect. 3.3) at both bony and soft tissue level. The position of the chin, gonial angles, mandibular inferior border and ascending mandibular rami are evaluated towards the horizontal and medial 3D PHP references planes of the patient (◘ Fig. 3.60).

It can sometimes be necessary to redefine the "virtual occlusal definition" to fine-tune facial symmetry. This can be done by additional virtual occlusal grinding or by virtual opening the occlusion at specific levels.

It is also important to understand that after "virtual occlusal definition", the maxilla and the distal mandibular segment are fused together as the "maxillo-mandibular complex in final virtual occlusion". Therefore, from now on any 3D virtual modification of the maxillary position in the next virtual planning steps (4–10) will automatically be transmitted virtually to the mandible.

Limit and Pitfall
Since there are currently no evidence-based data available on the accuracy of 3D soft tissue simulation in the frontal plane, the clinician should not rely on 3D soft tissue simulation.

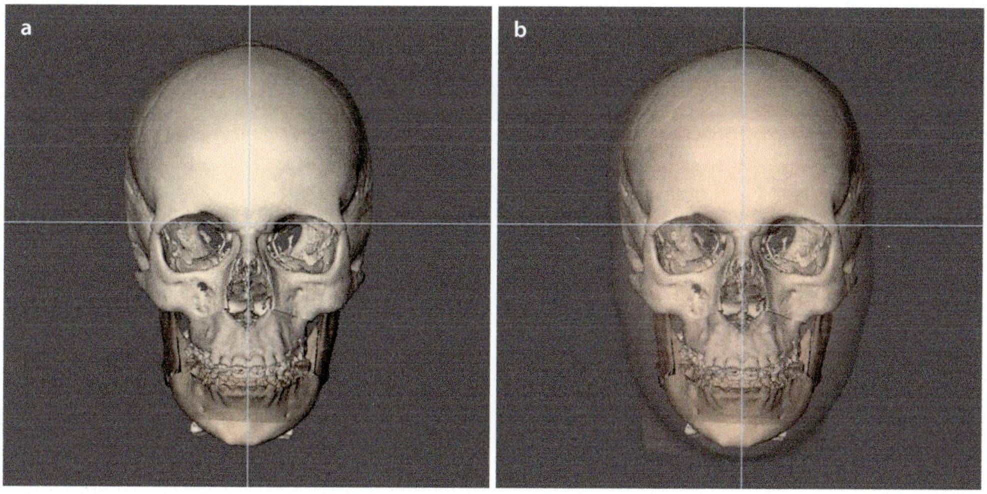

◘ **Fig. 3.60** Overall facial asymmetry of the patient's skull and face is assessed after virtual occlusal definition in the frontal view towards both the horizontal and facial midline 3D PHP reference planes. Note the persistent chin asymmetry to the right (3D "surface-rendered" representations, patient V.E.W., Maxilim v. 2.3.0.3). (**a**) Frontal view (**b**) frontal view with soft tissues in transparency

"Step 3": Overall Evaluation of Facial Asymmetry After Virtual Occlusal Definition

Towards overall assessment of facial symmetry and balance, it is helpful to virtually evaluate the mandibular border contour towards the contour of the zygomatic arches and the zygomatic bones (Fig. 3.61).

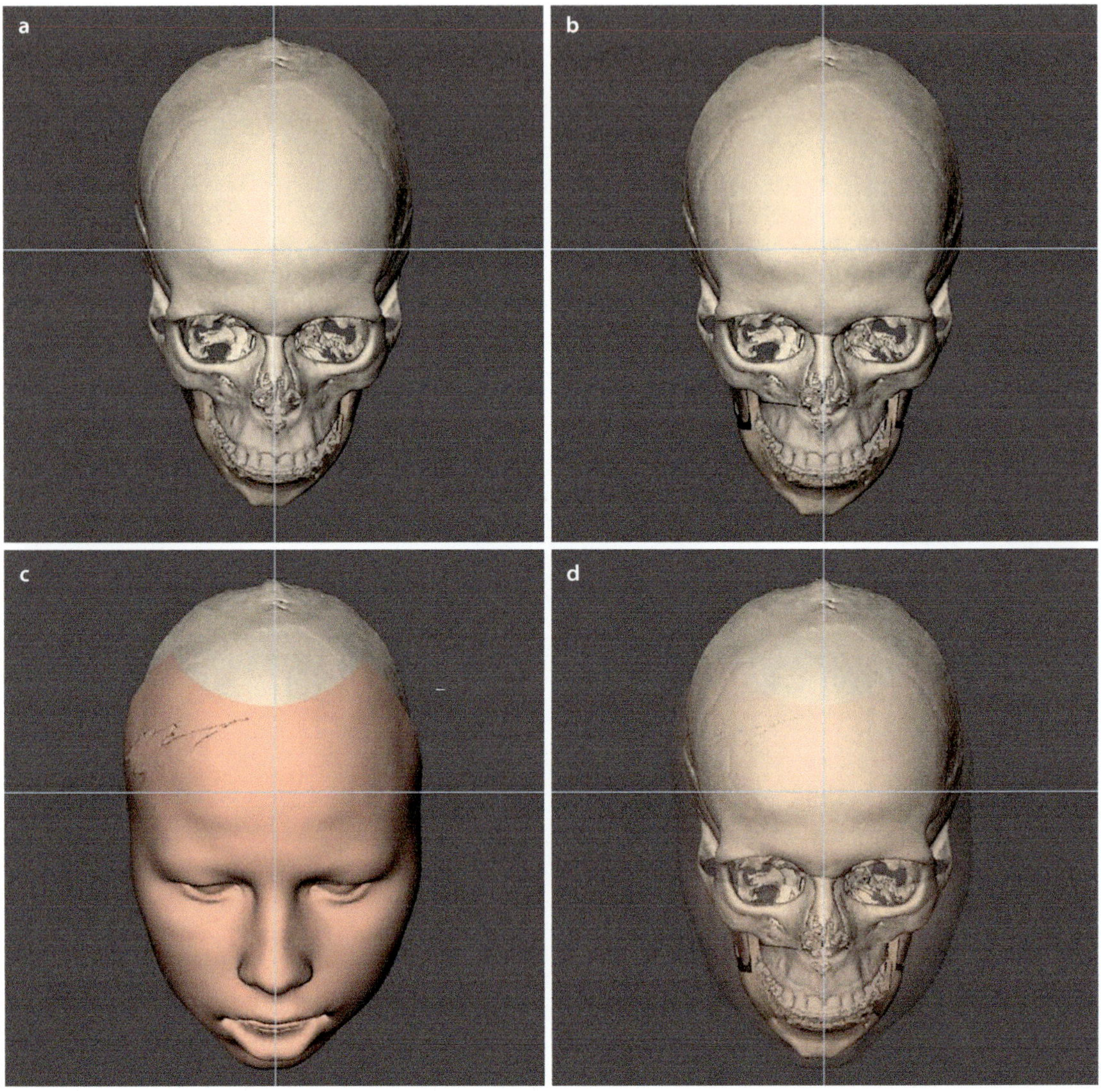

Fig. 3.61 To evaluate overall facial asymmetry after "virtual occlusal definition", the mandibular contour is evaluated virtually towards the contour of the zygomatic arches and zygomatic bones (3D "surface-rendered" representations, patient V.E.W., Maxilim v. 2.3.0.3) (**a**) 2/3 downward inclined view without virtual planning performed (**b**) 2/3 downward inclined view after step 1-3. (**c**) 2/3 downward inclined view after step 1-3 with 3D soft tissues (**d**) 2/3 downward inclined view with 3D soft tissues in transparency

3.5.4 "Step 4": Evaluation/ Correction of Flaring ("Yaw")

Compared to model articulator surgery in conventional treatment planning, the 3D virtual approach has the unprecedented potential in "Step 4" to virtually show the clinician, what is skeletally happening at (1) the bony osteotomy gaps, at both the mandible and the maxilla level and also (2) at the gonial angles and paranasal. This 3D virtual feature offers a huge advantage and benefit in treatment planning both functionally and aesthetically.

1. **From a functional point of view**, this is of clinical importance towards the mandible since flaring of the distal fragment can create torque on the ipsilateral proximal fragment leading to condylar torque, eventual compression and ultimately condylar resorption. Moreover, flaring could create additional compression on the inferior alveolar nerve (IAN) at both sides.
2. **From an aesthetic point of view**, this is of clinical importance towards both the mandible and the maxilla. Flaring of the condylar-ramus unit can cause gonial angle asymmetry and widening of the lower face (Go-Go). In the midface, flaring could cause paranasal asymmetry.

In bimaxillary surgery, flaring of the mandible can be corrected by a rotation in the base plane ("Yaw"), keeping the dental midlines aligned with the facial midline. Moreover, eventual bone collision can virtually be detected in order to be removed during the actual surgery. In most clinical cases, additional infracture osteotomies of the proximal portion of the distal ipsilateral fragment can be avoided by the virtual "Yaw" correction. (◘ Figs. 3.62, 3.63 and 3.64)

In mono-maxillary surgery, the 3D virtual approach makes the clinician aware of the potential flaring. It therefore shows where bone can be removed or additional infracturing of the proximal portion of the distal ipsilateral segment should be performed, in order to decrease the flaring.

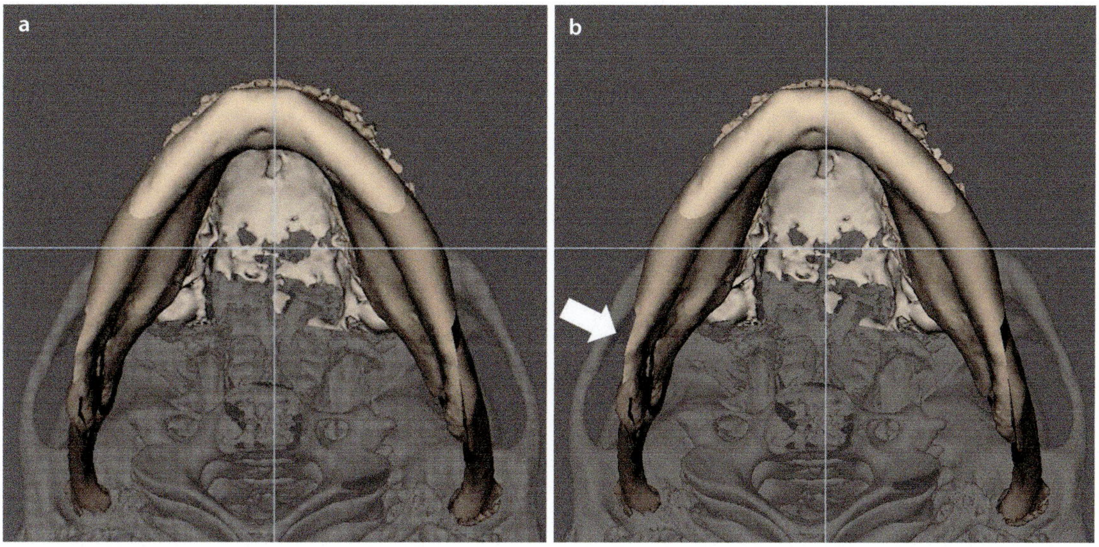

◘ **Fig. 3.62** The base views show lateral flaring of the right proximal segment of the mandible (3D "surface-rendered" representations, patient V.E.W., Maxilim v. 2.3.0.3). The base view (**a**) shows lateral flaring of the distal mandibular fragment to the right (**b**) highlighted by the arrow

"Step 4": Evaluation/Correction of Flaring ("Yaw")

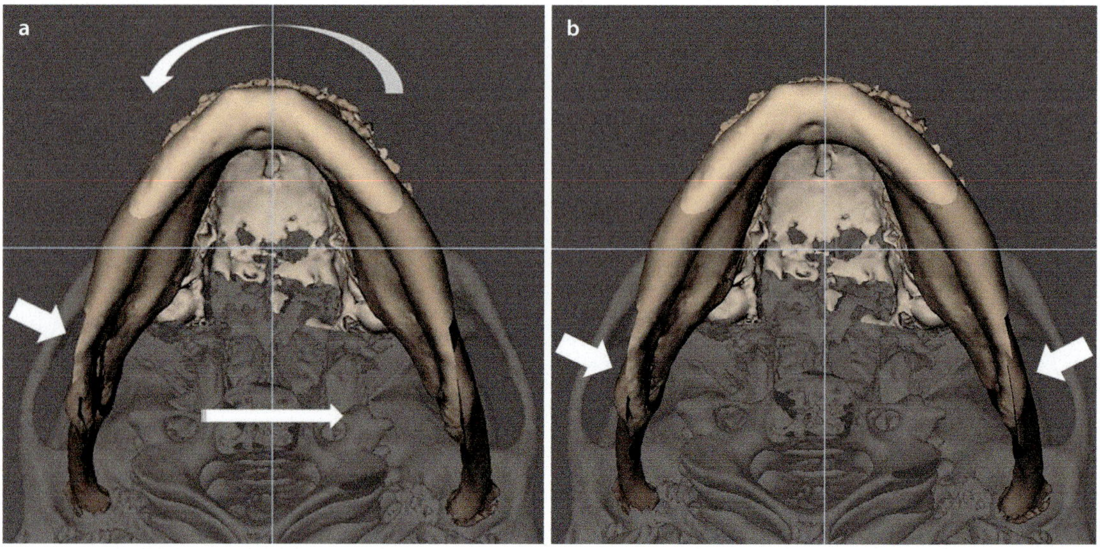

Fig. 3.63 The flaring of the mandible to the right side has been virtually corrected by a CCW "Yaw" rotational movement. Note that the distal mandibular segment has been parallelized to both proximal segments. Moreover 3D virtual planning shows the location of potential bone contacts that might need to be adjusted, during the actual surgery. However, the actual thickness of the bone cuts that will be performed during the clinical surgery needs to be considered (3D "surface-rendered" representations, patient V.E.W., Maxilim v. 2.3.0.3). (**a**) Before correction (**b**) after correction

The surgeon must consider the thickness of the actual clinical bone cuts during the virtual adaptation of the proximal and distal mandibular segments.

This important clinical surgical variable has not been incorporated yet in the 3D virtual osteotomy design and 3D virtual planning.

"Step 4": Evaluation/Correction of Flaring ("Yaw")

In some clinical cases, a certain extent of flaring can be created on purpose: unilaterally to correct a gonial angle asymmetry or bilaterally to widen the lower face width, by increasing the intergonial distance. By removing bone contacts or making the sagittal split shorter, the lower face can be narrowed unilaterally or bilaterally. However, it remains crucial to minimise any surgical movement of the proximal segment to prevent any deleterious effect on the condyles.

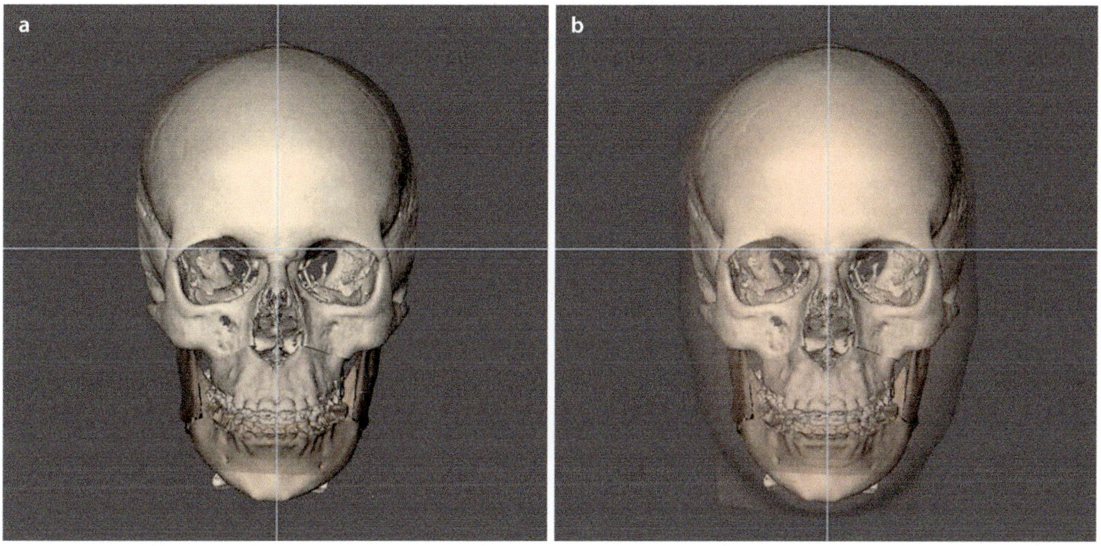

Fig. 3.64 Overall assessment of facial contour after correction of flaring to the right side by a "Yaw" movement of the maxillo-mandibular complex to the left (3D "surface-rendered" representations, patient V.E.W., Maxilim v. 2.3.0.3). (**a**) Frontal view (**b**) frontal view with soft tissues in transparency

3.5.5 "Step 5": Upper Vertical Incisal Position Evaluation/Correction

In "Step 5", the vertical upper incisal position is evaluated in the frontal plane as in conventional treatment planning, by clinical examination of upper incisal/gingival exposure in rest (Fig. 3.1b) and during spontaneous smiling (Fig. 3.52c), ideally at different time points.

In bimaxillary surgery, the vertical upper incisal position is corrected virtually, if needed, by a pure vertical translation movement of the "maxillo-mandibular complex in final occlusion", at the upper incisal level (▶ see also Case 1 in this Chapter) (Fig. 3.65).

In isolate Le Fort I surgery, the vertical upper incisal position is virtually corrected by a combination of vertical translation of the maxilla at the upper incisal level and CW or CCW autorotation of the mandible (▶ see also Case 7, Chap. 6).

The amount (in mm) of vertical virtual upward or downward upper incisal translation is purely based on clinical examination and clinical decision-making.

Limit
3D soft tissue simulation is currently not accurate at the level of the lips.

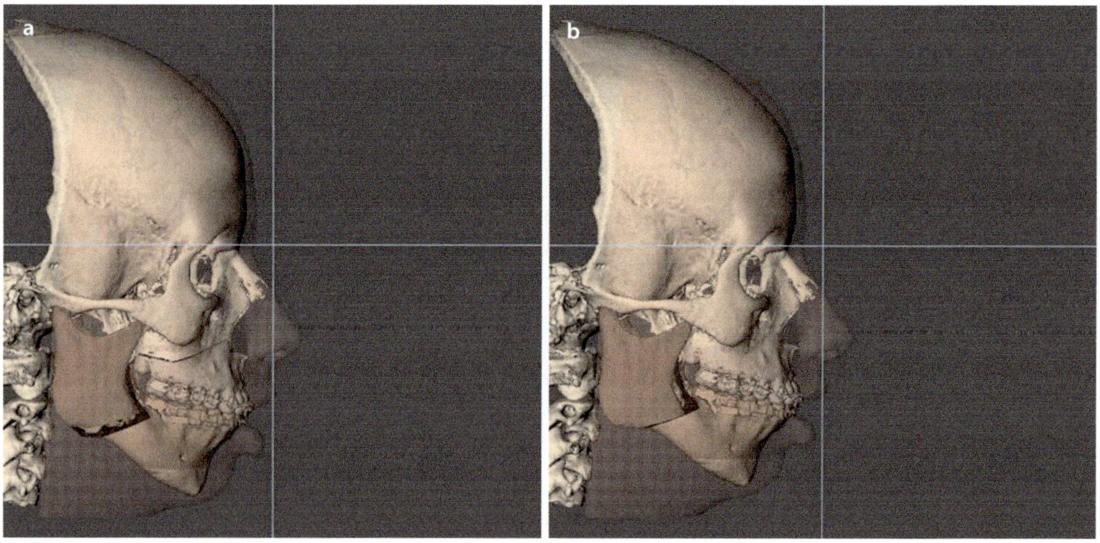

Fig. 3.65 Since the patient has an upper incisal exposure in rest of 8 mm and a gingival exposure of 4 mm, it was decided clinically at this stage to virtually intrude the maxilla 4 mm at the upper incisal level. Note the current limit of 3D soft tissue simulation: despite a vertical incisal intrusion of 4 mm, there is no change in lip morphology and interlabial distance (3D "surface-rendered" representations, patient V.E.W., Maxilim v. 2.3.0.3). (**a**) Before correction (**b**) after correction.

3.5.6 "Step 6": Sagittal Upper Incisal Position Evaluation/Correction

In "Step 6", the sagittal upper incisal position needs to be evaluated and eventually corrected (mostly by an advancement and rarely by a setback) as in conventional treatment planning, based on the clinical examination of the patient in rest (Figs. 3.1, 3.9 and 3.11) and during smiling (Fig. 3.52b–d).

The sagittal horizontal upper incisal position is corrected virtually, if needed, by a pure horizontal translation movement of the "maxillo-mandibular complex in final virtual occlusion", at the upper incisal level (Fig. 3.66).

The amount (in mm) of horizontal virtual forward or backward upper incisal translation is purely based on clinical examination.

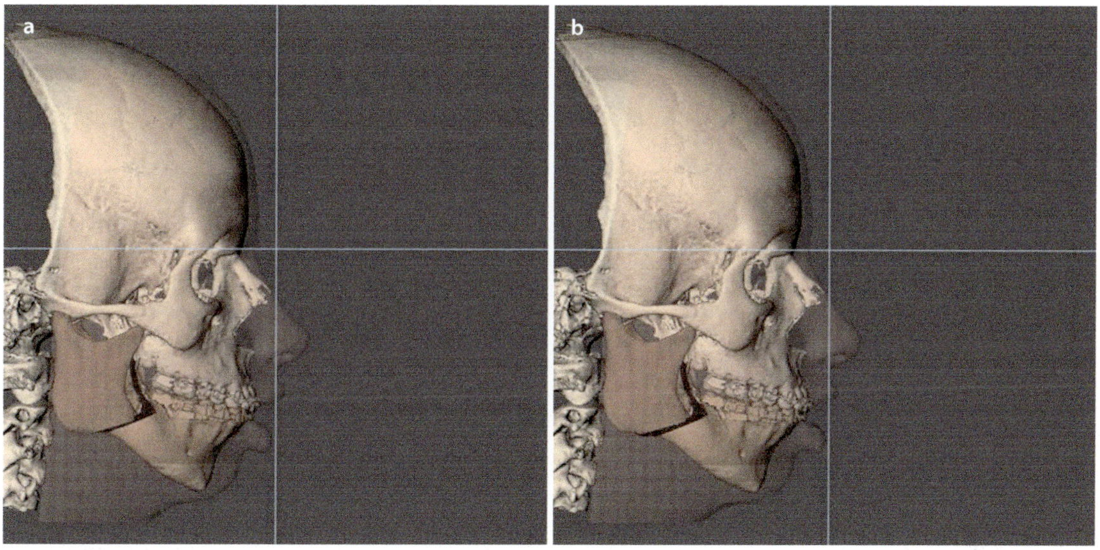

Fig. 3.66 From especially clinical examination but also 3D cephalometric analysis, it was decided to advance the "maxillo-mandibular complex in final occlusion" 2 mm at the upper incisal level (3D "surface-rendered" representations, patient V.E.W., Maxilim v. 2.3.0.3). (**a**) Before correction (**b**) after correction

3.5.7 "Step 7": Profile Evaluation/ Occlusal Plane Correction ("Pitch")

In "Step 7", the profile is evaluated, as in conventional treatment planning by evaluation of the right (◘ Fig. 3.9) and left (◘ Fig. 3.11) clinical profile views towards the TVL.

In the 3D virtual approach, a "Pitch" movement (CW or CCW) of the "maxillo-mandibular complex in final virtual occlusion" towards the vertical 3D PHP reference plane or TVP can be performed in the profile views. This rotational "Pitch" movement is associated with a CW or CCW rotation of the occlusal plane, decreasing or increasing chin projection/upper lip support and last but not least improving overall smile aesthetics (more or less anterior or posterior teeth exposure in the frontal and 2/3 profile views) (◘ Fig. 3.67).

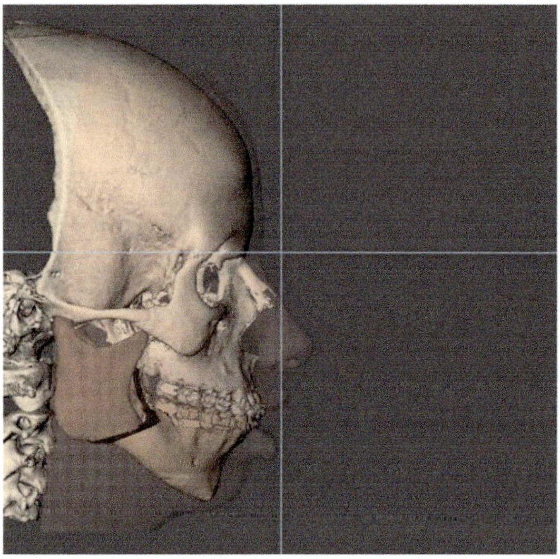

◘ **Fig. 3.67** At this stage (Step 7), it was clinically decided not to alter the occlusal plane and therefore no "Pitch" movement was performed (3D "surface-rendered" representations, patient V.E.W., Maxilim v. 2.3.0.3)

3.5.8 "Step 8": 3D Chin Position Evaluation/Correction

The final chin position is evaluated in "Step 8" in the frontal, profile and base views towards the 3D reference PHP planes of the patient (◘ Figs. 3.68 and 3.69).

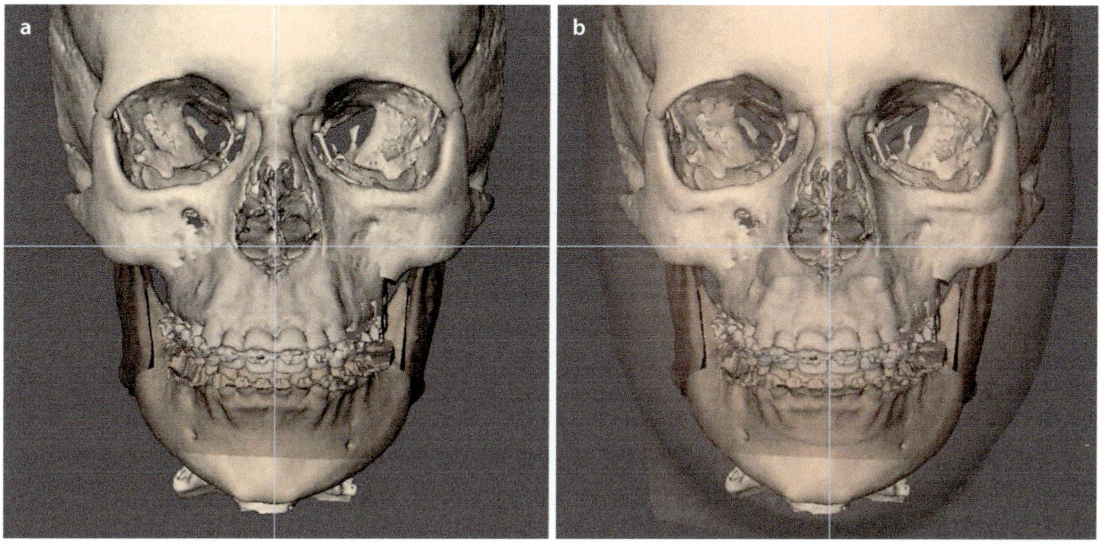

◘ **Fig. 3.68** Evaluation of the chin position in the frontal plane without (**a**) and with (**b**) the patient's 3D facial soft tissue mask in transparency (3D "surface-rendered" representations, patient V.E.W., Maxilim v. 2.3.0.3). Note the persistent cant of the mandibular symphysis and chin point deviation to the right

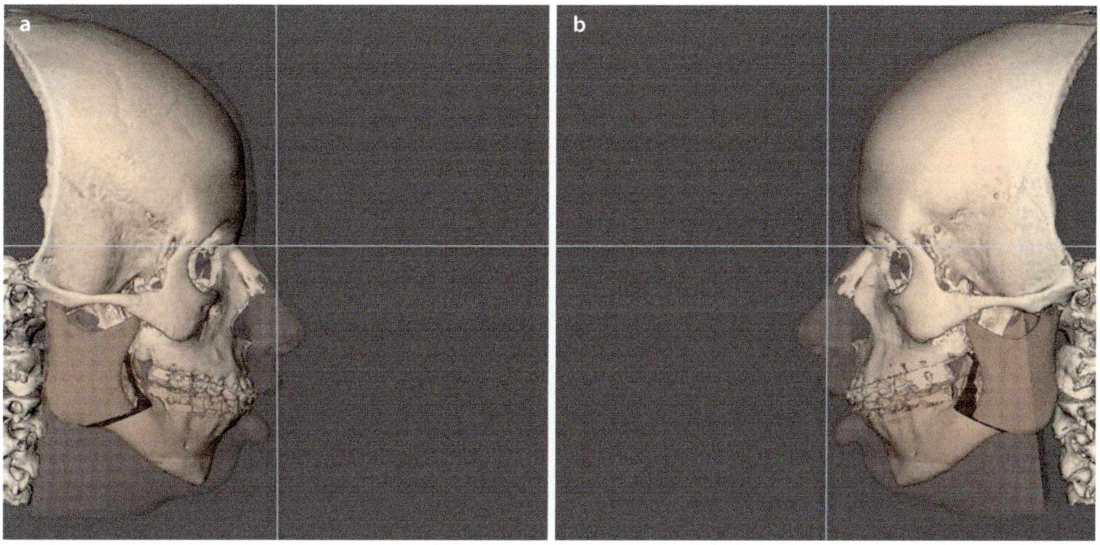

◘ **Fig. 3.69** Evaluation of the sagittal chin position in the right (**a**) and left profile (**b**) views which need to be individually assessed (3D "surface-rendered" representations, patient V.E.W., Maxilim v. 2.3.0.3). Note the retruded chin with absence of a well-defined plica labio-mentalis

"Step 8": 3D Chin Position Evaluation/Correction

The chin can be corrected by (1) a "Roll", (2) a "Yaw", (3) a "Pitch", (4) an advancement (or rarely a setback), (5) a translation to the right or left, (6) an intrusion or extrusion or (7) a combination of several of these movements. Moreover, it is important to additionally evaluate the chin also in the base, 2/3 downward and 2/3 upward rotated frontal views (◘ Figs. 3.70 and 3.71).

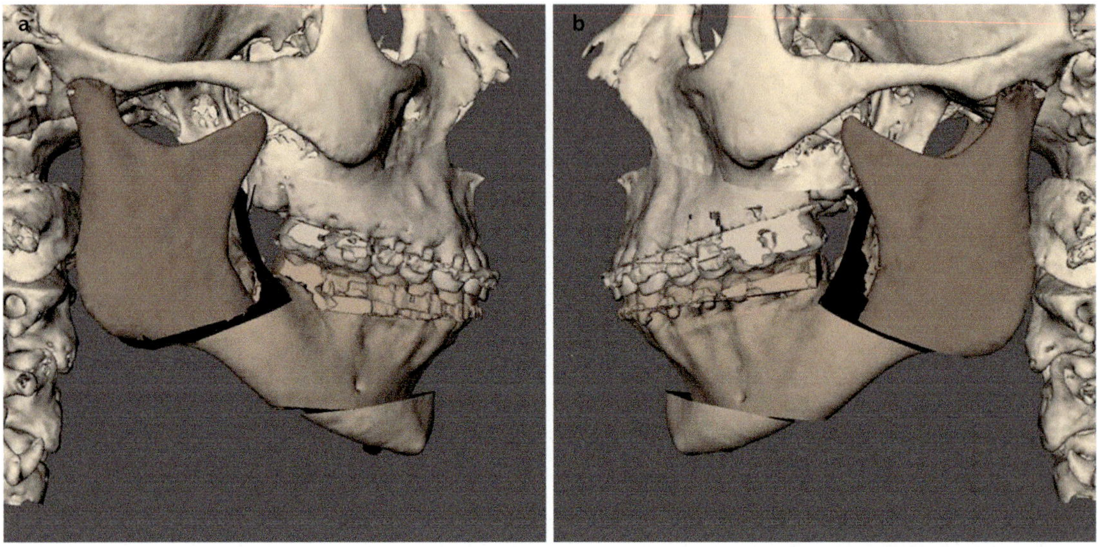

◘ **Fig. 3.70** In the profile planes, a chin advancement of 6 mm, with an anterior intrusion of 2 mm and a CCW "Pitch" rotation was virtually planned, in order to align the bony segments at the inferior mandibular border level (3D "surface-rendered" representations, patient V.E.W., Maxilim v. 2.3.0.3). (**a**) Profile right view (**b**) profile left view

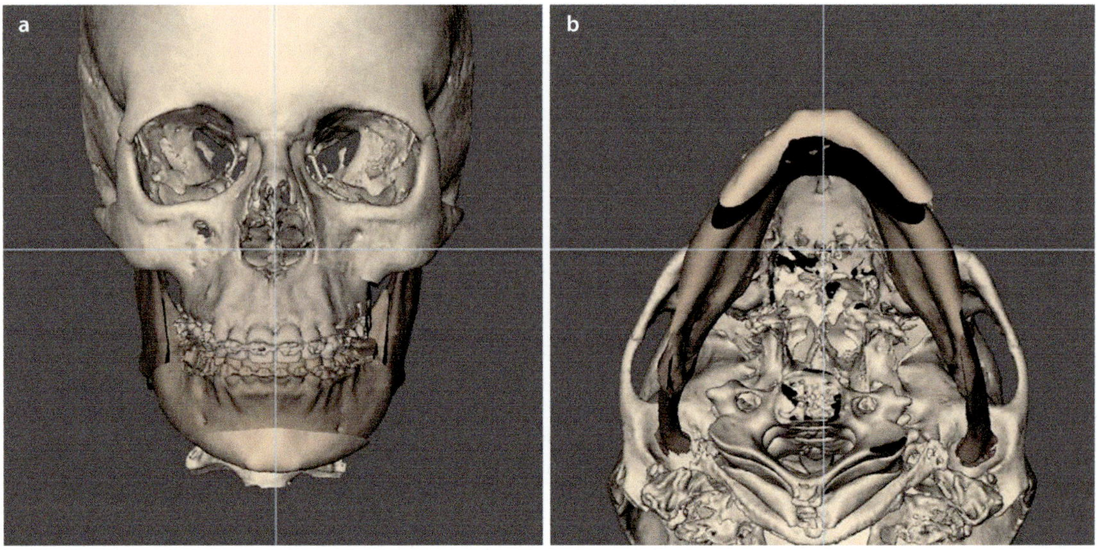

◘ **Fig. 3.71** In the frontal plane, a midline correction of 2 mm to the left combined with a CCW "Roll" movement was virtually planned to correct the mandibular symphysis deviation and cant. Additional, a CW "Yaw" correction was virtually planned in the base plane (3D "surface-rendered" representations, patient V.E.W., Maxilim v. 2.3.0.3). (**a**) Frontal view (**b**) base view

3.5.9 "Step 9": Patient Communication of the Individualised Treatment Plan

In "Step 9" the integrated "individualised 3D virtual treatment plan" is discussed with the patient and additional modifications can be decided on by the ortho-surgical team to meet the patient's expectations. The limitations of 3D soft tissue simulation, especially regarding the nasolabial aesthetic unit, must be considered by the clinician and well explained to the patient to avoid miscommunication.

Moreover, as far as education is concerned, in Step 9, the patient's "individualised 3D virtual treatment plan" can be discussed with residents, fellows and other staff members (◘ Figs. 3.72 and 3.73).

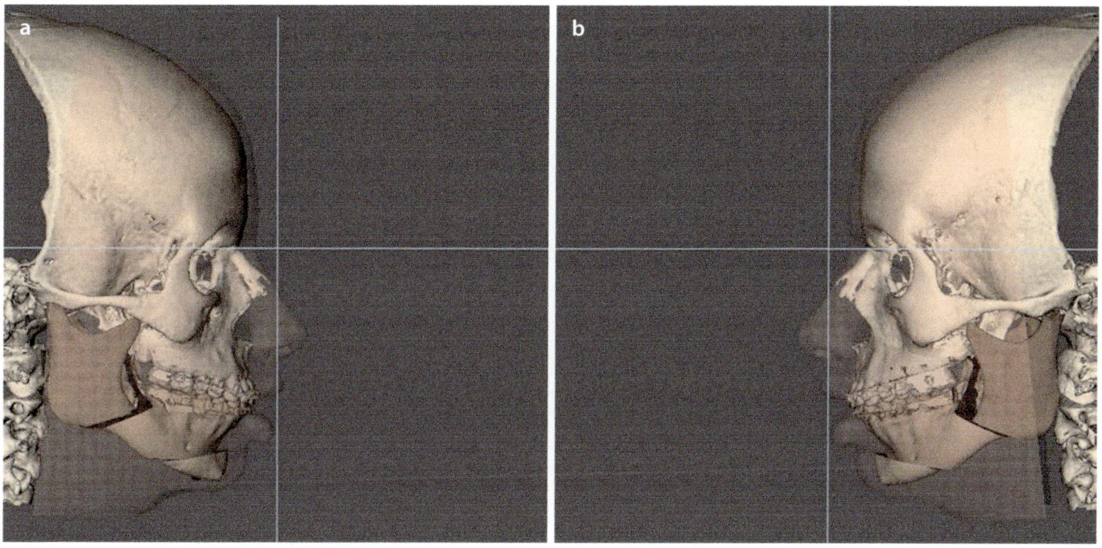

◘ **Fig. 3.72** "Individualised 3D virtual treatment plan", as presented to the patient, before the actual surgery. At this moment, it is still possible to adjust the planning to meet the patient's expectations (3D "surface-rendered" representations, patient V.E.W., Maxilim v. 2.3.0.3). Note the limit of the soft tissue simulation at the level of the lips. (**a**) Profile right view (**b**) profile left view

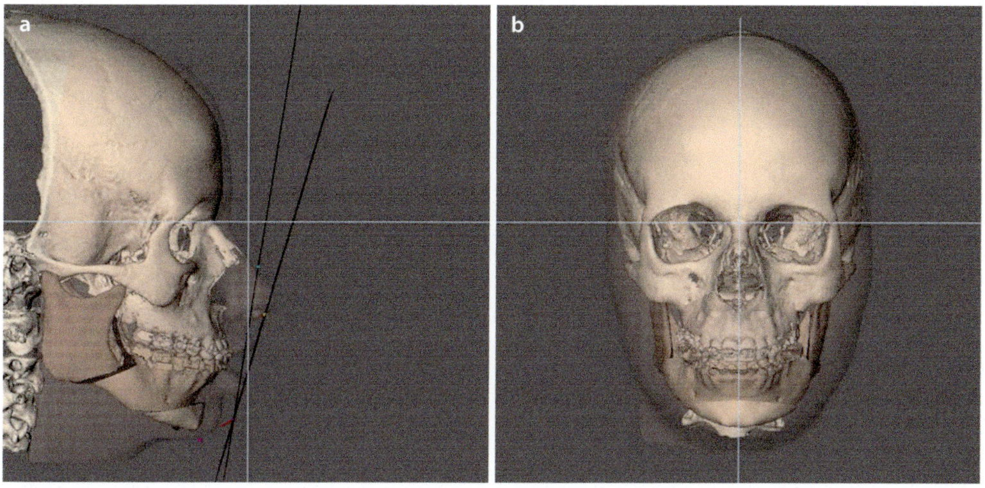

◘ **Fig. 3.73** "Individualised 3D virtual treatment plan", as presented to the patient, before the actual surgery. At this moment, it is still possible to adjust the planning to meet the patient's expectations. Besides the TVP and the horizontal PHP reference plane, the ideal profile plane and ideal lip plane according to the 3D Bruges facial mask analysis are visualised (► see also Sect. 2.2) (3D "surface-rendered" representations, patient V.E.W., Maxilim v. 2.3.0.3). Note the limit of the soft tissue simulation at the level of the lips. (**a**) Profile right view (**b**) frontal view

3.5.10 "Step 10": Final Adjustments of the 3D Virtual Treatment Plan

After having discussed the integrated "individualised 3D virtual treatment plan" in "Step 9" with the patient and the ortho-surgical team, final adjustments can be made in order to further enhance and optimise the surgical outcome towards the patient's expectations.

Again, it is imperative to consider the actual important and clinical relevant limits of 3D soft tissue simulation limits, especially in cases of lip incompetency and atonic lower lip. Additional manual morphing of the lips is possible, but it remains very subjective (Figs. 3.74, 3.75, 3.76, 3.77, 3.78 and 3.79).

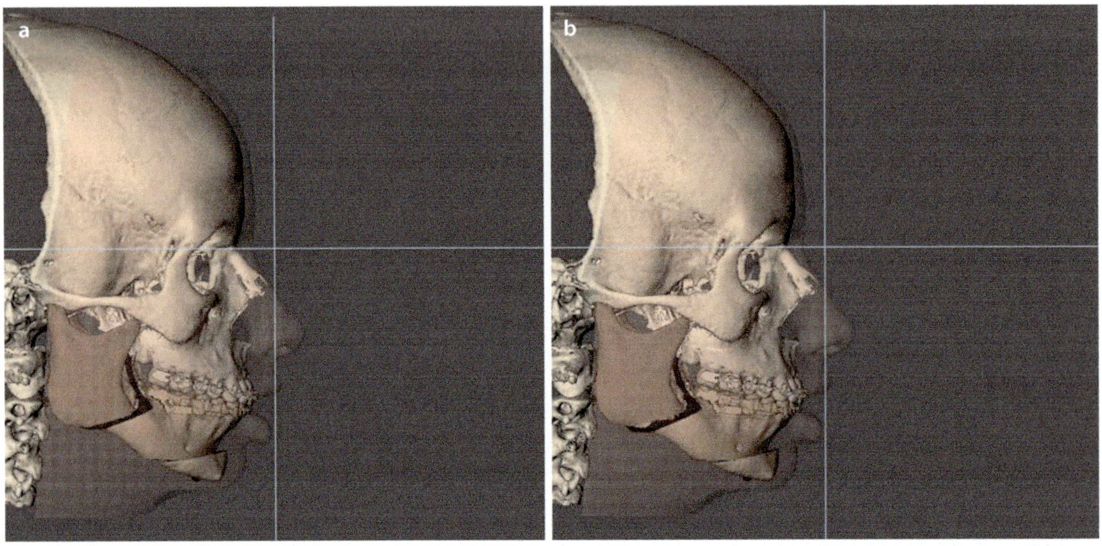

Fig. 3.74 Final adjustments of the "individualised 3D virtual treatment plan". It was decided to perform more CCW "Pitch" movement of the maxillo-mandibular complex, to provide more chin advancement (3D "surface-rendered" representations, patient V.E.W., Maxilim v. 2.3.0.3). Note the limit of the soft tissue simulation at the level of the lips. (**a**) Before correction (**b**) after correction

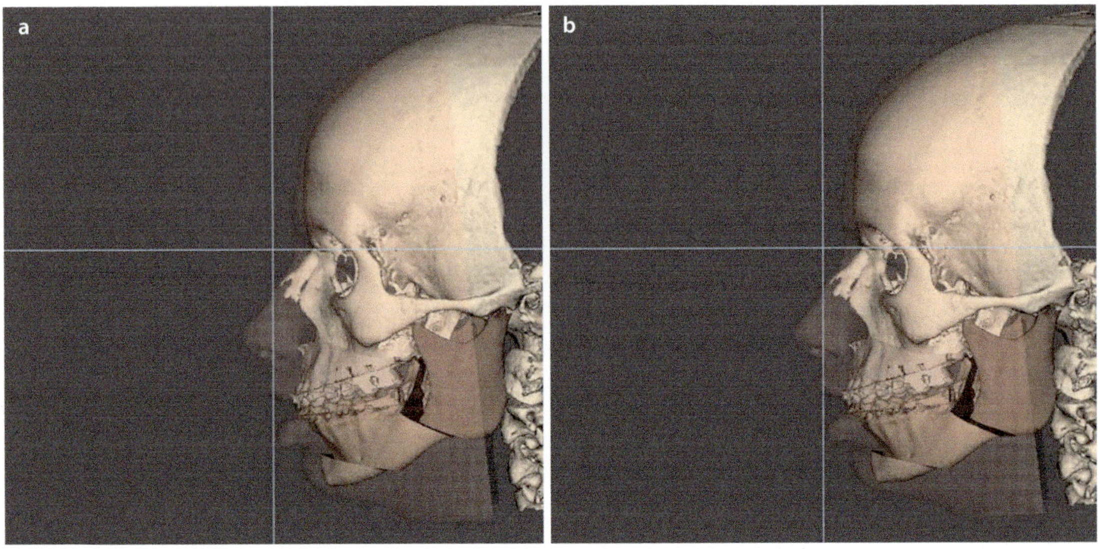

Fig. 3.75 Final adjustments of the "individualised 3D virtual treatment plan". It was decided to perform more CCW "Pitch" movement of the maxillo-mandibular complex, to provide more chin advancement (3D "surface-rendered" representations, patient V.E.W., Maxilim v. 2.3.0.3). Note the limit of the soft tissue simulation at the level of the lips. (**a**) Before correction (**b**) after correction

Final integrated "Individualised 3D Virtual Treatment Plan" (Patient V.E.W.)

The transfer and outcome evaluation of the "individualised 3D virtual treatment plan" of Case 1 (Patient V.E.W.) are explained and elaborated on in detail in Chap. 4 and Chap. 5, respectively.

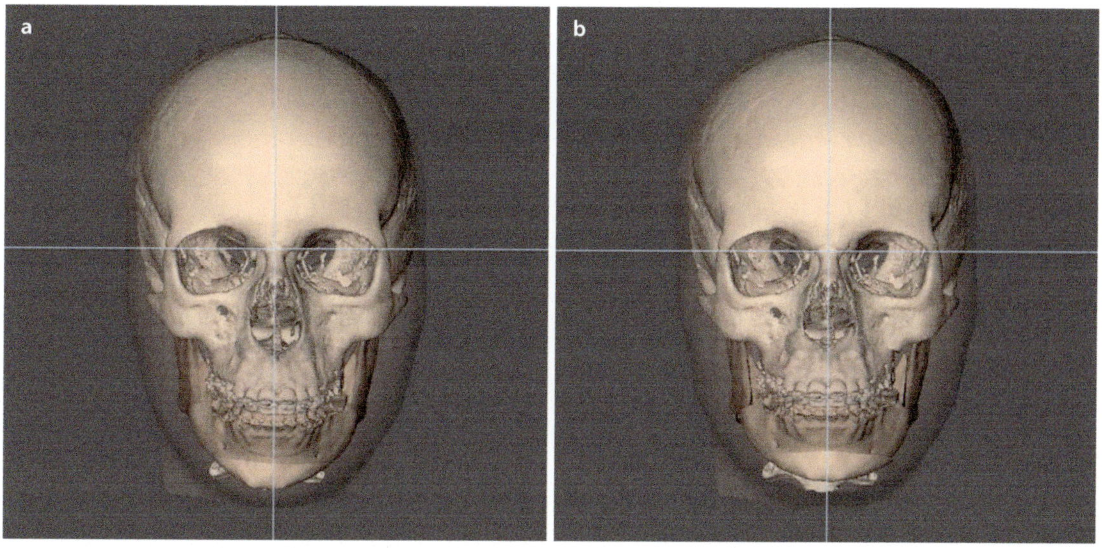

Fig. 3.76 Initial situation (**a**) and final "individualised 3D virtual treatment plan" (**b**), in the frontal plane (3D "surface-rendered" representations, patient V.E.W., Maxilim v. 2.3.0.3)

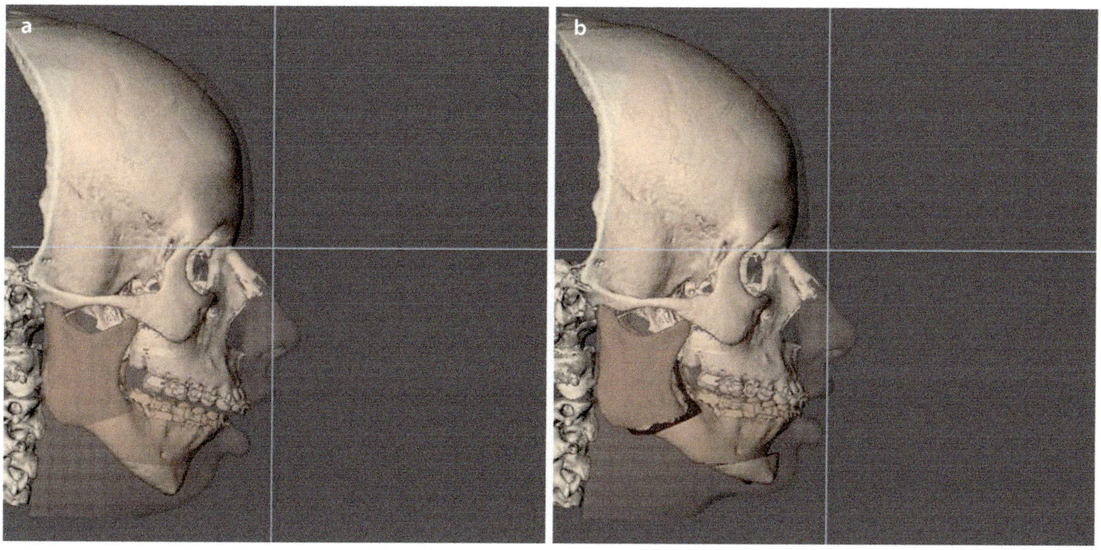

Fig. 3.77 Initial situation (**a**) and final "individualised 3D virtual treatment plan" (**b**), in the right profile plane (3D "surface-rendered" representations, patient V.E.W., Maxilim v. 2.3.0.3)

Final integrated "Individualised 3D Virtual Treatment Plan" (Patient V.E.W.)

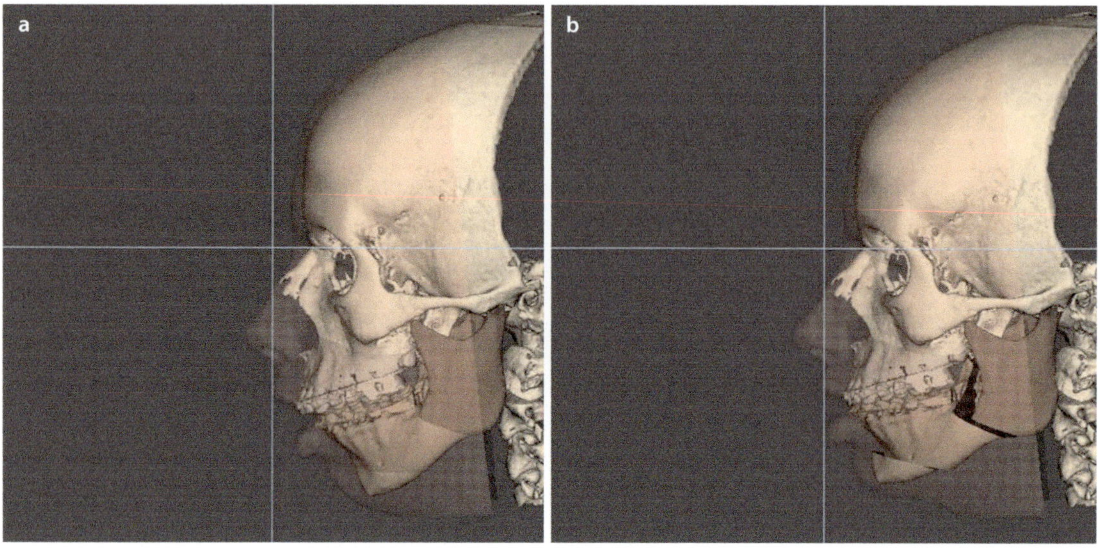

Fig. 3.78 Initial situation (**a**) and final "individualised 3D virtual treatment plan" (**b**), in the left profile plane (3D "surface-rendered" representations, patient V.E.W., Maxilim v. 2.3.0.3)

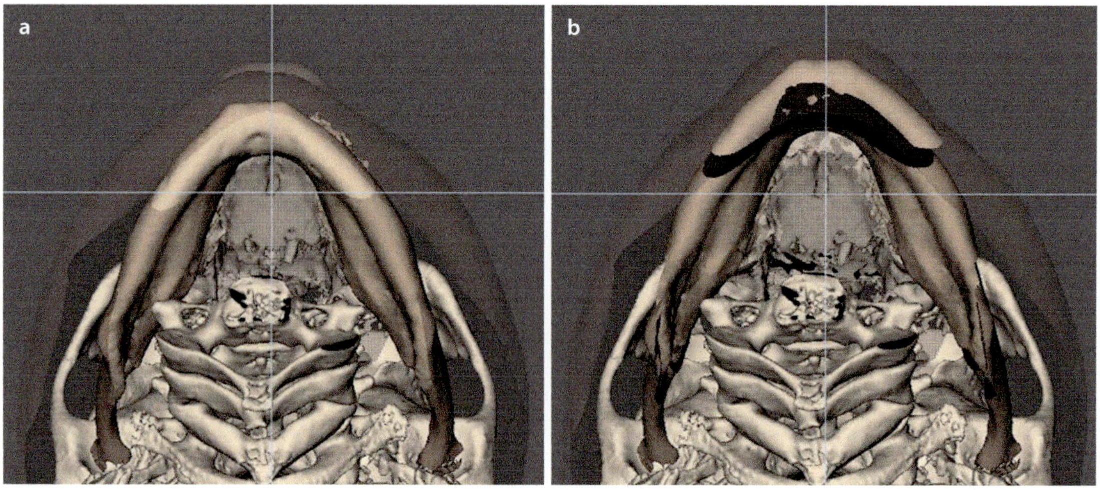

Fig. 3.79 Initial situation (**a**) and final "individualised 3D virtual treatment plan" (**b**), in the base plane (3D "surface-rendered" representations, patient V.E.W., Maxilim v. 2.3.0.3)

Additional Recommended Reading

Aboul-Hosn Centenero S, Hernández-Alfaro F (2012) 3D planning in orthognathic surgery: CAD/CAM surgical splints and prediction of the soft and hard tissues results - our experience in 16 cases. J Craniomaxillofac Surg 40:162–168
Ackerman JL, Proffit WR, Sarver DM, Ackerman MB, Kean MR (2007) Pitch, roll, and yaw: describing the spatial orientation of dentofacial traits. Am J Orthod Dentofac 131:305–310
Arnett GW, McLaughlin RP (2004) Facial and dental planning for orthodontists and oral surgeons. Mosby, Elsevier Limited. Philadelphia, USA
Arnett GW, Gunson MJ (2004) Facial planning for orthodontists and oral surgeons. Am J Orthod Dentofac 126:290–295
Bjerin R (1957) A comparison between the Frankfort horizontal and the Sella turcica-nasion as reference planes in cephalometric analysis. Acta Odontologica Scandinavia 15:1–12
Bobek S, Farrell B, Choi C, Farrell B, Weimer K, Tucker M (2015) Virtual surgical planning for orthognathic surgery using digital data transfer and an intraoral fiducial marker: the charlotte method. J Oral Maxillofac Surg. 73:1143–1158
Cevidanes L, Oliveira AEF, Motta A, Phillips C, Burke B, Tyndall D (2009) Head orientation in CBCT-generated cephalograms. Angle Orthod 79:971–977
Cooke MS (1990) Five-year reproducibility of natural head posture: a longitudinal study. Am J Orthod Dentofac Orthop Off Publ Am Assoc Orthod 97:489–494
Cooke MS, Wei SH (1988) The reproducibility of natural head posture: a methodological study. Am J Orthod Dentofac Orthop 93:280–288
Damstra J, Fourie Z, Ren Y (2010) Simple technique to achieve a natural position of the head for cone beam computed tomography. Br J Oral Maxillofac Surg 48:236–238
De Paula LK, Ackerman JL, Carvalho FdeAR, Eidson L, Cevidanes LHS (2012) Digital live-tracking 3-dimensional minisensors for recording head orientation during image acquisition. Am J Orthod Dentofac Orthop 141:116–123
Downs WB (1956) Analysis of the dento-facial profile. Angle Orthod 4:191–212
Farrell BB, Franco PB, Tucker MR (2014) Virtual surgical planning in orthognathic surgery. Oral Maxillofac Surg Clin N Am 26:459–473
Gateno J, Xia JJ, Teichgraeber JF (2011) New methods to evaluate craniofacial deformity and to plan surgical correction. Semin Orthod 17:225–234
Lundström A, Lundström F, Lebret LM, Moorrees CF (1995) Natural head position and natural head orientation: basic considerations in cephalometric analysis and research. Eur J Orthod 17:111–120
Lundström F, Lundström A (1992) Natural head position as a basis for cephalometric analysis. Am J Orthod Dentofac Orthop 101:244–247
Marchetti C, Bianchi A, Bassi M, Gori R, Lamberti C, Sarti A (2007) Mathematical modeling and numerical simulation in maxillo-facial virtual surgery (VISU). J Craniofac Surg 18:826–832
Marchetti C, Bianchi A, Muyldermans L, Di Martino M, Lancellotti L, Sarti A (2011) Validation of new soft tissue software in orthognathic surgery planning. Int J Oral Maxillofac Surg 40:26–32
Mollemans W, Schutyser F, Nadjmi N, Maes F, Suetens P (2007) Predicting soft tissue deformations for a maxillofacial surgery planning system: from computational strategies to a complete clinical validation. Med Image Anal 11:282–291
Moorrees CFA, Kean MR (1958) Natural head position, a basic consideration in the interpretation of cephalometric radiographs. Am J Phys Anthropol 16:213–234
Nadjmi N, Defrancq E, Mollemans W, Hemelen GV, Bergé S (2014) Quantitative validation of a computer-aided maxillofacial planning system, focusing on soft tissue deformations. Ann Maxillofac Surg 4:171–175
Nadjmi N, Mollemans W, Daelemans A, Van Hemelen G, Schutyser F, Bergé S (2010) Virtual occlusion in planning orthognathic surgical procedures. Int J Oral Maxillofac Surg 39:457–462
Peng L, Cooke MS (1999) Fifteen-year reproducibility of natural head posture: a longitudinal study. Am J Orthod Dentofac Orthop 116:82–85
Quevedo LA, Ruiz JV, Quevedo CA (2011) Using a clinical protocol for orthognathic surgery and assessing a 3-dimensional virtual approach: current therapy. J Oral Maxillofac Surg 69:623–637
Solow B, Tallgren A (1971) Natural head position in standing subjects. Acta Odontol Scand 29:591–607
Swennen GRJ, Schutyser F (2007) Three-dimensional virtual approach to diagnosis and treatment planning of maxillo-facial deformity. In: Bell WH, Guerrero CA, eds. Distraction osteogenesis of the facial skeleton. BC Decker Inc., Hamilton; 2007. p 6
Swennen GRJ, Mommaerts MY, Abeloos J, De Clercq C, Lamoral P, Neyt N, Casselman J, Schutyser F (2009a) A cone-beam CT based technique to augment the 3D virtual skull model with a detailed dental surface. Int J Oral Maxillofac Surg 38:48–57
Swennen GRJ, Mollemans W, Schutyser F (2009b) Three-dimensional treatment planning of orthognathic surgery in the era of virtual imaging. J Oral Maxillofac Surg 67:2080–2092
Swennen GRJ (2014) Timing of three-dimensional virtual treatment planning of orthognathic surgery: a prospective single-surgeon evaluation on 350 consecutive cases. Oral Maxillofac Surg Clin N Am 26:475–485
Xia JJ, Gateno J, Teichgraeber JF (2009) New clinical protocol to evaluate craniomaxillofacial deformity and plan surgical correction. J Oral Maxillofac Surg 67: 2093–2106
Xia JJ, McGrory JK, Gateno J, Teichgraeber JF, Dawson BC, Kennedy KA, Lasky RE, English JD, Kau CH, McGrory KR (2011) A new method to orient 3-dimensional computed tomography models to the natural head position: a clinical feasibility study. J Oral Maxillofac Surg 69:584–591

3D Virtual Treatment Planning Transfer in the Operation Theatre

Gwen R.J. Swennen and Martin Gaboury

G.R.J. Swennen (ed.), *3D Virtual Treatment Planning of Orthognathic Surgery*,
DOI 10.1007/978-3-662-47389-4_4

4.1 3D Virtual Treatment Planning Transfer

In "conventional treatment planning of orthognathic surgery", both model surgeries performed on mounted dental casts to mimic the planned movements and fabrication of intermediate splints for planning transfer, although well established, are prone to error (Ellis 1990). In the era of 2D imaging and conventional planning, however, most of the jaw movements were limited to linear antero-posterior, medio-lateral and infero-superior translations, therefore suitable to model articulator surgery.

"3D virtual treatment planning of orthognathic surgery" truly initiated a major paradigm shift. A prerequisite for accurate "3D Virtual Treatment Planning" is proper image acquisition (► see also Sect. 1.1) and accurate processing of the acquired image data towards an accurate 3D virtual augmented model of the patient's head (► see also Sect. 1.2). In contrast to "conventional treatment planning", "3D Virtual Treatment Planning" allows to precisely plan complex 3D geometric "Pitch", "Roll" and "Cant" (► see also Sect. 3.4) corrections in the "3D virtual scene". With such complex 3D movements in space, conventional model articulator surgery, which remains a multiple-step process and hence inherently prone to incorporate a vast array of errors, cannot be considered a valid option anymore.

After "Step-by-Step Individualised 3D Virtual Treatment Planning (3D-VPS$_5$)" (► see Sect. 3.5), the "3D virtual treatment plan" needs to be accurately transferred towards the patient in the operation theatre. For that purpose the bridge between conventional and 3D Virtual Treatment Planning is made by means of a combination of:

1. 3D surgical splints/3D templates (► Sect. 4.1.1)
2. Internal/external references for vertical repositioning (► Sect. 4.1.2)

Compared to conventional planning, the "3D Virtual Visualisation Paradigm" offers a major advantage since it allows the clinician to decide how in bimaxillary surgery he wants to transfer his "Final Integrated and Individualised 3D Virtual Treatment Plan" to the patient in the operation theatre depending on the clinical situation or his personal philosophy:

1. By a **"Maxilla-first" sequence** (◘ Figs. 4.1, 4.2, 4.3 and 4.4)
2. Or by a **"Mandible-first" sequence** (◘ Figs. 4.5, 4.6, 4.7 and 4.8)

The intra-operative transfer of the "3D virtual treatment plan" by means of a dental-borne 3D surgical splint, however, still relies on appropriate vertical measuring, condylar seating and autorotation of the mandible, a concept still prone to error and highly dependent on the experience of the surgeon.

More recently, innovative technologies, like patient-specific implants (PSIs) (► see also Sect. 4.1.3), navigation surgery (► see also Sect. 4.2.1) and augmented reality (AR) (► see also Sect. 4.2.2) emerged from the concept of "Waferless Orthognathic Surgery" in order to try to eliminate the potential errors associated with condylar seating and autorotation of the mandible.

4.1.1 3D Surgical Splint/Template Manufacturing

After "Step-by-Step Individualised 3D Virtual Treatment Planning (3D-VPS$_5$)" (► see Sect. 3.5), dental-borne wafers, consisting of an intermediate and a final surgical splint, are used to reposition the maxilla and the mandible.

The "3D virtual splints" need to be designed and consequently processed to "3D surgical splints" by CAD/CAM (Computer-Aided Design/Computer-Aided Manufacturing) technologies. In case a "Maxilla-first" sequence is adopted, a "3D virtual intermediate splint" (◘ Fig. 4.2a) will be designed to first reposition the maxilla (◘ Fig. 4.1a), while in a "Mandible-first" sequence, a "3D virtual intermediate splint" (◘ Fig. 4.6a) will be designed to first reposition the mandible (◘ Fig. 4.5a). The "3D final virtual splint" remains the same whenever a "Maxilla-first" (◘ Fig. 4.2b) or "Mandible-first" (◘ Fig. 4.6b) sequence is desired.

CAD/CAM technologies allow the production of highly precise dental-borne "3D surgical splints" (◘ Figs. 4.9 and 4.10) but also "3D templates" (e.g. for chin repositioning (◘ Figs. 4.13, 4.14 and 4.15) that can be used during the actual surgery. With CAD/CAM technologies, the "3D surgical splints" can be either processed by subtractive (e.g. milling) or additive manufacturing (e.g. stereolithography, 3D printing). These two rapid prototyping techniques (RPTs) have shown similar results in terms of accuracy in planning transfer and precision of fit. It remains however the responsibility of the clinician to examine the final product and especially verify that the "3D surgical splints" do not contact the orthodontic brackets in order to prevent errors in the surgical repositioning of the jaws (◘ Figs. 4.11 and 4.12). The actual 3D workflows are mostly based on "out-office" processing and subsequent shipping of the "3D surgical splints" and "3D templates" to the clinician which remains a significant disadvantage regarding efficiency and cost. "In-office" processing by RPT technologies could solve this problem towards the clinician in the future.

The concept of "3D surgical splints" and "3D templates" is illustrated by Case 1, patient V.E.W. which is used throughout the book (▶ Chaps. 1, 2, 3, 5 and 6).

■ **3D Virtual Splints: "Maxilla-First" Sequence**

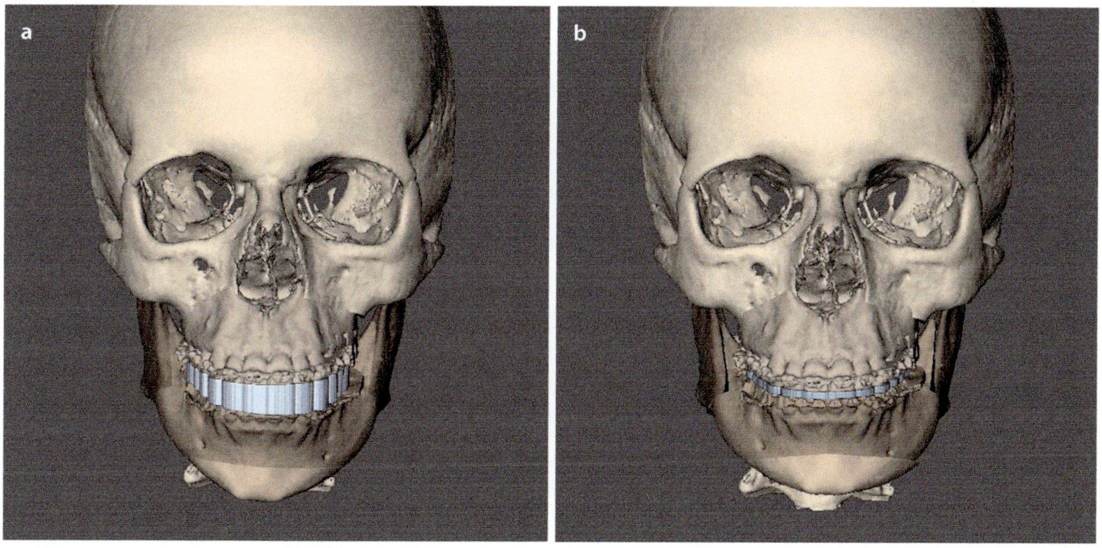

◘ **Fig. 4.1** Frontal views of the 3D virtual intermediate (**a**) and final (**b**) splints, when a "Maxilla-first" sequence is chosen (3D "surface-rendered" representations, patient V.E.W. Maxilim v. 2.3.0.3.). Note that the 3D virtual final splint is the same whenever a "Maxilla-first" or "Mandible-first" sequence is chosen

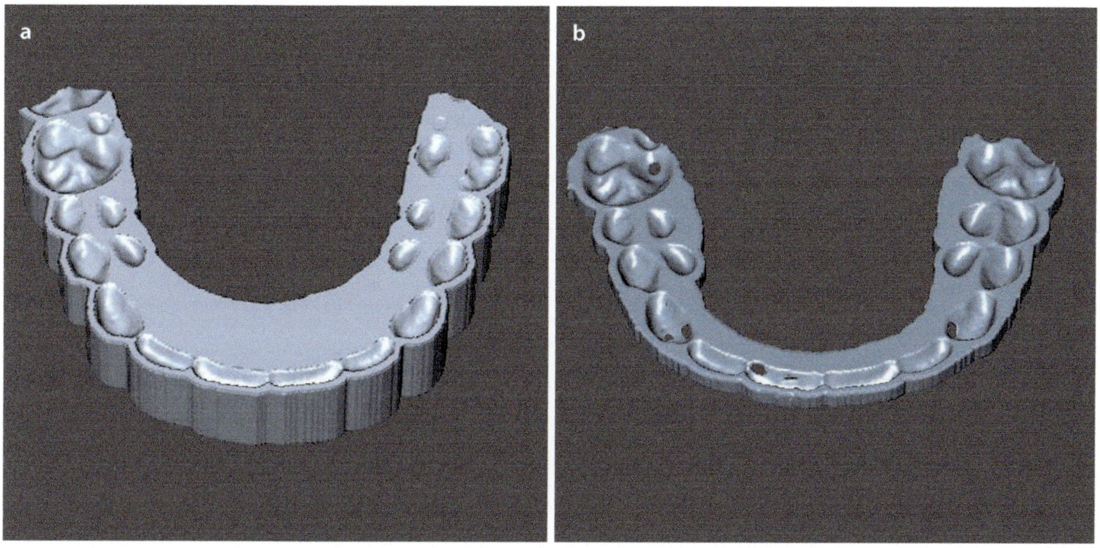

◘ **Fig. 4.2** 3D virtual intermediate (**a**) and final (**b**) splints, when a "Maxilla-first" sequence is chosen (3D "surface-rendered" representations, patient V.E.W. Maxilim v. 2.3.0.3.). Note that the 3D virtual final splint is the same whenever a "Maxilla-first" or "Mandible-first" sequence is chosen

3D Virtual Splints: "Maxilla-First" Sequence

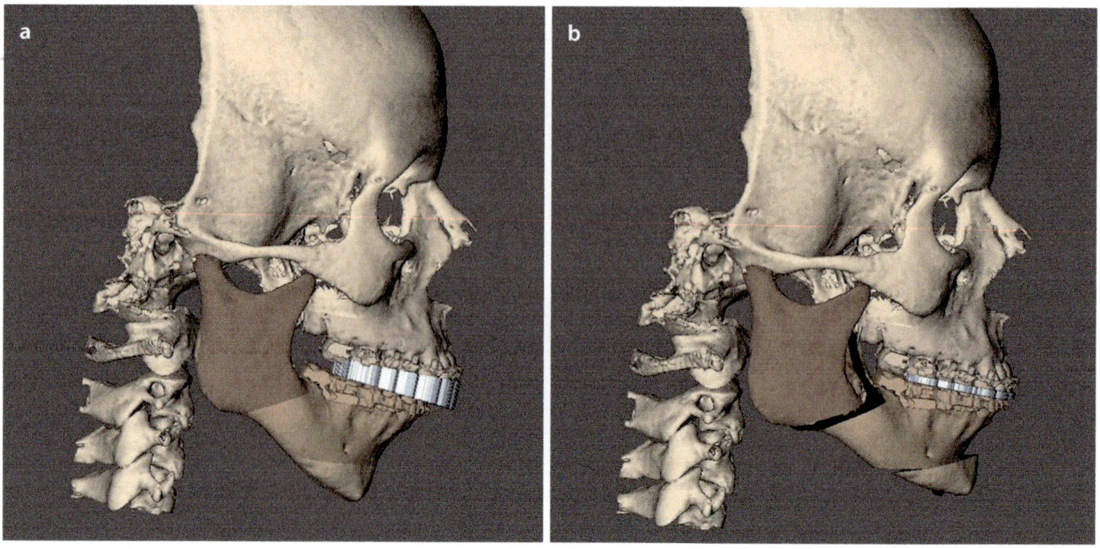

Fig. 4.3 Right profile views of the 3D virtual intermediate (**a**) and final (**b**) splints, when a "Maxilla-first" sequence is chosen (3D "surface-rendered" representations, patient V.E.W. Maxilim v. 2.3.0.3.)

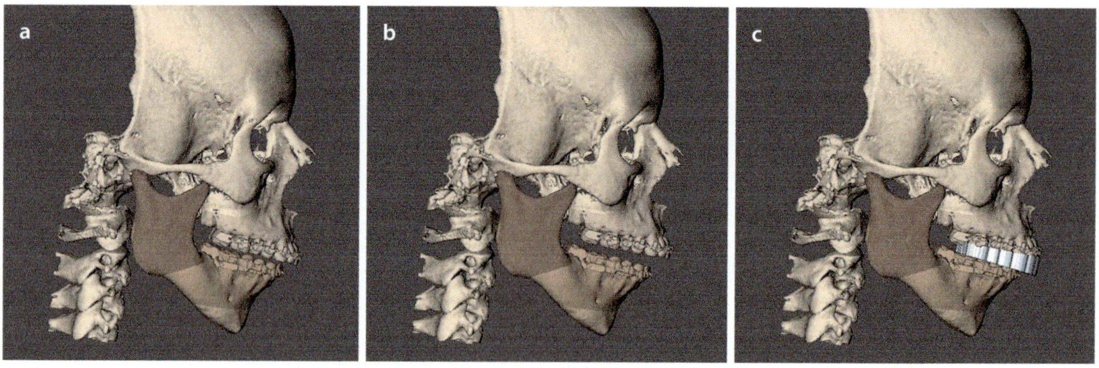

Fig. 4.4 Right profile views of the preoperative situation in CR (**a**), after virtual repositioning of the maxilla following a virtual non-segmental Le Fort I osteotomy (**b**) and with the 3D virtual intermediate splint in place to reposition the maxilla (**c**) when a "Maxilla-first" sequence is chosen (3D "surface-rendered" representations, patient V.E.W. Maxilim v. 2.3.0.3.). Note that due to the individual mandibular anatomy and the 3D virtual Le Fort I osteotomy movements, especially vertical impaction, the 3D virtual intermediate splint in this case was designed to avoid any autorotation of the mandible, which is still prone to errors. In some cases, it might be necessary to virtually autorotate (▶ see also Sect. 1.3) the mandible (CW or CCW) to allow the necessary space for the manufacturing of the 3D virtual intermediate splint

■ 3D Virtual Splints: "Mandible-First" Sequence

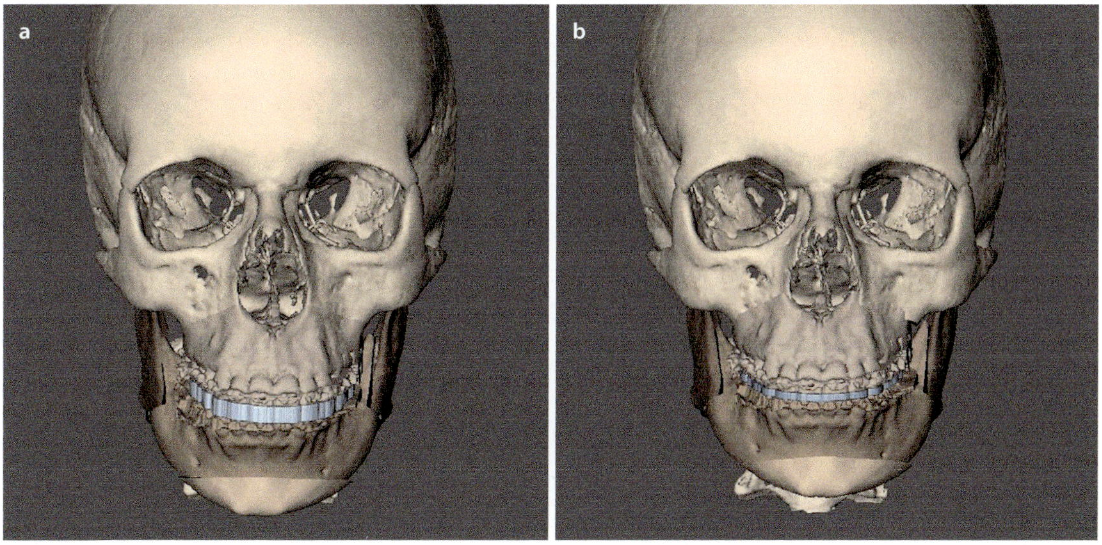

Fig. 4.5 Frontal views of the 3D virtual intermediate (**a**) and final (**b**) splints, when a "Mandible-first" sequence is chosen (3D "surface-rendered" representations, patient V.E.W. Maxilim v. 2.3.0.3.). Note that the 3D virtual final splint is the same whenever a "Mandible-first" or "Maxilla-first" (Fig. 4.1b) sequence is desired

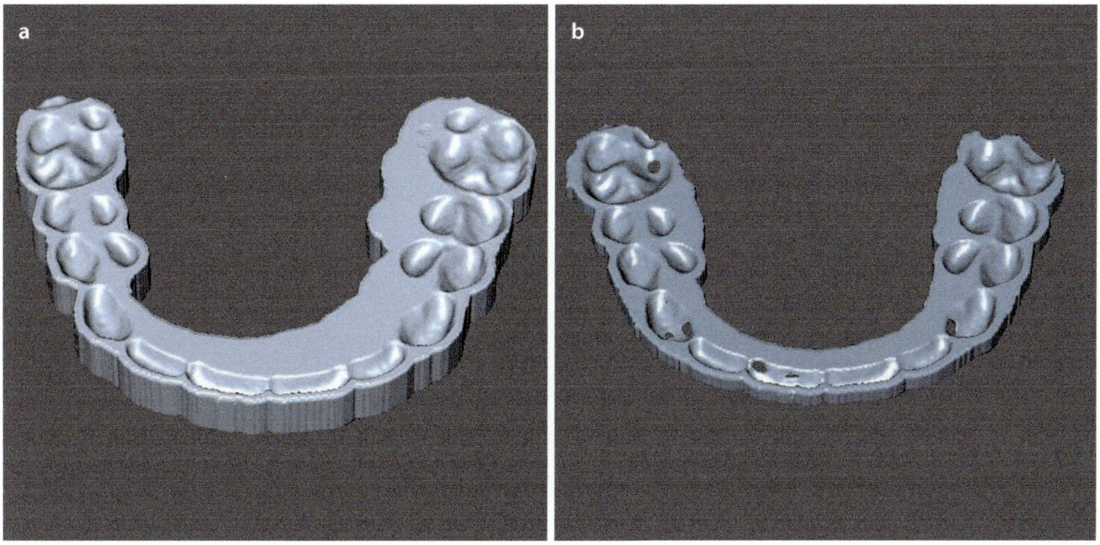

Fig. 4.6 3D virtual intermediate (**a**) and final (**b**) splints, when a "Mandible-first" sequence is chosen (3D "surface-rendered" representations, patient V.E.W. Maxilim v. 2.3.0.3.). Note that the 3D virtual final splint is the same whenever a "Mandible-first" or "Maxilla-first" (Fig. 4.2b) sequence is desired

3D Virtual Splints: "Mandible-First" Sequence

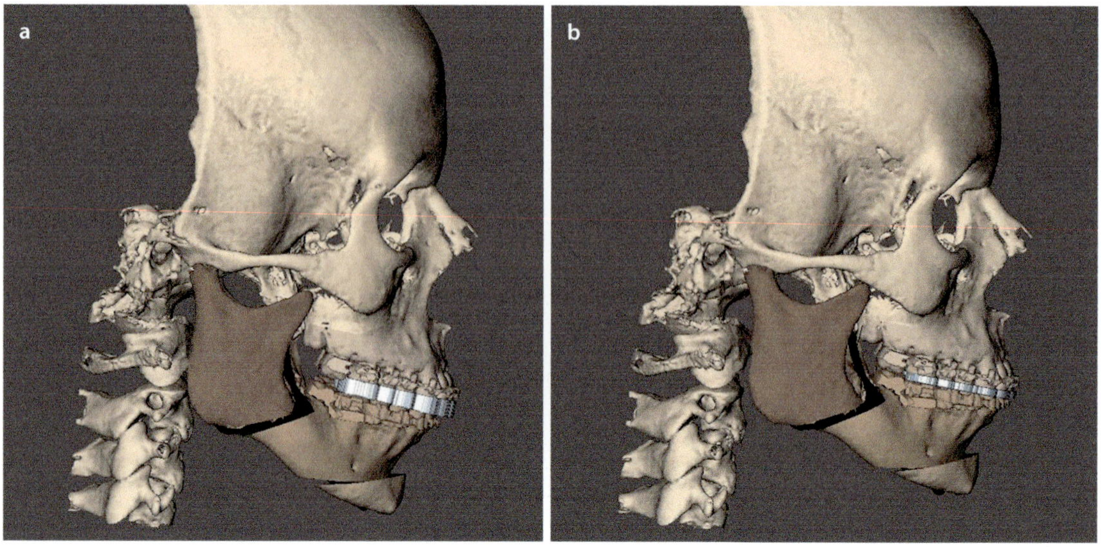

Fig. 4.7 Right profile views of the 3D virtual intermediate (**a**) and final (**b**) splints, when a "Mandible-first" sequence is chosen (3D "surface-rendered" representations, patient V.E.W. Maxilim v. 2.3.0.3.). Note that in order to manufacture a 3D virtual intermediate splint of adequate thickness, the mandible needs to be autorotated (**a**) in a CW fashion compared to a "Maxilla-first" sequence (Fig. 4.3a)

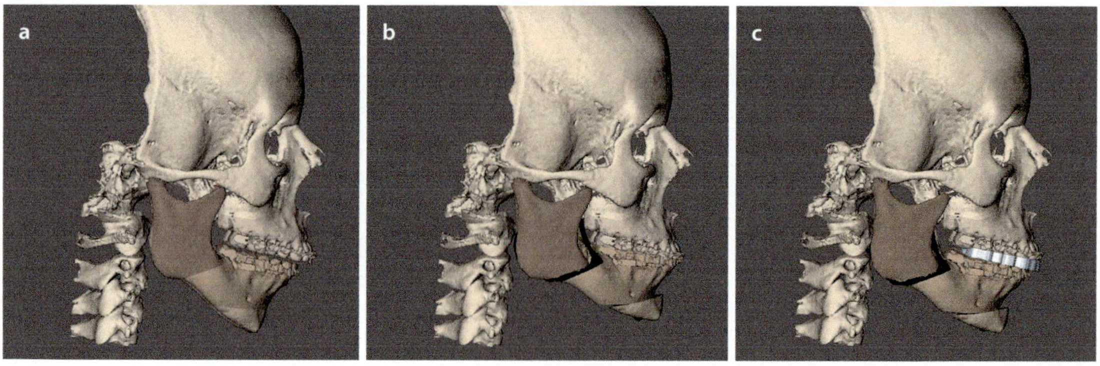

Fig. 4.8 Right profile views of the preoperative situation in CR (**a**), after virtual repositioning of the mandible following a virtual BSSO (**b**) and with the 3D virtual intermediate splint to reposition the mandible after a virtual BSSO (**c**), when a "Mandible-first" sequence is chosen (3D "surface-rendered" representations, patient V.E.W. Maxilim v. 2.3.0.3.). Note the virtual collision between the upper and lower dental arches after 3D virtual BSSO repositioning (**b**), due to the CCW pitch rotation and the vertical impaction of the maxilla. In order to allow the necessary space for the virtual intermediate splint, the mandible had to be autorotated in a CW fashion (**c**), a process which is still prone to errors

CAD/CAM Manufacturing of 3D Surgical Splints

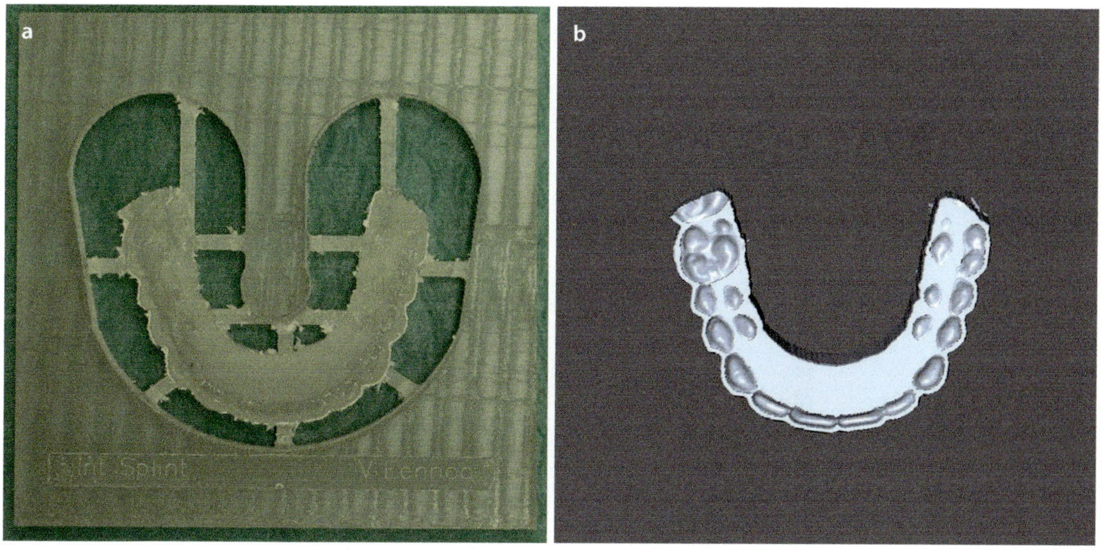

Fig. 4.9 3D CAD/CAM intermediate surgical splint manufactured from subtractive technologies by means of a milling process, when a "Maxilla-first" sequence is chosen (**a**) and its 3D surface representation (**b**) (patient V.E.W. Medicim, Belgium, Maxilim v. 2.3.0.3.). Note that the extensions still need to be trimmed before clinical usage

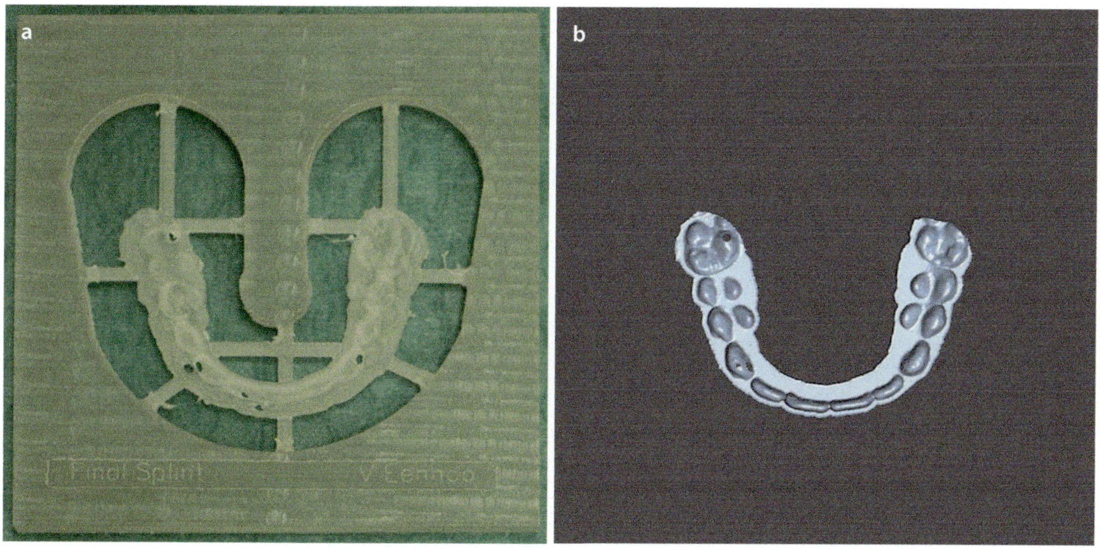

Fig. 4.10 3D CAD/CAM final surgical splint manufactured from subtractive technologies by means of a milling process, when a "Maxilla-first" sequence is chosen (**a**) and its 3D surface representation (**b**) (patient V.E.W. Medicim, Belgium, Maxilim v. 2.3.0.3.). Note that the extensions still need to be trimmed before clinical usage. Also note that the final 3D CAD/CAM splint is the same whenever a "Maxilla-first" or "Mandible-first" sequence is chosen

CAD/CAM Manufacturing of 3D Surgical Splints

The CAD/CAM surgical splints can be manufactured by either **ADDITIVE** (stereolithography/3D printing) or **SUBTRACTIVE** (milling) technologies.

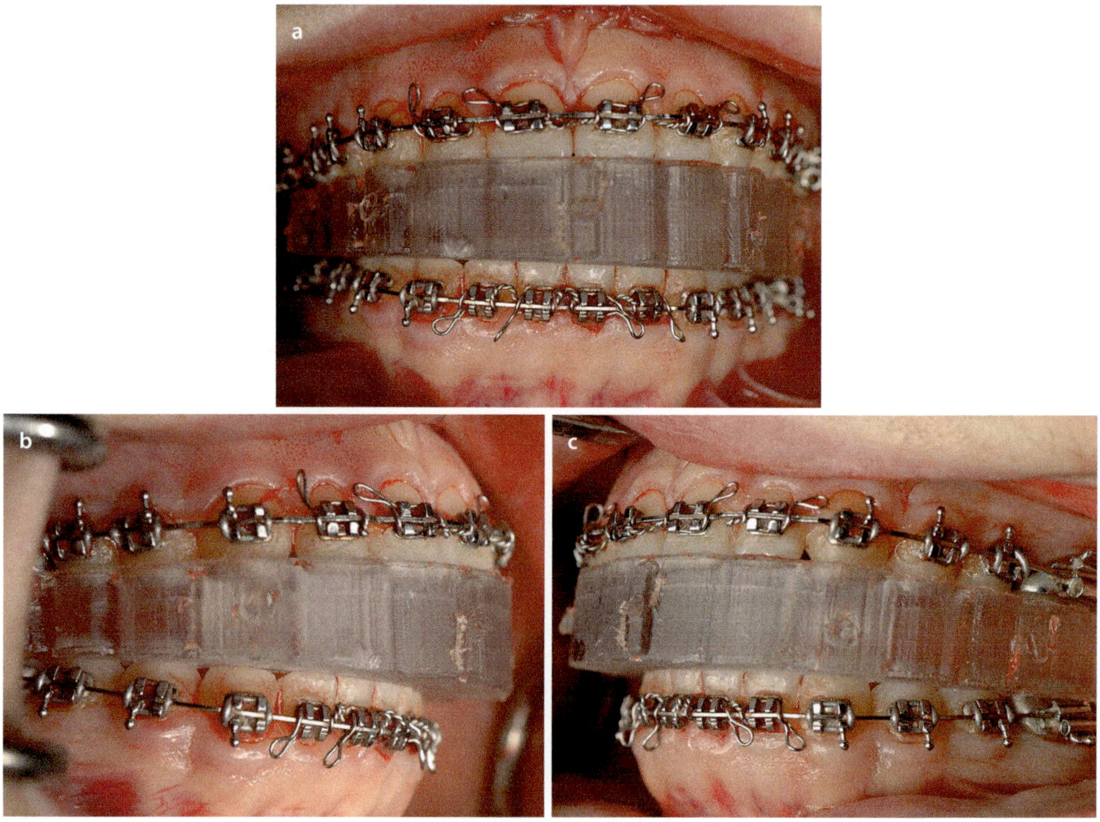

Fig. 4.11 Intra-oral frontal (**a**), profile right (**b**) and left (**c**) views of the 3D CAD/CAM intermediate surgical splint in place, when a "Maxilla-first" sequence is chosen (patient V.E.W. Medicim, Belgium). Note that the transparency of the surgical splint produced by a milling process allows to verify the correct fitting of the dental arches into the intermediate splint. Moreover the indentations incorporated in the splint must be deep enough to ensure a precise and stable fit. It is of paramount importance that the orthodontic brackets are not in contact with the splint, which would inevitably lead to errors in the surgical repositioning of the maxilla. Also note that the extensions (Fig. 4.9a) of the splint have been removed

CAD/CAM Manufacturing of 3D Surgical Splints

Attention
It is of paramount importance that the surgical splints do not contact the orthodontic brackets, to prevent any errors in the surgical repositioning of the jaws.

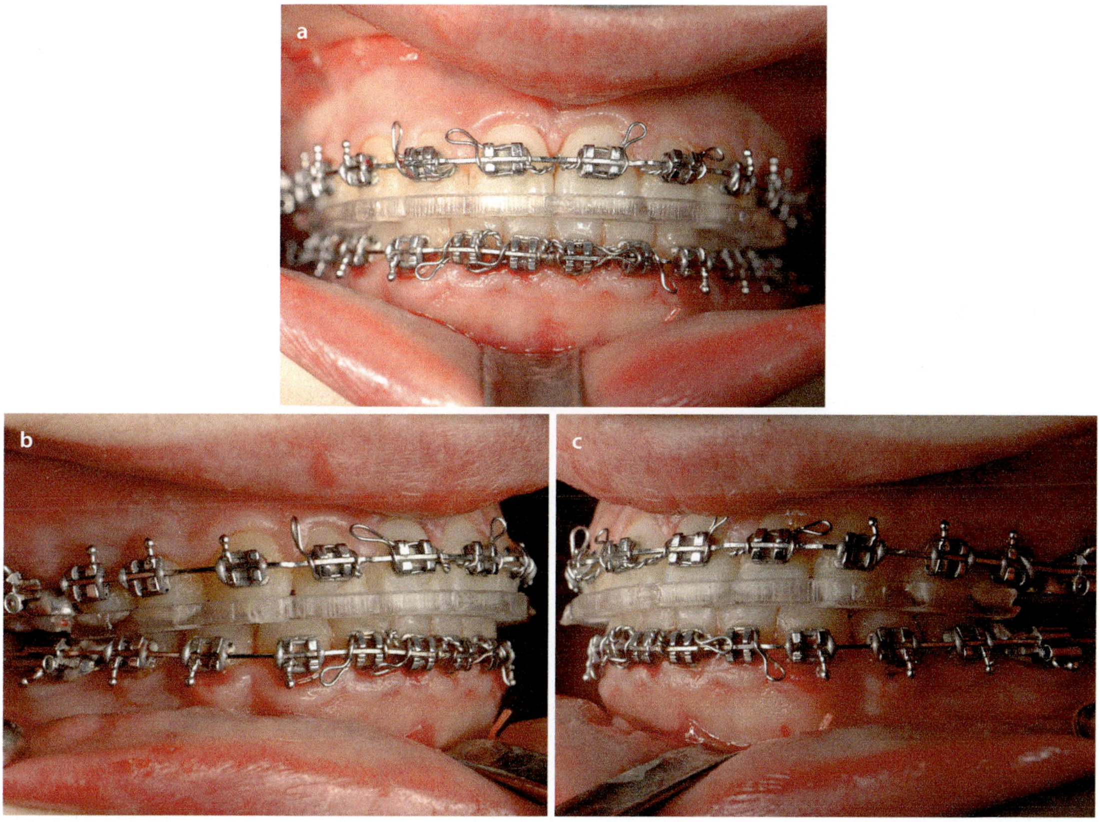

Fig. 4.12 Intra-oral frontal (**a**), profile right (**b**) and left (**c**) views of the 3D CAD/CAM final surgical splint in place, when a "Maxilla-first" sequence is chosen. However, the final 3D CAD/CAM splint is the same whenever a "Maxilla-first" or "Mandible-first" sequence is planned (patient V.E.W. Medicim, Belgium). Note that the transparency of the surgical splint produced by a milling process allows to verify the correct fitting of the dental arches into the final splint. Moreover the indentations incorporated in the splint must be deep enough to ensure a precise and stable fit. It is of paramount importance that the orthodontic brackets are not in contact with the splint, which would inevitably lead to errors in the surgical repositioning of the maxilla. Also note that the extensions (Fig. 4.10a) of the splint have been removed

3D Virtual Templates: "Chin Cutting and Repositioning" Guides

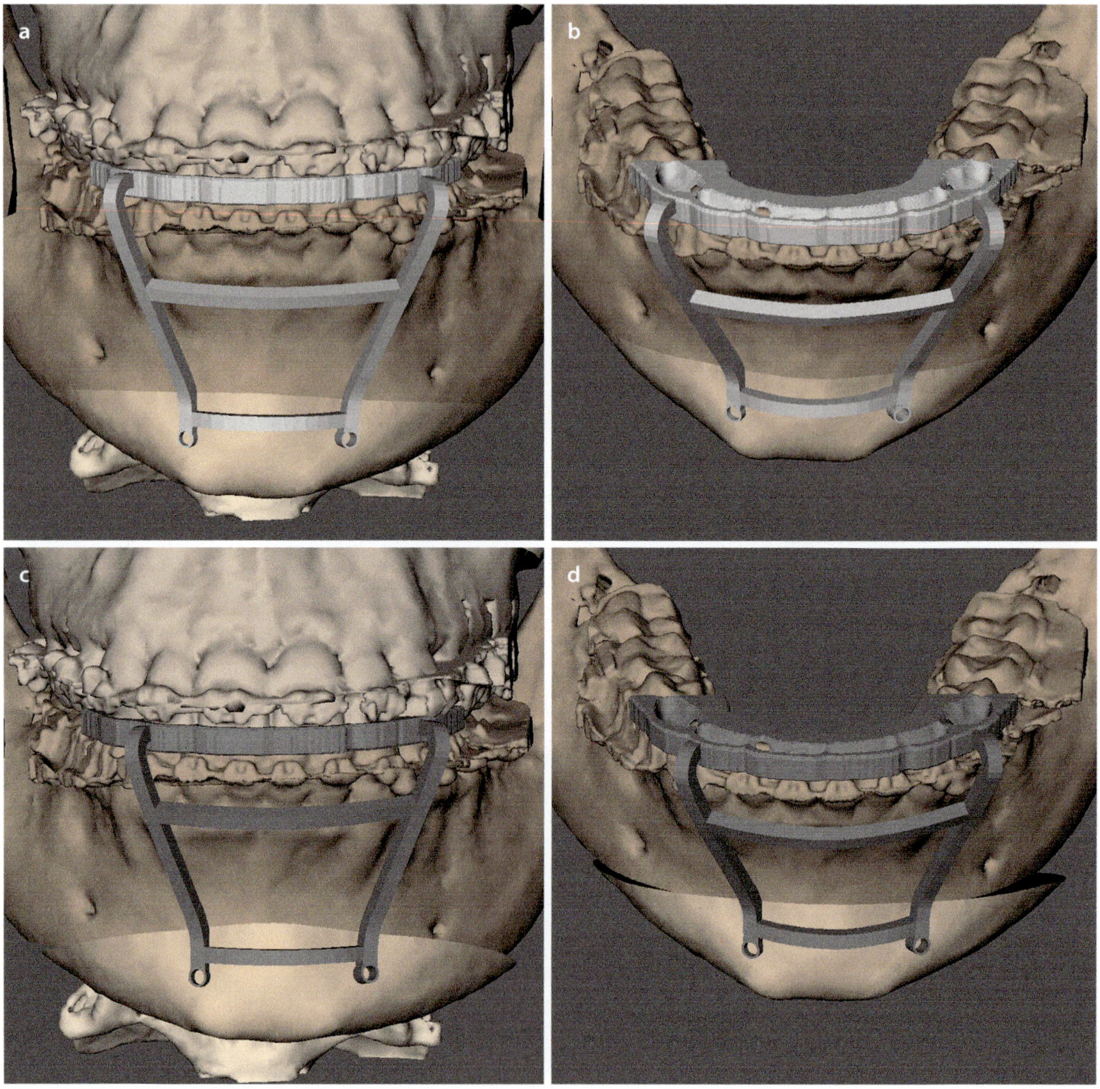

Fig. 4.13 Frontal and downward inclined views of the 3D CAD/CAM chin cutting (**a**–**b**) and repositioning (**c**–**d**) guides. These guides are based on the upper and lower dentition, and a temporary intermaxillary fixation is needed to accurately position and stabilise the guides. The cutting guide provides the position of two drill holes that will later be used by the repositioning guide to accurately transfer the final chin movements. The level of the chin osteotomy is provided by the cutting guide, where it contacts the symphysis bone. More restricted guides can also be designed and manufactured, with lateral wings or sluts, but the size of the guide will therefore inevitably be enlarged (3D "surface-rendered" representations, patient V.E.W. Maxilim v. 2.3.0.3.)

3D Virtual Templates: "Chin Cutting and Repositioning" Guides

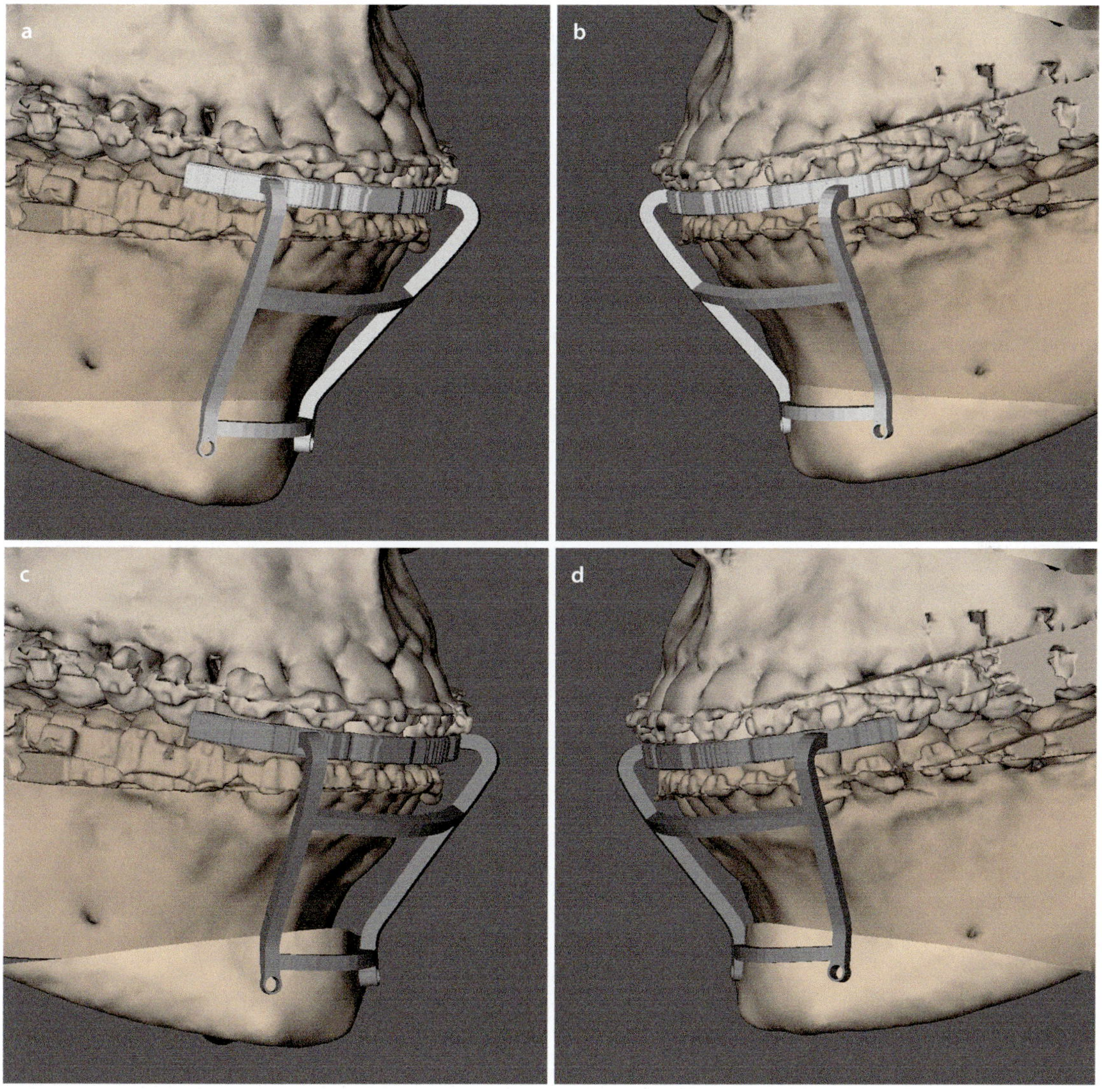

Fig. 4.14 Left and right 2/3 views of the 3D CAD/CAM chin cutting (**a**–**b**) and repositioning (**c**–**d**) guides. These guides are based on the upper and lower dentition, and a temporary intermaxillary fixation is needed to accurately position the guides. The cutting guide provides the position of two drill holes that will later be used by the repositioning guide, to accurately transfer the final distal chin segment movements. The level of the chin osteotomy is provided by the cutting guide, where it contacts the symphysis bone. More restricted guides can also be designed and manufactured, with lateral wings or sluts, but the size of the guide will therefore inevitably be enlarged (3D "surface-rendered" representations, patient V.E.W. Maxilim v. 2.3.0.3.)

CAD/CAM Manufacturing of 3D Templates

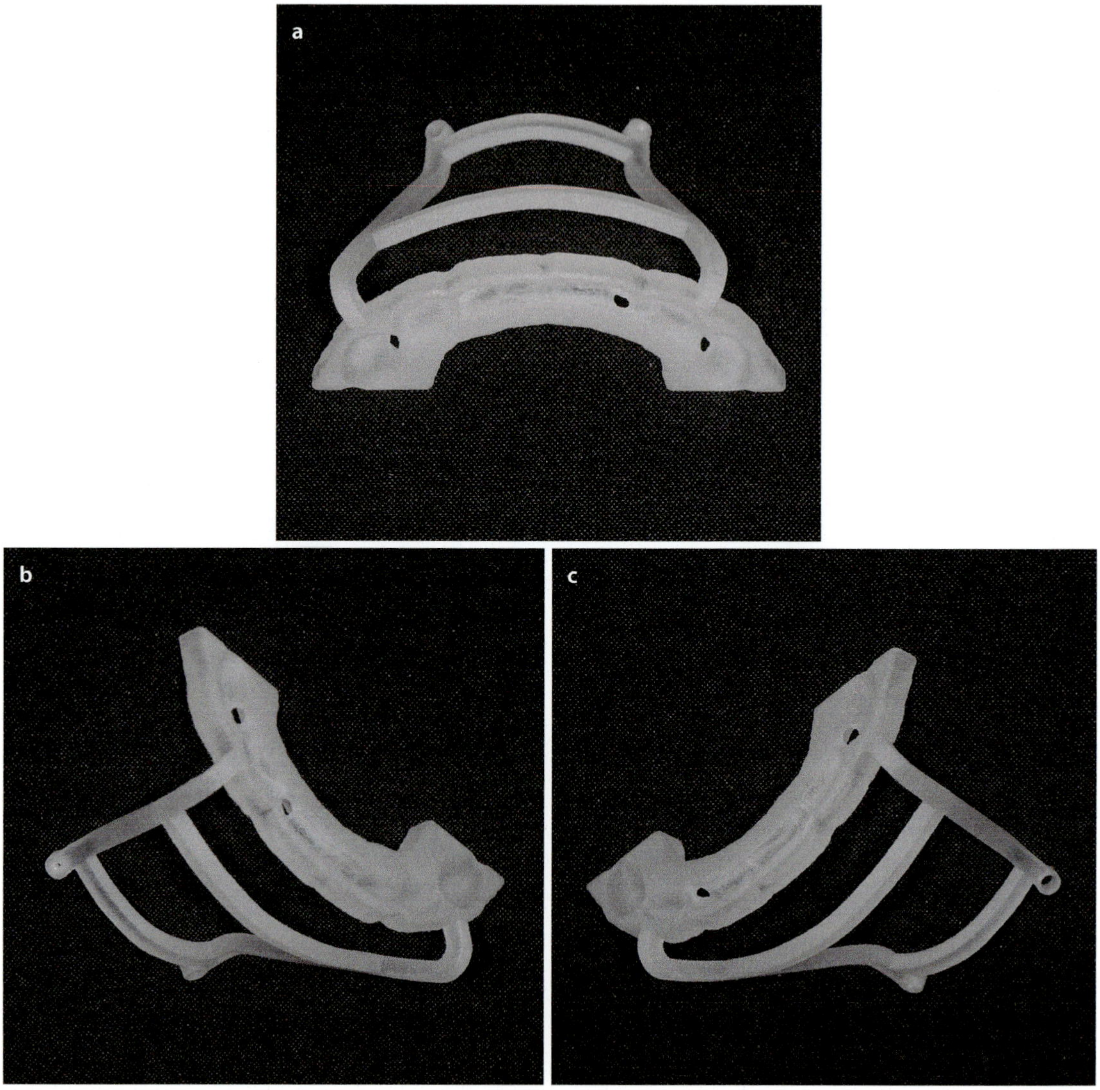

Fig. 4.15 Downward inclined frontal view (**a**) of the 3D CAD/CAM chin cutting guide and 2/3 left (**b**) and right (**c**) views of the 3D CAD/CAM chin repositioning guide made by 3D printing (patient V.E.W. Medicim, Belgium)

4.1.2 Internal/External References for Vertical Repositioning

In order to transfer the "Individualised 3D Virtual Treatment Plan" (▶ see Sect. 3.5) to the actual patient in the operation theatre, 3D CAD/CAM interdental surgical splints (▶ see also Sect. 4.1.1) are used in combination with internal or external anatomic reference landmarks for precise repositioning of the jaws:

1. Maxillary Le Fort I – repositioning
2. Mandibular – repositioning
3. Chin – repositioning

Since the authors do not use external reference landmarks in the clinical routine, the concept of "3D Virtual Treatment Planning Transfer" will be illustrated in this section by a combination of internal bony reference landmarks and 3D interdental surgical splints on **Case 1** (patient V.E.W.) which is used throughout this book (▶ Chaps. 1, 2, 3, 5 and 6).

The clinician nevertheless can easily modify the described concept by the use of external reference landmarks or by combined dental and bony internal reference landmarks according to his personal treatment planning philosophy.

▪ 3D Virtual Treatment Planning Transfer: Maxillary Le Fort I – Repositioning

The actual "3D virtual maxillary Le Fort I repositioning" towards the patient in the operation theatre depends on both the type and sequence of surgery:

1. Bimaxillary surgery following a "Maxilla-first" sequence
2. Bimaxillary surgery following a "Mandible-first" sequence
3. Monomaxillary Le Fort I surgery

In "bimaxillary surgery" following a "Mandible-first" sequence and in "monomaxillary Le Fort I surgery", "maxillary Le Fort I repositioning" is determined by the final occlusion (both in non-segmental and segmental cases) and CCW or CW mandibular autorotation with upper incisor vertical control.

In "maxillary (non-extrusion) Le Fort I repositioning" following a "Maxilla-first" sequence, all the virtual planned surgical movements of the maxilla, besides its vertical repositioning, are incorporated in the 3D intermediate surgical splint. These movements include (◘ Figs. 4.16, 4.17 and 4.18):

1. Maxillary occlusal cant correction ("Roll")
2. Upper dental midline deviation correction
3. Correction of flaring ("Yaw")
4. Upper sagittal incisal position correction
5. Occlusal plane correction ("Pitch")

Moreover, during vertical "maxillary Le Fort I repositioning", the following three types of vertical movements can occur separately or in combination (◘ Fig. 4.16):

1. Upper vertical incisal position correction
2. Maxillary occlusal cant correction ("Roll")
3. Occlusal plane correction ("Pitch")

From a theoretical standpoint, the "3D virtual maxillary (non-extrusion) Le Fort I repositioning" by means of a 3D intermediate surgical splint necessitates verification of the vertical position of the "surgically repositioned maxillary Le Fort I" only at one point, and either an internal or external reference landmark could be used under the following conditions:

1. Precise fit of the 3D intermediate surgical splint with IMF fixation (▶ see also Sect. 4.1.1)
2. Bilateral appropriate condylar seating without autorotation
3. Accurate vertical measuring

The authors, however, advocate the use of four vertical measurements (◘ Fig. 4.19) at the level of the upper canines and mesial buccal cusp of the first upper molars to have additional control on proper condylar seating and autorotation. The vertical measurements are extracted from "3D Cephalometry of the Patient's Hard Tissues and Teeth (3D-VPS$_2$)" (▶ see Sect. 2.2.2) after "Step-by-Step Individualised 3D Virtual Treatment Planning (3D-VPS$_5$)" (▶ see Sect. 3.5).These numbers can be precisely transferred in the operating theatre with commercially available callipers, using internal bony reference landmarks (◘ Figs. 4.20, 4.21, 4.22, 4.23 and 4.24). Using this concept, Swennen et al. (2010) reported a high accuracy of maxillary repositioning in 40 consecutive, non-segmental, non-extrusion, "Maxilla-first" cases: 0.48 mm ±1.00 mm in the x-axis (sagittal), 0.52 mm ±0.98 mm in the z-axis (transversal) and 1.02 mm ±1.94 mm in the y-axis (vertical).

In case of "maxillary (extrusion) Le Fort I repositioning" following a "Maxilla-first" sequence, additional CW autorotation of the mandible needs to be taken additionally into account, a concept still prone to error.

3D Virtual Treatment Planning Transfer: Maxillary Le Fort I – Repositioning

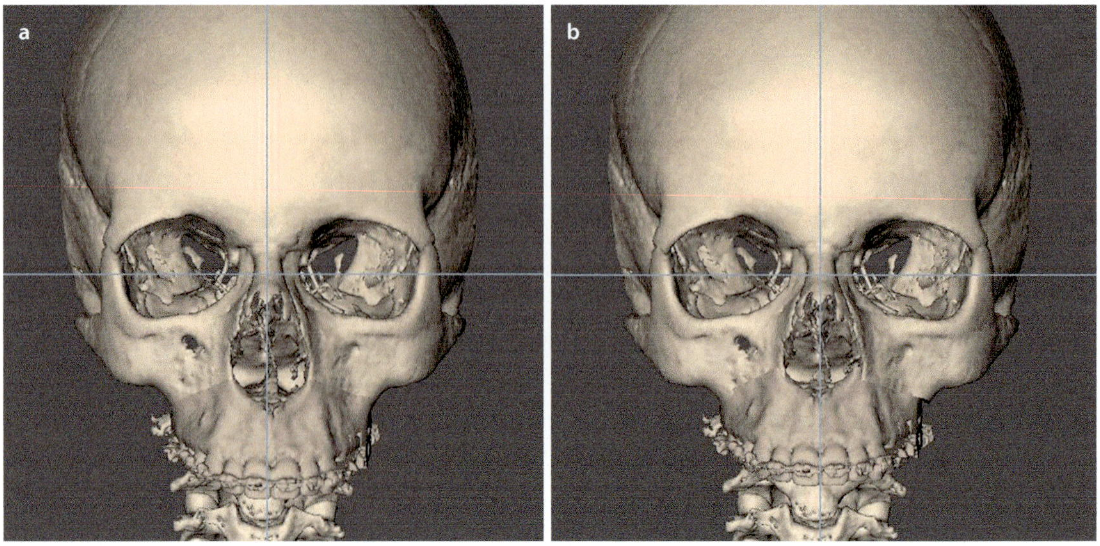

Fig. 4.16 Frontal views of the preoperative virtual situation (**a**) and after "3D virtual maxillary Le Fort I repositioning" (**b**) (3D "surface-rendered" representations, patient V.E.W. Maxilim v. 2.3.0.3.). Note the correction of the maxillary occlusal cant ("Roll"), the upper dental midline and the upper vertical incisal position

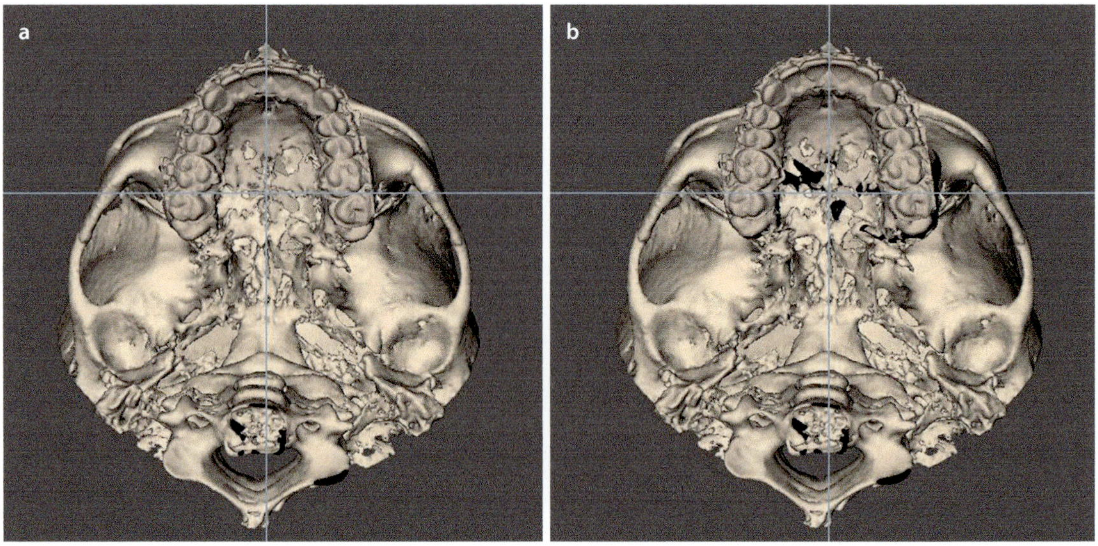

Fig. 4.17 Base views of the preoperative virtual situation (**a**) and after "3D virtual maxillary Le Fort I repositioning" (**b**) (3D "surface-rendered" representations, patient V.E.W. Maxilim v. 2.3.0.3.). Note the correction of the upper dental midline and flaring ("Yaw")

3D Virtual Treatment Planning Transfer: Maxillary Le Fort I – Repositioning

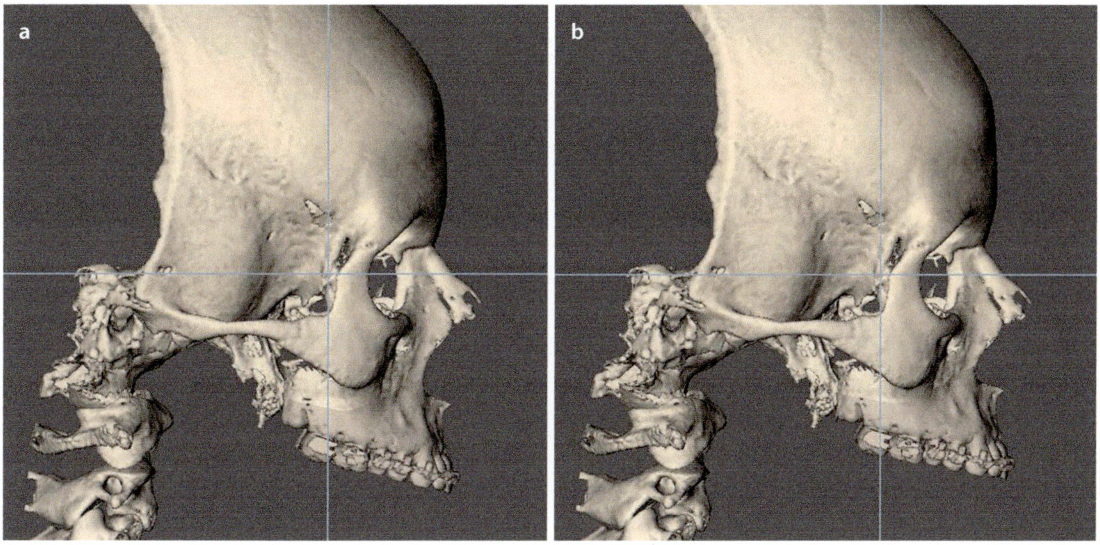

▫ **Fig. 4.18** Right profile views of the preoperative virtual situation (**a**) and after "3D virtual maxillary Le Fort I repositioning" (**b**) (3D "surface-rendered" representations, patient V.E.W. Maxilim v. 2.3.0.3.). Note the correction of the upper vertical and sagittal incisal position and the maxillary occlusal plane ("Pitch")

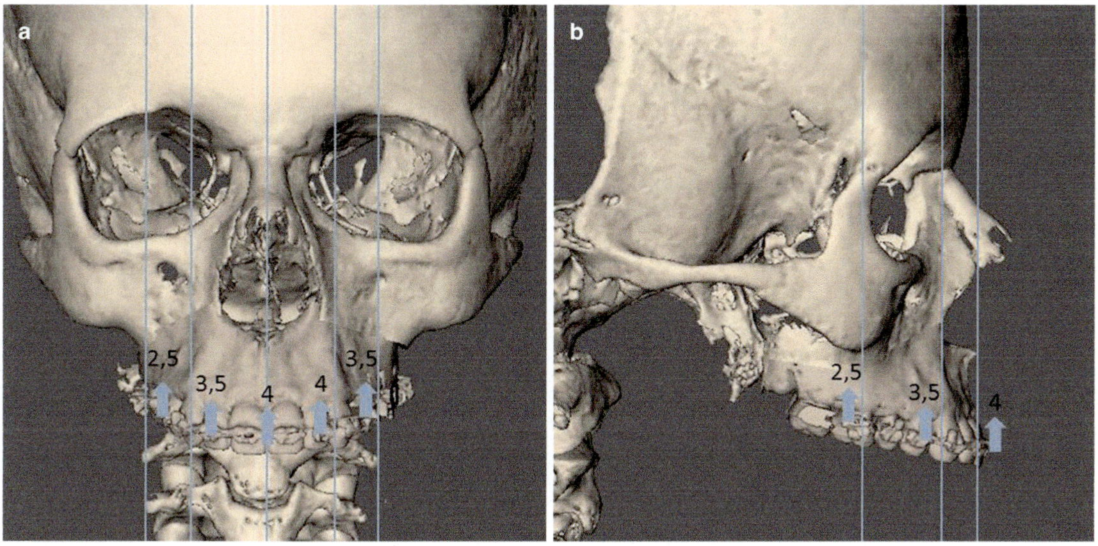

▫ **Fig. 4.19** Frontal (**a**) and right profile (**b**) views. During "3D virtual maxillary Le Fort I repositioning", three types of vertical movements can be combined: upper vertical incisal position, maxillary occlusal cant ("Roll") and occlusal plane ("Pitch") corrections. The final vertical movements can be extracted from the "3D Cephalometry of the Patient's Hard Tissues and Teeth (3D-VPS$_2$)" (► see Sect. 2.2.2) at the level of each upper canine and mesial buccal cusp of the first upper molars after "Step-by-Step Individualised 3D Virtual Treatment Planning (3D-VPS$_5$)" (► see Sect. 3.5). These numbers can be precisely transferred in the operating theatre with commercially available callipers, using internal bony reference landmarks (3D "surface-rendered" representations, patient V.E.W. Maxilim v. 2.3.0.3.)

3D Virtual Treatment Planning Transfer: Maxillary Le Fort I – Repositioning

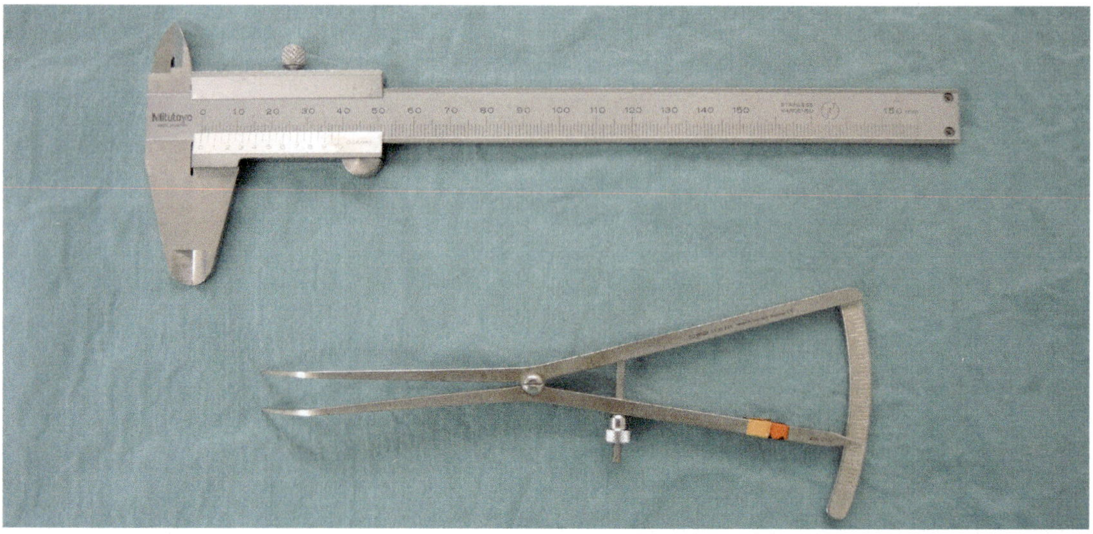

Fig. 4.20 Commercially available callipers used for vertical "3D virtual maxillary Le Fort I repositioning" during actual surgery. An inframillimetric calliper (superior calliper) is used to ensure adequate precision. Note also the use of a curved calliper (inferior calliper) to ease the manipulations during the actual surgery and to allow parallel measurements to the facial midline with the surgeon sitting at the head of the patient

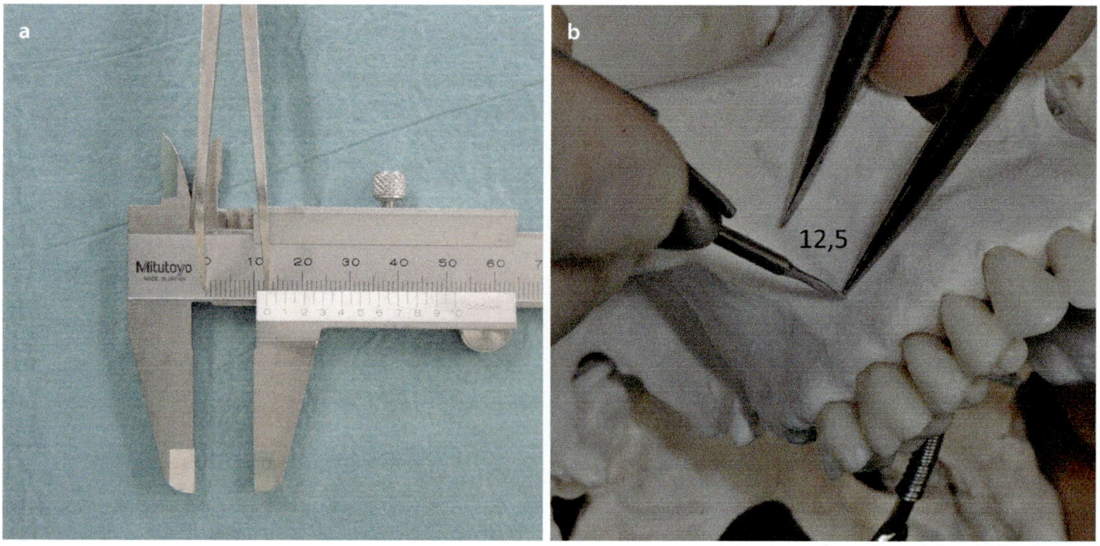

Fig. 4.21 In this particular case (patient V.E.W.), an impaction of 2.5 mm is planned at the mesial buccal cusp of the first upper right molar. The calliper is therefore set at 12.5 mm on the inframillimetric calliper (**a**) to transfer this measurement in the operating theatre, hereby demonstrated on a synthetic skull (**b**). A small fissure burr is used to mark two vertical bony landmarks at a vertical distance of 12.5 mm at the level of the mesial buccal cusp of the first upper right molar. It is crucial that theses bony landmarks are marked parallel to the facial midline to ensure adequate vertical repositioning of the maxilla

3D Virtual Treatment Planning Transfer: Maxillary Le Fort I – Repositioning

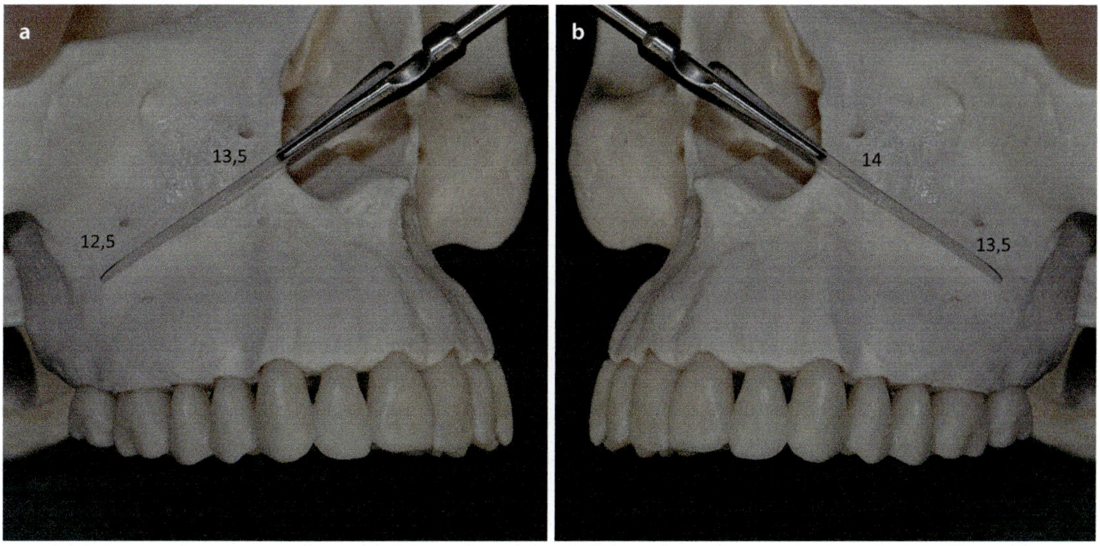

Fig. 4.22 2/3 right (**a**) and left (**b**) profile views demonstrating the vertical markings and measurements on a synthetic skull in the case of patient V.E.W. These internal bony vertical landmarks are precisely identified at each upper canine and mesial buccal cusp of the first upper molars based on "3D Cephalometry of the Patient's Hard Tissues and Teeth (3D-VPS_2)" (► see Sect. 2.2.2) after "Step-by-Step Individualised 3D Virtual Treatment Planning (3D-VPS_5)" (► see Sect. 3.5). It is crucial that these internal bony vertical landmarks are marked and well positioned above and below the Le Fort I osteotomy

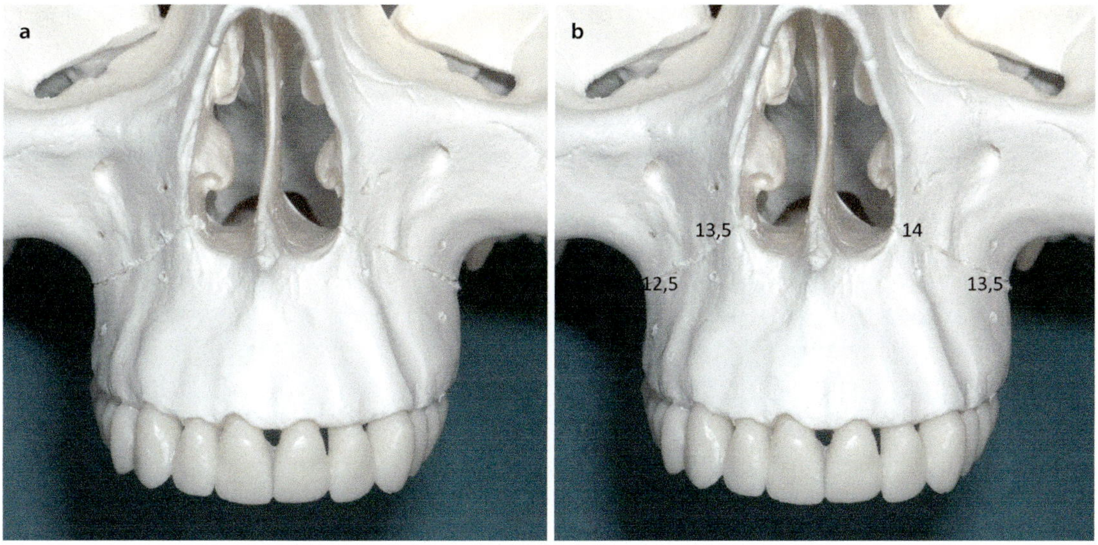

Fig. 4.23 Frontal views without (**a**) and with (**b**) 3D cephalometric vertical measurements demonstrating the vertical markings on a synthetic skull in the case of patient V.E.W. In this case, an impaction of 2.5 mm is planned at the right first molar and of 3.5 mm at the left first molar, while an impaction of 3.5 mm and 4 mm is, respectively, planned at the right and left canines (**b**). It is crucial that theses bony vertical landmarks are marked above and below the Le Fort I osteotomy before the down fracture of the maxilla and parallel to the facial midline to ensure adequate vertical repositioning of the maxilla

3D Virtual Treatment Planning Transfer: Maxillary Le Fort I – Repositioning

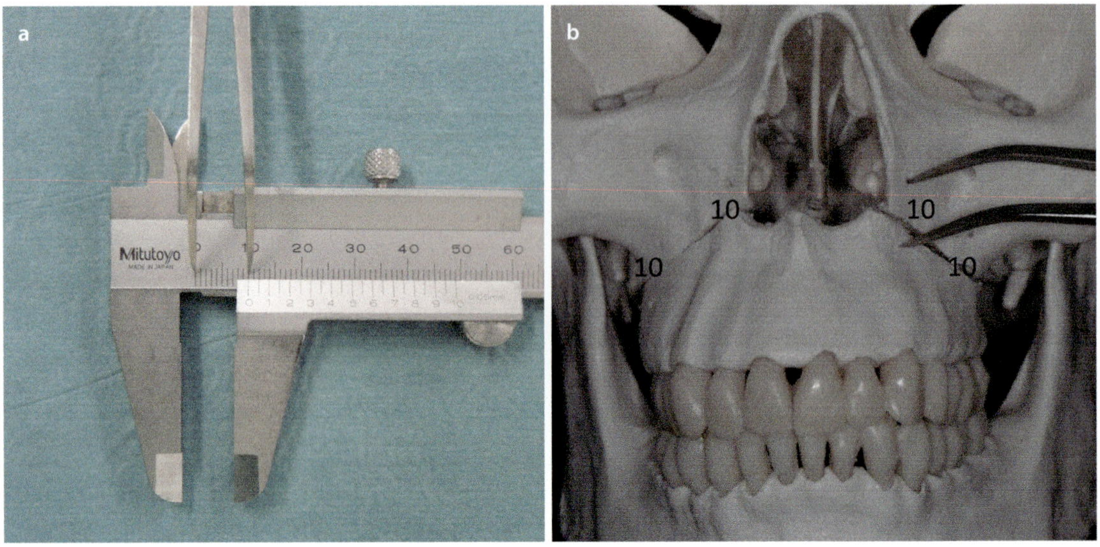

Fig. 4.24 For adequate transfer of "3D virtual maxillary Le Fort I repositioning" during actual surgery, the maxilla must be vertically repositioned using the 3D surgical intermediate splint (placed in correct IMF) (Fig. 4.11) and according to the internal bony landmarks previously identified. The calliper is set at 10 mm on the inframillimetric calliper (**a**) to verify the correct distance of 10 mm at the four levels (**b**) after adequate adaptation of the bony contacts. It is crucial that the surgeon is situated at the head of the patient to ensure that all measurements are made parallel to the facial midline for adequate vertical surgical repositioning of the maxilla. The curved calliper (**a**) is hereby of great help to the surgeon. Once precise surgical vertical repositioning of the maxilla is achieved, it can be rigidly fixed with titanium plates and screws as routinely. Demonstration of the particular case of patient V.E.W. on a synthetic skull (**b**)

Attention

Although with a 3D intermediate surgical splint vertical verification of "maxillary Le Fort I repositioning" from a theoretical standpoint is only necessary at one point, the use of four vertical measurements is advocated in order to have additional control on proper condylar seating and autorotation, during actual surgery.

- **3D Virtual Treatment Planning Transfer: Mandibular – Repositioning**

The actual transfer of "3D mandibular repositioning" towards the patient in the operation theatre depends as for "3D virtual maxillary Le Fort I repositioning" on both the type and sequence of surgery:

1. Bimaxillary surgery following a "Mandible-first" sequence
2. Bimaxillary surgery following a "Maxilla-first" sequence
3. Isolate mandibular bilateral or unilateral surgery

In "bimaxillary surgery" following a "Maxilla-first" sequence and in "isolate mandibular surgery" after bilateral or unilateral sagittal split or vertical ramus osteotomies, "mandibular repositioning" of the distal fragment is only determined by the final occlusion if preoperative condylar seating is respected.

In "mandibular repositioning surgery" following a "Mandible-first" sequence after bilateral or unilateral sagittal split or vertical ramus osteotomies, all the following virtual planned movements of the distal fragment of the mandible are incorporated in the 3D intermediate surgical splint:

1. Mandibular occlusal cant correction ("Roll")
2. Lower dental midline deviation correction
3. Correction of flaring ("Yaw")
4. Lower sagittal incisal position correction
5. Occlusal plane correction ("Pitch")

For proper manufacturing of the 3D CAD-CAM intermediate surgical splint, however, in some cases, additional (CW or CCW) virtual mandibular autorotation is necessary towards "mandibular repositioning surgery" following a "Mandible-first" sequence (e.g. Fig. 4.8), a concept still prone to error.

In case, additional "Pitch", "Roll" or "Yaw" rotations (▶ see also Sect. 3.4) of one or both proximal mandibular fragments are incorporated in the 3D virtual treatment plan (e.g. in case of mandibular narrowing with an additional mandibular midline split, in case of mandibular widening with or without additional mandibular midline split, in case of unilateral or bilateral gonial angle corrections, etc.), the clinician needs to be aware that he will inherently alter preoperative condylar seating at one or both sides.

Pitfall

Although the "3D Virtual Scene Approach" can be helpful in positioning the proximal mandibular fragments …., the surgical adaptation of the proximal and distal mandibular segments remains a technical manipulation and a clinical feeling based on surgical experience.

Whatever a "Maxilla-first" or "Mandible-first" sequence (with respectively a "final" and "intermediate" 3D surgical interdental splint) is chosen by the ortho-surgical team based on the actual clinical situation and their treatment philosophy, the actual surgical adaptation of the distal and proximal mandibular fragments remains a crucial technical surgical manipulation that remains sometimes a challenge for even the most experienced surgeons. A passive adaptation between both the proximal and distal segments is of paramount importance to minimise any undesirable movements of the proximal segments and its potential deleterious effects on the mandibular condyles.

Compared towards "conventional treatment planning", "3D Virtual Treatment Planning" offers the surgeon valuable information towards "mandibular repositioning surgery" especially regarding seating of the proximal fragments following the authors' next proposed steps:

Step 1: The sagittal split osteotomy (SSO) needs to be individually virtual designed, especially the buccal corticotomy, according to the specific surgical movement, the amount of surgical movement, the patient's distinct anatomy and the surgeon's personal philosophy (◘ Figs. 4.25a and 4.26a).

Step 2: The surgeon attempts to reproduce especially the angulation and position of the buccal corticotomy of the SSO during the actual surgery (◘ Figs. 4.25b and 4.26b).

Step 3: The surgeon correlates during surgery the actual clinical situation with the virtual position and adaptation of the proximal and distal mandibular segments (◘ Figs. 4.27 and 4.28). Although the surgical adaptation of the proximal and distal segments remains a technical manipulation and a clinical feeling based on experience, undesirable movements of the proximal segment can be potentially minimised. It is crucial, however, that the surgeon considers the thickness of the actual clinical bone cuts during the adaptation of the proximal and distal mandibular segments since current available commercial software do not take the latter important issue into account. Therefore, the bony osteotomy gaps will always be more pronounced in the clinical setting, compared to the "Individualised 3D Virtual Treatment Plan" (► see Sect. 3.5).

Attention
The surgeon must consider the thickness of the actual clinical bone cuts during the virtual adaptation of the proximal and distal mandibular segments. This important clinical surgical variable has not been incorporated yet in the 3D virtual osteotomy design and 3D virtual planning.

3D Virtual Treatment Planning Transfer: Mandibular Sagittal Split – Repositioning

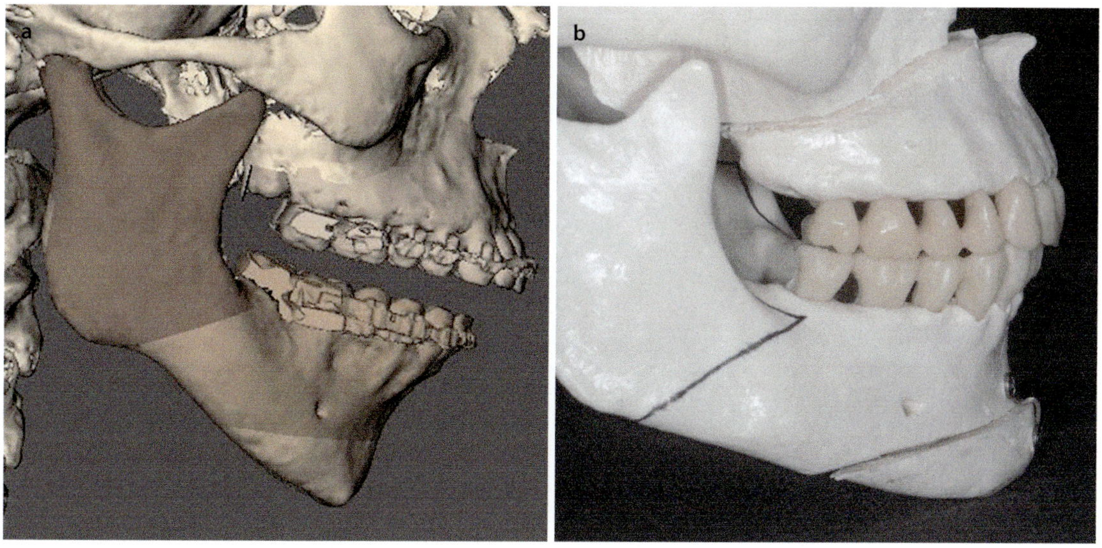

Fig. 4.25 During a sagittal split osteotomy (SSO), the "first step" is to individually virtual design the SSO, especially its buccal corticotomy. In the particular case of patient V.E.W. an oblique vertical buccal corticotomy was virtually planned at the right side from the antegonial notch to the middle of the second molar (3D "surface-rendered" representations, patient V.E.W. Maxilim v. 2.3.0.3.) (**a**). In the "second step", both the angulation and position of the virtual SSO design are reproduced during the actual surgery, hereby demonstrated on a synthetic skull (**b**)

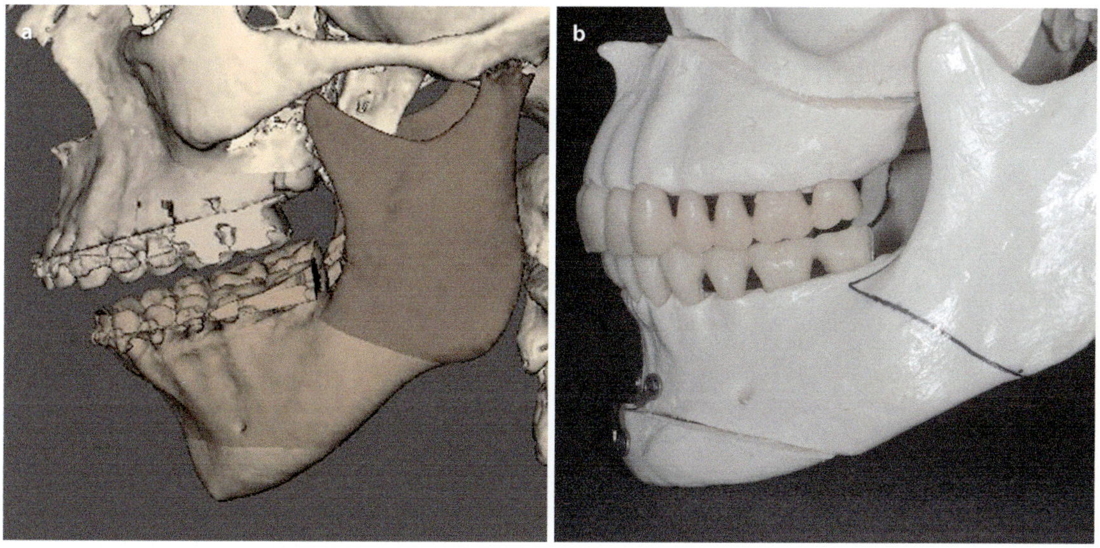

Fig. 4.26 During a sagittal split osteotomy (SSO), the "first step" is to individually virtual design the SSO, especially its buccal corticotomy. In the particular case of patient V.E.W. an oblique vertical buccal corticotomy was virtually planned at the left side from the antegonial notch to the middle of the second molar (3D "surface-rendered" representations, patient V.E.W. Maxilim v. 2.3.0.3.) (**a**). In the "second step", both the angulation and position of the virtual SSO design are reproduced during the actual surgery, hereby demonstrated on a synthetic skull (**b**)

3D Virtual Treatment Planning Transfer: Mandibular Sagittal Split – Repositioning

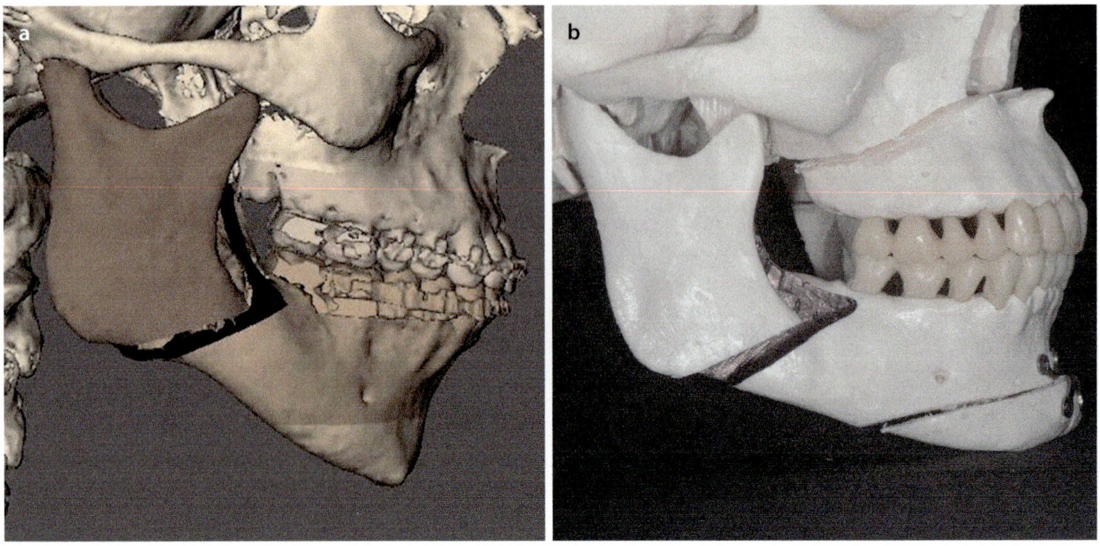

Fig. 4.27 In the "third step", the surgeon can correlate during actual surgery the virtual position and adaptation of the right proximal and distal mandibular segments (3D "surface-rendered" representations, patient V.E.W. Maxilim v. 2.3.0.3.) (**a**) with the clinical adaptation, hereby illustrated in the particular case of patient V.E.W. on a synthetic skull (**b**). Note especially the correlation of the CCW opening and positioning of the right proximal fragment both at the level of the right mandibular border as in the retro-molar region

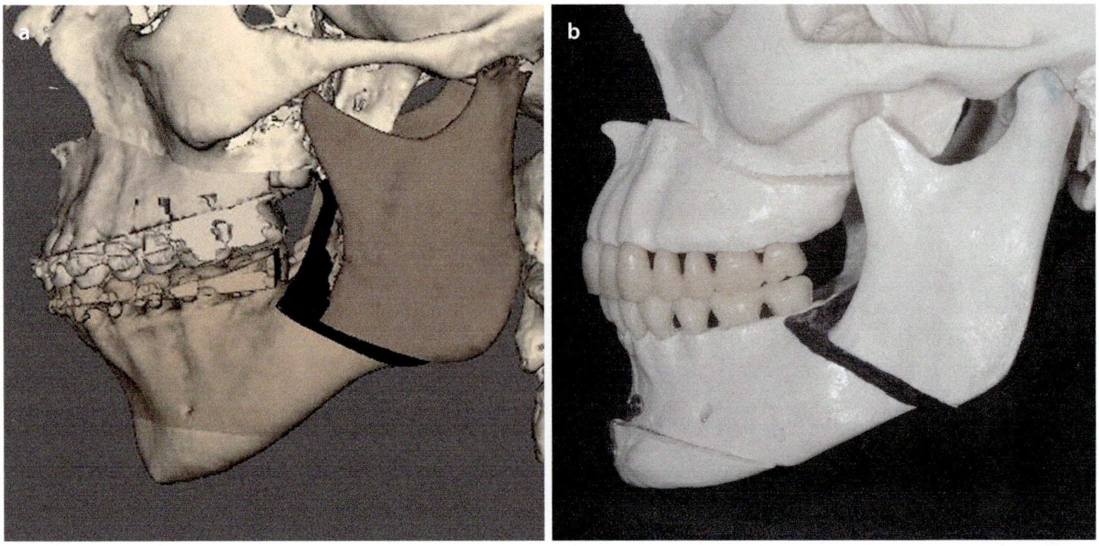

Fig. 4.28 In the "third step", the surgeon can correlate during actual surgery the virtual position and adaptation of the left proximal and distal mandibular segments (3D "surface-rendered" representations, patient V.E.W. Maxilim v. 2.3.0.3.) (**a**) with the clinical adaptation, hereby illustrated in the particular case of patient V.E.W. on a synthetic skull (**b**). Note especially the correlation of less CCW opening between the proximal and distal segments and a small step at the level of the left mandibular border compared to the right side as a consequence of maxillary cant correction (▶ see also Sect. 3.5)

3D Virtual Treatment Planning Transfer: Chin – Repositioning

"3D virtual treatment planning of orthognathic surgery" does not only allow to precisely plan and transfer more complex 3D geometric "Pitch", "Roll" and "Cant" corrections of the bimaxillary complex but also allows the clinician to accurately and reliably three-dimensionally analyse the chin deformity, virtually design the chin osteotomy and virtually plan its surgical movements (Figs. 4.29, 4.30 and 4.31).

The final "Individualised 3D Virtual Treatment Plan (► see Sect. 3.5)" of the patient regarding "chin repositioning" can include the following virtual planned movements:

1. Advancement (or rarely a setback)
2. Midline deviation correction
3. Intrusion or extrusion
4. Cant correction ("Roll")
5. Profile correction ("Pitch")
6. Correction of flaring ("Yaw")
7. A combination of several of the these movements

The actual transfer of "3D virtual chin repositioning" towards the patient in the operation theatre can be performed by:

1. "The use of pre-bent titanium mini-plates in combination with bony internal reference landmarks and calliper measuring".

   Especially if the "virtual chin repositioning" is composed of simple surgical movements, like sagittal advancement (or rarely a setback), vertical intrusion or extrusion or minimal midline corrections, it can consistently be transferred towards the patient in the operating theatre in a precise way using internal bony reference landmarks and calliper measuring in combination with prebent titanium mini-plates. Also minimal cant corrections can be effectively transferred following this concept (Figs. 4.32, 4.33 and 4.34).
2. "The use of 3D templates – chin cutting and repositioning guides" (► see also Sect. 4.1.1).

   In case "virtual chin repositioning" is composed of more complex movements with significant "Roll" and "Yaw" (Fig. 4.35) corrections or major asymmetry corrections, the use of 3D CAD/CAM "chin cutting and repositioning guides" should be considered for accurate transfer of the virtual treatment plan. Moreover, in such cases there is a potential for PSIs (► see also Sect. 4.1.3) in the future.

Currently, in the era of virtual imaging, intra-operative imaging with low-dose radiation CBCT (► see also Sect. 4.2.2) allows the surgeon to verify "surgical chin repositioning" during actual surgery and carry out modifications before the final closure of the wound, if necessary.

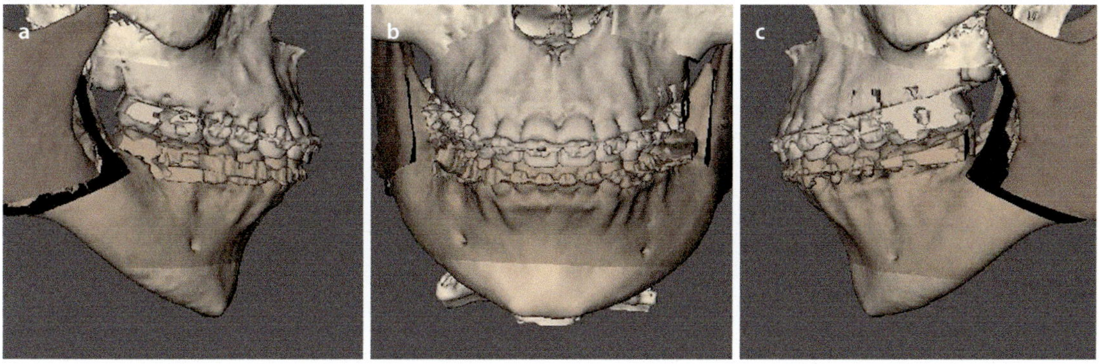

Fig. 4.29 Profile right (**a**), frontal (**b**) and profile left (**c**) views after "Step 7 of 3D-VPS$_5$ – Individualised 3D Virtual Treatment Planning" (► see Sect. 3.5), prior to "Step 8: 3D Chin Position Evaluation/Correction" (3D "surface-rendered" representations, patient V.E.W. Maxilim v. 2.3.0.3.)

3D Virtual Treatment Planning Transfer: Chin - Repositioning

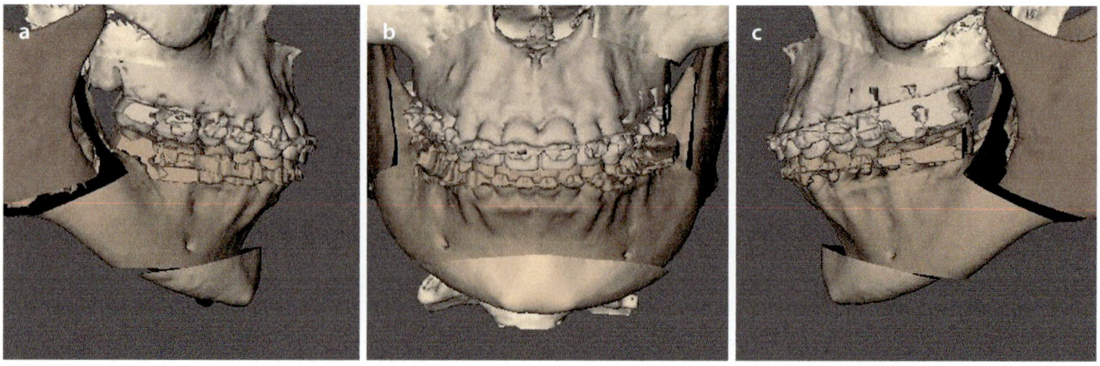

Fig. 4.30 Profile right (**a**), frontal (**b**) and profile left (**c**) views after "Step 8 of 3D-VPS$_5$ – Chin Position Evaluation/Correction" (► see Sect. 3.5) (3D "surface-rendered" representations, patient V.E.W. Maxilim v. 2.3.0.3.)

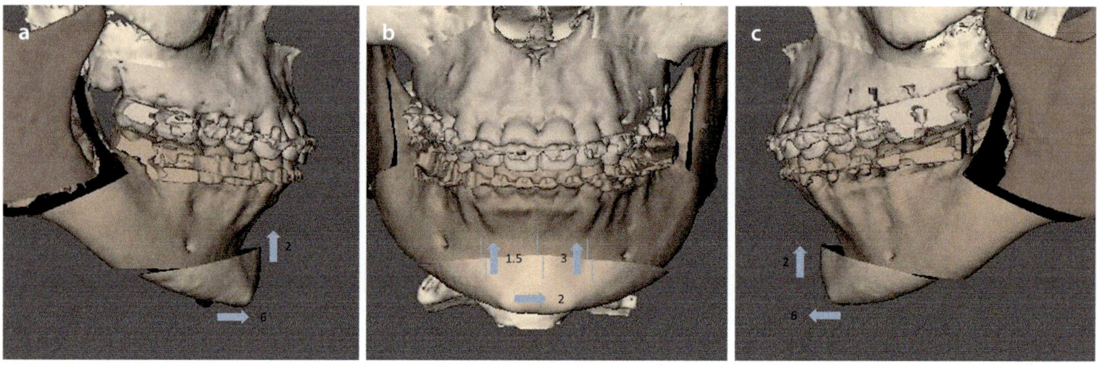

Fig. 4.31 Profile right (**a**), frontal (**b**) and profile left (**c**) views after "3D virtual chin repositioning ("Step 8") with the exact vertical and horizontal surgical movements: sagittal advancement of 6 mm, anterior midline intrusion of 2 mm, cant correction ("Roll") with 1.5 mm intrusion at the right lower canine and *3* mm intrusion at the left lower canine level, midline correction of 2 mm to the left and CCW ("Pitch") rotation (3D "surface-rendered" representations, patient V.E.W. Maxilim v. 2.3.0.3.)

3D Virtual Treatment Planning Transfer: Chin – Repositioning

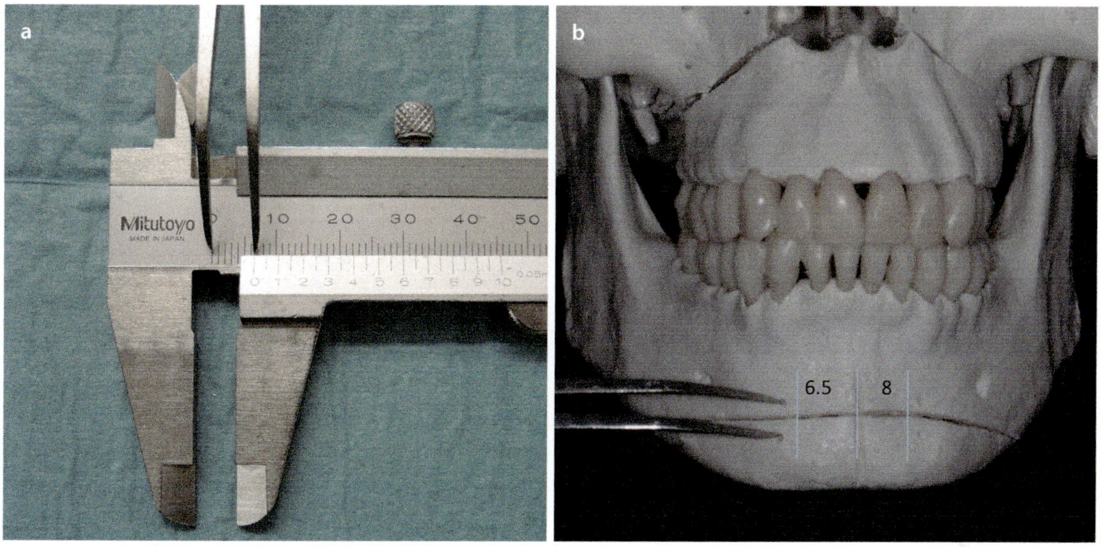

Fig. 4.32 In the particular case of patient V.E.W. an anterior midline intrusion of 2 mm is planned with a cant ("Roll") correction. The calliper is therefore set at *6.5* mm, on the inframillimetric calliper (**a**), at the right canine level, and *8* mm at the left canine level to transfer the intrusion with cant correction towards the patient in the operating theatre, hereby illustrated on a synthetic skull (**b**). A small burr is used to identify the above-mentioned vertical landmarks, on each side of the genioplasty osteotomy. It is crucial that these landmarks are placed parallel to the facial midline, to ensure adequate repositioning of the chin

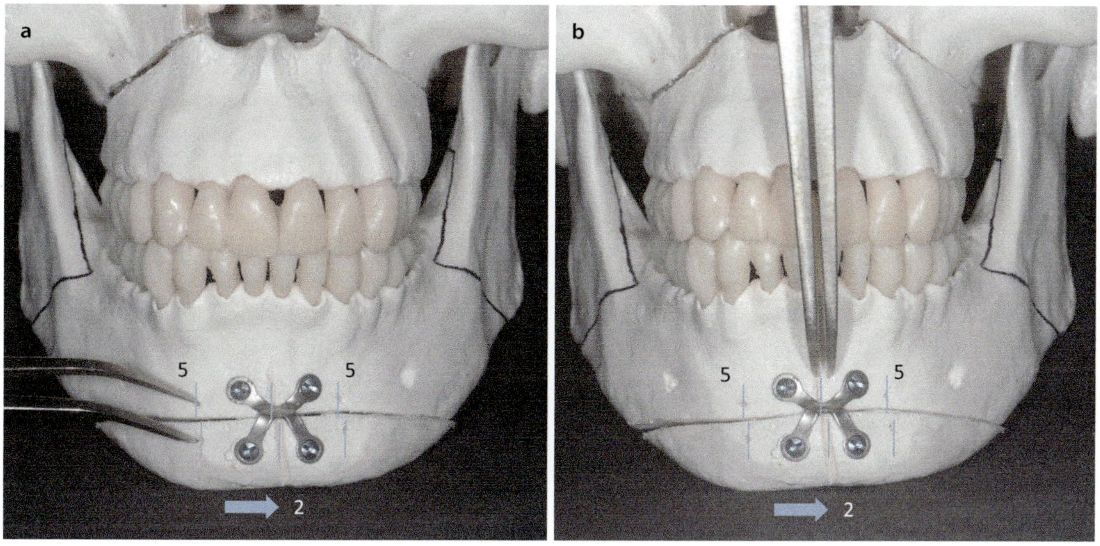

Fig. 4.33 For adequate transfer of "3D virtual chin repositioning", a pre-bent titanium chin mini-plate ("Arnett chin plate", KLS Martin, Germany) is used in combination with internal vertical measurements after adequate adaptation of the bony contacts. The calliper is set at *5* mm, on the inframillimetric calliper, to verify the correct intrusion at both canine levels (**a**). The calliper is then set at *2* mm, on the inframillimetric calliper, to transfer and verify the *2* mm midline correction to the left. Note that a midline vertical line is also marked with the burr, to assist in midline correction. Note that the advancement of 6 mm is incorporated in the pre-bent titanium chin mini-plate. The particular case of patient V.E.W. is simulated for illustration on a synthetic skull (**b**)

3D Virtual Treatment Planning Transfer: Chin – Repositioning

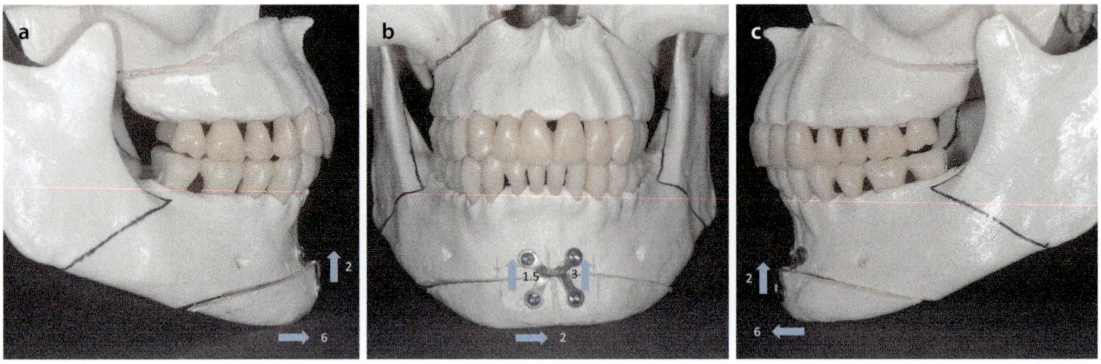

Fig. 4.34 Profile right (**a**), frontal (**b**) and profile left (**c**) views after "surgical chin repositioning" ("Step 8") by the use of a pre-bent titanium chin mini-plate ("Arnett chin plate", KLS Martin) in combination with internal bony references. Note the precise transfer of a *6* mm sagittal advancement (incorporated in the pre-bent chin plate), an anterior midline intrusion of *2* mm, cant correction ("Roll") with *1.5* mm intrusion at the right lower canine and *3* mm intrusion at the left lower canine level, midline correction of *2* mm to the left and CCW ("Pitch") rotation. The particular case of patient V.E.W. is simulated for illustration on a synthetic skull

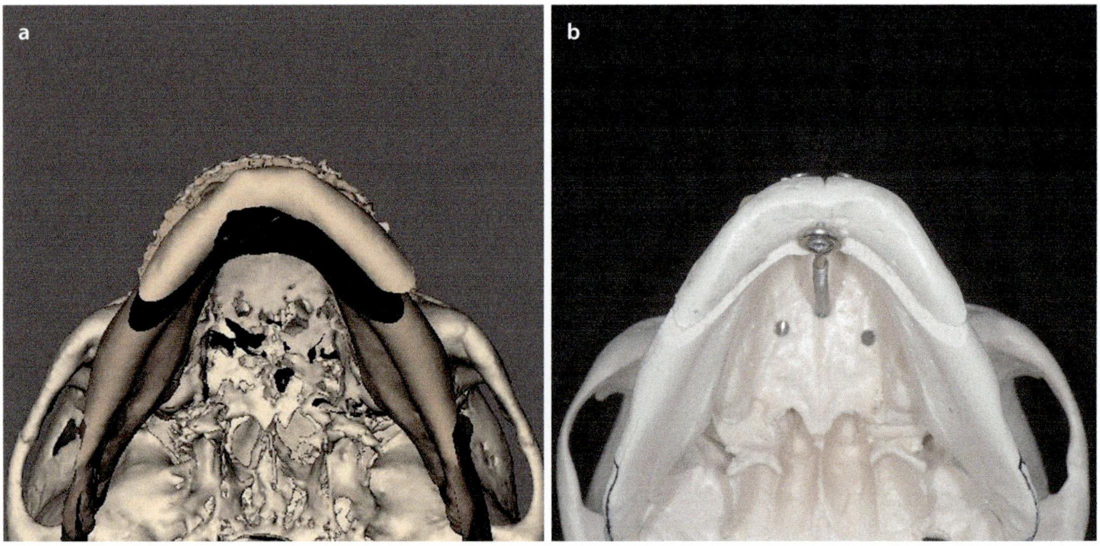

Fig. 4.35 In case "3D virtual chin repositioning" (3D "surface-rendered" representations, patient V.E.W. Maxilim v. 2.3.0.3.) (**a**) includes a ("Yaw") correction, this particular movement is more difficult to adequately transfer in the operating theatre, hereby demonstrated on a synthetic skull (**b**)

4.1.3 Potential of Patient Specific Implants (PSI) for Transfer Without Splint

Recent developments in computer-assisted manufacturing of implantable osteosynthesis material, like rigid titanium, actually allow the application of patient-specific implants (PSIs) in orthognathic surgery towards potential "Waferless Orthognathic Surgery" (▶ see also Sect. 4.2.2) in the future.

The "3D Imaging Workflow" (▶ see Chap. 1) and "3D Virtual Treatment Planning" (▶ see Sect. 3.5), in this concept, remain the same, but instead of using "3D surgical splints" and "3D templates" (▶ see Sect. 4.1.1), the following PSIs are used for the transfer of the "Individualised 3D Virtual Treatment Plan" towards the patient in the operation theatre:

1. PSI – "cutting and jaw repositioning" transfer guides (◘ Figs. 4.36 and 4.37)
2. PSI – 3D customised osteosynthesis plates (◘ Figs. 4.38 and 4.39)

This concept implements that there is no need any more for interdental surgical splints and intermaxillary fixation neither internal nor external references for vertical repositioning. Moreover, surgical repositioning of the jaws no longer relies on condylar seating neither on autorotation of the mandible which remains difficult to reproduce virtually (▶ see also Sect. 1.3). "3D maxillary Le Fort I repositioning surgery" with PSIs becomes completely independent of condylar seating, while during "3D mandibular repositioning surgery", the positioning of the proximal segments and condylar seating is transferred by the PSIs. Finally, another advantage of this concept is that there is no need any more for intra-operative osteosynthesis plate bending, since PSIs are fully 3D customised to rigidly fixate the maxilla and mandible towards their new 3D virtually planned position.

However, although very promising, the actual limits and drawbacks of this concept are still numerous and raise the following important challenging concerns to cope with in the future:

1. Although the clinical time necessary for "Step-by-Step Individualised 3D Virtual Treatment Planning (3D-VPS_5)" (▶ see Sect. 3.5) remains the same, relevant additional planning time for designing and manufacturing the above PSIs, which can never be performed by the clinician himself, currently jeopardises the efficiency of the clinical workflow and inherently increases costs.
2. The actual PSIs being larger in nature, especially the "cutting and jaw repositioning" transfer guides cannot be used in "minimal invasive surgical approaches", inevitably increase the surgical operation time and raising important concerns in case "plate removal" or "redo orthognathic surgery" would be necessary.
3. In case bone quality (especially in "maxillary Le Fort I repositioning surgery") is not sufficient for screw placement in the pre-identified drill holes, there is an important lack of freedom to the surgeon for intra-operative modification or adaptation with inappropriate transfer of the 3D virtual treatment plan as a clinical important consequence.
4. Towards "mandibular repositioning surgery", PSIs force the surgeon to adapt the proximal segments towards the distal segment only based on the PSI instead of the position dictated by the clinical situation and last but not the least the surgeon's experience.
5. Finally, since any intra-operative intermaxillary fixation is used, the accuracy and precision of the final occlusion, the accuracy of the 3D virtual planning transfer and the final outcome especially towards the condyles need to be investigated in the future.

■ PSIs: "3D Osteotomy Cutting and Jaw Repositioning" Transfer Guides

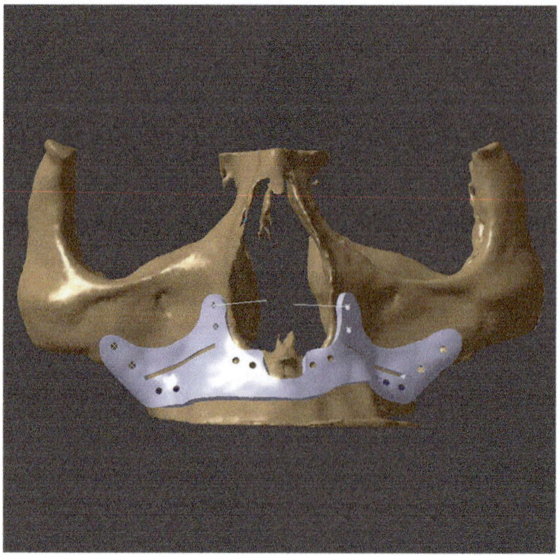

Fig. 4.36 Virtual Le Fort I "3D Osteotomy Cutting and Jaw Repositioning" PSI transfer guide (3D "surface-rendered" representation, iPlan v. 3.0.5., Brainlab Catia V5/Dassault Systèmes) (with courtesy to Harald Essig). Note the position of the virtual drill holes for precise transfer of maxillary repositioning following a "Maxilla-first" sequence with a "waferless" approach by means of "3D Customised Osteosynthesis Plates" (Fig. 4.38)

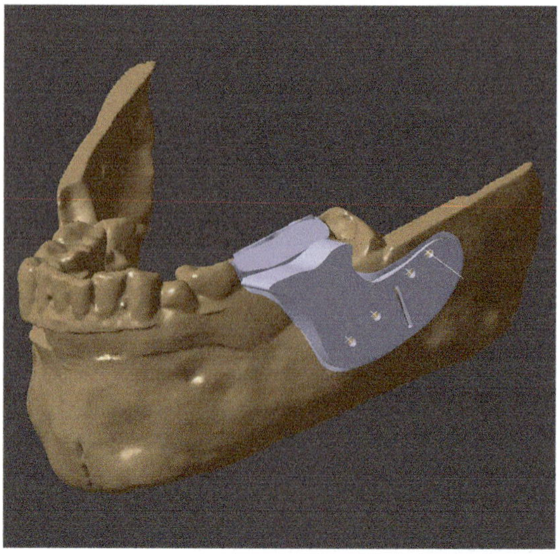

Fig. 4.37 Virtual left SSO "3D Osteotomy Cutting and Jaw Repositioning" PSI transfer guide (3D "surface-rendered" representation, iPlan v. 3.0.5., Brainlab Catia V5/Dassault Systèmes) (with courtesy to Harald Essig). Note the position of the virtual drill holes for precise transfer of mandibular repositioning with a "waferless" approach by means of "3D Customised Osteosynthesis Plates" (Fig. 4.39)

PSIs: "3D Customised Osteosynthesis Plates" for "Maxillary Le Fort I" Repositioning

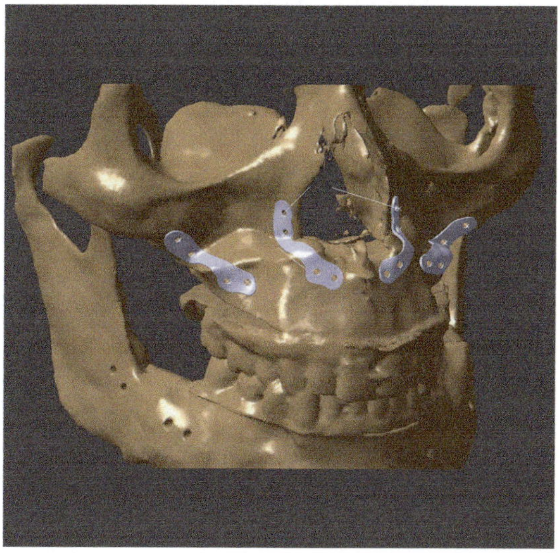

Fig. 4.38 Virtual maxillary repositioning following a "Maxilla-first" sequence with a "waferless" approach by means of "3D Customised Osteosynthesis Plates" which incorporate all surgical movements (3D "surface-rendered" representation, iPlan v. 3.0.5., Brainlab Catia V5/Dassault Systèmes) (with courtesy to Harald Essig). Note that there is no need any more for internal or external vertical reference landmarks, neither intermaxillary fixation (IMF)

Pitfall

Although "PSIs" in "maxillary Le Fort I repositioning surgery" certainly have a potential …., their actual weakness is their lack of freedom to the surgeon to intra-operatively modify or adapt in case bone quality is not sufficient for screw placement in the pre-identified holes with inappropriate planning transfer as a consequence.

▪ PSIs: "3D Customised Osteosynthesis Plates" for "Mandibular" Repositioning

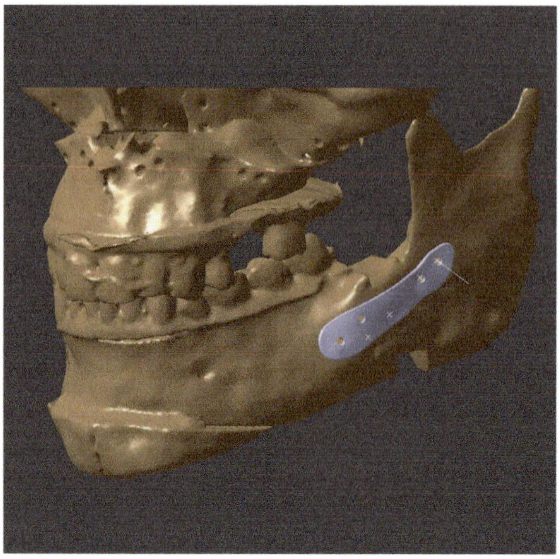

Fig. 4.39 Virtual mandibular repositioning following a "waferless" approach by means of "3D Customised Osteosynthesis Plates" which incorporate all surgical movements of the mandible, obviating the need for any intermaxillary fixation (IMF) (3D "surface-rendered" representation, iPlan v. 3.0.5., Brainlab Catia V5/Dassault Systèmes) (with courtesy to Harald Essig). Note that the crosses illustrate the original position

Pitfall

Although "PSIs" in "mandibular repositioning surgery" have a potential towards positioning the proximal mandibular fragments …., the delicate surgical adaptation of the proximal and distal mandibular segments remains a clinical feeling based on surgical experience.

4.2 Intra-operative Control of the Planning Transfer

Besides "3D Virtual Imaging (▶ Chap. 1), 3D Virtual Diagnosis (▶ Chap. 2) and 3D Virtual Treatment Planning (▶ Chap. 3)", new technologies are continuously changing the major paradigm shift that happened in orthognathic surgery.

Even if the actual standards towards both precision of planning transfer (▶ see also Sect. 4.1) and accuracy of final treatment outcome assessment (▶ see also Chap. 5) have been brought to a higher level compared to the conventional approach, the demand for intra-operative control of the "Individualised 3D Virtual Treatment Plan" becomes more and more obvious.

In order to allow immediate intra-operative evaluation and eventual correction of inadequate bony segment repositioning, the following technologies need to be further explored by different research groups in order to prevent potential additional surgery and further optimise the final surgical treatment outcome:

1. Intra-operative low-dose Cone-Beam CT (IO-CBCT) imaging (▶ see also Sect. 4.2.1)
2. Navigation surgery (▶ see also Sect. 4.2.2)
3. Augmented virtual reality (▶ see also Sect. 4.2.2)

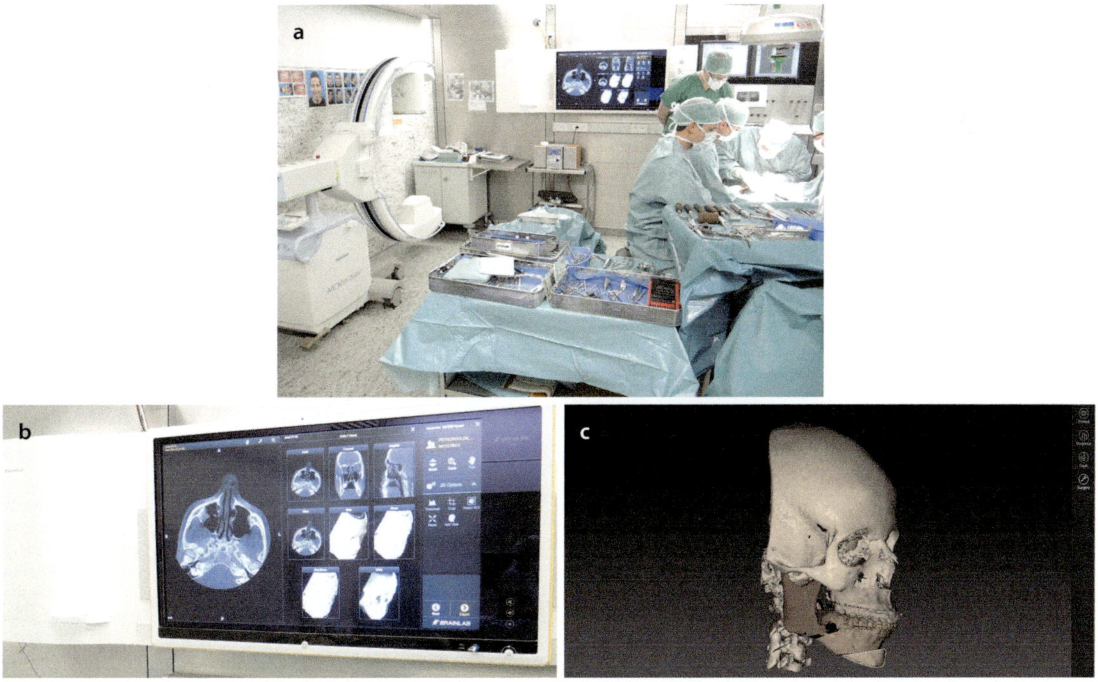

Fig. 4.40 Current orthognathic set-up in the operation theatre at the GH St. John, Bruges, Belgium. Note the C-arm of the intra-operative CBCT apparatus (Arcadis® Orbic 3D C-arm, Siemens Healthcare GmbH) on the *left* (**a**), the central multimodality touch screen (Buzz® Digital O.R., Brainlab) in the *back* (**b**) and the multiple computer screens visualising the patient's "Individualised 3D Virtual Treatment Plan (▶ see Sect. 3.5) IPS CaseDesigner" (**c**) during surgery

4.2.1 The Use of Intra-operative CBCT (IO-CBCT)

Intra-operative imaging, initially limited to 2D C-arm fluoroscopic evaluation, evolved towards 3D evaluation based on Multi-Slice CT (MSCT) and more recently towards Cone-Beam CT (CBCT) technology which allows low-dose radiation image acquisition and intra-operative rendering of high-contrast structures, like facial bones (◘ Figs. 4.47–4.60).

Compared towards conventional MSCT apparatus or technology for intra-operative imaging, IO-CBCT offers numerous advantages:

1. Image quality almost similar
2. Less radiation
3. Faster and less complicated image acquisition
4. Lower level of metal artefacts from osteosynthesis material and orthodontic brackets
5. Smaller apparatus (C-arm VS O-arm) with easier manipulation
6. Lower cost

Nevertheless, the main disadvantage of current IO-CBCT versus IO-MSCT remains its limited field of view (FOV) (◘ Fig. 4.46).

The clinical routine use of IO-CBCT imaging necessitates some changes in the conventional surgical set-up in the operation theatre:

1. Extra space needs to be provided for the presence of the IO-CBCT C-arm and its multimodality workstation in the operating theatre (◘ Figs. 4.40 and 4.41).
2. A "radiolucent carbon headrest" is a prerequisite for appropriate IO-CBCT image acquisition to avoid metal artefacts that would be inevitably caused by a conventional headrest (◘ Fig. 4.42a).
3. The regular surgical table must be adapted towards the "radiolucent carbon headrest" by a cephalad extension in most cases to allow adequate support of the patient's shoulders and back (◘ Fig. 4.42b).
4. Prior to surgery, care should be taken to avoid any collision between the IO-CBCT C-arm and the "radiolucent carbon headrest" mounted on the surgical table.

Since the main advantage of IO-CBCT imaging in orthognathic surgery is the potential towards the surgeon to immediately evaluate the transfer of the virtual planning and eventually correct the position of the bony segments, it is crucial that the operative field remains sterile during the entire process of IO-CBCT image acquisition in order not to lose additional time during surgery. Based on their personal experience, the authors propose the following guidelines:

1. Temporary IMF fixation prior to IO-CBCT imaging
2. Placement of a sterile surgical drape (◘ Fig. 4.43a) over the sterile operative field, secured with non-sterile tape (◘ Fig. 4.43b–c)
3. Marking of the volume of interest (VOI) (e.g. the chin) to be scanned on the surgical drape (◘ Fig. 4.43c)
4. Manual positioning of the IO-CBCT C-arm in the profile (◘ Fig. 4.43d) and frontal (◘ Fig. 4.43e) planes with the aid of laser light localisers
5. Scout views are then taken in these two planes to ensure that the VOI is well positioned in the FOV of the IO-CBCT apparatus (◘ Fig. 4.44)

Our personal experience (Kurihara et al. 2015) has shown that for proper IO-CBCT image acquisition with the Arcadis® Orbic 3D C-arm (Siemens Healthcare GmbH), the profile FOV should be centred in the profile scout view on the crown of the lower first molar (◘ Fig. 4.45).

■ Intra-operative Cone-Beam CT (IO-CBCT)

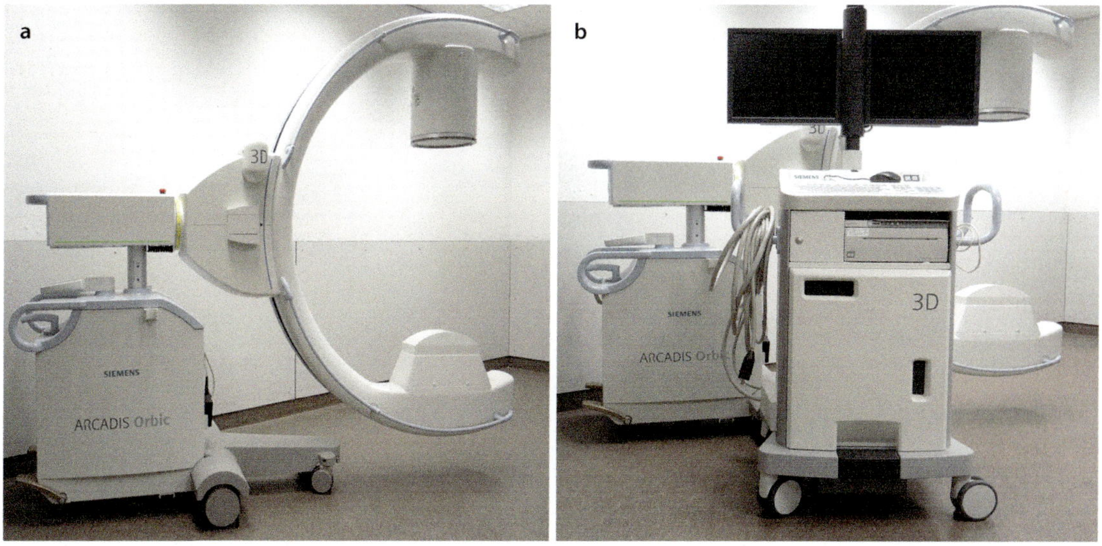

Fig. 4.41 Intra-operative CBCT apparatus: C-arm (**a**) and mutimodality workstation and C-arm (**b**) (Arcadis® Orbic 3D C-arm, Siemens Healthcare GmbH)

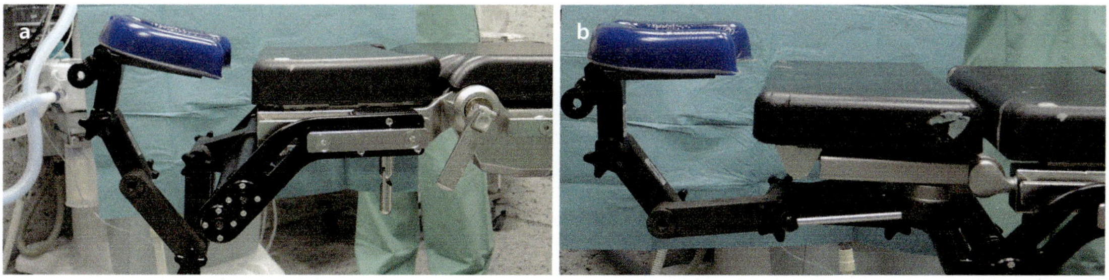

Fig. 4.42 For proper intra-operative CBCT image acquisition, a "radiolucent carbon headrest" (**a**) is mandatory to avoid metal artefacts. It is crucial that the latter headrest must be set up at its full horizontal extension (**b**) to allow free circular rotation of the IO-CBCT C-arm during image acquisition to avoid potential collision and subsequent movement artefacts. Note also the surgical table's extension to support the patient's shoulders and back, when the "radiolucent carbon headrest" headrest is fully extended

Intra-operative Cone-Beam CT (IO-CBCT)

Temporary IMF is advocated prior to IO-CBCT image acquisition to allow appropriate scanning towards the "volume of interest (VOI)" determined by the clinician.

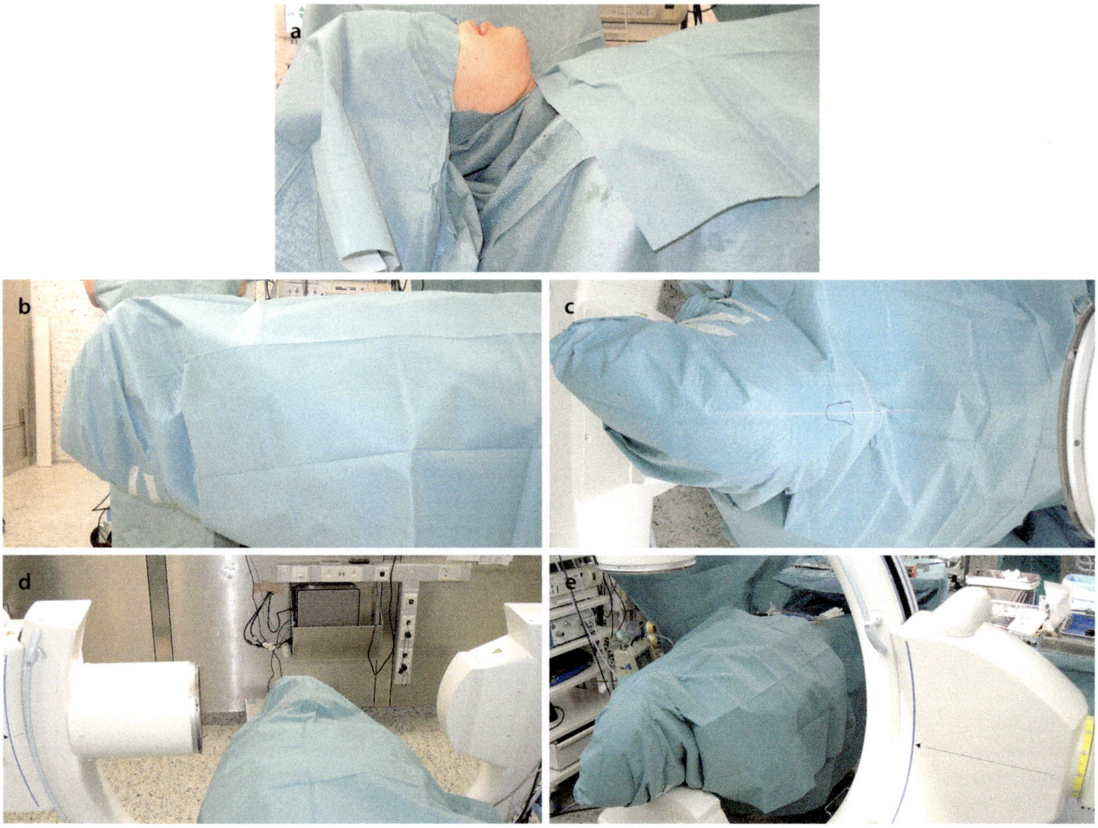

Fig. 4.43 During IO-CBCT imaging, it is important that the operative field remains sterile during image acquisition (**a**). A sterile surgical drape is therefore placed over the operative field and secured with non-sterile tape (**b**). The VOI (e.g. the chin) is then marked on the surgical drape (**c**). Subsequently the IO-CBCT C-arm is manually positioned in the profile (**d**) and frontal (**e**) planes with the aid of laser light localisers. A radiation-free manual "test run" should then ensure that no collision will occur between the C-arm of the IO-CBCT apparatus and the "radiolucent carbon headrest" mounted on the surgical table during IO-CBCT scanning. In this case, the C-arm was touching the inferior portion of the "radiolucent carbon headrest" (**e**). The surgical table was therefore consequently moved superiorly (Arcadis® Orbic 3D c-arm, Siemens Healthcare GmbH)

Intra-operative Cone-Beam CT (IO-CBCT)

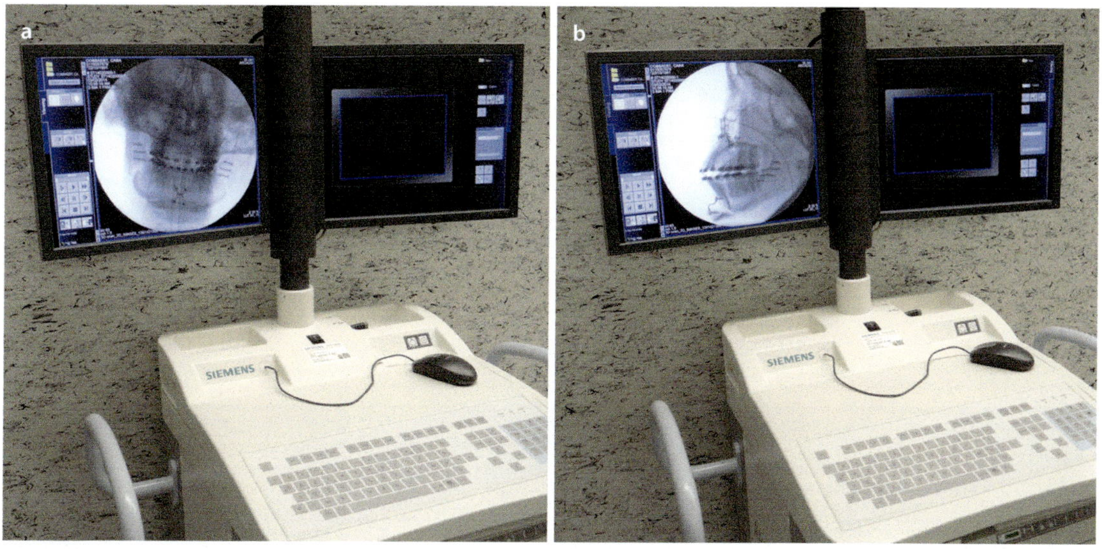

Fig. 4.44 Scout views are taken and visualised on the multimodality workstation in the frontal (**a**) and profile (**b**) planes prior to IO-CBCT image acquisition, since the FOV is still limited in the current IO-CBCT apparatus (Arcadis® Orbic 3D c-arm, Siemens Healthcare GmbH)

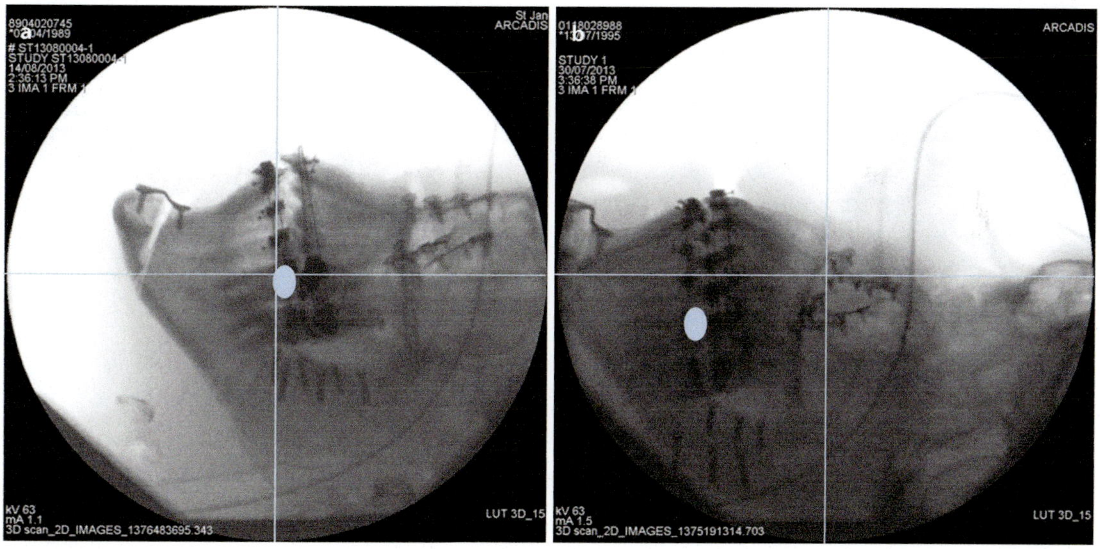

Fig. 4.45 Scout views in the profile plane prior to IO-CBCT scanning (Arcadis® Orbic 3D c-arm, Siemens Healthcare GmbH) of two different patients. According to our personal experience with the Arcadis® Orbic 3D IO-CBCT apparatus, the profile FOV should be centered on the crown of the lower first molar (**a**) for appropriate imaging in orthognathic surgery taking into account the current limited FOV. The scout view of another patient (**b**) shows inappropriate positioning of the C-arm during IO-CBCT imaging. Note that the "shaded circle" shows that the profile FOV should ideally be centered on the crown of the first lower molar

Intra-operative Cone-Beam CT (IO-CBCT)

> Non-published data of an in-house study on 15 consecutive orthognathic patients revealed a mean time of 6 minutes needed for the entire workflow for IO-CBCT image acquisition and image processing, from the moment the sterile drape was put over the patient until the moment that actual surgery could start again with eventual modifications or immediate final wound closure.

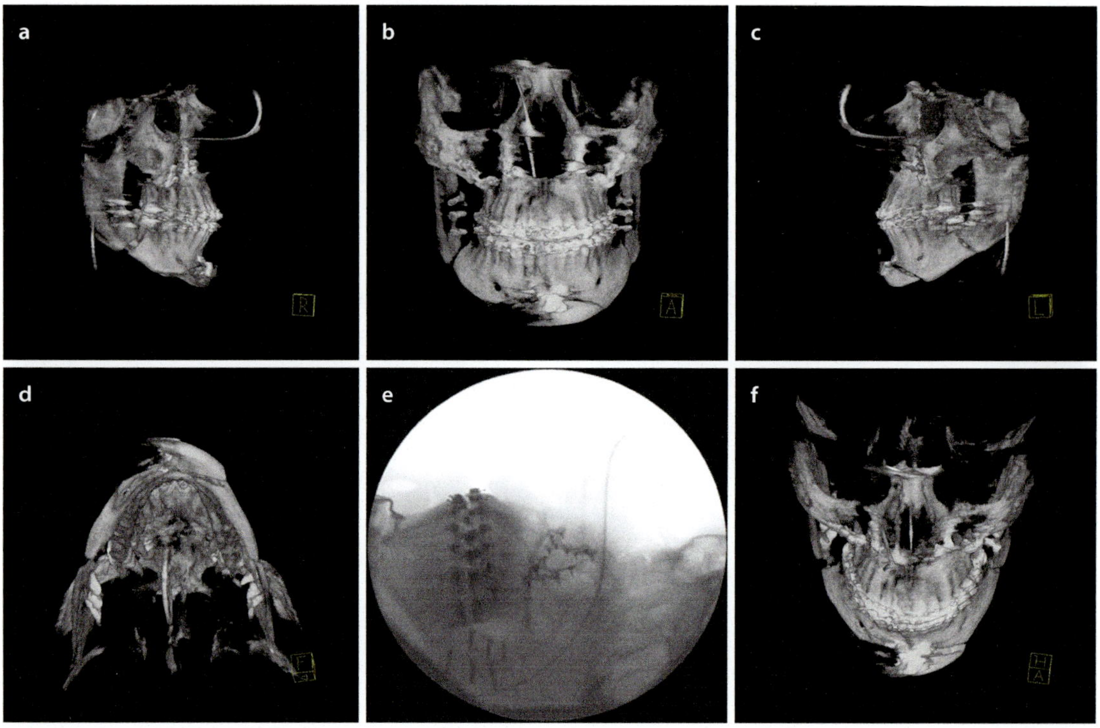

Fig. 4.46 Profile right (**a**), frontal (**b**), profile left (**c**), base (**d**), scout (**e**) and downward inclined (**f**) views of IO-CBCT imaging after surgical repositioning of the maxilla, mandible and chin. Example of a clinical case where the VOI was clearly out of the FOV during IO-CBCT image acquisition (3D "volume-rendered" representations, Arcadis® Orbic 3D C-arm, Siemens Healthcare GmbH). Note on the profile scout view (**e**) that the FOV was not centred on the crown of the lower first molar, therefore positioning the chin outside of the FOV

▪ Intra-operative Cone-Beam CT: "Chin Repositioning" Transfer Control – Patient C.C.

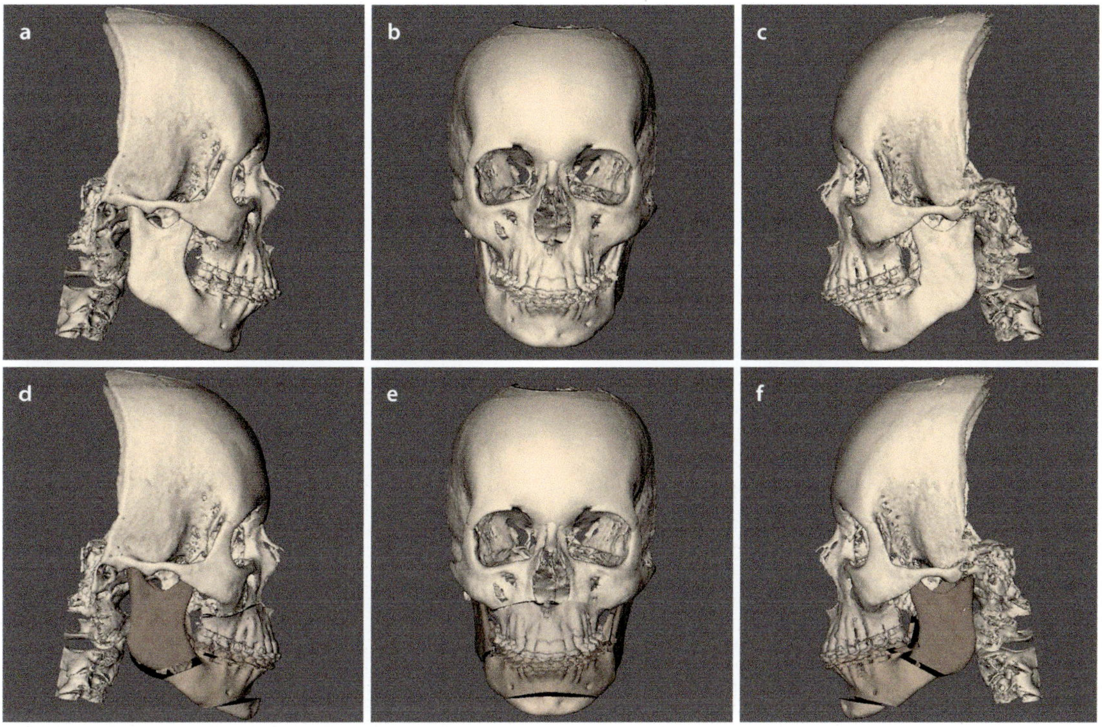

▫ **Fig. 4.47** Profile right (**a**), frontal (**b**) and profile left (**c**) views of the patient's AUM prior to virtual planning. Profile right (**d**), frontal (**e**) and profile left (**f**) views after virtual repositioning of the maxilla, mandible and chin. In this particular case, "virtual chin repositioning" included a sagittal advancement of 6 mm and an anterior extrusion of 4 mm to allow a clockwise ("Pitch") rotation of the chin in order to increase the inferior third of the anterior facial vertical height (3D "surface-rendered" representations, patient C.C., Maxilim v. 2.3.0.3.)

Intra-operative Cone-Beam CT: "Chin Repositioning" Transfer Control – Patient C.C.

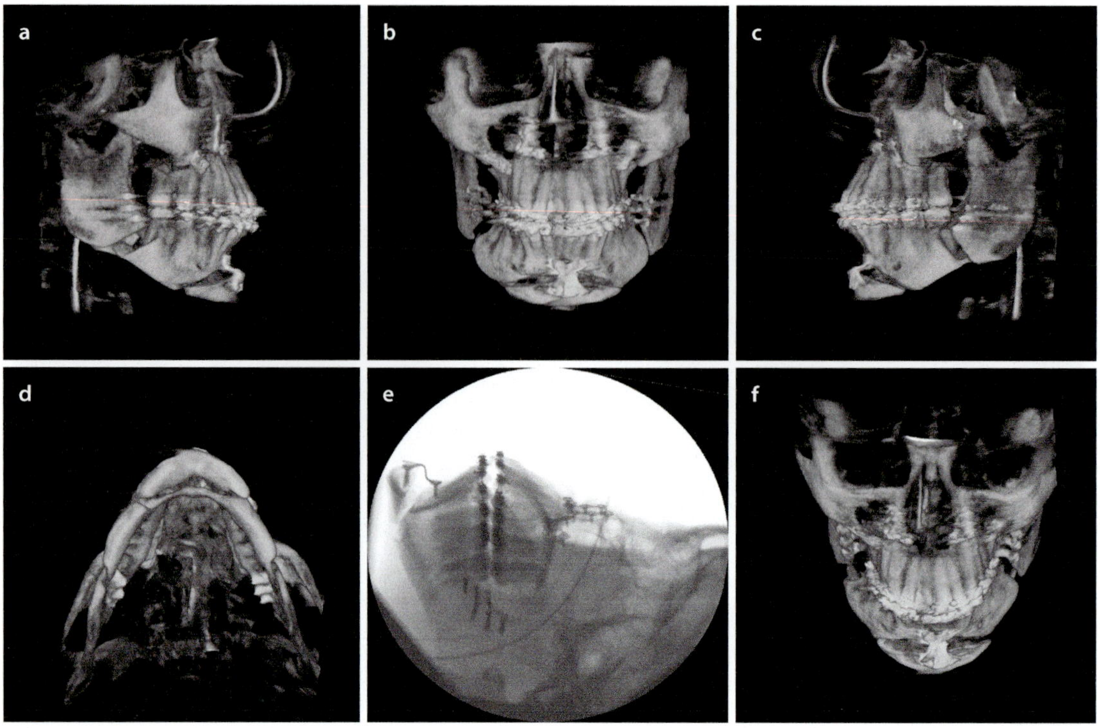

Fig. 4.48 Profile right (**a**), frontal (**b**), profile left (**c**), base (**d**), scout (**e**) and downward inclined (f) views of IO-CBCT imaging after surgical repositioning of the maxilla, mandible and chin (3D "volume-rendered" representations, patient C.C., Arcadis® Orbic 3D C-arm, Siemens Healthcare GmbH). Note the adequate chin advancement and anterior extrusion while avoiding any undesirable midline and yaw movements

Intra-operative Cone-Beam CT: "Chin Repositioning" Transfer Control – Patient C.C.

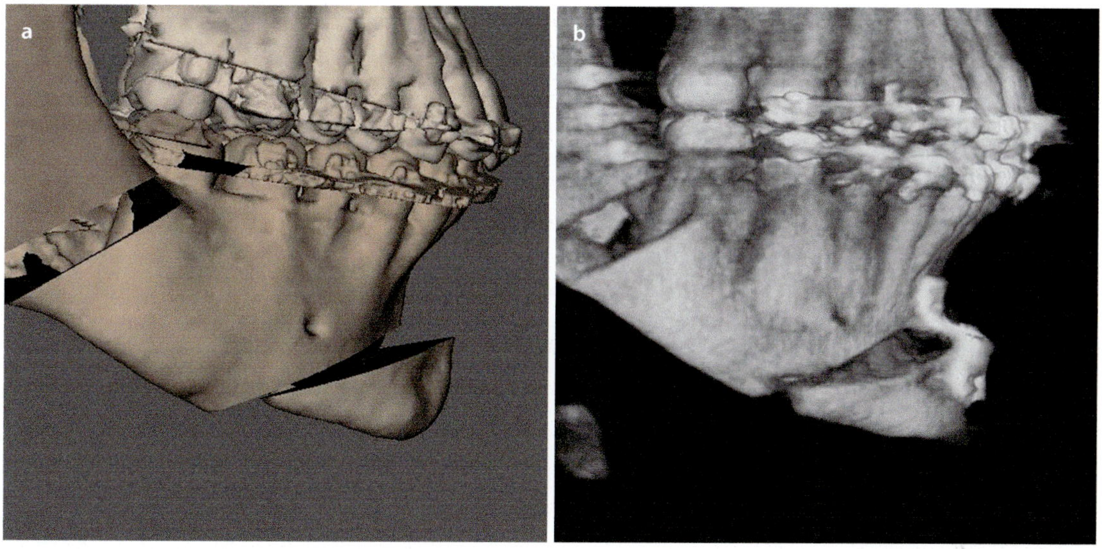

Fig. 4.49 Profile right views of "3D virtual chin repositioning" (3D "surface-rendered" representation, patient C.C., Maxilim v. 2.3.0.3.) (**a**) and IO-CBCT imaging after "surgical chin repositioning" (3D "volume-rendered" representation, patient C.C., Arcadis® Orbic 3D C-arm, Siemens Healthcare GmbH) (**b**). Note that the radiopaque bone graft (Fig. 4.50) is visible on the IO-CBCT image. Also note the similar angulation of the right buccal corticotomy as well as the comparable but slightly larger bony gap between the right proximal and distal mandibular segments due to the buccal cut of the SSO performed with a Lindemann burr

Intra-operative Cone-Beam CT: "Chin Repositioning" Transfer Control – Patient C.C.

Attention
After IO-CBCT imaging and image processing, modifications can be performed if necessary prior to the final wound closure.

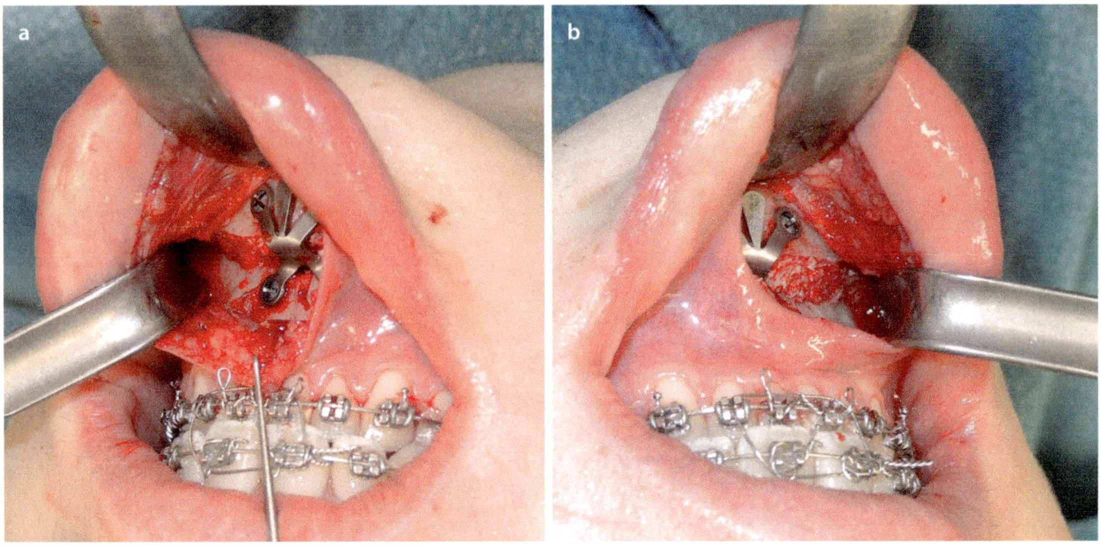

Fig. 4.50 Clinical intra-operative right (**a**) and left (**b**) intra-oral views after surgical repositioning of the chin according to the Individualised 3D Virtual Treatment Plan including 4 mm anterior extrusion and 6 mm advancement prior to IO-CBCT scanning (patient C.C.). Note that a bone graft was placed in the bone gap to promote bony healing

Intra-operative Cone-Beam CT: "Chin Repositioning" Transfer Control – Patient V.T.H.

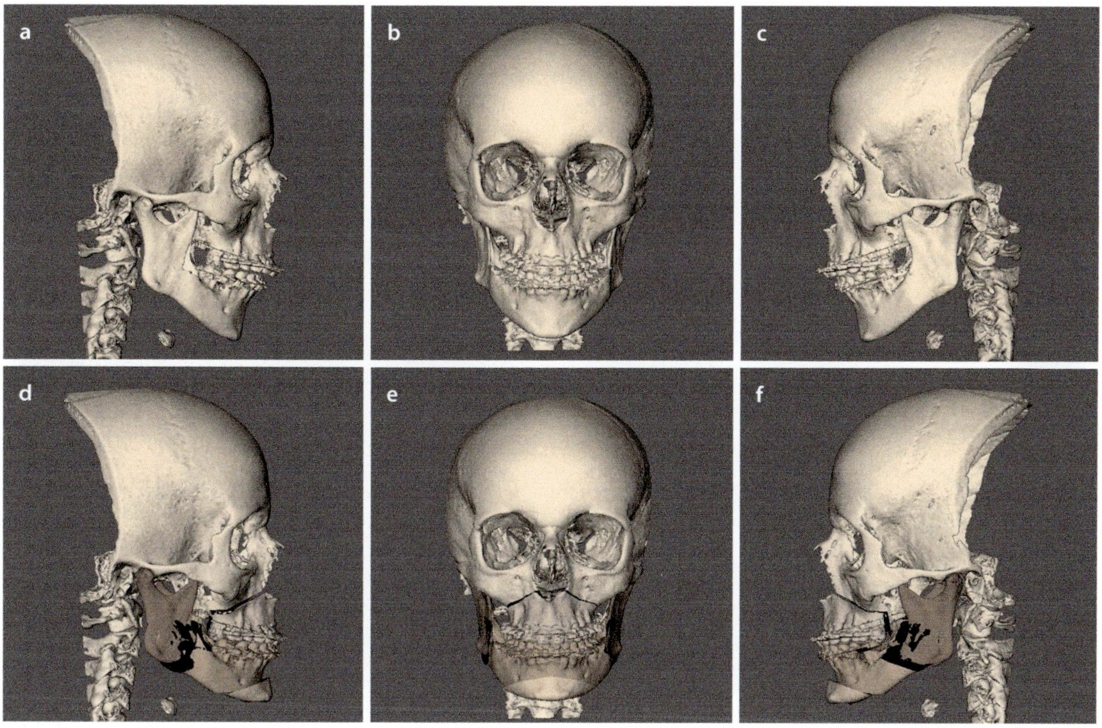

Fig. 4.51 Profile right (**a**), frontal (**b**) and profile left (**c**) views of the patient's AUM prior to virtual planning. Profile right (**d**), frontal (**e**) and profile left (**f**) views after virtual repositioning of the maxilla, mandible and chin. In this particular case, "virtual chin repositioning" included a sagittal advancement of 6 mm and an anterior impaction of 4 mm to allow a CCW rotation ("Pitch") for more chin projection and in order to decrease the bony steps at the inferior mandibular border (3D "surface-rendered" representations, patient V.T.H., Maxilim v. 2.3.0.3.)

Intra-operative Cone-Beam CT: "Chin Repositioning" Transfer Control – Patient V.T.H.

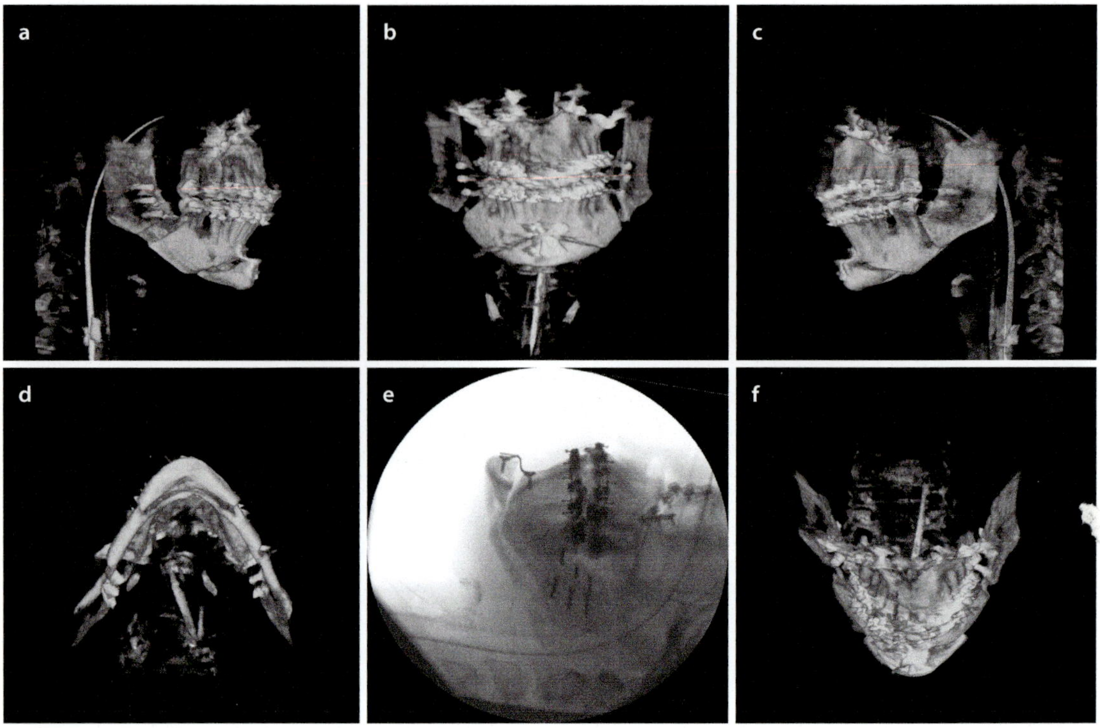

Fig. 4.52 Profile right (**a**), frontal (**b**), profile left (**c**), base (**d**), scout (**e**) and downward inclined (**f**) views of IO-CBCT imaging after surgical repositioning of the maxilla, mandible and chin (3D "volume-rendered" representations, patient V.T.H., Arcadis® Orbic 3D C-arm, Siemens Healthcare GmbH). Note the adequate chin advancement and anterior impaction, while avoiding any midline asymmetry neither inadvertent "Yaw" rotation

Intra-operative Cone-Beam CT: "Chin Repositioning" Transfer Control – Patient V.T.H.

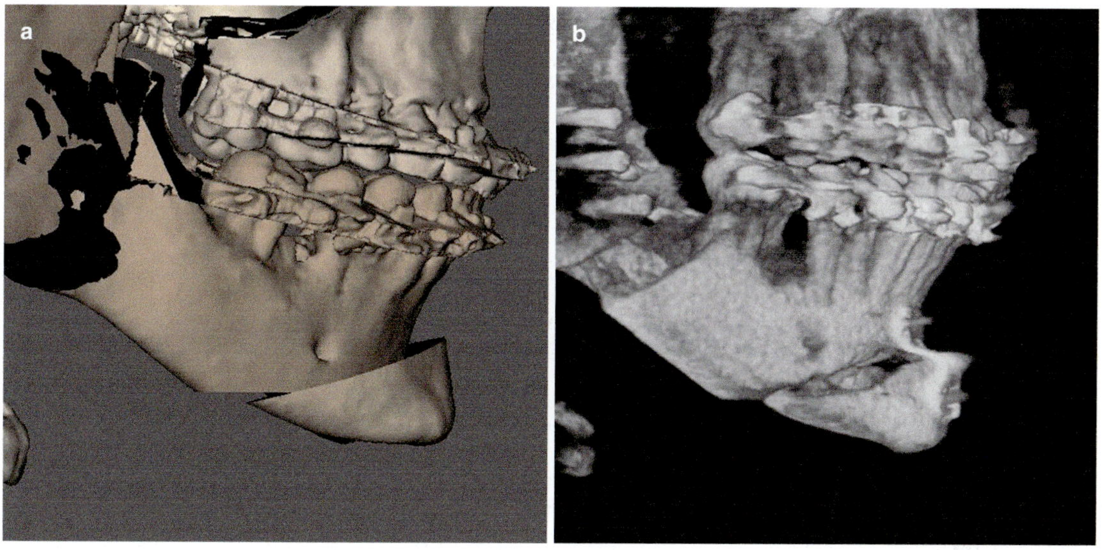

Fig. 4.53 Profile right views of "3D virtual chin repositioning" (3D "surface-rendered" representation, patient C.C., Maxilim v. 2.3.0.3.) (**a**) and IO-CBCT imaging after "surgical chin repositioning" (3D "volume-rendered" representation, patient C.C., Arcadis® Orbic 3D C-arm, Siemens Healthcare GmbH) (**b**). Note the precise transfer of chin repositioning

Intra-operative Cone-Beam CT: "Gonial Angle Reduction" Transfer Control – Patient L.F.

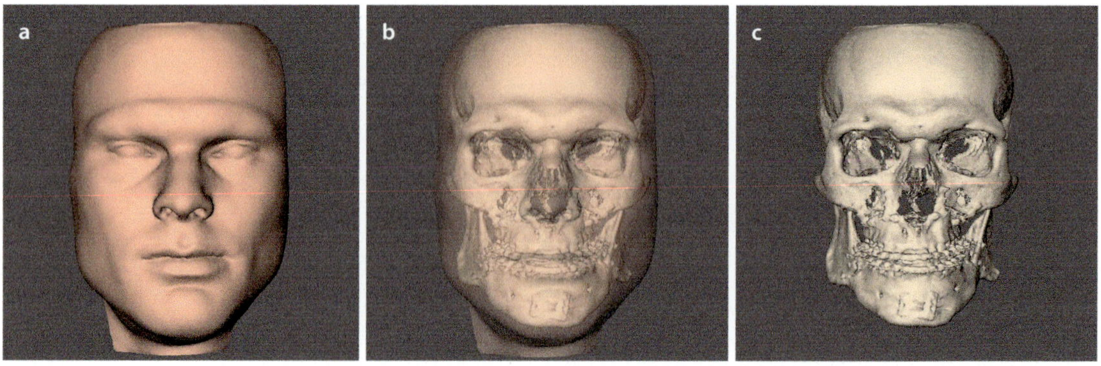

Fig. 4.54 Frontal views of the soft tissue (**a**), hard and semitransparent soft tissue (**b**) and hard tissue (**c**) 3D "surface-rendered" representations of the head of the patient as acquired during CBCT imaging (i-CAT^{TM}, Imaging Sciences International, Inc., Hatfield, USA, Maxilim v. 2.3.0.3. patient L.F.). Note the asymmetric gonial angles after a previous orthognathic surgery performed by another surgeon, where the right gonial angle is projecting more laterally and more inferiorly. In order to meet the patient's expectations, it was decided to surgically reduce the right gonial angle, to achieve facial symmetry

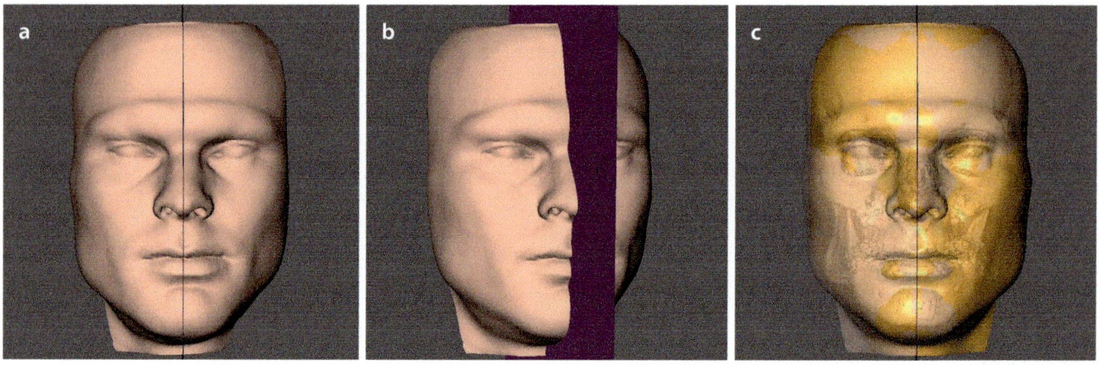

Fig. 4.55 After virtual modification of the patient's head position towards its individual "PHP" (► see also Sect. 2.2.1), the facial midline is identified (**a**), the "3D Virtual Mirror Plane" is set up (**b**) and the facial soft tissue mask is mirrored (**c**) (► see also Sect. 2.3) (3D "surface-rendered" representations, patient L.F., Maxilim v. 2.3.0.3.). Note that the right side of the face is mirrored on the left side (yellow), while the left side of the face is mirrored on the right side (transparent pink), and take special attention to the relation of the bony gonial angles towards the related soft tissues comparing to Fig. 4.54

Intra-operative Cone-Beam CT: "Gonial Angle Reduction" Transfer Control – Patient L.F.

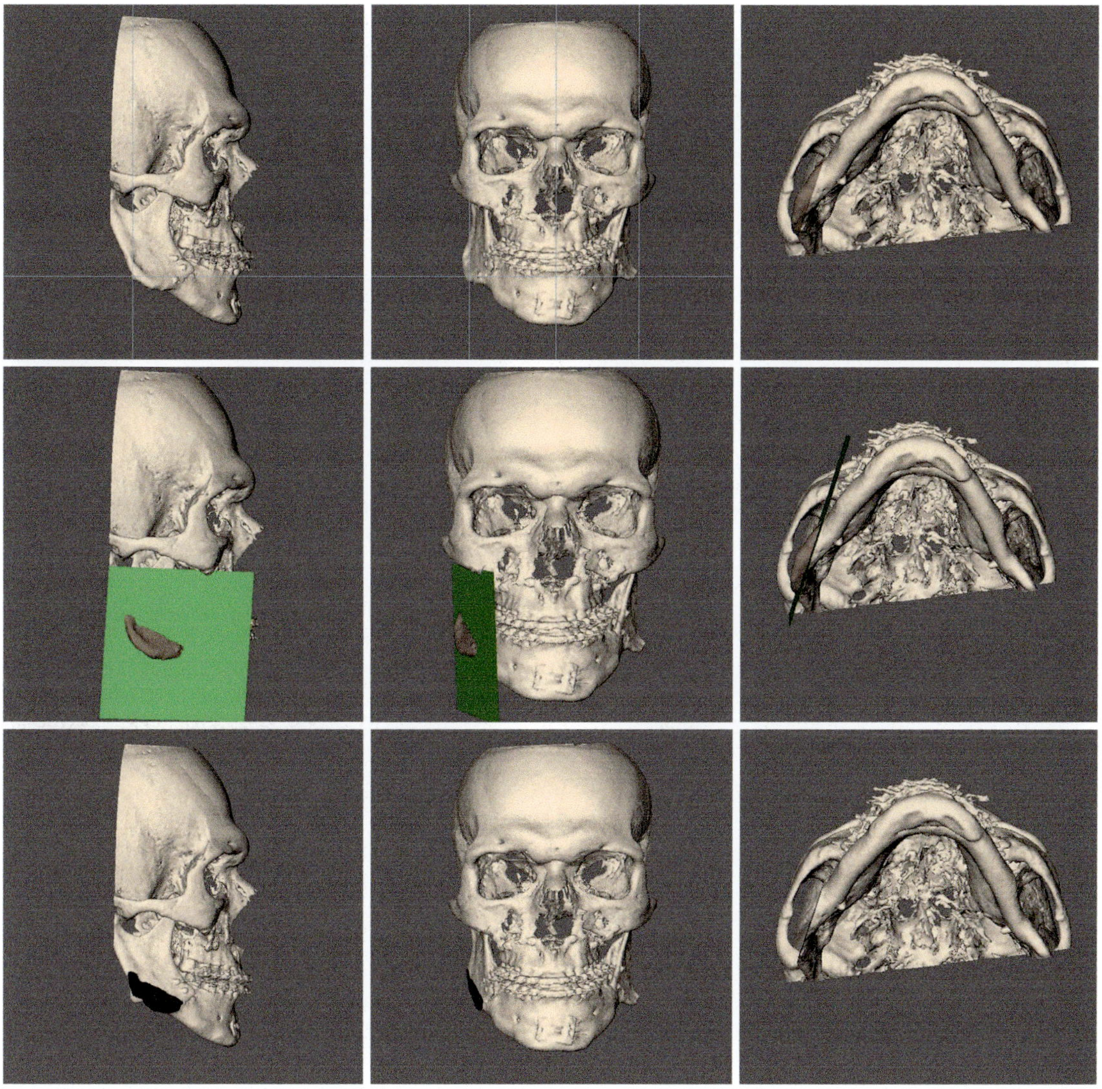

Fig. 4.56 Profile right (**a**), frontal (**b**) and base (**c**) views of the patient's AUM prior to virtual planning of right gonial angle reduction. Profile right (**d**), frontal (**e**) and base (**f**) views visualising the 3D osteotomy plane for right gonial angle reduction. Profile right (**g**), frontal (**h**) and base (**i**) views after virtual right gonial angle reduction (3D "surface-rendered" hard tissue representations, patient L.F., Maxilim v. 2.3.0.3.). Note that using an individualised grid (**a**–**b**), the right gonial angle reduction can be precisely virtually planned, based on the individual anatomy of the left gonial angle

Intra-operative Cone-Beam CT: "Gonial Angle Reduction" Transfer Control – Patient L.F.

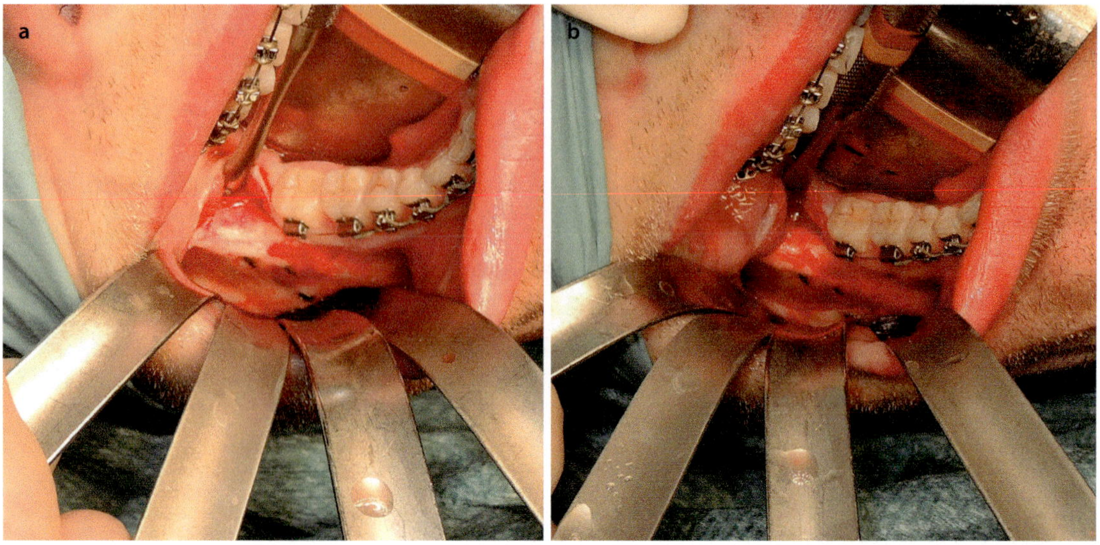

Fig. 4.57 Clinical intra-operative intra-oral views before (**a**) and after (**b**) right gonial angle reduction performed by a reciprocating saw prior to IO-CBCT scanning (patient L.F.). Note that no 3D template (cutting guide) was used but transfer of the virtual right gonial angle reduction was performed by means of direct measurements

Intra-operative Cone-Beam CT: "Gonial Angle Reduction" Transfer Control – Patient L.F.

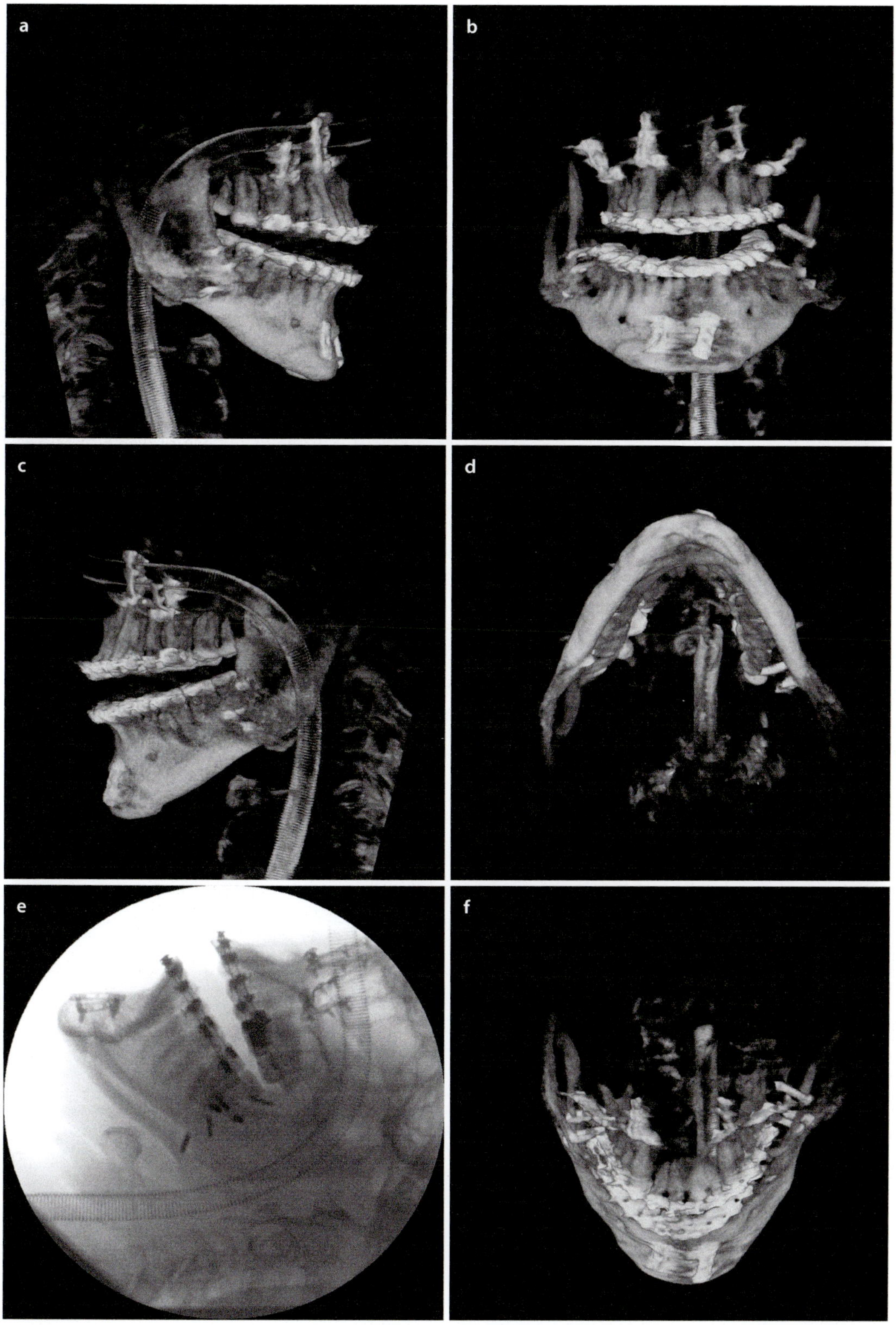

Fig. 4.58 Profile right (**a**), frontal (**b**), profile left (**c**), base (**d**), scout (**e**) and downward inclined (**f**) views of IO-CBCT imaging after right gonial angle reduction (3D "volume-rendered" representations, patient L.F., Arcadis® Orbic 3D C-arm, Siemens Healthcare GmbH)

Intra-operative Cone-Beam CT: "Gonial Angle Reduction" Transfer Control – Patient L.F.

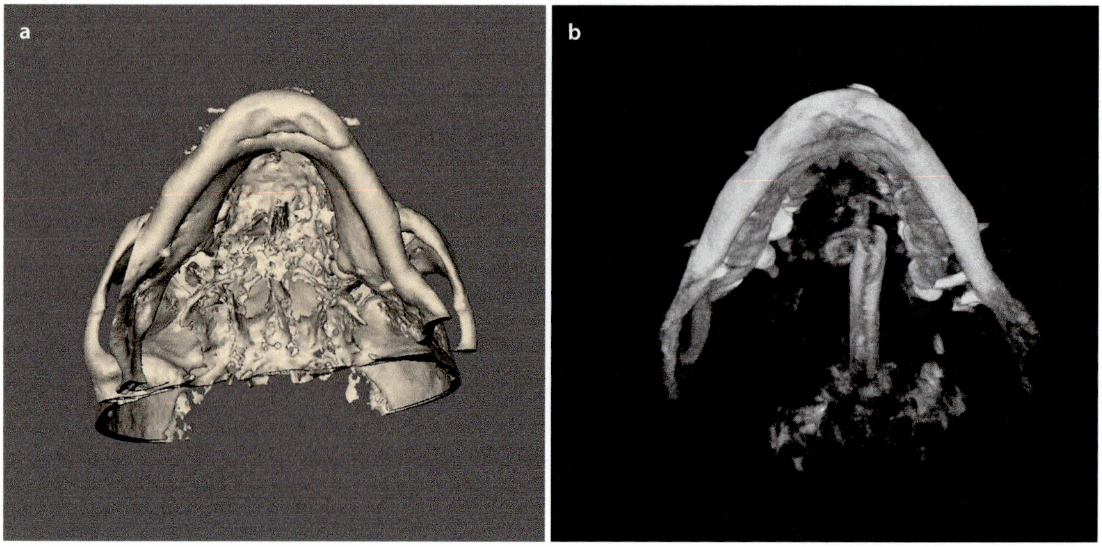

Fig. 4.59 Base views of "3D virtual right gonial angle reduction" (3D "surface-rendered" representation, patient C.C., Maxilim v. 2.3.0.3.) (**a**) and IO-CBCT imaging after "surgical right gonial angle reduction" (3D "volume-rendered" representation, patient L.F., Arcadis® Orbic 3D C-arm, Siemens Healthcare GmbH) (**b**). Note that right gonial angle reduction could be precisely and efficiently performed

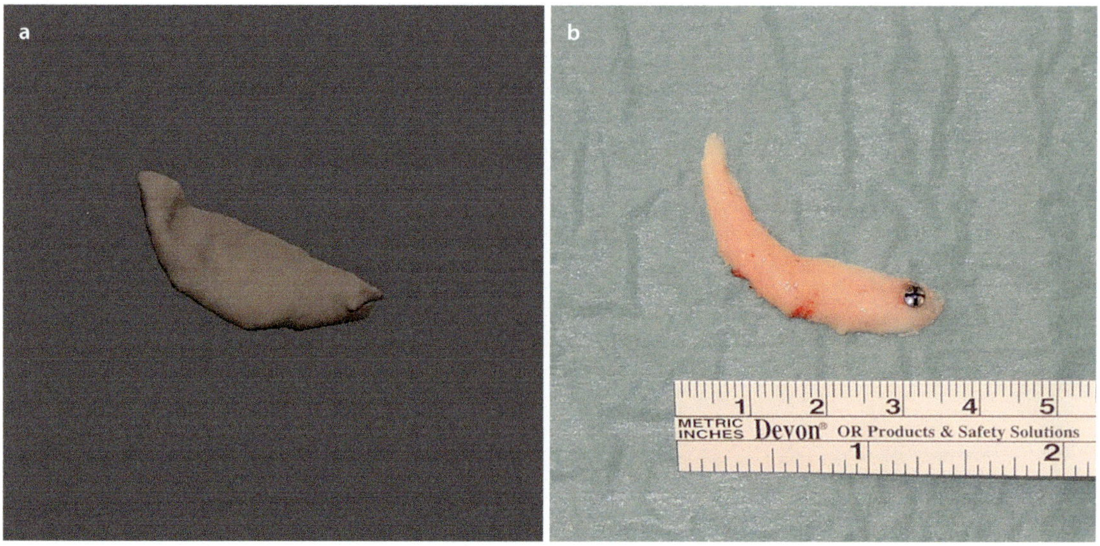

Fig. 4.60 Virtual (3D "surface-rendered" representation, Maxilim v. 2.3.0.3.) (**a**) and actual surgically removed bony segment (**b**) after right gonial angle reduction (patient L.F.)

4.2.2 Potential of Navigation and Augmented Virtual Reality

In the quest for "Waferless Orthognathic Surgery" in order to exclude potential errors induced by inappropriate condylar seating and mandibular autorotation, the following two potential alternatives are currently being explored besides the use of "patient-specific implants (PSIs)" (▶ see also Sect. 4.1.3):

1. Navigational surgery
2. Augmented virtual reality

"Navigational Surgery" has initially being used in orthognathic surgery for intra-operative control of planning transfer and to confirm the spatial relationship of skeletal and dental structures. Different research groups are nowadays exploring its usability towards "Waferless Orthognathic Surgery". However, despite the potential of surgical navigated translocation of bony segments in orthognathic surgery, the registration process remains the critical point. Despite recent technological advances, "Navigational Surgery" especially in orthognathic surgery, where the spatial position of bone is altered during surgery, remains prone to error. Moreover, navigating a mobile structure like the mandible still deserves additional consideration.

"Augmented Virtual Reality" which integrates and complements "Navigational Surgery" might be the next significant technological advancement towards "Waferless Orthognathic Surgery". "Augmented Virtual Reality" is an innovative technology allowing co-registration of data from the real environment with virtual information, creating a hybrid world which is simultaneously visualised on a stereoscopic video display. It can be displayed on a conventional monitor or on a wearable head-mounted display, thereby increasing the surgeon's 3D perception. In other words, "Augmented Virtual Reality" can be considered as the fusion of "Navigational Surgery" and "3D Virtual Treatment Planning" to enable the transfer to the real surgical field. The important potential of the interactive display consists in allowing intra-operative control of jaw repositioning by "real-time" superimposition and visualisation through a video display camera of the virtually planned jaw position (e.g. the maxilla in a "Maxilla-first" sequence or the mandible in a "Mandible-first" sequence) and the actual obtained clinical position of the jaw during surgery.

Although both "Navigational Surgery" and "Augmented Virtual Reality" have certainly a promising potential towards orthognathic surgery, the more complex clinical workflow, increasing operating time and high cost currently do not allow their use in routine clinical practice.

Additional Recommended Reading

Aboul-Hosn Centenero S, Hernández-Alfaro F (2012) 3D planning in orthognathic surgery: CAD/CAM surgical splints and prediction of the soft and hard tissues results – our experience in 16 cases. J Craniomaxillofac Surg 40:162–168

Badiali G, Ferrari V, Cutolo F, Freschi C, Caramella D, Bianchi A, Marchetti C (2014) Augmented reality as an aid in maxillofacial surgery: validation of a wearable system allowing maxillary repositioning. J Craniomaxillofac Surg 42:1970–1976

Bai S, Bo B, Bi Y, Wang B, Zhao J, Liu Y, Feng Z, Shang H, Zhao Y (2010) CAD/CAM surface templates as an alternative to the intermediate wafer in orthognathic surgery. Oral Surg Oral Med Oral Pathol Oral Radiol Endod 110:1–7

Bell RB (2010) Computer planning and intraoperative navigation in cranio-maxillofacial surgery. Oral Maxillofac Surg Clin North Am 22:135–156

Bobek SL (2014) Applications of navigation for orthognathic surgery. Oral Maxillofac Surg Clin North Am 26:587–598

Borumandi F, Brandtner C, Krenkel C, Gaggl A (2013) Navigated repositioning of the maxilla: technical note. Br J Oral Maxillofac Surg 51:568–569

Dobbe JG, Curnier F, Rondeau X, Streekstra GJ (2015) Precision of image-based registration for intraoperative navigation in the presence of metal artifacts: application to corrective osteotomy surgery. Med Eng Phys 37:524–530

Ellis E 3rd (1990) Accuracy of model surgery: evaluation of an old technique and introduction of a new one. J Oral Maxillofac Surg 48:1161–1167

Füglein A, Riediger D (2012) Exact three-dimensional skull-related repositioning of the maxilla during orthognathic surgery. Br J Oral Maxillofac Surg 50:614–616

Gander T, Bredell M, Eliades T, Rücker M, Essig H (2015) Splintless orthognathic surgery: a novel technique using patient-specific implants (PSI). J Craniomaxillofac Surg 43:319–322

Gateno J, Xia J, Teichgraeber JF, Rosen A, Hultgren B, Vadnais T (2003) The precision of computer-generated surgical splints. J Oral Maxillofac Surg 61:814–817

Heiland M, Schmelzle R, Hebecker A, Schulze D (2004) Intraoperative 3D imaging of the facial skeleton using the SIREMOBIL Iso-C3D. Dentomaxillofac Radiol 33:130–132

Kang SH, Kim MK, Choi YS, Park W, Lee SH (2011) Navigation-assisted intraoral vertical ramus osteotomy. J Oral Maxillofac Surg 69:931–934

KuriharaY, Boeckx P, Shirota T, Gaboury M, Swennen GRJ (2015) Prospective evaluation of the potential of intraoperative Cone-Beam CT (IO-CBCT) imaging towards genioplasty in orthognathic surgery. Unpublished

Li B, Zhang L, Sun H, Yuan J, Shen SG, Wang X (2013) A novel method of computer aided orthognathic surgery using individual CAD/CAM templates: a combination of osteotomy and repositioning guides. Br J Oral Maxillofac Surg 51:239–244

Li B, Zhang L, Sun H, Shen SG, Wang X (2014) A new method of surgical navigation for orthognathic surgery: optical tracking guided free-hand repositioning of the maxillomandibular complex. J Craniofac Surg 25:406–411

Lin HH, Chang HW, Wang CH, Kim SG, Lo LJ (2015) Three-dimensional computer-assisted orthognathic surgery: experience of 37 patients. Ann Plast Surg 74:118–126

Lo J, Xia JJ, Zwahlen RA, Cheung LK (2010) Surgical navigation in correction of hemimandibular hyperplasia: a new treatment strategy. J Oral Maxillofac Surg 68:1444–1450

Marmulla R, Mühling J (2007) Computer-assisted condyle positioning in orthognathic surgery. J Oral Maxillofac Surg 65:1963–1968

Mazzoni S, Badiali G, Lancellotti L, Babbi L, Bianchi A, Marchetti C (2010) Simulation-guided navigation: a new approach to improve intraoperative three-dimensional reproducibility during orthognathic surgery. J Craniofac Surg 21:1698–1705

Mazzoni S, Bianchi A, Schiariti G, Badiali G, Marchetti C (2015) Computer-aided design and computer-aided manufacturing cutting guides and customized titanium plates are useful in upper maxilla waferless repositioning. J Oral Maxillofac Surg 73:701–707

Mischkowski RA, Zinser MJ, Kübler AC, Krug B, Seifert U, Zöller JE (2006) Application of an augmented reality tool for maxillary positioning in orthognathic surgery – a feasibility study. J Craniomaxillofac Surg 34:478–483

Metzger MC, Hohlweg-Majert B, Schwarz U, Teschner M, Hammer B, Schmelzeisen R (2008) Manufacturing splints for orthognathic surgery using a three-dimensional printer. Oral Surg Oral Med Oral Pathol Oral Radiol Endod 105:1–7

Polley JW, Figueroa AA (2013) Orthognathic positioning system: intraoperative system to transfer virtual surgical plan to operating field during orthognathic surgery. J Oral Maxillofac Surg 71:911–920

Reichert C (2014) CAD/CAM and surgical navigation splints versus intermaxillary occlusal splints. J Orofac Orthop 75:164–166

Sadiq Z, Collyer J, Sneddon K, Walsh S (2012) Orthognathic treatment of asymmetry: two cases of "waferless" stereotactic maxillary positioning. Br J Oral Maxillofac Surg 50:27–29

Seeberger R, Thiele OC, Mertens C, Hoffmann J, Engel M (2013) Proximal segment positioning with high oblique sagittal split osteotomy: indications and limits of intraoperative mobile cone-beam computerized tomography. Oral Surg Oral Med Oral Pathol Oral Radiol 115:731–736

Shim BK, Shin HS, Nam SM, Kim YB (2013) Real-time navigation-assisted orthognathic surgery. J Craniofac Surg 24:221–225

Swennen GRJ, Schutyser F (2007) Three-dimensional virtual approach to diagnosis and treatment planning of maxillo-facial deformity. In: Bell WH, Guerrero CA (eds) Distraction osteogenesis of the facial skeleton, vol 6. BC Decker Inc, Hamilton, pp 55–79

Swennen GRJ, Mollemans W, Schutyser F (2009) Three-dimensional treatment planning of orthognathic surgery in the era of virtual imaging. J Oral Maxillofac Surg 67:2080–2092

Swennen G, Mollemans W, Schutyser F, Lamoral P (2010) Evaluation of the accuracy of maxillary repositioning after 3D virtual planning of orthognathic surgery: a prospective study. Abstract book of the 20th EACMFS Congress

Sun Y, Luebbers HT, Agbaje JO, Schepers S, Vrielinck L, Lambrichts I, Politis C (2013) Evaluation of 3 different registration techniques in image-guided bimaxillary surgery. J Craniofac Surg 24:1095–1099

Wagner A, Rasse M, Millesi W, Ewers R (1997) Virtual reality for orthognathic surgery: the augmented reality environment concept. J Oral Maxillofac Surg 55: 456–462

Xia JJ, Gateno J, Teichgraeber JF (2009) New clinical protocol to evaluate craniomaxillofacial deformity and plan surgical correction. J Oral Maxillofac Surg 67: 2093–2106

Ye N, Long H, Zhu S, Yang Y, Lai W, Hu J (2014) The accuracy of computer image-guided template for Mandibular Angle Ostectomy. Aesthetic Plast Surg 39:117–123

Zinser MJ, Mischkowski RA, Sailer HF, Zöller JE (2012) Computer-assisted orthognathic surgery: feasibility study using multiple CAD/CAM surgical splints. Oral Surg Oral Med Oral Pathol Oral Radiol 113:673–687

Zinser MJ, Sailer HF, Ritter L, Braumann B, Maegele M, Zöller JE (2013a) A paradigm shift in orthognathic surgery? A comparison of navigation, computer-aided designed/computer-aided manufactured splints, and "classic" intermaxillary splints to surgical transfer of virtual orthognathic planning. J Oral Maxillofac Surg 71:2151–2152

Zinser MJ, Mischkowski RA, Dreiseidler T, Thamm OC, Rothamel D, Zöller JE (2013b) Computer-assisted orthognathic surgery: waferless maxillary positioning, versatility, and accuracy of an image-guided visualisation display. Br J Oral Maxillofac Surg 51:827–833

Zhu M, Chai G, Zhang Y, Ma X, Gan J (2011) Registration strategy using occlusal splint based on augmented reality for mandibular angle oblique split osteotomy. J Craniofac Surg 22:1806–1809

Zizelmann C, Hammer B, Gellrich NC, Schwestka-Polly R, Rana M, Bucher P (2012) An evaluation of face-bow transfer for the planning of orthognathic surgery. J Oral Maxillofac Surg 70:1944–1950

3D Virtual Evaluation of Treatment Outcome of Orthognathic Surgery

Gwen R.J. Swennen

G.R.J. Swennen (ed.), *3D Virtual Treatment Planning of Orthognathic Surgery*,
DOI 10.1007/978-3-662-47389-4_5

5.1 Systematic Virtual Evaluation of Treatment Outcome

There is no doubt that "3D virtual evaluation of treatment outcome" will bring new substantial knowledge and insights (e.g. on long-term stability, airway, condylar changes, facial harmony and aesthetics, etc.) and moreover will initiate innovative concepts in orthognathic surgery that will further improve care of the patient with "dento-maxillo-facial deformity".

Towards "Systematic Virtual Evaluation of Treatment Outcome", the same standardised "step-by-step" approach based on the "3D Virtual Visualisation Paradigm" (Swennen and Schutyser 2007) can be used as for "systematic virtual diagnosis of the patient's deformity, anatomy and pathology (▶ see also Sect. 2.1)":

1. Dento-maxillo-facial
2. Airway
3. TMJ

The systematic approach towards individualised patient's treatment outcome assessment in this section is illustrated on Case 1 Patient (V.E.W.), which is used throughout this book (▶ Chaps. 1, 2, 3, 4 and 6). Patient V.E.W. underwent a combined Le Fort I osteotomy, BSSO, genioplasty and rhinoplasty (dorsal hump reduction) for the correction of her Class II long-face deformity (▶ see also Chap. 6). The "step-by-step individualised 3D virtual treatment planning ($3D\text{-}VPS_5$) (▶ see Sect. 3.5)" and "3D virtual treatment planning transfer (▶ see Sect. 4.1)" of patient V.E.W. have been outlined in detail in this book.

Virtual evaluation of treatment outcome of other clinical cases with other types of "dento-maxillo-facial deformity" is demonstrated in Chap. 6.

> 3D Virtual Evaluation of Treatment Outcome has the unprecedented potential to provide new evidence-based data to further improve care of the patient with dento-maxillo-facial deformity.

5.1.1 Dento-maxillo-facial

After appropriate post-surgical CBCT image acquisition and consecutive 3D rendering (▶ see also Sect. 1.1.1), the 3D soft and hard tissue surface representations of the patient's head can be systematically evaluated in the "3D virtual scene" towards the patient's individual dento-maxillo-facial treatment outcome:

1. Frontal view (◘ Fig. 5.1)
2. Profile view right/left (◘ Figs. 5.2 and 5.3)
3. Base view (◘ Fig. 5.4)
4. Cranial view (◘ Fig. 5.5)
5. Posterior view (◘ Fig. 5.6)

Towards virtual "dento-maxillo-facial" treatment outcome analysis, "volume rendering" is more appropriate compared to "surface rendering" since it allows more detailed visualisation of the patient's occlusion and dentition.

Systematic Virtual Treatment Outcome Evaluation: Dento-maxillo-facial

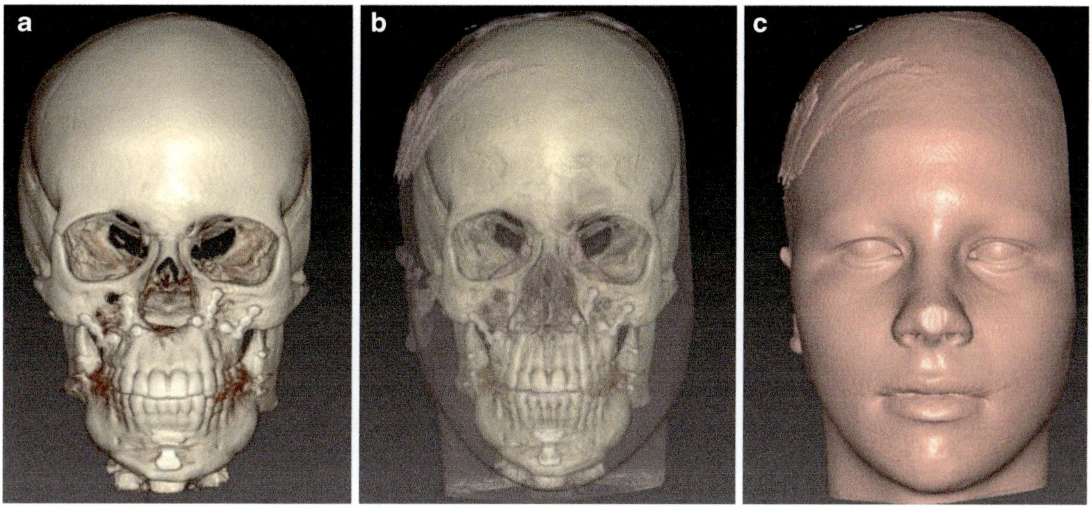

Fig. 5.1 One-year post-surgical frontal views of 3D "volume-rendered" hard (**a**), hard and transparent soft tissue (**b**) and soft tissue (**c**) surface representations of the patient's head (i-CAT, Imaging Sciences International Inc, IPS CaseDesigner ALPHA version) (patient V.E.W.). Note that parts of the 3D facial soft tissues (tip of the nose/left temporo-parietal region) were out of the FOV during scanning. Note pre-surgical views (Fig. 2.1)

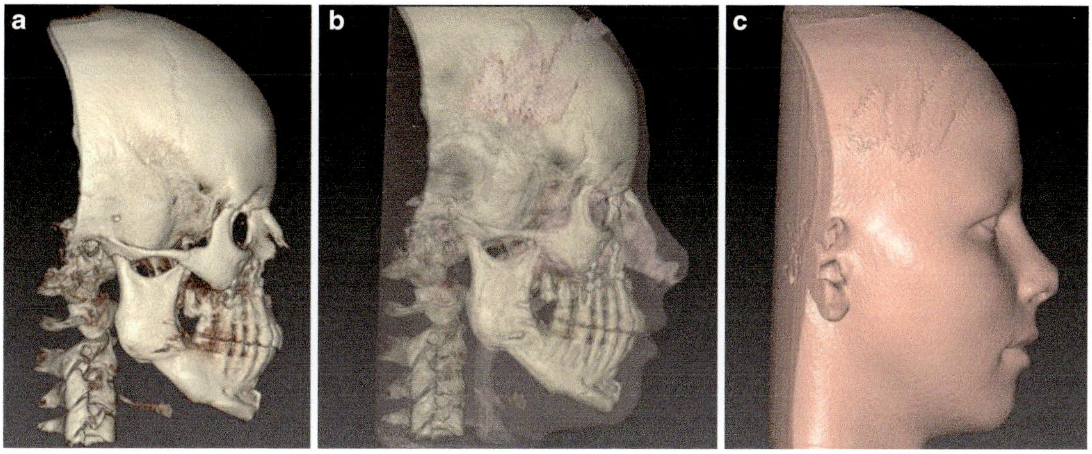

Fig. 5.2 One-year post-surgical right profile views of 3D "volume-rendered" hard (**a**), hard and transparent soft tissue (**b**) and soft tissue (**c**) surface representations of the patient's head (i-CAT, Imaging Sciences International Inc, IPS CaseDesigner ALPHA version) (patient V.E.W.). Note that parts of the 3D facial soft tissues (tip of the nose) were out of the FOV during scanning. Note pre-surgical views (Fig. 2.2)

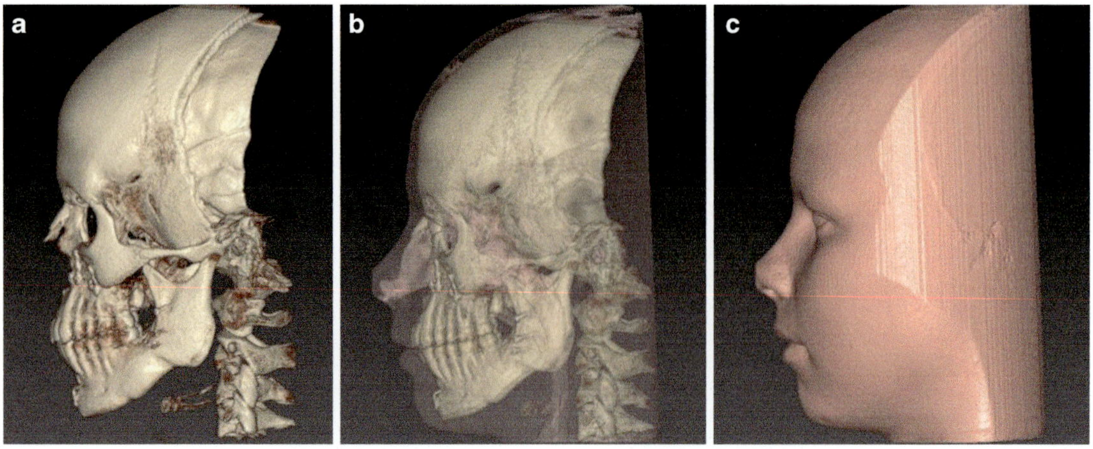

Fig. 5.3 One-year post-surgical left profile views of 3D "volume-rendered" hard (**a**), hard and transparent soft tissue (**b**) and soft tissue (**c**) surface representations of the patient's head (i-CAT, Imaging Sciences International Inc, IPS CaseDesigner ALPHA version) (patient V.E.W.). Note that parts of the 3D facial soft tissues (tip of the nose/left temporo-parietal region) were out of the FOV during scanning. Note pre-surgical views (Fig. 2.3)

Systematic Virtual Treatment Outcome Evaluation: Dento-maxillo-facial

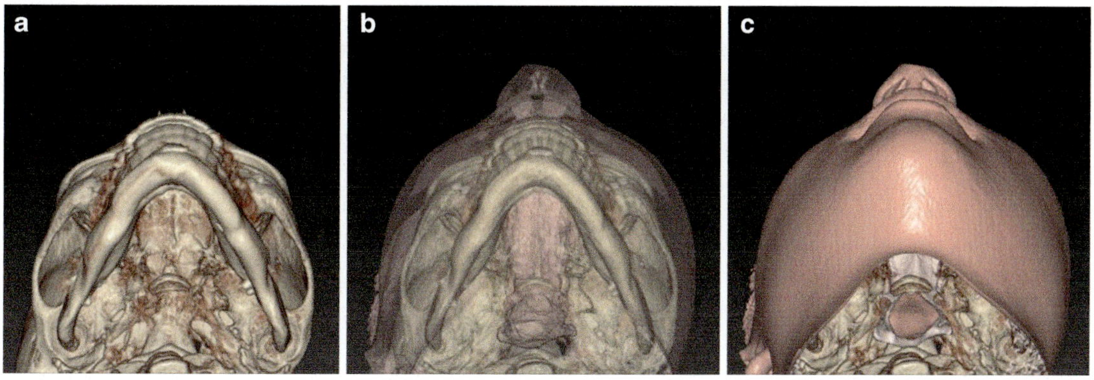

Fig. 5.4 One-year post-surgical base views of 3D "volume-rendered" hard (**a**), hard and transparent soft tissue (**b**) and soft tissue (**c**) surface representations of the patient's head (i-CAT, Imaging Sciences International Inc, IPS CaseDesigner ALPHA version) (patient V.E.W.). Note that parts of the 3D facial soft tissues (tip of the nose) were out of the FOV during scanning. Note pre-surgical views (Fig. 2.4)

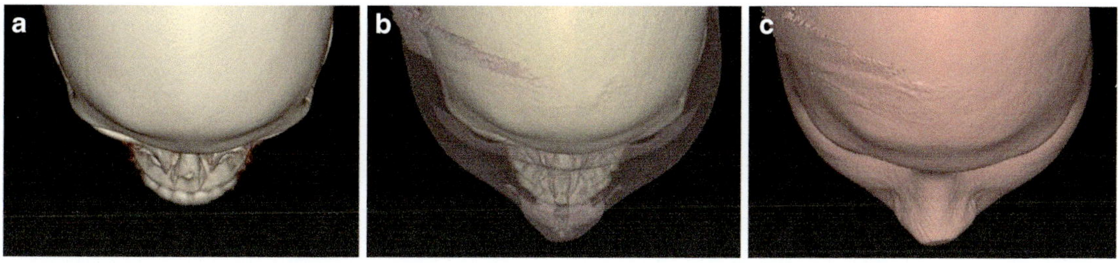

Fig. 5.5 One-year post-surgical cranial views of 3D "volume-rendered" hard (**a**), hard and transparent soft tissue (**b**) and soft tissue (**c**) surface representations of the patient's head (i-CAT, Imaging Sciences International Inc, IPS CaseDesigner ALPHA version) (patient V.E.W.). Note that parts of the 3D facial soft tissues (tip of the nose/left temporo-parietal region) were out of the FOV during scanning. Note pre-surgical views (Fig. 2.5)

Fig. 5.6 One-year post-surgical posterior views of 3D "volume-rendered" hard (**a**), hard and transparent soft tissue (**b**) surface representations of the patient's head (i-CAT, Imaging Sciences International Inc, IPS CaseDesigner ALPHA version) (patient V.E.W.). Note that parts of the 3D facial soft tissues (left temporo-parietal region) were out of the FOV during scanning. Note pre-surgical views (Fig. 2.6)

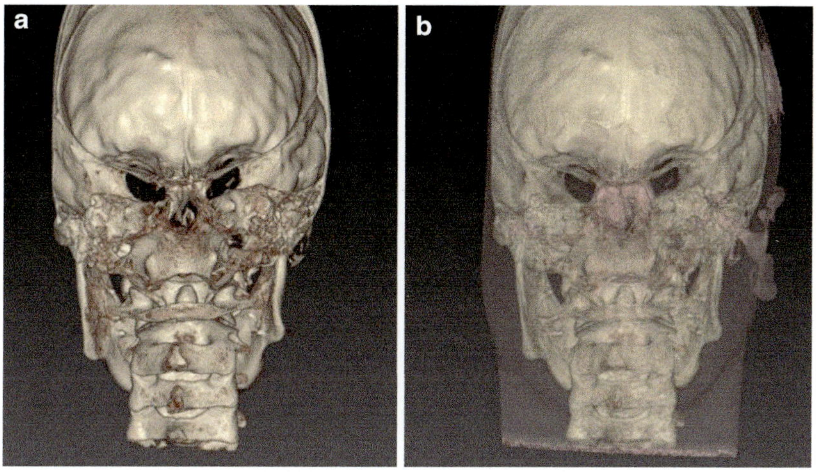

5.1.2 Airway

After "systematic virtual evaluation" of the patient's dento-maxillo-facial treatment outcome (▶ Sect. 5.1.1), the "3D Virtual Visualisation Paradigm" allows more enhanced post-surgical evaluation of the patient's upper airway in the "3D virtual scene".

The post-surgical upper pharyngeal airway and its subregions (the "nasopharyngeal", "oropharyngeal" and "hypopharyngeal" airway) can be evaluated in an accurate and reliable way following a standardised protocol (Guijarro-Martínez and Swennen 2013) (▶ see also Sect. 5.1.2):

1. Standardised CBCT scanning of the patient's head
2. Verification of the patient's head position by measuring the "cranio-cervical inclination" in the sagittal plane (◘ Figs. 5.7 and 5.8)
3. Virtual reorientation of the patient's head with the set-up of an "upper airway 3D coordinate system"
4. Segmentation of the upper pharyngeal airway by "thresholding"
5. 3D CBCT definition of the anatomical boundaries of the upper pharyngeal airway and its subregions (◘ Fig. 5.9)

Towards virtual "airway" treatment outcome analysis, "surface rendering" is more appropriate compared to "volume rendering" since it allows segmentation of the upper pharyngeal airway and its subregions.

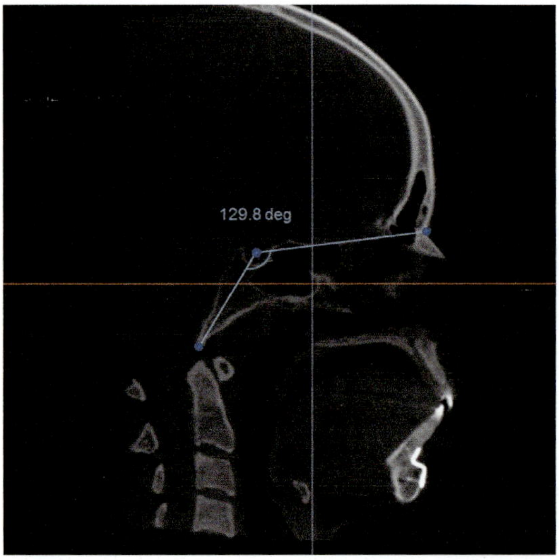

◘ **Fig. 5.7** One-year post-surgical sagittal slice illustrating the "cranio-cervical inclination" (i-CAT, Imaging Sciences International Inc, IPS CaseDesigner Alpha version) (patient V.E.W.). Note that the "cranio-cervical inclination" is slightly less compared to the pre-operative inclination of 98.1 °degrees (◘ Fig. 2.60)

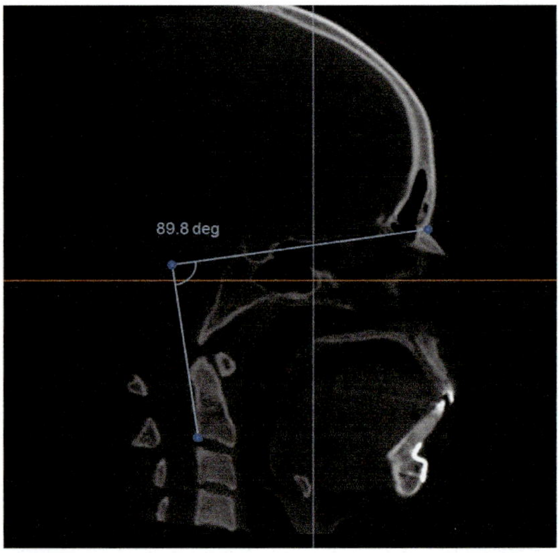

◘ **Fig. 5.8** One-year post-surgical sagittal slice illustrating the "cranial base angle" (i-CAT, Imaging Sciences International Inc, IPS CaseDesigner Alpha version) (patient V.E.W.), which is the same as the pre-operative inclination (◘ Fig. 2.61)

Systematic Virtual Treatment Outcome Evaluation: Airway

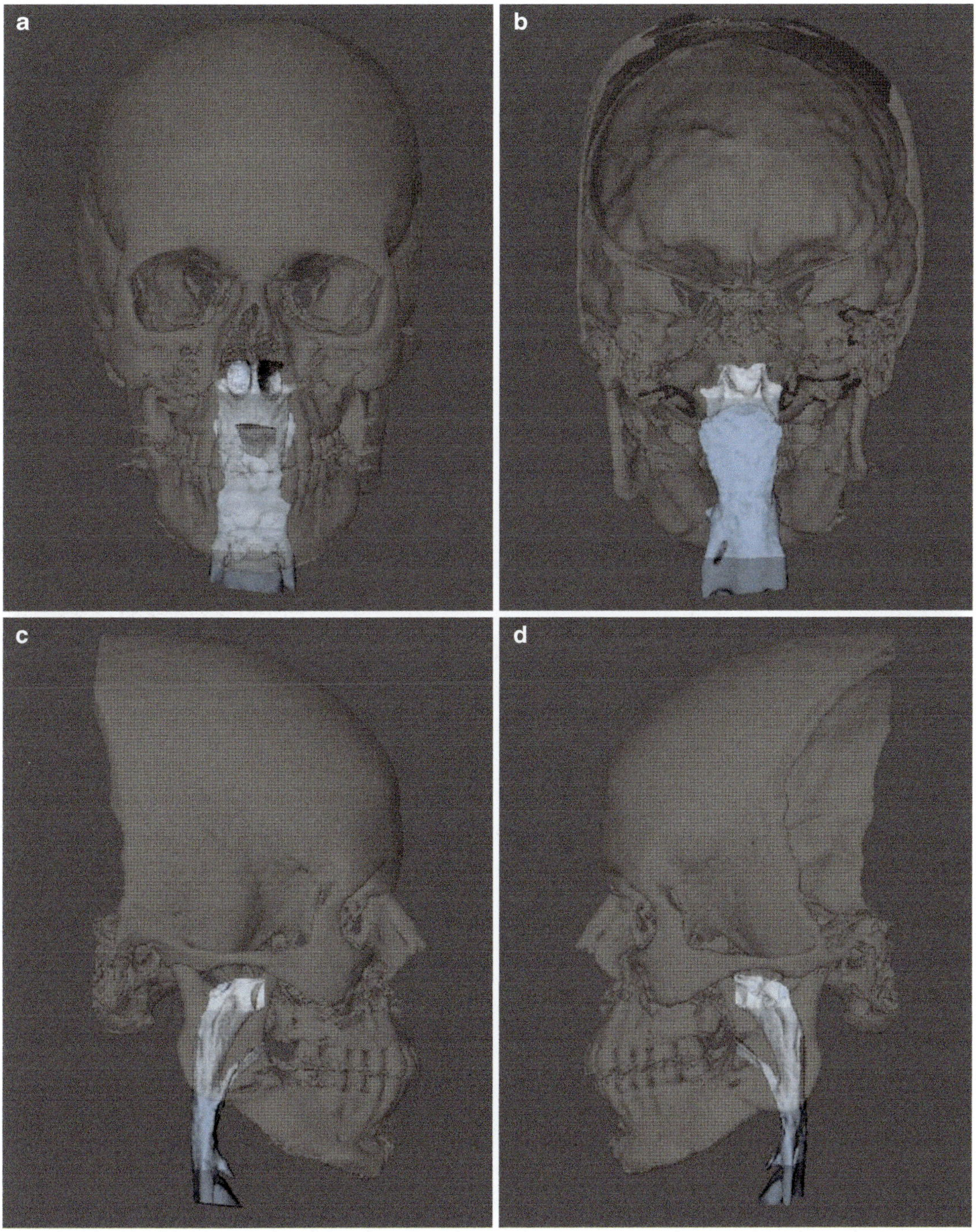

Fig. 5.9 Visualisation of the post-surgical 3D nasopharyngeal (2854,89 mm^3), the 3D oropharyngeal (14.434,38 mm^3) and 3D hypopharyngeal (3500,31 mm^3) subvolumes of the upper pharyngeal airway on semi-transparent "surface-rendered" hard tissue representations of the patient's head: (**a**) frontal view, (**b**) posterior view, (**c**) right profile view and (**d**) left profile view (i-CAT, Imaging Sciences International Inc, Maxilim v. 2.3.0.3) (patient V.E.W.) Note the major expansion of both the 3D oropharyngeal and hypopharyngeal subvolumes of the upper pharyngeal airway and the decrease of the nasopharyngeal airway due to maxillary impaction compared to the pre-operative upper pharyngeal airway volumes (Fig. 2.70)

5.1.3 TMJ

Finally, after standardised "step-by-step" systematic virtual evaluation of the patient's "dento-maxillo-facial" treatment outcome (▶ Sect. 5.1.1), the patient's post-surgical "upper airway" (▶ Sect. 5.1.2), the "3D Virtual Visualisation Paradigm" allows more enhanced post-surgical evaluation of the patient's TMJ in the "3D virtual scene".

The post-surgical "condyle-fossa units" (▶ see also Sect. 2.1.4) can be evaluated using a:

1. "Individual Condylar 2D Coordinate System" (◘ Figs. 5.10 and 5.11)
2. "Individual Condylar 3D Coordinate System" (◘ Figs. 5.12, 5.13, 5.14, and 5.15)

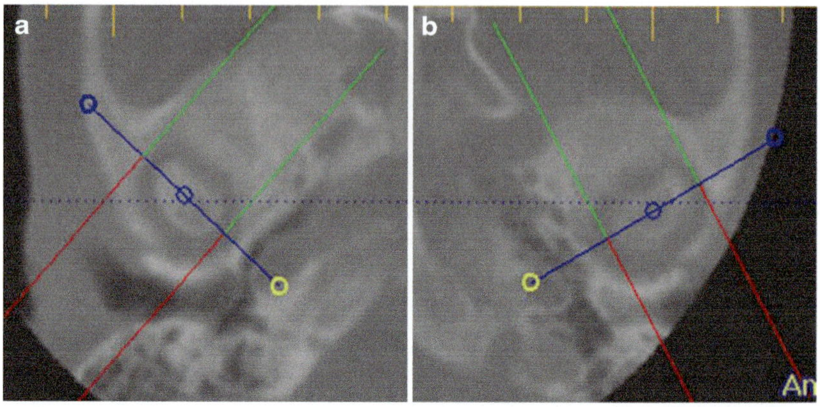

◘ **Fig. 5.10** One-year post-surgical axial views at the level of the right (**a**) and left (**b**) condyles demonstrating the individual set-up of a 2D coordinate system for generation of multiplanar coronal and sagittal slices, using the CBCT apparatus software (i-CAT, Imaging Sciences International Inc, i-CAT Vision™ software) (patient V.E.W.)

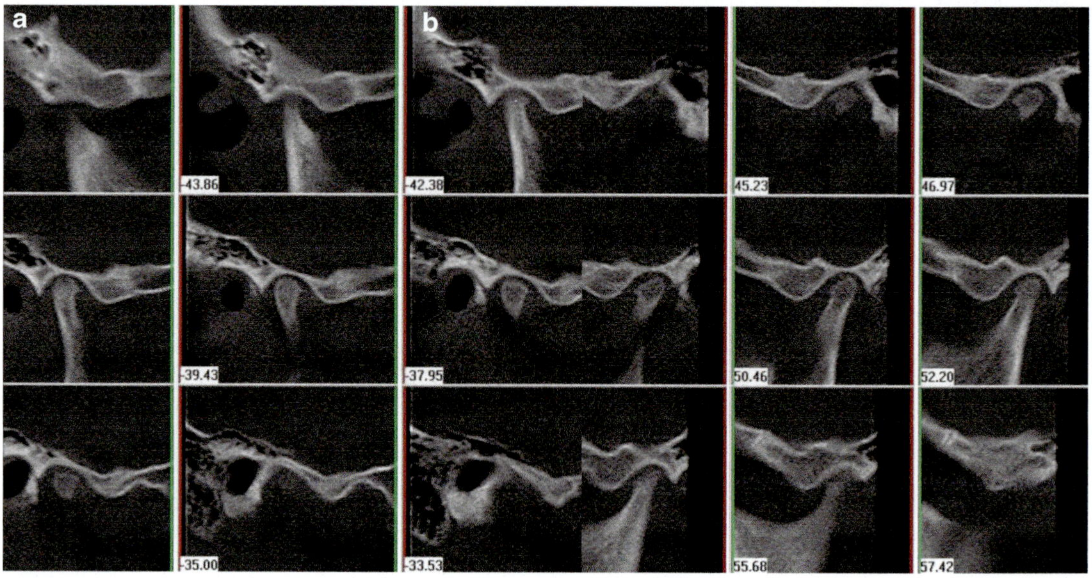

◘ **Fig. 5.11** One-year post-surgical multiple reconstructed sagittal views of the right (**a**) and left (**b**) condyle/fossa units using the CBCT apparatus software based on an "Individual Condylar 2D Coordinate System" (i-CAT, Imaging Sciences International Inc, i-CAT Vision™ software) (patient V.E.W.). Note that comparison with the pre-operative slices (◘ Fig. 2.72) does not show significant alterations of the TMJ

Systematic Virtual Treatment Outcome Evaluation: TMJ

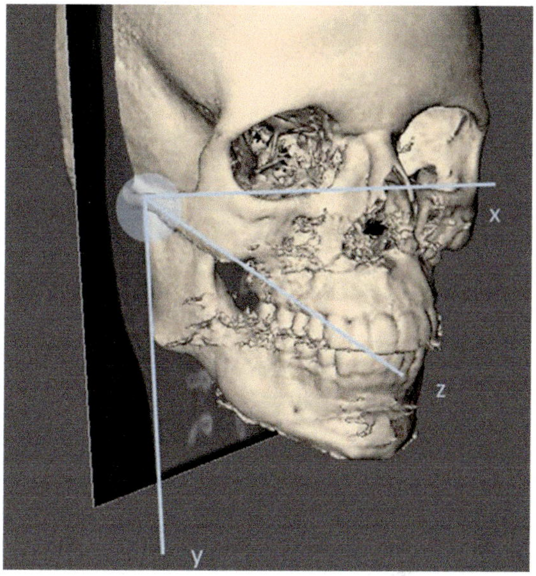

Fig. 5.12 One-year post-surgical "Individual Condylar 3D Coordinate System" based on the individual anatomy of the right "ramus-condyle-fossa unit" to generate multiplanar reslices that allow adequate and objective evaluation (i-CAT, Imaging Sciences International Inc, Maxilim v. 2.3.0.3) (patient V.E.W.)

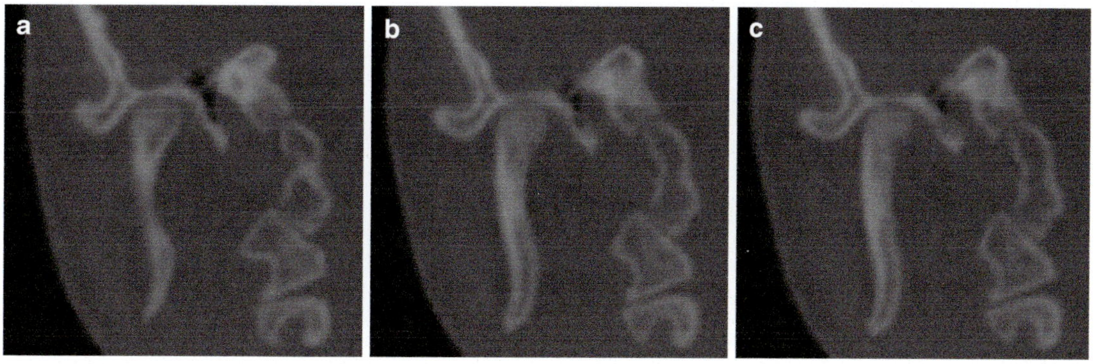

Fig. 5.13 One-year post-surgical coronal slices (a, b and c) of the right ramus-condyle-fossa unit generated from the "Individual Condylar 3D Coordinate System" (patient V.E.W., i-CAT, Imaging Sciences International Inc, Maxilim v. 2.3.0.3). Note that comparison with the pre-operative slices (Fig. 2.75) does not show significant alterations of the right ramus-condyle-fossa unit

Systematic Virtual Treatment Outcome Evaluation: TMJ

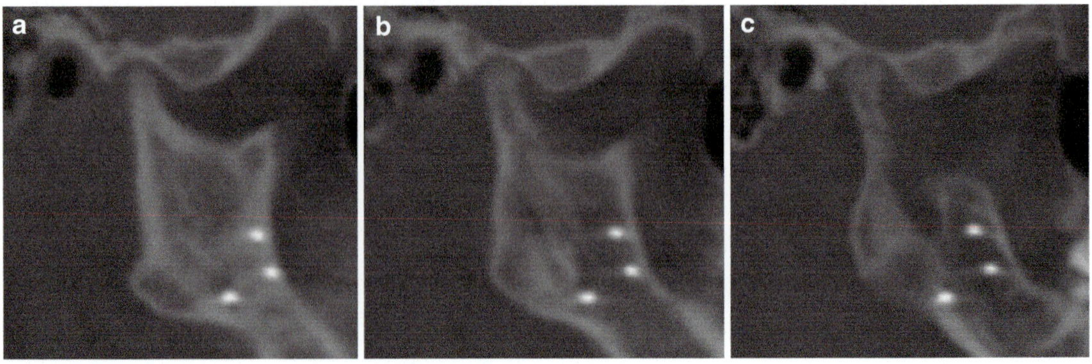

Fig. 5.14 One-year post-surgical sagittal slices (a, b and c) of the right ramus-condyle-fossa unit generated from the "Individual Condylar 3D Coordinate System" (patient V.E.W., i-CAT, Imaging Sciences International Inc, Maxilim v. 2.3.0.3). Note that comparison with the pre-operative slices (Fig. 2.76) does not show significant alterations of the right ramus-condyle-fossa unit

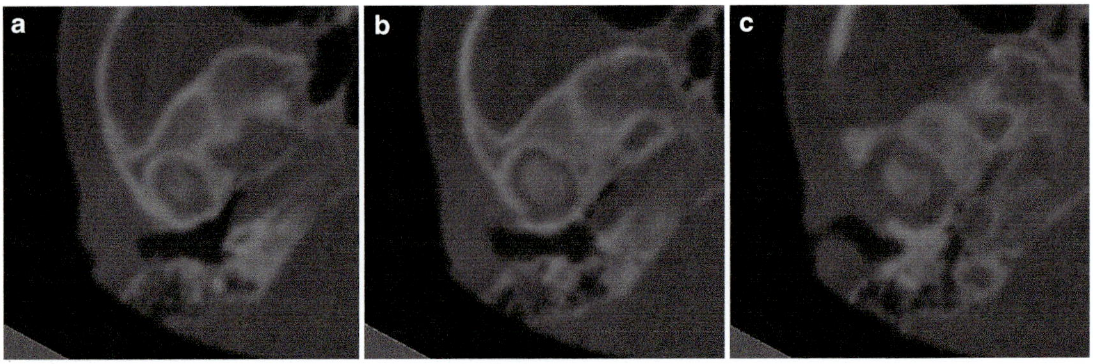

Fig. 5.15 One-year post-surgical axial slices (a, b and c) of the right ramus-condyle-fossa unit generated from the "Individual Condylar 3D Coordinate System" (patient V.E.W., i-CAT, Imaging Sciences International Inc, Maxilim v. 2.3.0.3). Note that comparison with the pre-operative slices (Fig. 2.77) does not show alterations of the right condyle

5.2 3D Cephalometric Analysis and 3D Virtual Superimposition

After systematic post-surgical virtual evaluation of the patient's dento-maxillo-facial treatment outcome, upper airway and TMJ (▶ Sect. 5.1), the "3D Virtual Visualisation Paradigm" offers the clinician (both orthodontists and surgeons) more objective analysing tools for standardised virtual evaluation of treatment outcome in the daily clinical routine:

1. 3D cephalometry of the patient's hard, soft tissues and teeth
2. Voxel-based superimposition

In this section, both "3D cephalometry of the patient's hard, soft tissues and teeth" (▶ Sect. 5.2.1) and "voxel-based superimposition" (▶ Sect. 5.2.2) are illustrated on Case 1 Patient (V.E.W.), which is used throughout this book (▶ Chaps. 1, 2, 3, 4 and 6).

5.2.1 3D Cephalometry of the Patient's Hard, Soft Tissues and Teeth

In 2005, Swennen, Schutyser and Hausamen made the bridge between conventional 2D and 3D cephalometric analysis by introducing an innovative "3D Virtual Scene Approach" towards 3D cephalometry. Moreover, the potential of 3D virtual superimposition on a 3D cephalometric reference system as a registration method was demonstrated. By superimposing cadaver skulls of a newborn, a 6-year-old child and an adult, some of the concepts of Enlow's counterpart theory on facial growth could be three-dimensionally visualised based on 3D virtual superimposition on a 3D cephalometric reference frame.

In 2006, Swennen et al., validated an "anatomic Cartesian 3D reference system" that proved to be accurate and reliable for 3D cephalometric hard and soft tissue analysis in the clinical routine.

In 2007, Swennen and Schutyser demonstrated the clinical application of "3D virtual superimposition on the anatomic Cartesian 3D cephalometric reference frame".

Towards 3D virtual evaluation of treatment outcome of orthognathic surgery, "3D cephalometry of the patient's hard, soft tissues and teeth" consists of:

1. "Generation of a 3D cephalometric reference frame". In case the "3D PHP cephalometric reference frame (▶ see Sect. 2.2.1)" is used, it is crucial that the scanned post-surgical head position of the patient is modified towards its individual PHP ("planning head position") prior to surgery. Using "voxel-based superimposition (▶ see Sect. 5.2.2)" on the cranial base, this can be accomplished in a fast and reliable way. The alternative is the use of an "anatomic Cartesian 3D reference system" for pre- and post-surgical 3D cephalometric analysis as introduced and validated by Swennen in 2005 and 2006, respectively.
2. "Step-by-step" 3D virtual definition of the hard tissue, teeth (▶ see Sect. 2.2.2) and soft tissue (▶ see Sect. 2.2.3) 3D cephalometric landmarks that were used for 3D virtual diagnosis of the orthognathic patient prior to surgery. (◘ Figs. 5.16, 5.17, 5.18, 5.19 and 5.20)
3. Automated set-up of 3D cephalometric planes and 3D cephalometric analysis of hard tissues, teeth (▶ see Sect. 2.2.2) and soft tissues (▶ see Sect. 2.2.3) used for 3D virtual diagnosis of the patient prior to surgery.

■ 3D Cephalometry of the Patient's Hard, Soft Tissues and Teeth: Outcome Analysis

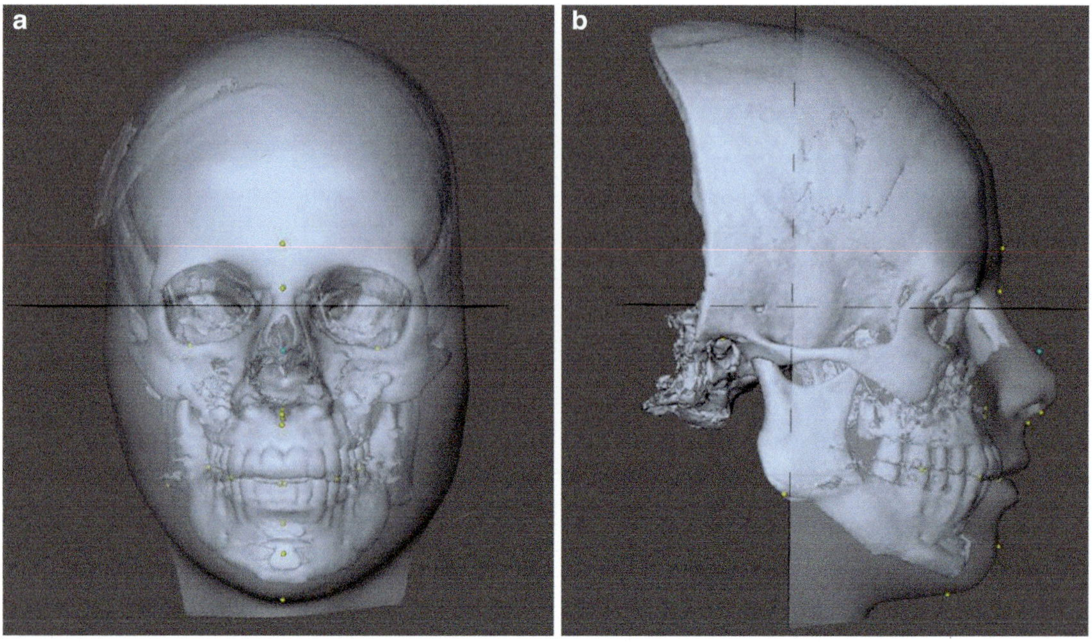

Fig. 5.16 One-year post-surgical frontal (**a**) and right profile (**b**) views. Set-up of 3D hard, soft tissue and teeth cephalometric landmarks of the "Bruges Target Facial Mask" 3D cephalometric analysis. 3D "surface-rendered" hard tissue representations with transparent soft tissues of the patient's head (i-CAT, Imaging Sciences International Inc, Maxilim v. 2.3.0.3, patient V.E.W.). Note pre-surgical views (Figs. 2.146, 2.147, 2.214 and 2.215)

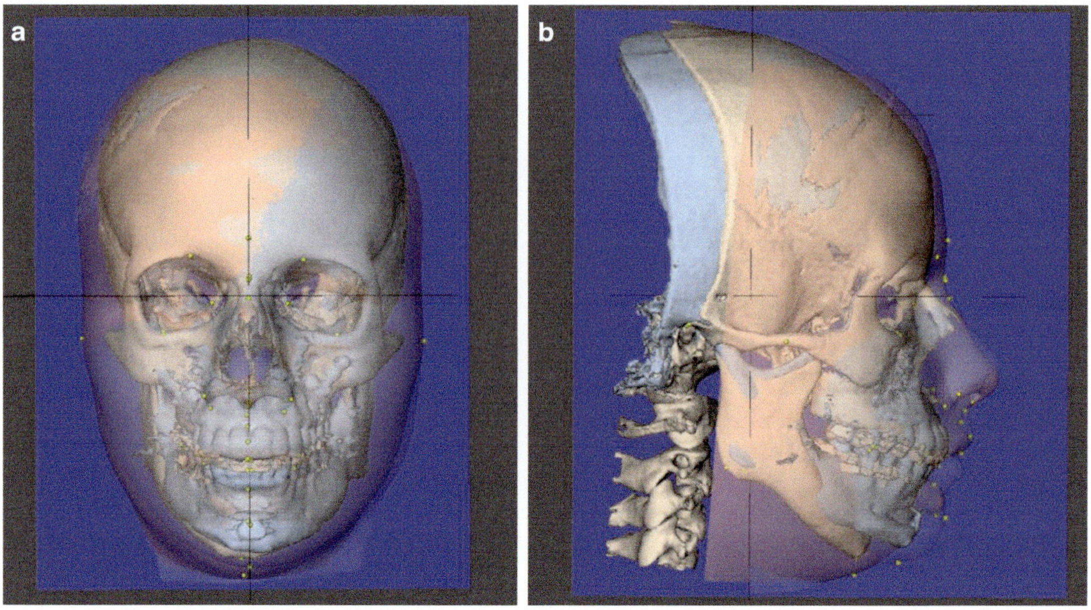

Fig. 5.17 Frontal (**a**) and right profile (**b**) pre-surgical and 1-year post-surgical 3D cephalometric analysis and 3D superimposition visualising the "3D PHP cephalometric reference frame" with set-up of 3D hard, soft tissue and teeth cephalometric landmarks of the "Bruges Target Facial Mask" and "Bruges 3D Soft Tissue" 3D cephalometric analyses. 3D "surface-rendered" hard tissue representations of the patient's head with transparent soft tissues (i-CAT, Imaging Sciences International Inc, Maxilim v. 2.3.0.3, patient V.E.W.). Note that the tip of the nose was out of the FOV during post-surgical CBCT scanning. Note pre-surgical views (Figs. 2.146, 2.147, 2.214 and 2.215)

3D Cephalometry of the Patient's Hard, Soft Tissues and Teeth: Outcome Analysis

3D cephalometry analysis (3D-VPS$_1$) report			
"Bruges Target Facial Mask" 3D cephalometric analysis			
Patient name: V.E.W.			
Physician name: GS			
Linear measurement analysis (mm)			
Morphological height of the face (n-gn)	113.3		
Height of the face (gl-gn)	129.1		
Morphological height of the midface (n-sn)	50.6		
Height of the midface (gl-sn)	64.2		
Overjet	2.6		
Overbite	1.0		
Angular measurement analysis (deg)			
Upper incisor inclination (Mx-Pl/Ulapex-UI)	111.5		
Lower incisor inclination (Md-Pl/Llapex-LI)	94.5		
Frontal inclination of the upper occlusal plane – x-Pl	0.0		
Frontal inclination of the lower occlusal plane – x-Pl	0.6		
Frontal inclination of the mandibular plane – x-Pl	1.5		
Lateral inclination of the upper occlusal plane – x-Pl	8.3		
Lateral inclination of the lower occlusal plane – x-Pl	5.9		
Lateral inclination of the mandibular plane – x-Pl	28.0		
Proportional measurement Analysis (%)			
Morphological height of the midface/morphological height of the face (n-sn × 100/n-gn)	44.6		
Height of the midface/height of the face (gl-sn × 100/gl-gn)	49.7		
Orthogonal measurement analysis (mm)	x-Pl	y-Pl	z-Pl
UI_r	63.5	76.8	0.02
UI_l	63.5	76.8	−0.02
UC_r	61.7	68.6	18.5
UC_l	62.3	70.2	−19.2
$UMcusp_r$	58.9	48.2	25.4
$UMcusp_l$	59.2	49.6	−26.7

x-Pl horizontal plane, *y-Pl* vertical plane, *z-Pl* median plane

3D Cephalometry of the Patient's Hard, Soft Tissues and Teeth: Outcome Analysis

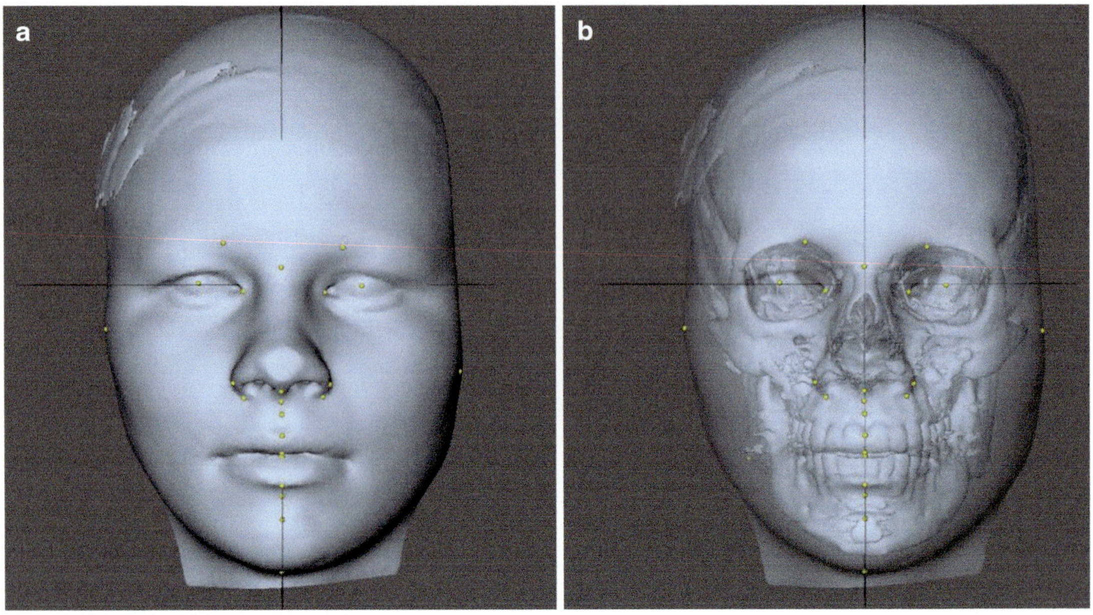

Fig. 5.18 One-year post-surgical frontal views. Set-up of 3D soft tissue cephalometric landmarks of the "Bruges 3D Soft Tissue" 3D cephalometric analysis. 3D "surface-rendered" soft tissue representations of the patient's head (**a**) with transparent soft tissues (**b**) (i-CAT, Imaging Sciences International Inc, Maxilim v. 2.3.0.3, patient V.E.W.). Note that parts of the 3D facial soft tissues (tip of the nose/left temporo-parietal region) were out of the FOV during post-surgical CBCT scanning. Note pre-surgical views (Figs. 2.146 and 2.214)

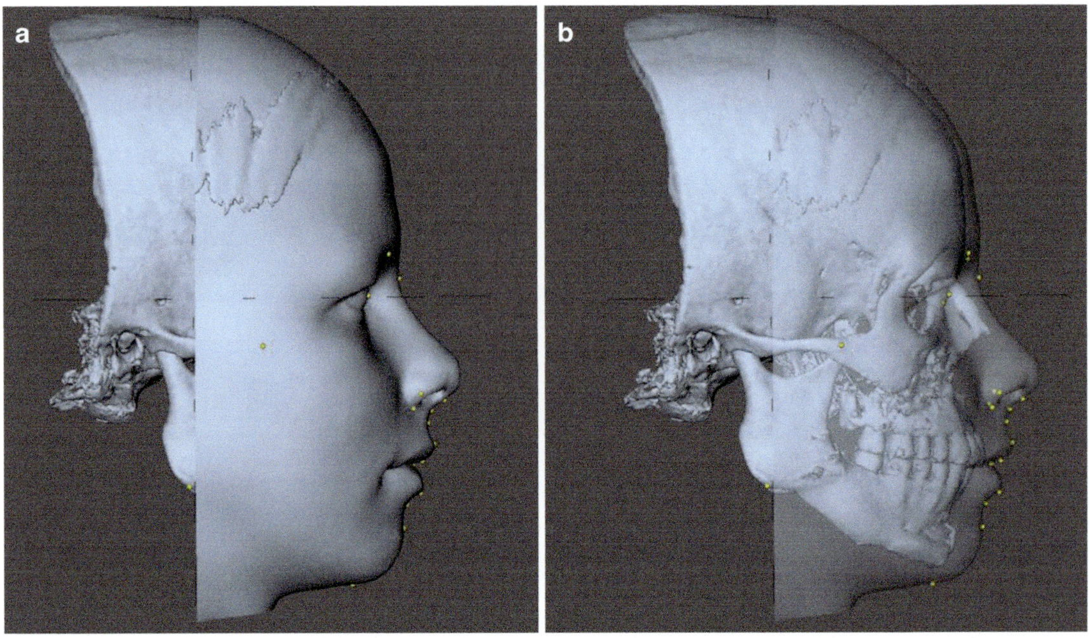

Fig. 5.19 One-year post-surgical right profile views. Set-up of 3D soft tissue cephalometric landmarks of the "Bruges 3D Soft Tissue" 3D cephalometric analysis. 3D "surface-rendered" soft tissue representations of the patient's head (**a**), with transparent soft tissues (**b**) (i-CAT, Imaging Sciences International Inc, Maxilim v. 2.3.0.3, patient V.E.W.). Note that the tip of the nose was out of the FOV during post-surgical CBCT scanning. Note pre-surgical views (Figs. 2.147 and 2.215)

3D Cephalometry of the Patient's Hard, Soft Tissues and Teeth: Outcome Analysis

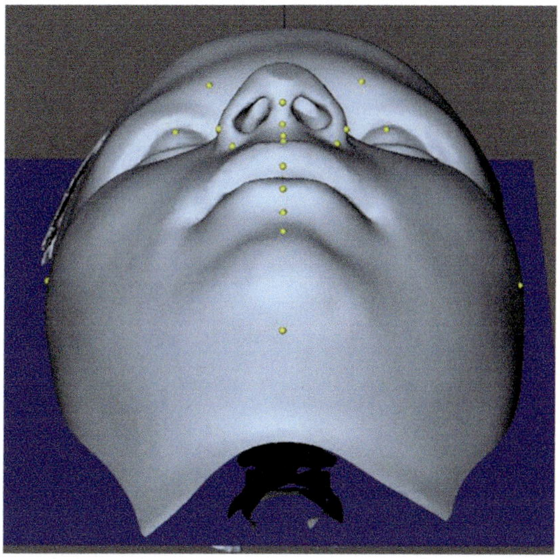

Fig. 5.20 One-year post-surgical base view. Set-up of 3D soft tissue cephalometric landmarks of the "Bruges 3D Soft Tissue" 3D cephalometric analysis. 3D "surface-rendered" soft tissue representation of the patient's head (i-CAT, Imaging Sciences International Inc, Maxilim v. 2.3.0.3, patient V.E.W.). Note that the tip of the nose was out of the FOV during post-surgical CBCT scanning. Note pre-surgical view Fig. 2.216

3D Cephalometry of the Patient's Hard, Soft Tissues and Teeth: Outcome Analysis

3D cephalometry analysis (3D-VPS$_2$) report	
"Bruges 3D soft tissue cephalometric analysis"	
Patient name: V.E.W.	
Physician name: GS	
Linear measurement analysis (mm)	
Height of the lower face (sn-gn)	64.3
Height of the face according to da Vinci (right) (os_r-gn)	122.3
Height of the face according to da Vinci (left) (os_l-gn)	120.6
Height of the skin portion of the upper lip (philtrum) (sn-ls)	12.5
Height of the upper lip (sn-sto_u)	18.9
Interlabial gap (ILG) (sto_{u-} sto_l)	1.4
Height of the mandible (sto_l-gn)	44.0
Interpupillary distance (IPD) (p_r-p_l)	60.1
Intercanthal width (en_r-en_l)	30.1
Upper face width (zy_r-zy_l) 135.5	
Morphological width of the nose according to Farkas (al_r-al_l)	35.0
Angular measurement analysis (deg)	
Nasolabial angle (c"-sn/ss-ls)	90.0
Mentolabial angle (li-sl-pg)	131.8
Proportional measurement analysis (%)	
Facial index (zy_r-zy_l) × 100/(sn-gn)	119.6
Bruges index (r) (p_r-p_l) × 100/(os_r-gn)	24.6
Bruges index (l) (p_r-p_l) × 100/(os_l-gn)	25.0
Height of the mandible/height of the lower face (sto_l-gn) × 100/(sn-gn)	68.4
Philtrum/height of the upper lip (sn-ls) × 100/(sn-sto_u)	65.9

5.2.2 Voxel-Based Superimposition

Objective and accurate 3D virtual evaluation of treatment outcome of orthognathic surgery is essential in a time of evidence-based medicine to improve care of the patient with maxillo-facial deformity.

Superimposition on 3D cone-beam CT models of orthognathic surgery patients has been pioneered by Cevidanes and co-workers (2005, 2006) who demonstrated its use and importance in bringing new insights towards mandibular changes after orthognathic surgery (2007), soft tissue changes (2010, 2011), evaluation of 3D virtual simulation (2010), mandibular and glenoid fossa changes (2012), temporomandibular joint (2014, 2015) and long-term outcomes of orthognathic surgery (2011, 2013a, b, c, 2015).

"3D Virtual Superimposition on an Anatomic Cartesian 3D Reference System (▶ Sect. 5.2.1)" remains from a technical point of view a smart application of "point-based rigid registration (▶ see Sect. 1.2.1)". The anatomic reference system is set up based on anatomical points and the translation and rotation between the pre- and post-surgical reference systems are computed in order to coincide them. With this type of registration, it is crucial that the points that define the reference system are indicated with the highest precision because it heavily influences the results of the 3D superimposition.

"Voxel-based superimposition" is a more preferred 3D virtual superimposition method since it is more accurate and less prone to observer error. It uses "voxel-based rigid registration (▶ see Sect. 1.2.1)" using the "Maximisation of Mutual Information (MI)" registration algorithm, developed by Maes and co-workers (1997) which has been shown to be very accurate and stable for registration of skull structures. Based on a subvolume (e.g. anterior cranial base, cranial base and cranial bones) that has not changed during orthognathic surgery, all image information within these subvolumes is used to automatically register the pre- and post-surgical volumes of the patient's head after a rough manual initialisation.

> Voxel-based superimposition provides objective and accurate 3D virtual evaluation of treatment outcome after orthognathic and orthofacial surgery.

■ Voxel-Based Superimposition on the Volume of Interest (VOI)

"Step-by-step" semi-automated "voxel-based superimposition" consists of the following five consecutive steps:

1. Definition of the pre-surgical "volume of interest (VOI)" (◘ Fig. 5.21)
2. Definition of the post-surgical "volume of interest (VOI)" (◘ Fig. 5.22)
3. Manual rough 3D alignment (◘ Fig. 5.23)
4. Automated "voxel-based" alignment (◘ Fig. 5.24)
5. Check final 3D alignment (◘ Fig. 5.25)

In this section, "voxel-based superimposition" is illustrated on Case 1 Patient (V.E.W.), in which a subvolume of the skull, the cranial base and the cranial bones was used "volume of interest (VOI)" for 3D alignment of the pre- and post-surgical hard tissue surface representations of the patient's head. (◘ Figs. 5.26, 5.27, 5.28, 5.29, 5.30, 5.31, 5.32 and 5.33)

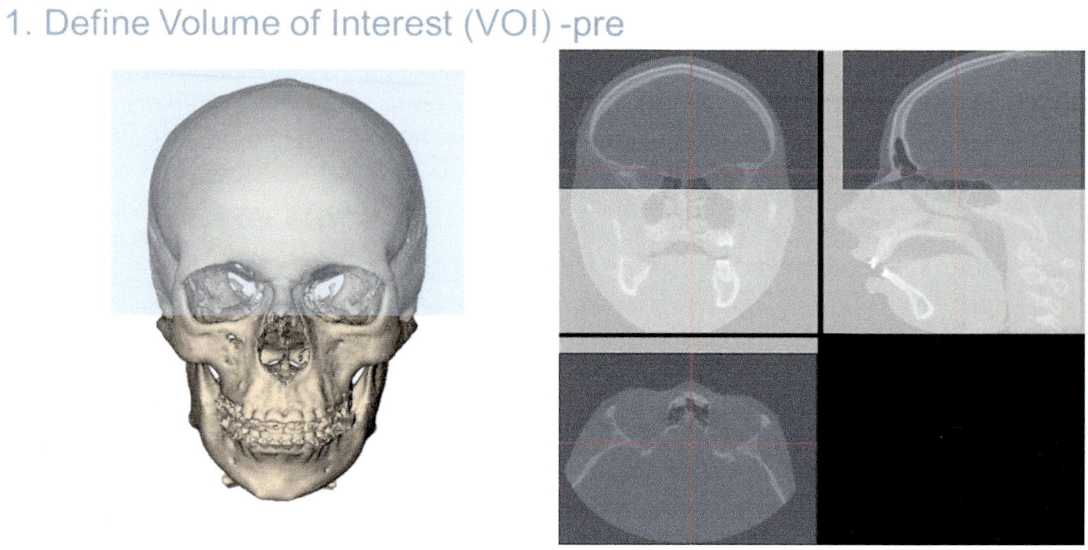

◘ **Fig. 5.21** "Step 1" of semi-automated voxel-based superimposition. The "volume of interest (*VOI*) (cranial base and cranial bones, marked *blue*)" is defined on the coronal, sagittal and axial slices of the "pre-surgical" DICOM dataset and visualised on the 3D "surface-rendered" hard tissue representation (i-CAT, Imaging Sciences International Inc, Maxilim v. 2.3.0.3) (patient V.E.W.)

Voxel-Based Superimposition on the Volume of Interest (VOI)

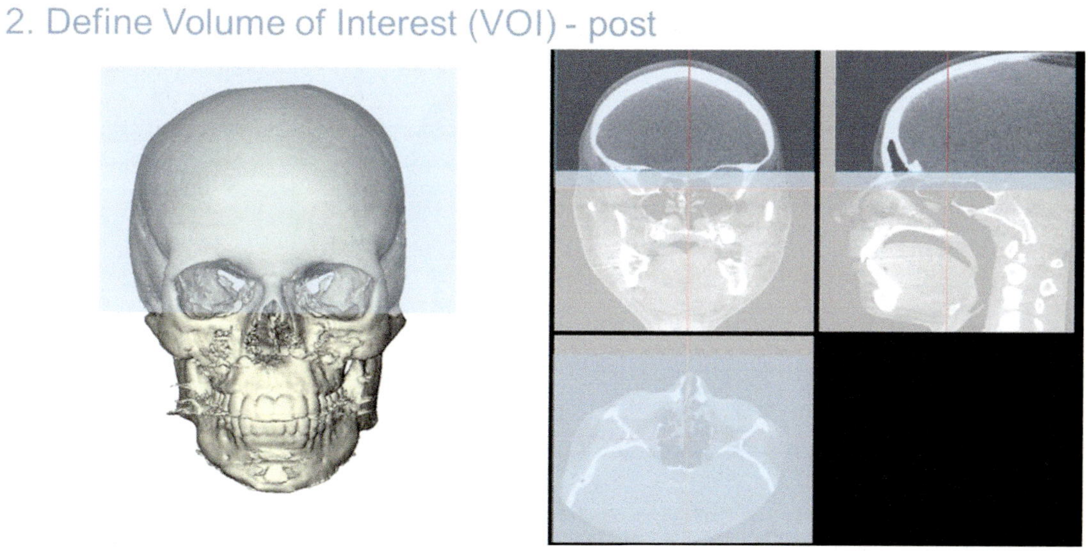

Fig. 5.22 "Step 2" of semi-automated voxel-based superimposition. The "volume of interest (*VOI*) (cranial base and cranial bones, marked *blue*)" is defined on the coronal, sagittal and axial slices of the "post-surgical" DICOM dataset and visualised on the 3D "surface-rendered" hard tissue representation (i-CAT, Imaging Sciences International Inc, Maxilim v. 2.3.0.3) (patient V.E.W.)

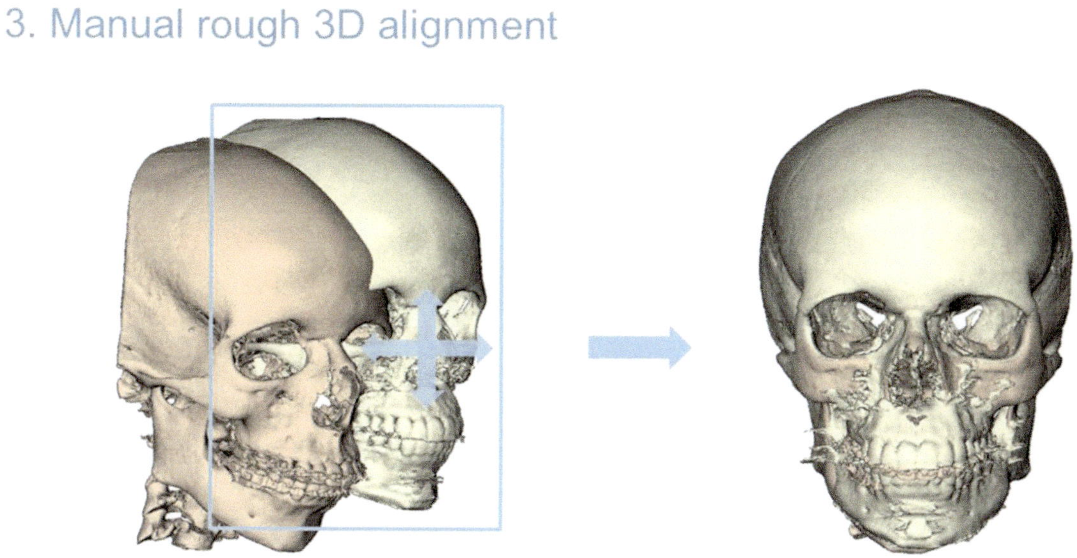

Fig. 5.23 "Step 3" of semi-automated voxel-based superimposition. Manual rough 3D alignment of the pre- and post-surgical 3D "surface-rendered" hard tissue representations of the patient's head (i-CAT, Imaging Sciences International Inc, Maxilim v. 2.3.0.3) (patient V.E.W.)

Voxel-Based Superimposition on the Volume of Interest (VOI)

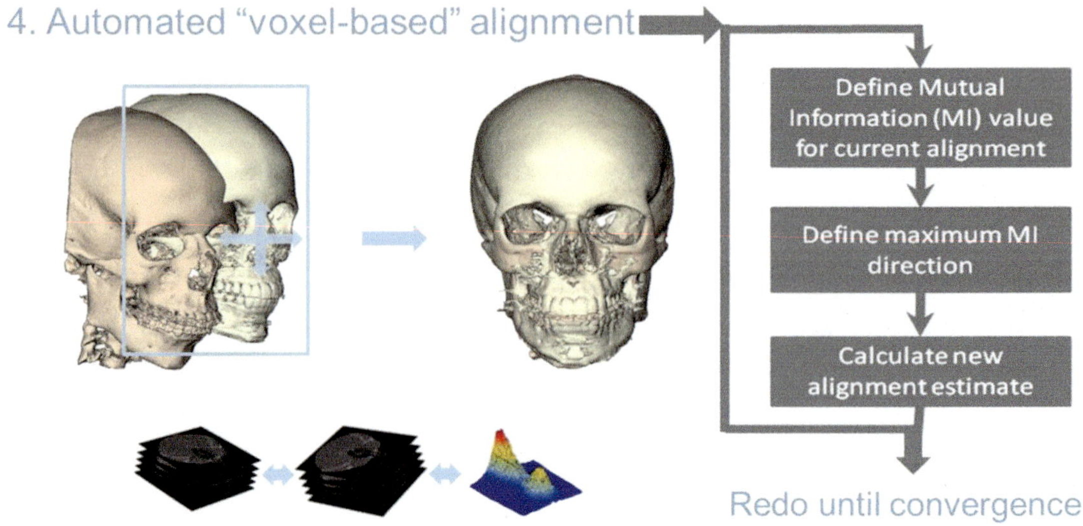

Fig. 5.24 "Step 4" of semi-automated voxel-based superimposition. Automated 3D alignment of the pre- and post-surgical 3D "surface-rendered" hard tissue representations of the patient's head, using voxel-based registration (based on the MI algorithm) of the pre- and post-surgical "volume of interests (*VOI's*)" (i-CAT, Imaging Sciences International Inc, Maxilim v. 2.3.0.3) (patient V.E.W.)

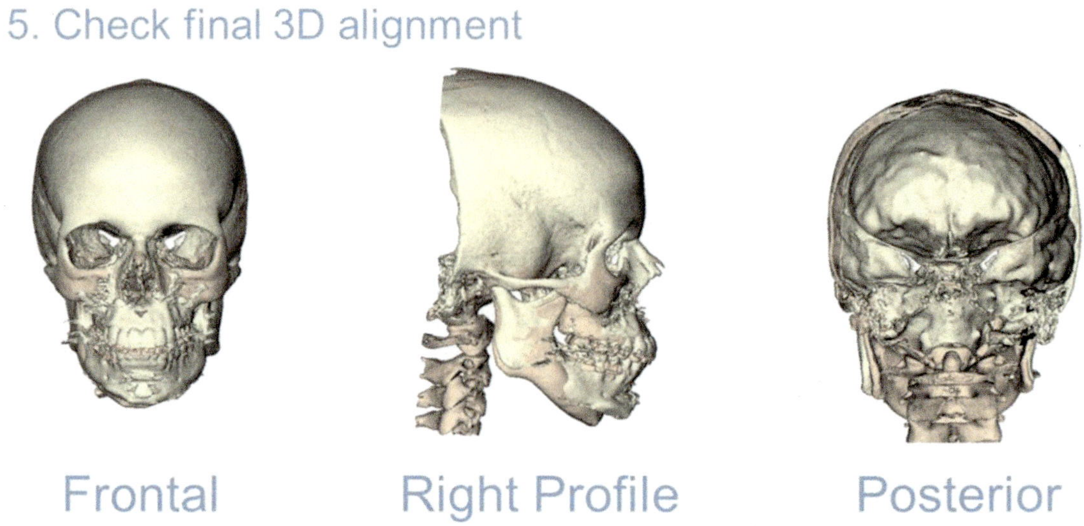

Fig. 5.25 "Step 5" of semi-automated voxel-based superimposition. Check of the final alignment by the clinician after automated voxel-based registration of the pre- and post-surgical 3D "surface-rendered" hard tissue representations of the patient's head (i-CAT, Imaging Sciences International Inc, Maxilim v. 2.3.0.3) (patient V.E.W.)

Voxel-Based Superimposition on the Cranial Base: Dento-maxillo-facial Outcome

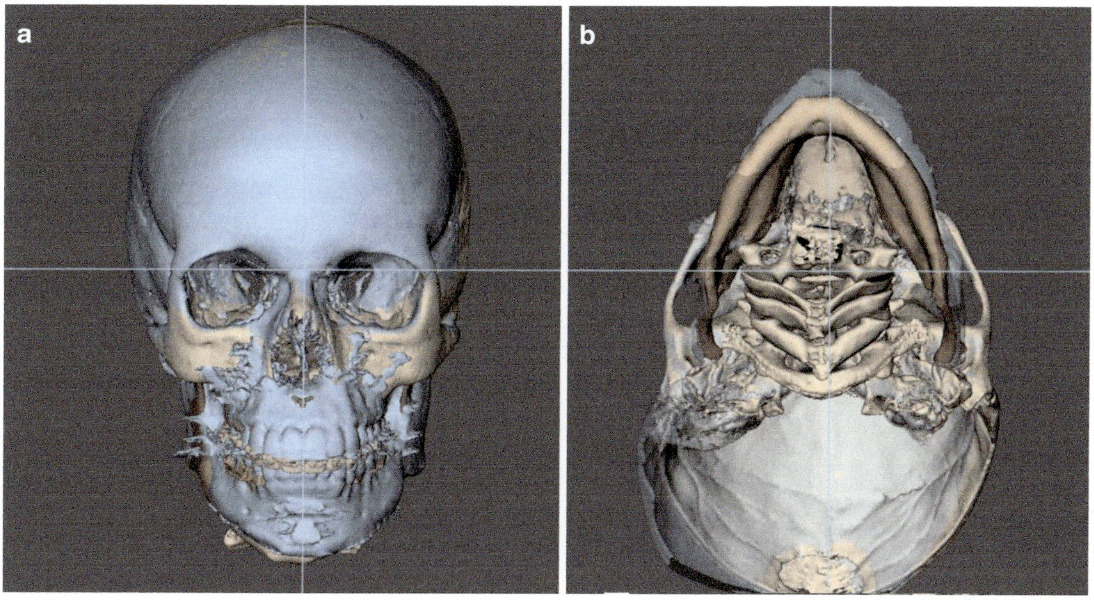

Fig. 5.26 Voxel-based superimposition on the cranial base of the pre-surgical and 1-year post-surgical 3D "surface-rendered" hard tissue representations of the patient's head. Frontal (**a**) and base (**b**) views (i-CAT, Imaging Sciences International Inc, Maxilim v. 2.3.0.3) (patient V.E.W.). Note the maxillary impaction, correction of the chin deviation and mandibular border asymmetry

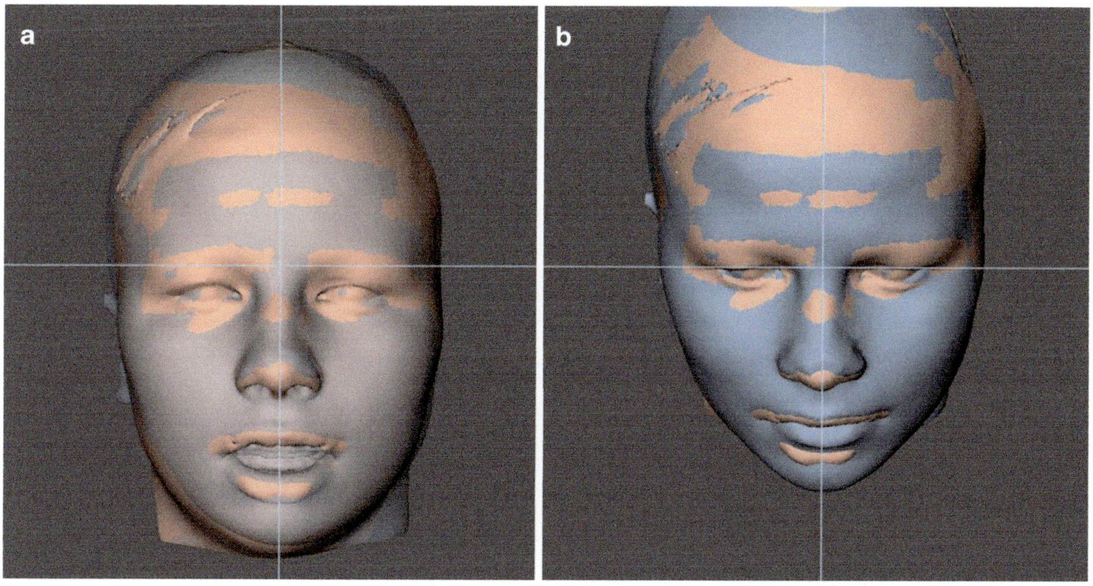

Fig. 5.27 Voxel-based superimposition on the cranial base of the pre-surgical and 1-year post-surgical 3D "surface-rendered" soft tissue representations. Frontal (**a**) and downward inclined (**b**) views (i-CAT, Imaging Sciences International Inc, Maxilim v. 2.3.0.3) (patient V.E.W.). Note the post-surgical (*blue*) facial symmetry and harmony

Voxel-Based Superimposition on the Cranial Base: Dento-maxillo-facial Outcome

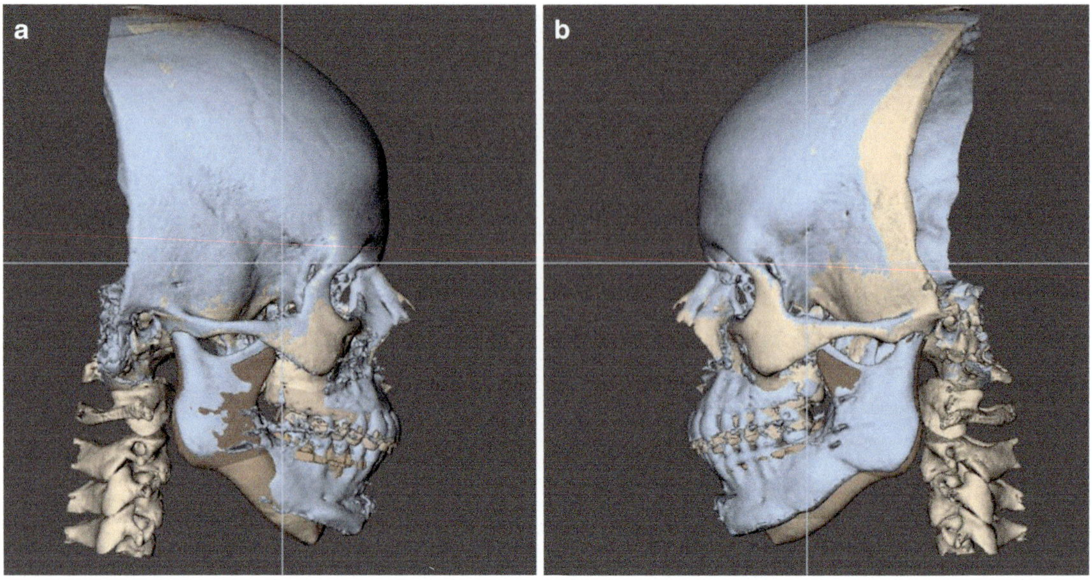

Fig. 5.28 Voxel-based superimposition on the cranial base of the pre-surgical and 1-year post-surgical 3D "surface-rendered" hard tissue representations. Right (**a**) and left (**b**) profile views (i-CAT, Imaging Sciences International Inc, Maxilim v. 2.3.0.3) (patient V.E.W.). Note the CCW rotation of the bimaxillary complex with maxillary impaction. Also note that a CCW rotation of both proximal fragments took place

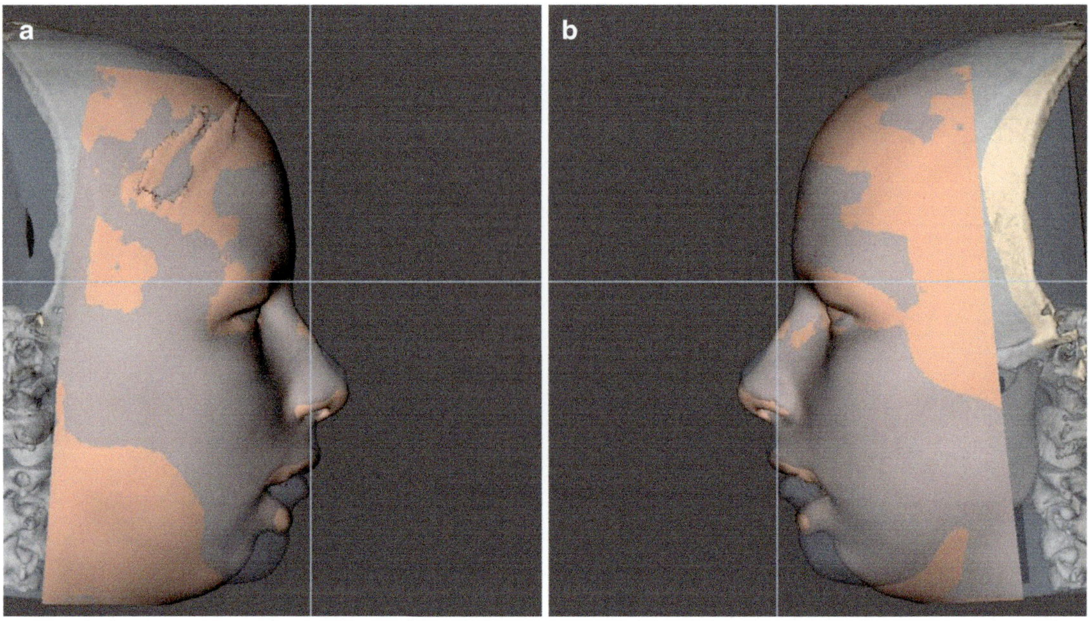

Fig. 5.29 Voxel-based superimposition on the cranial base of the pre-surgical and 1-year post-surgical 3D "surface-rendered" soft tissue representations. Right (**a**) and left (**b**) profile views (i-CAT, Imaging Sciences International Inc, Maxilim v. 2.3.0.3) (patient V.E.W.). Note especially the changes at the nasolabial aesthetic unit with nasal dorsum correction and post-surgical lip competence, besides the CCW "Pitch" profile changes

Voxel-Based Superimposition on the Cranial Base: Dento-maxillo-facial Outcome

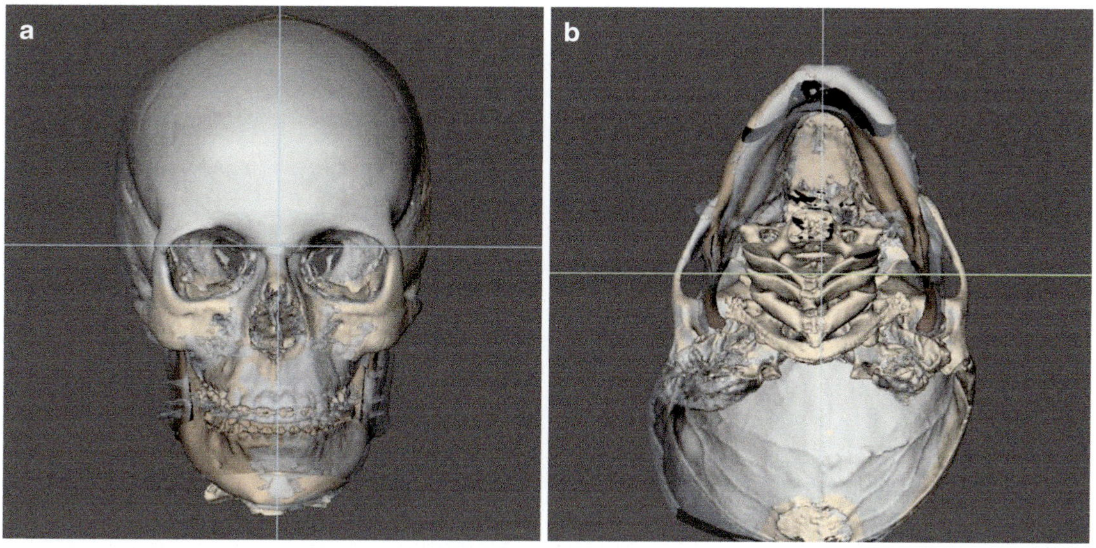

Fig. 5.30 Voxel-based superimposition on the cranial base of the 3D virtual planning and 1-year post-surgical 3D "surface-rendered" hard tissue representations. Frontal (**a**) and base (**b**) views (i-CAT, Imaging Sciences International Inc, Maxilim v. 2.3.0.3) (patient V.E.W.). Note the accurate midline correction of the chin. Also note the CCW "Roll" and "Yaw" movement of the left proximal fragment

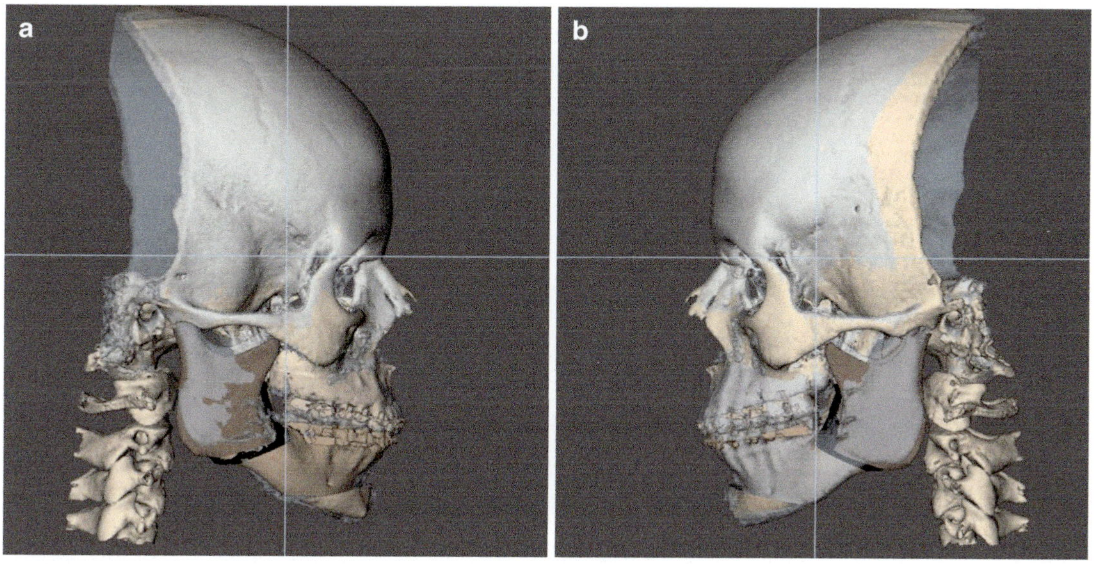

Fig. 5.31 Voxel-based superimposition on the cranial base of the 3D virtual planning and 1-year post-surgical 3D "surface-rendered" hard tissue representations. Right (**a**) and left (**b**) profile views (i-CAT, Imaging Sciences International Inc, Maxilim v. 2.3.0.3) (patient V.E.W.). Note the accurate maxillary repositioning. Also note that a CCW rotation of both proximal fragments took place. Towards the chin note the accurate sagittal repositioning with CCW "Pitch" rotation. Note that less anterior chin impaction was performed compared to the 3D virtual planning which remains a clinical decision on the operation table

■ Voxel-Based Superimposition on the Cranial Base: Upper Airway Outcome

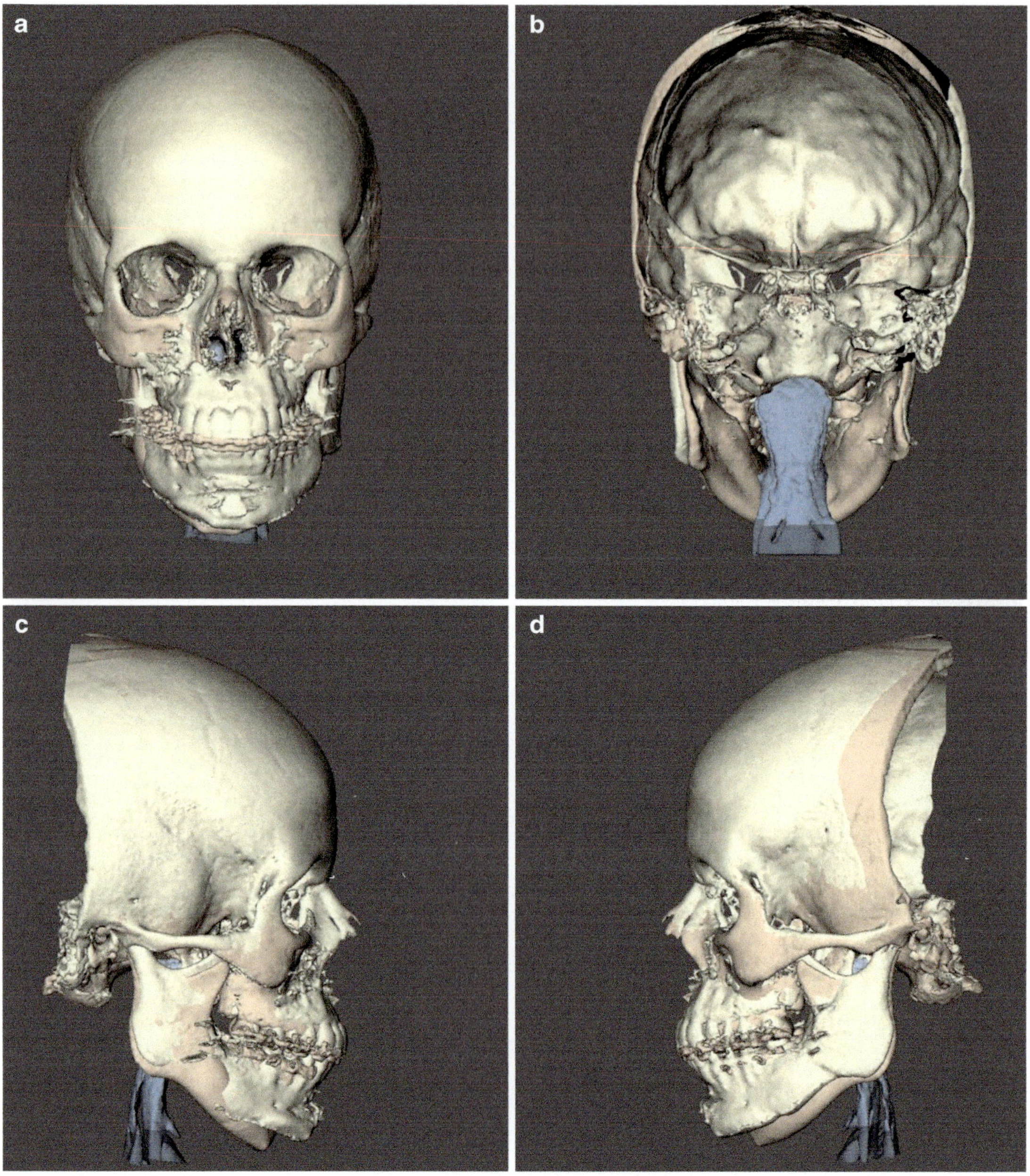

Fig. 5.32 Voxel-based superimposition on the cranial base of the pre-surgical and 1-year post-surgical 3D "surface-rendered" hard tissue representations visualising the 3D nasopharyngeal, the 3D oropharyngeal and 3D hypopharyngeal subvolumes of the upper pharyngeal airway. Frontal (**a**), posterior (**b**), left (**c**) and right profile (**d**) views (i-CAT, Imaging Sciences International Inc, Maxilim v. 2.3.0.3) (patient V.E.W.). Note the important volume expansion of both the 3D oropharyngeal and hypopharyngeal subvolumes and the overall post-surgical CCW "Pitch" rotation (**c–d**) of the upper pharyngeal airway

Voxel-Based Superimposition on the Cranial Base: Upper Airway Outcome

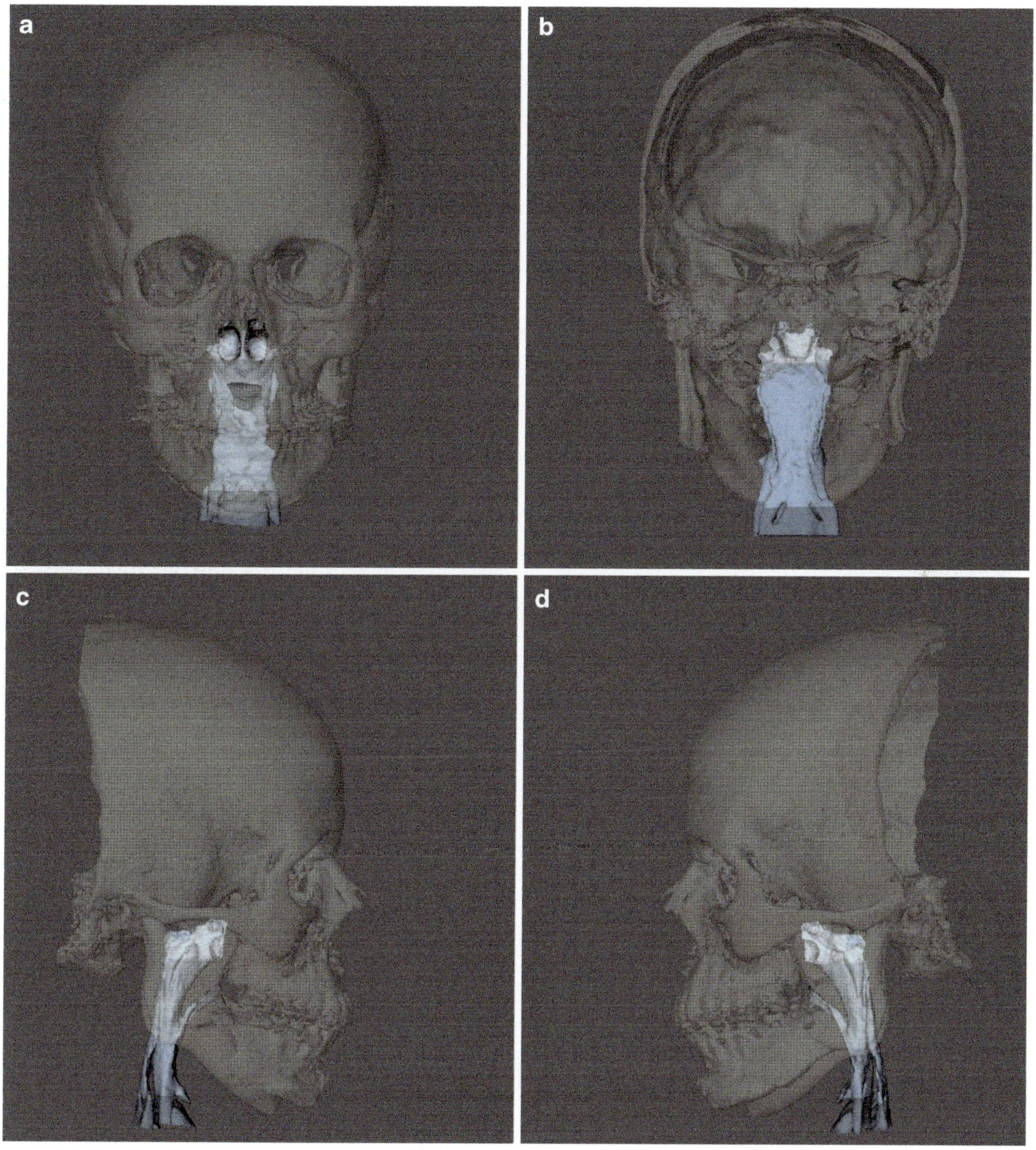

Fig. 5.33 Voxel-based superimposition on the cranial base of the pre-surgical and 1-year post-surgical 3D semi-transparent "surface-rendered" hard tissue representations visualising the 3D nasopharyngeal, the 3D oropharyngeal and 3D hypopharyngeal subvolumes of the upper pharyngeal airway. Frontal (**a**), posterior (**b**), left (**c**) and right profile (**d**) views (i-CAT, Imaging Sciences International Inc, Maxilim v. 2.3.0.3) (patient V.E.W.). Note the important volume expansion of both the 3D oropharyngeal and hypopharyngeal subvolumes and the overall post-surgical CCW "Pitch" rotation (**c–d**) of the upper pharyngeal airway

5.3 The Potential of Colour Distance Maps in Enhanced Treatment Outcome Evaluation

Towards more enhanced 3D virtual evaluation of treatment outcome of orthognathic surgery, the "3D Virtual Visualisation Paradigm" allows to visualise and to quantify differences between "rigid registered" surfaces of the patient's head by means of:

1. "Colour distance maps" between "surface-rendered" representations
2. "Calculation of the inter-surface distances" using the iterative closest point (ICP) technique to measure the root mean square (RMS) distance between "surface-rendered" representations

The pioneering work on this research has been done by Cevidanes and co-workers. In 2005, Cevidanes et al. used CBCT cranial base superimposition with a colour-coded method to display condylar changes and remodelling after orthognathic surgery and expected that this method could be used as a predictor for long-term condylar changes and adaptation.

"Colour distance maps" with subsequent "calculation of the inter-surface distances "can actually be computed based on:

1. Cone-beam CT (CBCT) data (► Sect. 5.3.1)
2. 3D photographs (► Sect. 5.3.2)

5.3.1 The Use of Colour Distance Maps Based on CBCT

"Colour distance maps based on CBCT" and "calculation of the inter-surface distances" after rigid registration can be used for evaluation of:

1. Pre-surgical towards post-surgical skeletal and dental 3D changes (◘ Figs. 5.34 and 5.35)
2. Pre-surgical towards post-surgical facial soft tissue 3D changes (◘ Fig. 5.36)
3. Accuracy of 3D virtual treatment planning (e.g. 3D maxillary repositioning, (◘ Fig. 5.37).

In this section, the use of "colour distance maps" based on CBCT is illustrated on Case 1 Patient (V.E.W.), which is used throughout this book (► Chaps. 1, 2, 3, 4 and 6).

■ 3D Virtual Voxel-Based Superimposition of CBCTs: Colour Distance Maps

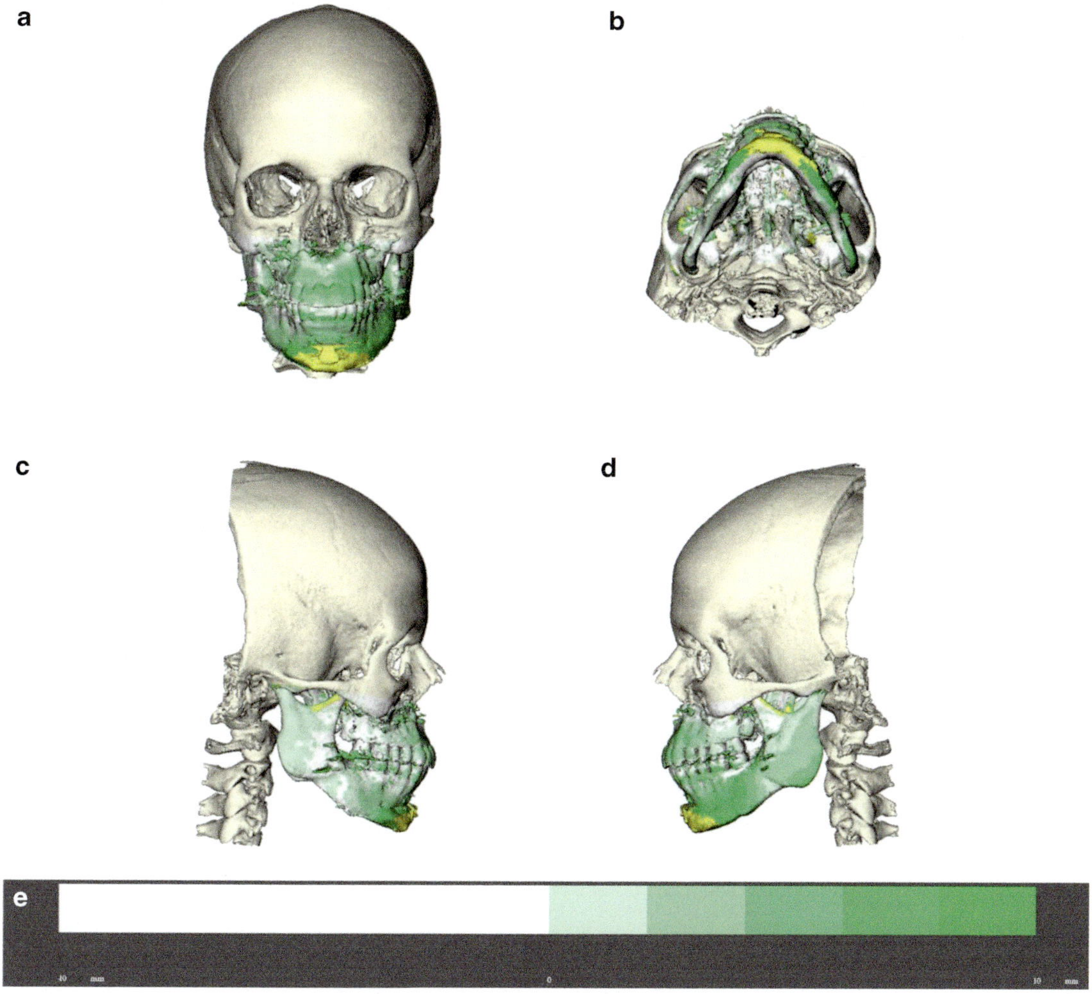

Fig. 5.34 Colour surface distance maps visualising the inter-surface distance between the "pre-surgical" and "1-year post-surgical" "surface-rendered" hard tissue representations of the patient's head after voxel-based superimposition on the cranial base and cranial bones, only showing the "post-operative" bimaxillary complex. Frontal (**a**), base (**b**), right (**c**) and left (**d**) profile views. (i-CAT, Imaging Sciences International Inc, Maxilim v. 2.3.0.3, patient V.E.W.). Note the applied colour scale (**e**). The yellow colour implies an inter-surface distance of more than 10 mm

3D Virtual Voxel-Based Superimposition of CBCTs: Colour Distance Maps

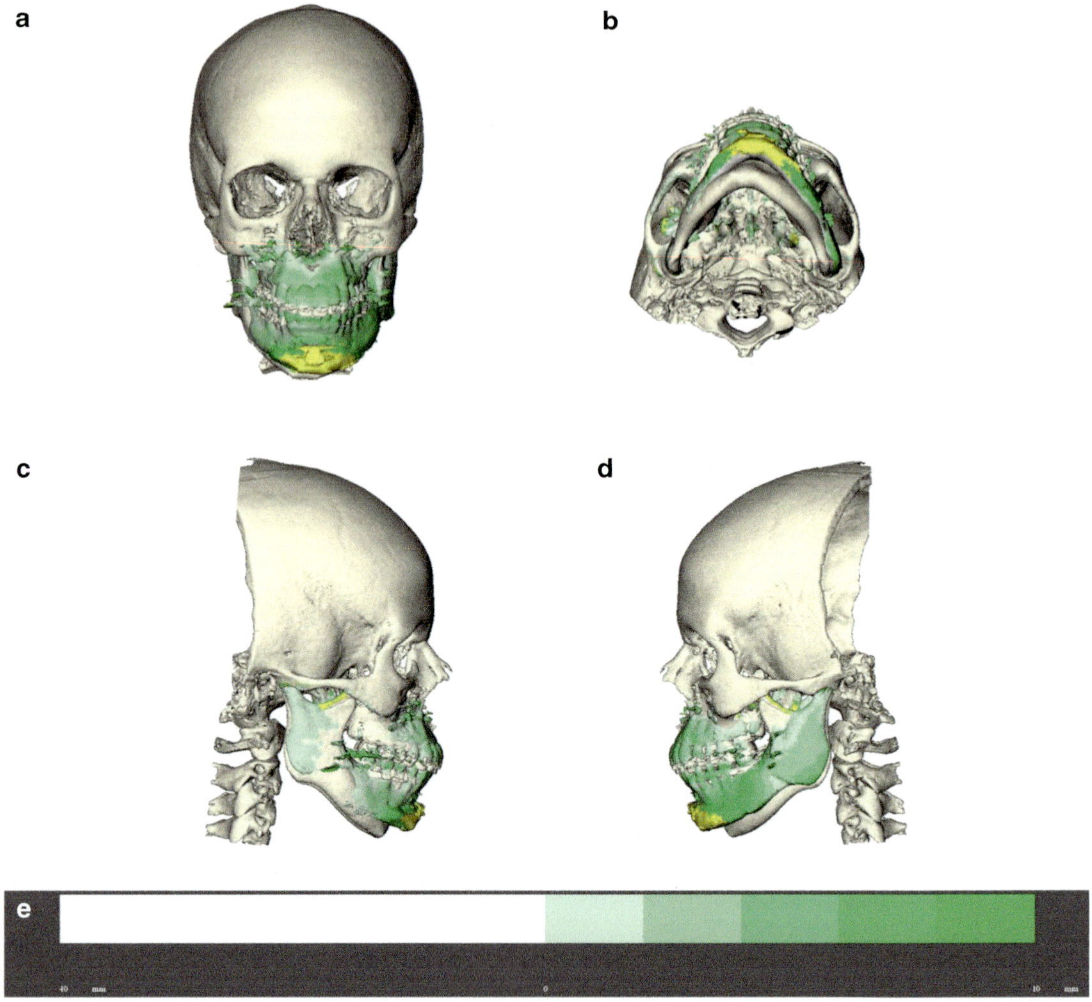

Fig. 5.35 Colour surface distance maps visualising the inter-surface distance between the "pre-surgical" and "1-year post-surgical" "surface-rendered" hard tissue representations of the patient's head after voxel-based superimposition on the cranial base and cranial bones with the "pre-surgical" bimaxillary complex visualised. Frontal (**a**), base (**b**), right (**c**) and left (**d**) profile views. (i-CAT, Imaging Sciences International Inc, Maxilim v. 2.3.0.3, patient V.E.W.). Note the applied colour scale (**e**). The *yellow* colour implies an inter-surface distance of more than 10 mm

3D Virtual Voxel-Based Superimposition of CBCTs: Colour Distance Maps

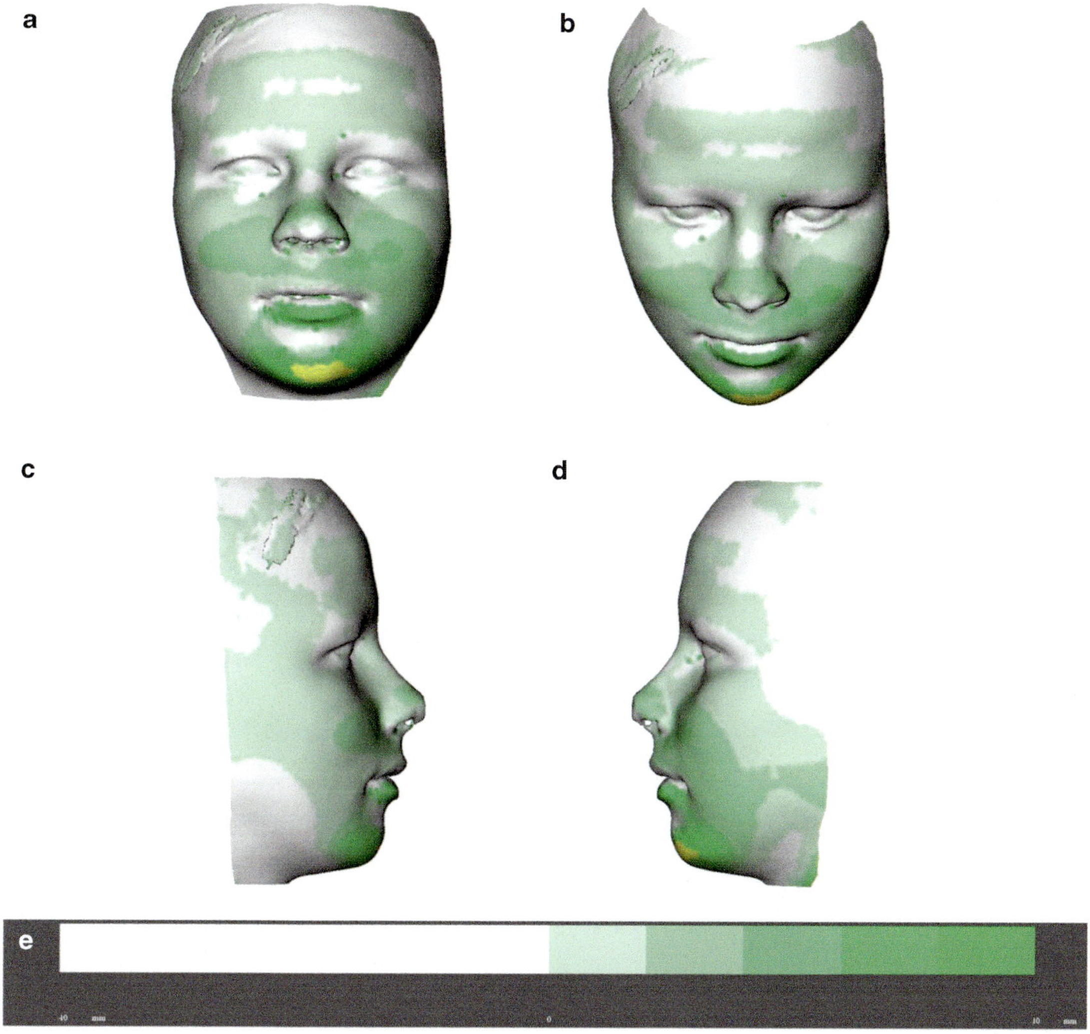

Fig. 5.36 Colour surface distance maps visualising the inter-surface distance between the "pre-surgical" and "1-year post-surgical" "surface-rendered" soft tissue representations of the patient's head after voxel-based superimposition on the cranial base and cranial bones. Frontal (**a**), frontal downward inclined (**b**), right (**c**) and left (**d**) profile views. (i-CAT, Imaging Sciences International Inc, Maxilim v. 2.3.0.3, patient V.E.W.). Note the applied colour scale (**e**). The *yellow* colour implies an inter-surface distance of more than 10 mm

Accuracy of 3D Maxillary Repositioning: Colour Distance Maps

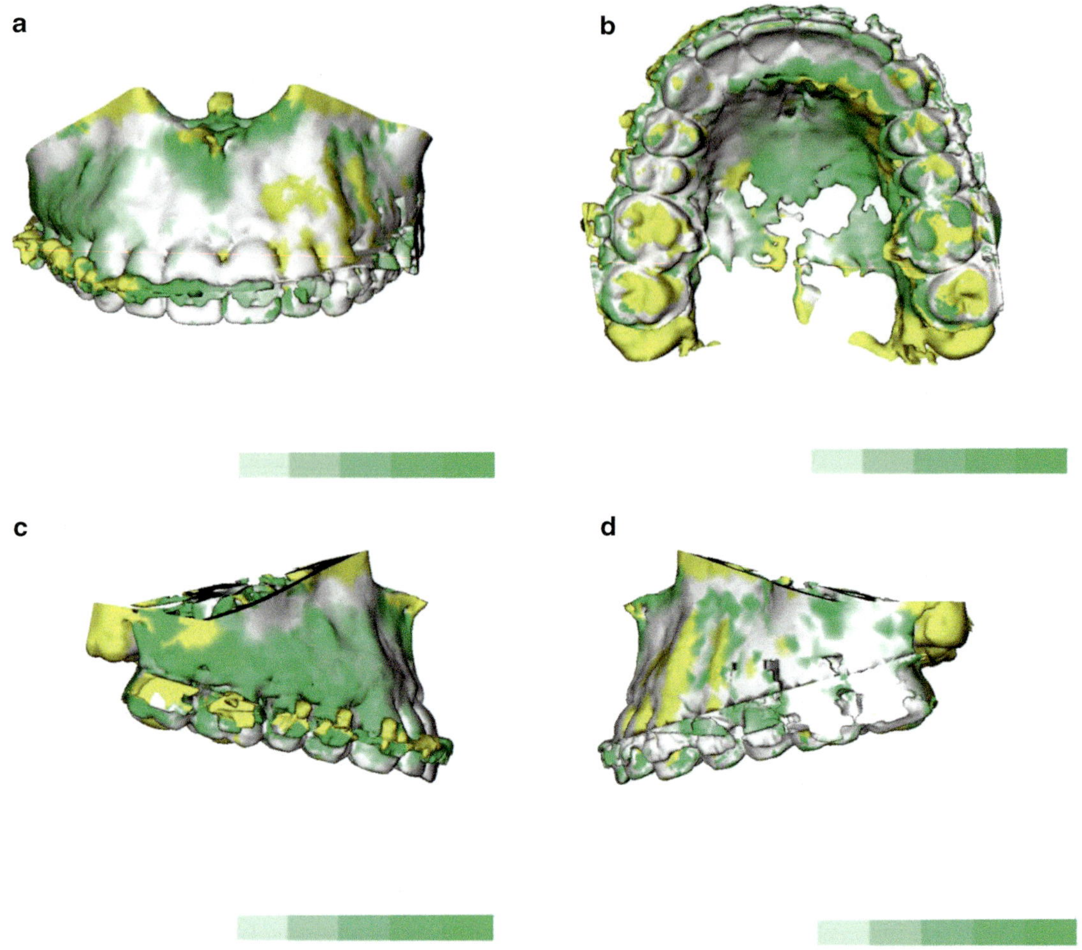

Fig. 5.37 Colour surface distance maps visualising the inter-surface distance between the "1-year post-surgical maxillary position" and the "3D virtual planned maxillary repositioning" after voxel-based superimposition. Frontal (**a**), base (**b**), right (**c**) and left (**d**) profile views of the "surface-rendered" hard tissue representations of the maxilla (i-CAT, Imaging Sciences International Inc, Maxilim v. 2.3.0.3, patient V.E.W.). The *yellow* colour implies an inter-surface distance of more than 1 mm. The root mean standard deviation (RMSD) of the maxillary virtual planning transfer was 0.48 mm for the combined "x", "y" and "z" axis values. Note that the vomer and anterior nasal spine partially colour *yellow* since these were partially removed during surgery. The same for the braces that were removed. Since the upper wisdom teeth are more erupted prior to surgery, these also colour *yellow*. Since the outline of the virtual maxillary osteotomy could not be identically reproduced on the 1-year post-surgical hard tissue representation of the maxilla, the upper border also partially colours *yellow*

5.3.2 The Use of Colour Distance Maps Based on 3D Photographs

3D photographs offer an important clinical relevant potential and benefit towards longitudinal non-ionising 3D virtual treatment outcome analysis (◘ Figs. 5.38 and 5.39). "Colour distance maps based on 3D photographs" with subsequent "calculation of the inter-surface distances" are computed after surface-base rigid registration on the forehead and can be used to evaluate facial soft tissue changes (◘ Fig. 5.40) after orthognathic surgery.

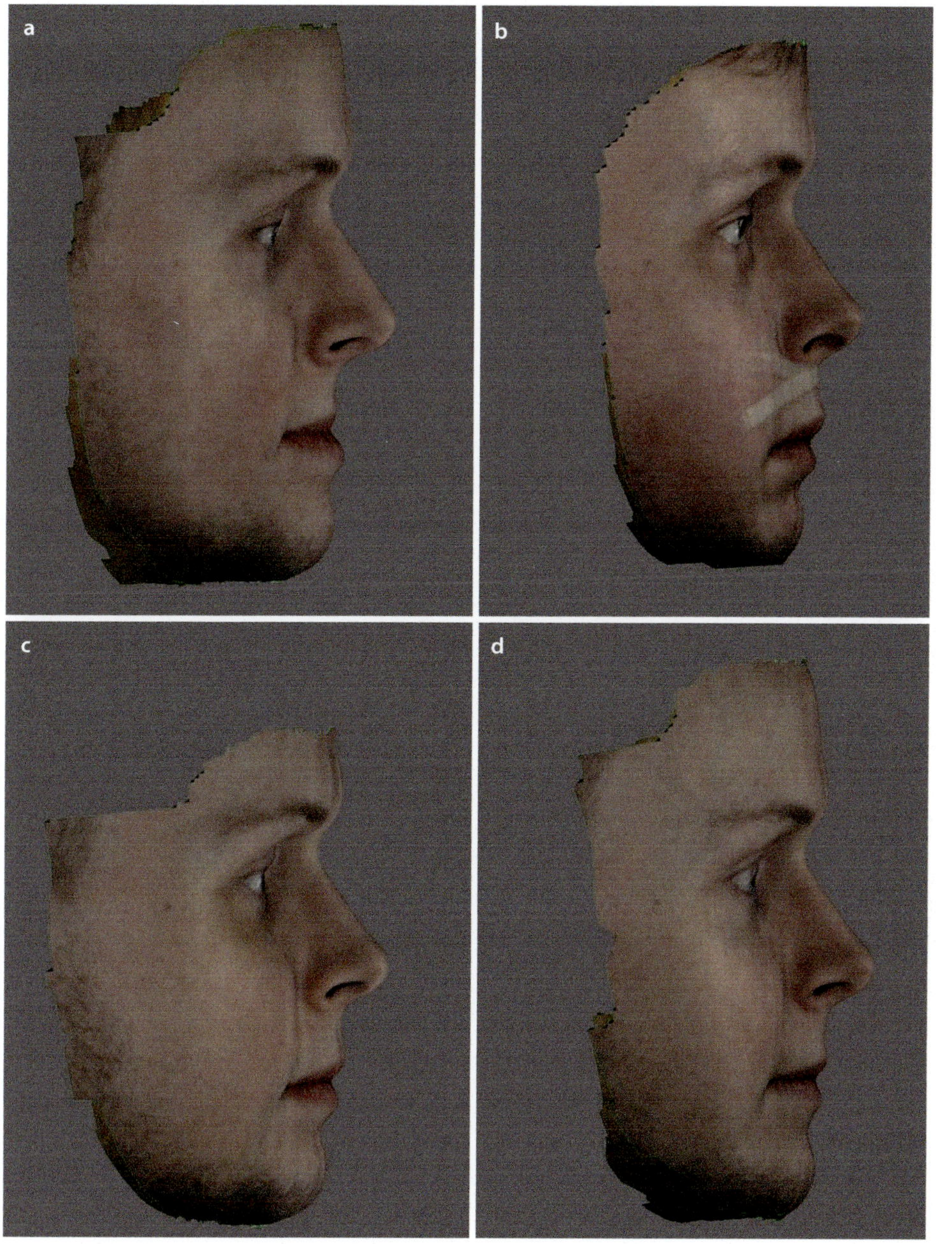

◘ **Fig. 5.38** Right profile views of 3D photographs of patient D.T. who underwent a Le Fort I advancement combined with a unilateral sagittal split (USSO) at the right side (Planmeca ProMax® 3D Max, ProFace™, Planmeca Oy, Helsinki, Finland): T0, prior to surgery (**a**); T1, 1 day after surgery at discharge from the hospital (**b**); T2, 10 days after surgery (**c**); and T3, 4 weeks after surgery (**d**) (With courtesy to orthodontist, Michael de Baets)

3D Virtual Surface-Based Superimposition of 3D Photographs

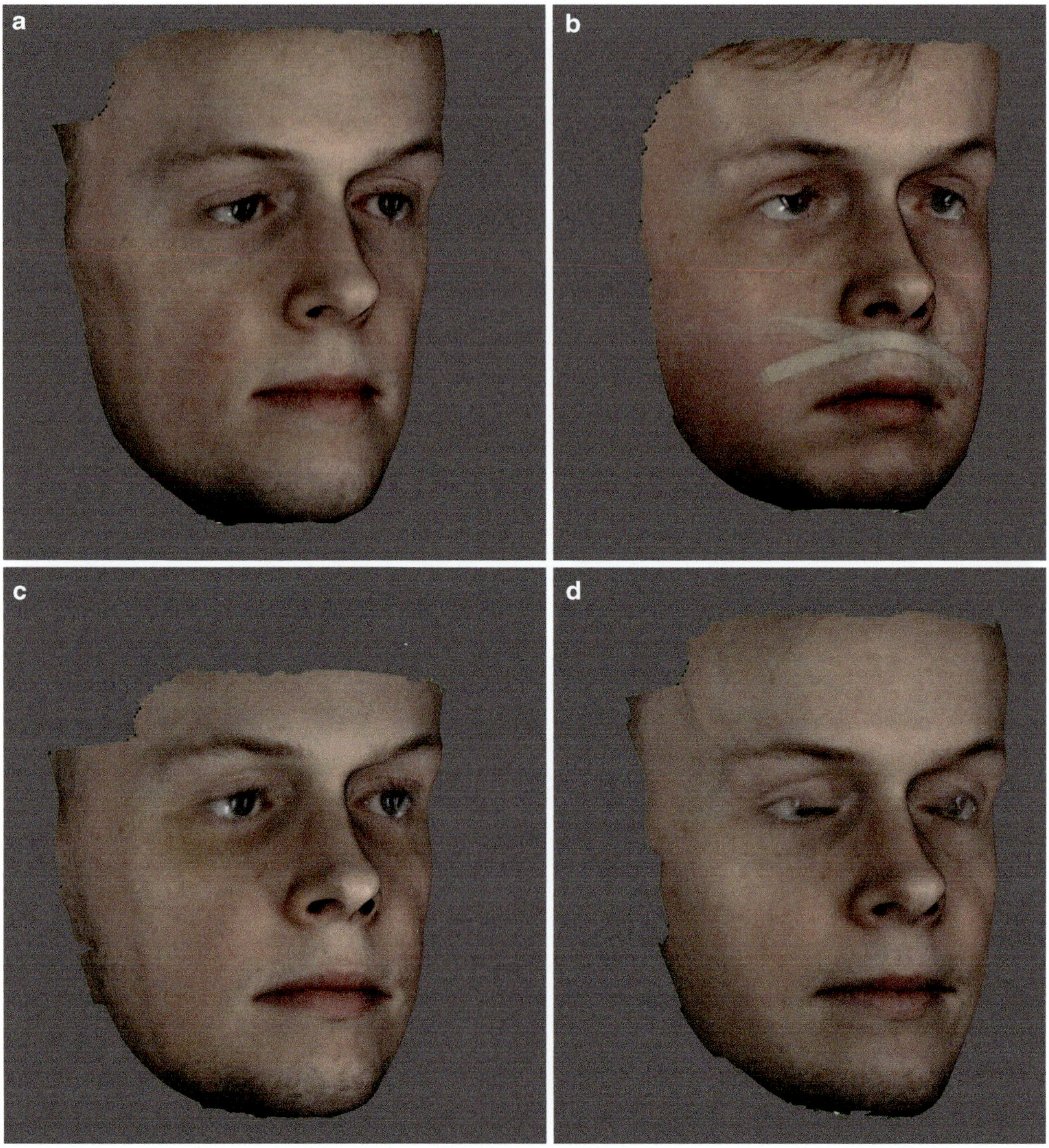

Fig. 5.39 2/3 right profile views of 3D photographs of patient D.T. who underwent a Le Fort I advancement combined with a unilateral sagittal split (USSO) at the right side (Planmeca ProMax® 3D Max, ProFace™, Planmeca Oy, Helsinki, Finland): T0, prior to surgery (**a**); T1, 1 day after surgery at discharge from the hospital (**b**); T2, 10 days after surgery (**c**); and T3, 4 weeks after surgery (**d**) (With courtesy to orthodontist, Michael de Baets)

3D Virtual Surface-Based Superimposition of 3D Photographs: Colour Distance Maps

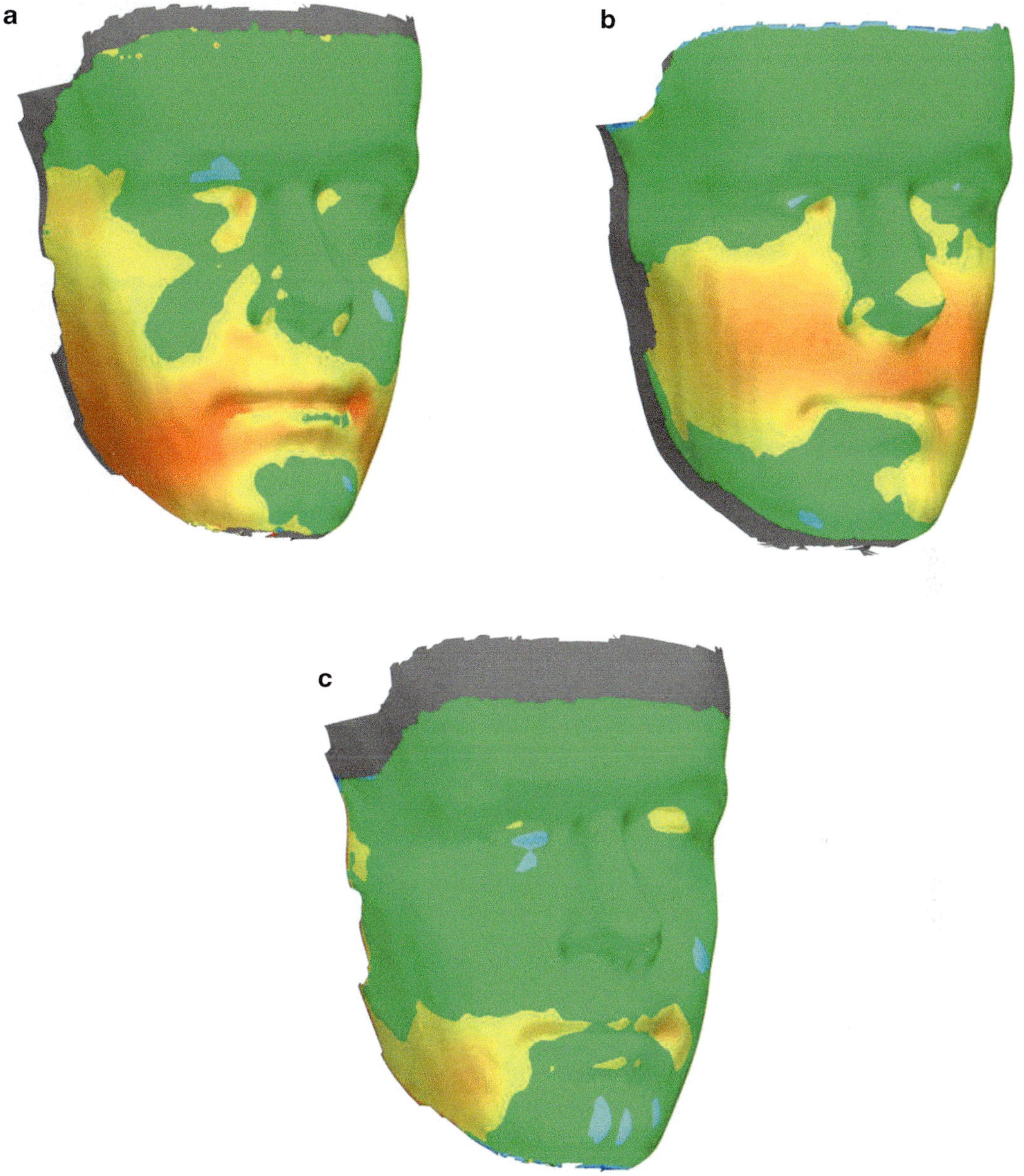

Fig. 5.40 2/3 right profile views of surface-based superimposition on the forehead of 3D photographs of patient D.T. who underwent a Le Fort I advancement combined with a unilateral sagittal split (USSO) at the right side (Planmeca ProMax® 3D Max, ProFace™, Planmeca Oy, Helsinki, Finland): T1, 1 day after surgery at discharge of the hospital superimposed on T3, 4 weeks after surgery (**a**); T0, prior to surgery superimposed on T3, 4 weeks after surgery (**b**); and T2, 10 days after surgery superimposed on T3, 4 weeks after surgery (**c**). Note that the superimposition of T3 on T0 clearly shows the advancement of the maxilla and the asymmetrical displacement (rotation of the mandible after a right USSO). Also note that the superimpositions of T1 on T3 and T2 on T3 show that the most important post-surgical swelling takes place in the lower jaw at the right side and not at the level of the maxilla (**c**). (With courtesy to orthodontist, Michael de Baets)

Additional Recommended Reading

Aboul-Hosn Centenero S, Hernández-Alfaro F (2012) 3D planning in orthognathic surgery, CAD/CAM surgical splints and prediction of the soft and hard tissues results – our experience in 16 cases. J Craniomaxillofac Surg 40:162–168

Alhadidi A, Cevidanes LH, Paniagua B, Cook R, Festy F, Tyndall D (2012) 3D quantification of mandibular asymmetry using the SPHARM-PDM tool box. Int J Comput Assist Radiol Surg 7:265–271

Almeida RC, Cevidanes LH, Carvalho FA, Motta AT, Almeida MA, Styner M, Turvey T, Proffit WR, Phillips C (2011) Soft tissue response to mandibular advancement using 3D CBCT scanning. Int J Oral Maxillofac Surg 4:353–359

Almukhtar A, Ju X, Khambay B, McDonald J, Ayoub A (2014) Comparison of the accuracy of voxel based registration and surface based registration for 3D assessment of surgical change following orthognathic surgery. PLoS One 9:93402

Badiali G, Roncari A, Bianchi A, Taddei F, Marchetti C, Schileo E (2015) Navigation in orthognathic surgery, 3D accuracy. Facial Plast Surg 31:463–473

Baik HS, Kim SY (2010) Facial soft-tissue changes in skeletal class III orthognathic surgery patients analyzed with 3-dimensional laser scanning. Am J Orthod Dentofacial Orthop 138:167–178

Bianchi A, Muyldermans L, Di Martino M, Lancellotti L, Amadori S, Sarti A, Marchetti C (2010) Facial soft tissue esthetic predictions, validation in craniomaxillofacial surgery with cone beam computed tomography data. J Oral Maxillofac Surg 68:1471–1479

Bianchi A, Betti E, Tarsitano A, Morselli-Labate AM, Lancellotti L, Marchetti C (2014) Volumetric three-dimensional computed tomographic evaluation of the upper airway in patients with obstructive sleep apnea syndrome treated by maxillomandibular advancement. Br J Oral Maxillofac Surg 52:831–837

Blockhaus M, Kochel J, Hartmann J, Stellzig-Eisenhauer A, Meyer-Marcotty P (2014) Three-dimensional investigation of facial surface asymmetries in skeletal malocclusion patients before and after orthodontic treatment combined with orthognathic surgery. J Orofac Orthop 75:85–95

Burkhard JP, Dietrich AD, Jacobsen C, Roos M, Lübbers HT, Obwegeser JA (2014) Cephalometric and three-dimensional assessment of the posterior airway space and imaging software reliability analysis before and after orthognathic surgery. Craniomaxillofac Surg 42:1428–1436

Cevidanes LH, Bailey LJ, Tucker GR Jr, Styner MA, Mol A, Phillips CL, Profitt WR, Turvey T (2005) Superimposition of 3D cone-beam CT models of orthognathic surgery patients. Dentomaxillofac Radiol 34:369–375

Cevidanes LH, Styner MA, Proffit WR (2006) Image analysis and superimposition of 3-dimensional cone-beam computed tomography models. Am J Orthod Dentofacial Orthop 129:611–618

Cevidanes LH, Bailey LJ, Tucker SF, Styner MA, Mol A, Phillips CL, Proffit WR, Turvey T (2007) Three-dimensional cone-beam computed tomography for assessment of mandibular changes after orthognathic surgery. Am J Orthod Dentofacial Orthop 131:44–50

Cevidanes LH, Motta A, Proffit WR, Ackerman JL, Styner M (2010) Cranial base superimposition for 3-dimensional evaluation of soft-tissue changes. Am J Orthod Dentofacial Orthop 137:S120–S129

Cevidanes LH, Gomes LR, Jung BT, Gomes MR, Ruellas AC, Goncalves JR, Schilling J, Styner M, Nguyen T, Kapila S, Paniagua B (2015) 3D superimposition and understanding temporomandibular joint arthritis. Orthod Craniofac Res 18:S18–S28

Choi JH, Mah J (2010) A new method for superimposition of CBCT volumes. J Clin Orthod 44:303–312

De Clerck H, Nguyen T, de Paula LK, Cevidanes L (2012) Three-dimensional assessment of mandibular and glenoid fossa changes after bone-anchored class III intermaxillary traction. Am J Orthod Dentofacial Orthop 14:25–31

de Paula LK, Ruellas AC, Paniagua B, Styner M, Turvey T, Zhu H, Wang J, Cevidanes LH (2013) One-year assessment of surgical outcomes in class III patients using cone beam computed tomography. Int J Oral Maxillofac Surg 42:780–789

de Souza Carvalho AC, Magro Filho O, Garcia IR Jr, Araujo PM, Nogueira RL (2012) Cephalometric and three-dimensional assessment of superior posterior airway space after maxillomandibular advancement. Int J Oral Maxillofac Surg 41:1102–1111

Franco AA, Cevidanes LH, Phillips C, Rossouw PE, Turvey TA, Carvalho FA, Paula LK, Quintão CC, Almeida MA (2013) Long-term 3-dimensional stability of mandibular advancement surgery. J Oral Maxillofac Surg 71:1588–1597

Gerbino G, Bianchi FA, Verzé L, Ramieri G (2014) Soft tissue changes after maxillo-mandibular advancement in OSAS patients, a three-dimensional study. J Craniomaxillofac Surg 42:66–72

Guijarro-Martínez R, Swennen GR (2013) Three-dimensional cone beam computed tomography definition of the anatomical subregions of the upper airway, a validation study. Int J Oral Maxillofac Surg 42:1140–1149

Hajeer MY, Ayoub AF, Millett DT, Bock M, Siebert JP (2002) Three-dimensional imaging in orthognathic surgery, the clinical application of a new method. Int J Adult Orthodon Orthognath Surg 17:318–330

Hajeer MY, Ayoub AF, Millett DT (2004) Three-dimensional assessment of facial soft-tissue asymmetry before and after orthognathic surgery. Br J Oral Maxillofac Surg 42:396–404

Hajeer MY, Mao Z, Millett DT, Ayoub AF, Siebert JP (2005) A new three-dimensional method of assessing facial volumetric changes after orthognathic treatment. Cleft Palate Craniofac J 42:113–120

Hatab NA, Konstantinović VS, Mudrak JK (2015) Pharyngeal airway changes after mono- and bimaxillary surgery in skeletal class III patients, cone-beam computed tomography evaluation. J Craniomaxillofac Surg 43:491–496

Hernández-Alfaro F, Guijarro-Martínez R, Mareque-Bueno J (2011) Effect of mono- and bimaxillary advancement on pharyngeal airway volume, cone-beam computed tomography evaluation. J Oral Maxillofac Surg 69:395–400

Hsu SS, Gateno J, Bell RB, Hirsch DL, Markiewicz MR, Teichgraeber JF, Zhou X, Xia JJ (2013) Accuracy of a computer-aided surgical simulation protocol for orthognathic surgery, a prospective multicenter study. J Oral Maxillofac Surg 71:128–142

Jabar N, Robinson W, Goto TK, Khambay BS (2015) The validity of using surface meshes for evaluation of three-dimensional maxillary and mandibular surgical changes. Int J Oral Maxillofac Surg 44:914–920

Kau CH, Cronin A, Durning P, Zhurov AI, Sandham A, Richmond S (2006) A new method for the 3D measurement of postoperative swelling following orthognathic surgery. Orthod Craniofac Res 9:31–37

Khambay B, Nebel JC, Bowman J, Walker F, Hadley DM, Ayoub A (2002) 3D stereophotogrammetric image superimposition onto 3D CT scan images, the future of orthognathic surgery. A pilot study. Int J Adult Orthodon Orthognath Surg 17:331–341

Kim YI, Jung YH, Cho BH, Kim JR, Kim SS, Son WS, Park SB (2010) The assessment of the short- and long-term changes in the condylar position following sagittal split ramus osteotomy (SSRO) with rigid fixation. J Oral Rehabil 37:262–270

Kim EJ, Choi JH, Kim YS, Kim TH, Lee SH, Lee HM, Shin C, Lee SH (2011a) Upper airway changes in severe obstructive sleep apnea, upper airway length and volumetric analyses using 3D MDCT. Acta Otolaryngol 131:527–532

Kim YI, Cho BH, Jung YH, Son WS, Park SB (2011b) Cone-beam computerized tomography evaluation of condylar changes and stability following two-jaw surgery. Le Fort I osteotomy and mandibular setback surgery with rigid fixation. Oral Surg Oral Med Oral Pathol Oral Radiol Endod 111:681–687

Kim DS, Huh KH, Lee SS, Heo MS, Choi SC, Hwang SJ, Yi WJ (2013) The relationship between the changes in three-dimensional facial morphology and mandibular movement after orthognathic surgery. J Craniomaxillofac Surg 41:686–693

Kim MA, Kim BR, Youn JK, Kim YJ, Park YH (2014) Head posture and pharyngeal airway volume changes after bimaxillary surgery for mandibular prognathism. J Craniomaxillofac Surg 42:531–535

Kim JW, Son WS, Kim SS, Kim YI (2015) Proximal segment changes after bilateral sagittal split ramus osteotomy in facial asymmetry patients. J Oral Maxillofac Surg 73:1592–1605

Koerich L, Ruellas AC, Paniagua B, Styner M, Turvey T, Cevidanes LH (2015) Three-dimensional regional displacement after surgical-orthodontic correction of class III malocclusion. Orthod Craniofac Res 19:65–73

Lee JH, Kim MJ, Kim SM, Kwon OH, Kim YK (2012) The 3D CT superimposition method 307 using image fusion based on the maximum mutual information algorithm for the assessment of oral and maxillofacial surgery treatment results. Oral Surg Oral Med Oral Pathol Oral Radiol 114:167–174

Li YM, Liu JL, Zhao JL, Dai J, Wang L, Chen JW (2014) Morphological changes in the pharyngeal airway of female skeletal class III patients following bimaxillary surgery, a cone beam computed tomography evaluation. Int J Oral Maxillofac Surg 43:862–867

Liebregts JH, Timmermans M, De Koning MJ, Bergé SJ, Maal TJ (2014) Three-dimensional facial simulation in bilateral sagittal split osteotomy, a validation study of 100 patients. J Oral Maxillofac Surg 73:961–970

Liebregts J, Xi T, Timmermans M, de Koning M, Bergé S, Hoppenreijs T, Maal T (2015) Accuracy of three-dimensional soft tissue simulation in bimaxillary osteotomies. J Craniomaxillofac Surg 43:329–335

Lin HH, Chang HW, Wang CH, Kim SG, Lo LJ (2015) Three-dimensional computer-assisted orthognathic surgery, experience of 37 patients. Ann Plast Surg 74:S118–S126

Maes F, Collignon A, Vandermeulen D, Marchal G, Suetens P (1997) Multimodality image -registration by maximization of mutual information. IEEE Trans Med Imaging 16:187–198

Marchetti C, Bianchi A, Muyldermans L, Di Martino M, Lancellotti L, Sarti A (2011) Validation of new soft tissue software in orthognathic surgery planning. Int J Oral Maxillofac Surg 40:26–32

Mazzoni S, Badiali G, Lancellotti L, Babbi L, Bianchi A, Marchetti C (2010) Simulation-guided navigation, a new approach to improve intraoperative three-dimensional reproducibility during orthognathic surgery. J Craniofac Surg 21:1698–1705

Meulstee J, Liebregts J, Xi T, Vos F, de Koning M, Bergé S, Maal T (2015) A new 3D approach to evaluate facial profile changes following BSSO. J Craniomaxillofac Surg 43:1994–1999

Mollemans W, Schutyser F, Nadjmi N, Maes F, Suetens P (2007) Predicting soft tissue deformations for a maxillofacial surgery planning system, from computational strategies to a complete clinical validation. Med Image Anal 11:282–301

Motta AT, de Assis Ribeiro Carvalho F, Oliveira AE, Cevidanes LH, de Oliveira Almeida MA (2010) Superimposition of 3D cone-beam CT models in orthognathic surgery. Dent Press J Orthod 15:39–41

Motta AT, Cevidanes LH, Carvalho FA, Almeida MA, Phillips C (2011) Three-dimensional regional displacements after mandibular advancement surgery, one year of follow-up. J Oral Maxillofac Surg 2011(69):1447–1457

Nada RM, Maal TJ, Breuning KH, Berge SJ, Mostafa YA, Kuijpers-Jagtman AM (2011) Accuracy and reproducibility of voxel based superimposition of cone beam computed tomography models on the anterior cranial base and the zygomatic arches. PLoS One 6:e16520

Nkenke E, Vairaktaris E, Kramer M, Schlegel A, Holst A, Hirschfelder U, Wiltfang J, Neukam FW, Stamminger M (2008) Three-dimensional analysis of changes of the malar-midfacial region after LeFort I osteotomy and maxillary advancement. Oral Maxillofac Surg 12:5–12

Oh KM, Seo SK, Park JE, Sim HS, Cevidanes LH, Kim YJ, Park YH (2013) Post-operative soft tissue changes in patients with mandibular prognathism after bimaxillary surgery. J Craniomaxillofac Surg 41:204–211

Paniagua B, Cevidanes L, Zhu H, Styner M (2011) Outcome quantification using SPHARM-PDM toolbox in orthognathic surgery. Int J Comput Assist Radiol Surg 6:617–626

Park SB, Kim YI, Son WS, Hwang DS, Cho BH (2012a) Cone-beam computed tomography evaluation of short- and long-term airway change and stability after orthognathic surgery in patients with class III skeletal deformities, bimaxillary surgery and mandibular setback surgery. Int J Oral Maxillofac Surg 41:87–93

Park SB, Yang YM, Kim YI, Cho BH, Jung YH, Hwang DS (2012b) Effect of bimaxillary surgery on adaptive condylar head remodeling, metric analysis and image interpretation using cone-beam computed tomography volume superimposition. J Oral Maxillofac Surg 70:1951–1959

Park SB, Yoon JK, Kim YI, Hwang DS, Cho BH, Son WS (2012c) The evaluation of the nasal morphologic changes after bimaxillary surgery in skeletal class III malocclusion by using the superimposition of cone-beam computed tomography (CBCT) volumes. J Craniomaxillofac Surg 40:87–92

Plooij JM, Naphausen MT, Maal TJ, Xi T, Rangel FA, Swennnen G, de Koning M, Borstlap WA, Bergé SJ (2009) 3D evaluation of the lingual fracture line after a bilateral sagittal split osteotomy of the mandible. Int J Oral Maxillofac Surg 38:1244–1249

Rana M, Gellrich NC, Joos U, Piffkó J, Kater W (2011) 3D evaluation of postoperative swelling using two different cooling methods following orthognathic surgery, a randomised observer blind prospective pilot study. Int J Oral Maxillofac Surg 40:690–696

Schendel SA, Jacobson R, Khalessi S (2013) 3-dimensional facial simulation in orthognathic surgery, is it accurate? J Oral Maxillofac Surg 71:1406–1414

Schendel SA, Broujerdi JA, Jacobson RL (2014) Three-dimensional upper-airway changes with maxillomandibular advancement for obstructive sleep apnea treatment. Am J Orthod Dentofacial Orthop 146:385–393

Schilling J, Gomes LC, Benavides E, Nguyen T, Paniagua B, Styner M, Boen V, Gonçalves JR, Cevidanes LH (2014) Regional 3D superimposition to assess temporomandibular joint condylar morphology. Dentomaxillofac Radiol 43:20130273

Schneider D, Kämmerer PW, Schön G, Bschorer R (2015) A three-dimensional comparison of the pharyngeal airway after mandibular distraction osteogenesis and bilateral sagittal split osteotomy. J Craniomaxillofac Surg 43:1632–1637

Shafi MI, Ayoub A, Ju X, Khambay B (2013) The accuracy of three-dimensional prediction planning for the surgical correction of facial deformities using Maxilim. Int J Oral Maxillofac Surg 42:801–806

Shimomatsu K, Nozoe E, Ishihata K, Okawachi T, Nakamura N (2012) Three-dimensional analyses of facial soft tissue configuration of Japanese females with jaw deformity – a trial of polygonal view of facial soft tissue deformity in orthognathic patients. J Craniomaxillofac Surg 40:559–567

Song WW, Kim SS, Sándor GK, Kim YD (2013) Maxillary yaw as the primary predictor of maxillary dental midline deviation; 3D analysis using cone-beam computed tomography. J Oral Maxillofac Surg 71:752–762

Sun Y, Luebbers HT, Agbaje JO, Schepers S, Vrielinck L, Lambrichts I, Politis C (2013) Accuracy of upper jaw positioning with intermediate splint fabrication after virtual planning in bimaxillary orthognathic surgery. J Craniofac Surg 24:1871–1876

Swennen GRJ (2005a) 3-D cephalometry and craniofacial growth. In: Swennen GRJ, Schutyser F, Hausamen JE (eds) Three-dimensional cephalometry, vol 8. Springer, Heidelberg, pp 289–306

Swennen GRJ (2005b) Clinical applications. In: Swennen GRJ, Schutyser F, Hausamen JE (eds) Three-dimensional cephalometry, vol 9. Springer, Heidelberg, pp 307–340

Swennen GR, Schutyser F (2007) Three-dimensional virtual approach to diagnosis and treatment planning of maxillo-facial deformity. In: Bell WH, Guerrero CA (eds) Distraction osteogenesis of the facial skeleton, vol 6. Decker Inc, Hamilton, pp 55–79

Swennen GRJ, Schutyser F, Hausamen JE (2005) Three-dimensional cephalometry. A color atlas and manual. Springer, Heidelberg

Swennen GRJ, Schutyser F, Barth EL, De Groeve P, De Mey A (2006) A new method of 3-D cephalometry. Part I. The anatomic cartesian 3-D reference system. J Craniofac Surg 17:314–325

Swennen GR, Mollemans W, Schutyser F (2009) Three-dimensional treatment planning of orthognathic surgery in the era of virtual imaging. J Oral Maxillofac Surg 67:2080–2092

Swennen G, Mollemans W, Schutyser F, Lamoral P (2010) Evaluation of the accuracy of maxillary repositioning after 3D virtual planning of orthognathic surgery, a prospective study. 20th EACMFS Congress, abstract book, Elsevier, UK.

Terzic A, Combescure C, Scolozzi P (2014) Accuracy of computational soft tissue predictions in orthognathic surgery from three-dimensional photographs 6 months after completion of surgery, a preliminary study of 13 patients. Aesthetic Plast Surg 38:184–191

Tucker S, Cevidanes LH, Styner M, Kim H, Reyes M, Proffit W, Turvey T (2010) Comparison of actual surgical outcomes and 3-dimensional surgical simulations. J Oral Maxillofac Surg 68:2412–2421

van Loon B, van Heerbeek N, Bierenbroodspot F, Verhamme L, Xi T, de Koning MJ, Ingels KJ, Bergé SJ, Maal TJ (2015) Three-dimensional changes in nose and upper lip volume after orthognathic surgery. Int J Oral Maxillofac Surg 44:83–89

Verdenik M, Ihan Hren N (2014) Differences in three-dimensional soft tissue changes after upper, lower, or both jaw orthognathic surgery in skeletal class III patients. Int J Oral Maxillofac Surg 43:1345–1351

Weissheimer A, Menezes LM, Sameshima GT, Enciso R, Pham J, Grauer D (2012) Imaging software accuracy for 3-dimensional analysis of the upper airway. Am J Orthod Dentofacial Orthop 142:801–813

Weissheimer A, Menezes LM, Koerich L, Pham J, Cevidanes LH (2015) Fast three-dimensional superimposition of cone beam computed tomography for orthopaedics and orthognathic surgery evaluation. Int J Oral Maxillofac Surg 44:1188–1196

Wermker K, Kleinheinz J, Jung S, Dirksen D (2014) Soft tissue response and facial symmetry after orthognathic surgery. J Craniomaxillofac Surg 42:339–345

Xi T, van Loon B, Fudalej P, Bergé S, Swennen G, Maal T (2013) Validation of a novel semi-automated method for three-dimensional surface rendering of condyles using cone beam computed tomography data. Int J Oral Maxillofac Surg 42:1023–1029

Xi T, de Koning M, Bergé S, Hoppenreijs T, Maal T (2015a) The role of mandibular proximal segment rotations on skeletal relapse and condylar remodelling following bilateral sagittal split advancement osteotomies. J Craniomaxillofac Surg 43:1716–1722

Xi T, Schreurs R, van Loon B, de Koning M, Bergé S, Hoppenreijs T, Maal T (2015b) 3D analysis of condylar remodelling and skeletal relapse following bilateral sagittal split advancement osteotomies. J Craniomaxillofac Surg 43:462–468

Xia JJ, Gateno J, Teichgraeber JF, Christensen AM, Lasky RE, Lemoine JJ, Liebschner MA (2007) Accuracy of the computer-aided surgical simulation (CASS) system in the treatment of patients with complex craniomaxillofacial deformity. A pilot study. J Oral Maxillofac Surg 65:248–254

Xia JJ, Shevchenko L, Gateno J, Teichgraeber JF, Taylor TD, Lasky RE, English JD, Kau CH, McGrory KR (2011) Outcome study of computer-aided surgical simulation in the treatment of patients with craniomaxillofacial deformities. J Oral Maxillofac Surg 69:2014–2024

Clinical Applications of 3D Virtual Treatment Planning of Orthognathic Surgery

Gwen R.J. Swennen

G.R.J. Swennen (ed.), *3D Virtual Treatment Planning of Orthognathic Surgery*,
DOI 10.1007/978-3-662-47389-4_6

▪ Case 1: Class II, Long Face, Video

Patient V.E.W. is a 16-year-old girl with a Class II/I long-face maxillofacial deformity due to a vertical maxillary excess (VME). In the frontal view, she is clinically not presenting any obvious facial asymmetries. In rest, she has an incisal display of 8 mm, while during spontaneous smiling, she has full incisal exposure with 4 mm gingival display at incisal level. In the profile view, she presents a dorsal nasal hump, a limited vermilion exposure, a significant lip incompetence, an atonic lower lip and a retruded mandible with poor chin definition. She has an Angle Class II malocclusion with adequate transversal relationship and a 1.5 mm lower dental midline deviation to the right. There is no history of TMJ dysfunction neither pain.

Patient V.E.W. is used throughout this book to illustrate all different aspects of 3D virtual treatment planning of orthognathic surgery.

"Imaging Workflow for 3D Virtual Treatment Planning of Orthognathic Surgery" and "3D Virtual Diagnosis of the Orthognathic Patient" of Case 1 (Patient V. E. W.) are illustrated extensively in Chapter 1 and Chapter 2, respectively.

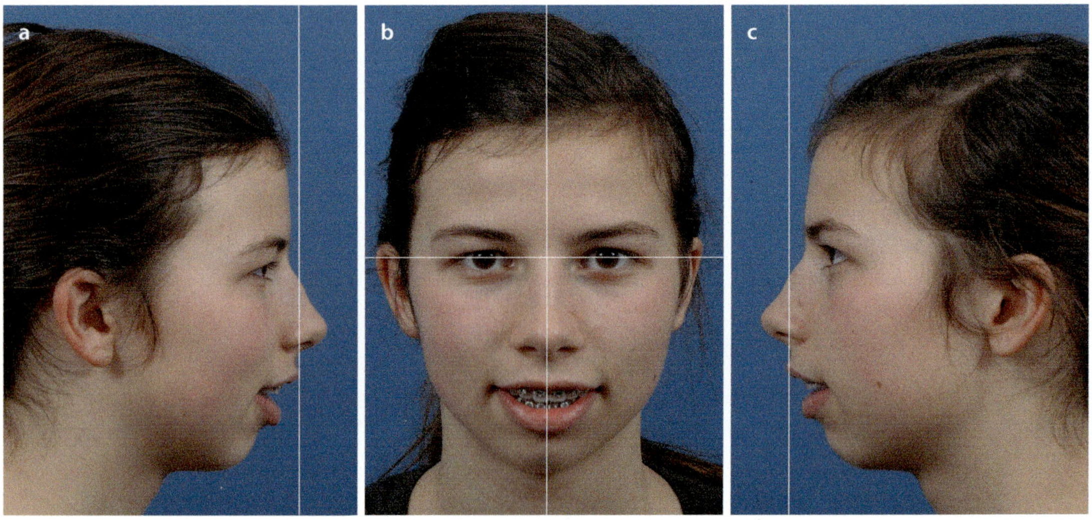

Fig. 6.1 Pre-surgical clinical right profile (**a**), frontal (**b**) and left profile (**c**) views of patient V.E.W. in *c*-NHP in rest, at the time of the workup, approximately 3 weeks prior to surgery. Note that clinically, she does not present any obvious cant of the maxilla neither of the mandible

Case 1: Class II, Long Face, v-NHP and PHP

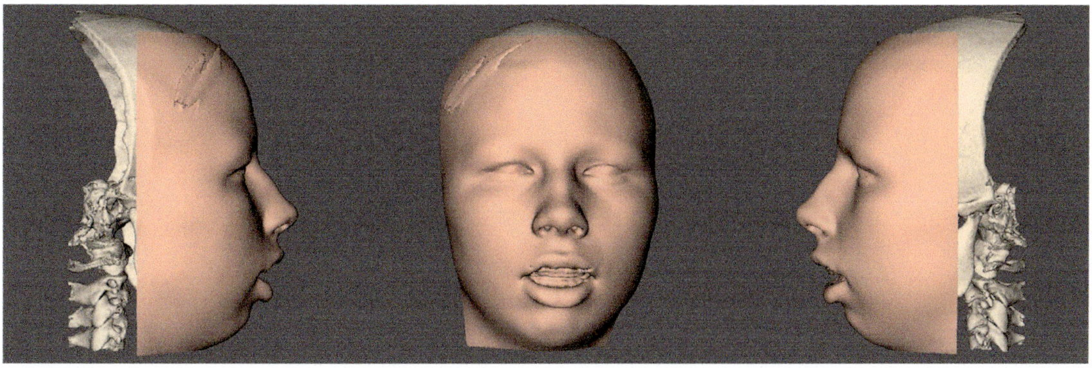

Fig. 6.2 Pre-surgical 3D "surface-rendered" right profile, frontal and profile left soft and hard tissue representations of the head of patient V.E.W., as generated during standardised CBCT image acquisition, at the time of the workup (Maxilim v. 2.3.0.3). Note the incorrect position and orientation of patient's V.E.W. virtual head compared to her clinical pictures (Fig. 6.1), although it was attempted to scan the patient in her correct *c*-NHP in rest

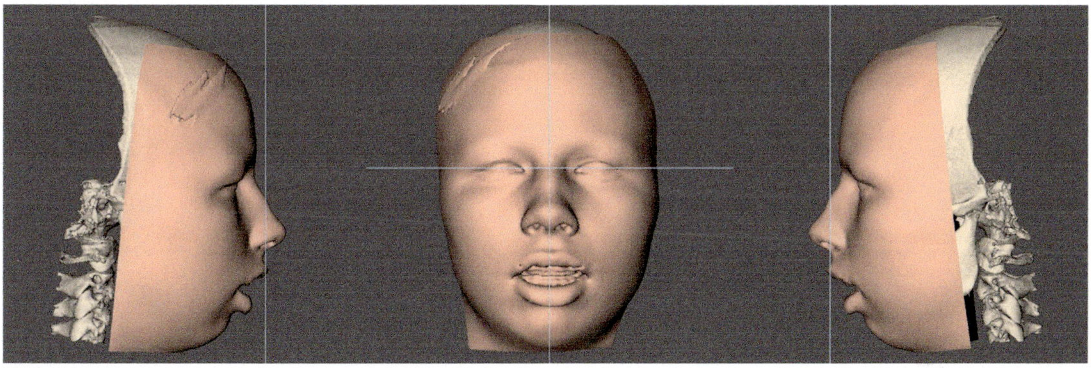

Fig. 6.3 Following a standardised "step-by-step" approach (▶ see Sect. 3.1), the scanned head position of patient V.E.W. (Fig. 6.2) was virtually modified towards her *c*-NHP (Fig. 6.1), which results in the *v*-NHP corresponding to her individual "Planning Head Position (PHP)" (3D "surface-rendered" representations, patient V.E.W., Maxilim v. 2.3.0.3)

Case 1: Class II, Long Face

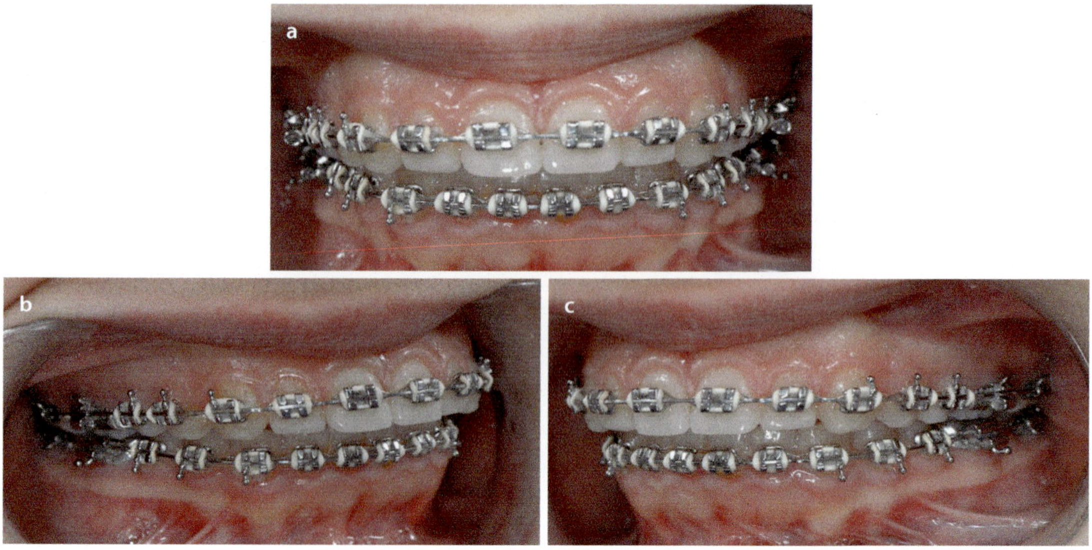

Fig. 6.4 Pre-surgical frontal (**a**), right (**b**) and left (**c**) intra-oral views of patient's V.E.W. occlusion at the time of the workup, approximately 3 weeks prior to surgery

"10 step-by-step integrated 3D virtual treatment planning", "3D virtual treatment planning transfer in the operation theatre" and "3D virtual evaluation of treatment outcome of orthognathic surgery" of Case 1 (patient V.E.W.) are thoroughly explained and illustrated in detail in Chaps. 3, 4 and 5, respectively.

Case 1: Class II, Long Face, "3D Virtual Treatment Planning, OR" Template

Maxillary osteotomy

■ Le Fort: ■I ☐II ☐III
■ One-piece
☐ Segmental:
Pieces: ....
Interdental: ....
■ Advancement: 2.0 mm
☐ Set-back : ....
■ Midline: 1.5 mm ■R ☐L
■ Midline after Le Fort 1: inbetween 31/41
■ Vertical: (➔)
■ "Yaw" correction: CCW to the left
☐ Other: ....

Planning Requirements

■ Maxilla first
☐ Mandible first
☐ Minimally Invasive Le Fort I
☐ IO-CBCT
☐ Kobayashi wires : ....
☐ Skeletal anchorage : ....
☐ Orthodontic buttons : ....
☐ Occlusal grinding : ....
☐ Other : ....

2.5 mm	3.5 mm	4.5 mm	4.5 mm	3.5 mm
16	13	11	23	26

"Roll" correction: ☐CW ■CCW

Mandibular osteotomy

■ SSO ■R ■L
☐ Inverted-L ☐R ☐L
☐ VRO ☐R ☐L
■ Advancement: R 6.0 mm L 5.0 mm
☐ Set-back: R .... L ....
☐ CW "Pitch" rotation
■ CCW "Pitch" rotation
☐ Midline split
■ IAN course: R lingual L lingual
☐ Midline after BSSO: ....
☐ Other: ....

Miscellaneous

■ Para-nasal cross sutures
☐ Alar cinch
■ Septoplasty
■ Inferior turbinectomy
■ ANS: ■Shortening ■Midline
■ Nasal base plasty ■R ■L
■ Lateral nasal wall plasty ■R ☐L
☐ Bone graft(s): ....
☐ Extraction(s): ....
☐ Other: ....

Chin osteotomy

■ Advancement: 6.0 mm
☐ Set-back: ....
■ Midline: 2.0 mm ☐R ■L
■ Intrusion:
■Anterior: 2.0 mm
■Posterior: R 1.0 L 2.5 mm
☐ Extrusion:
☐Anterior: ....
☐Posterior: R ...... L ......
☐ "Shield" osteotomy
☐ "Chin wing" osteotomy
Mental Foramen level:
☐ Symmetric
■ Asymmetric
■ Other: CCW "Roll" / CW "Yaw" rotation

Adjuvant Cosmetic Procedures

☐ Bichatectomy ☐R ☐L
☐ Zygoma osteotomies ☐R ☐L
Infraorbital Foramen level:
☐ Symmetric
☐ Asymmetric
☐ Otoplasty: ☐R ☐L
■ Rhinoplasty: Closed
☐ Browlift: ....
☐ Blepharoplasty: ....
☐Upper ☐Lower
☐ Facelift: ....
☐ Necklift: ....
☐ Liposuction: ....
☐ Lipofilling: ....
☐ Other: ....

Addendum Template. Prof. Gwen Swennen and Dr. Martin Gaboury, Maxillofacial and Facial Plastic Surgery.

Case 1: Class II, Long Face, Clinical Treatment Outcome

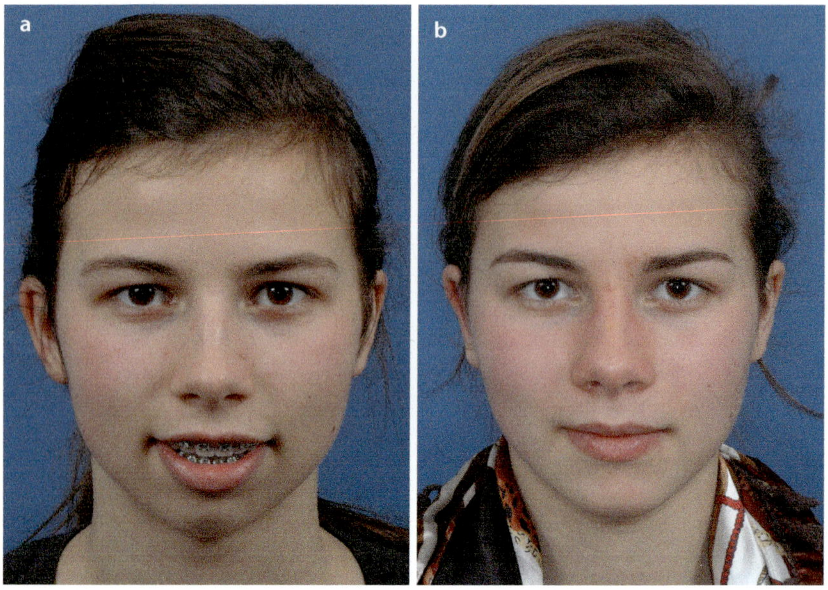

Fig. 6.5 Frontal clinical views in rest, pre-surgical (**a**) and 1 year after (**b**) combined orthodontic-surgical treatment and closed rhinoplasty of patient V.E.W

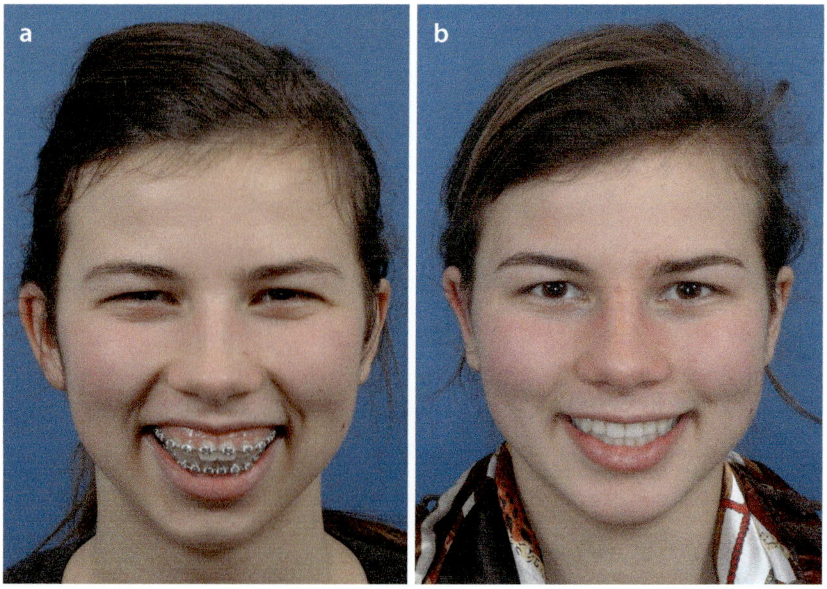

Fig. 6.6 Frontal clinical views during smiling, pre-surgical (**a**) and 1 year after (**b**) combined orthodontic-surgical treatment and closed rhinoplasty of patient V.E.W. Note that compared to her long-term result (Fig. 6.16a), the 1-year post-treatment smile (Fig. 6.6b) is not fully spontaneous

Case 1: Class II, Long Face, Clinical Treatment Outcome

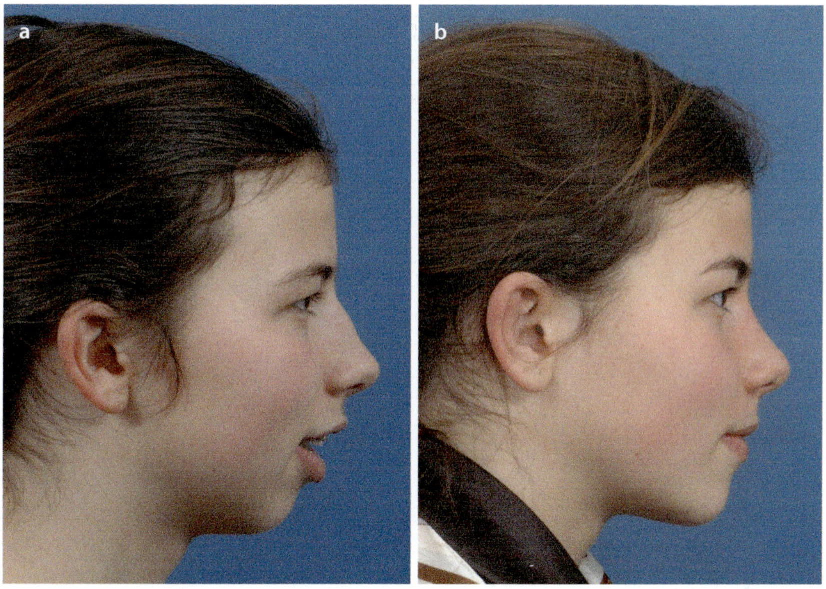

Fig. 6.7 Right profile clinical views in rest, pre-surgical (**a**) and 1 year after (**b**) combined orthodontic-surgical treatment and closed rhinoplasty of patient V.E.W.

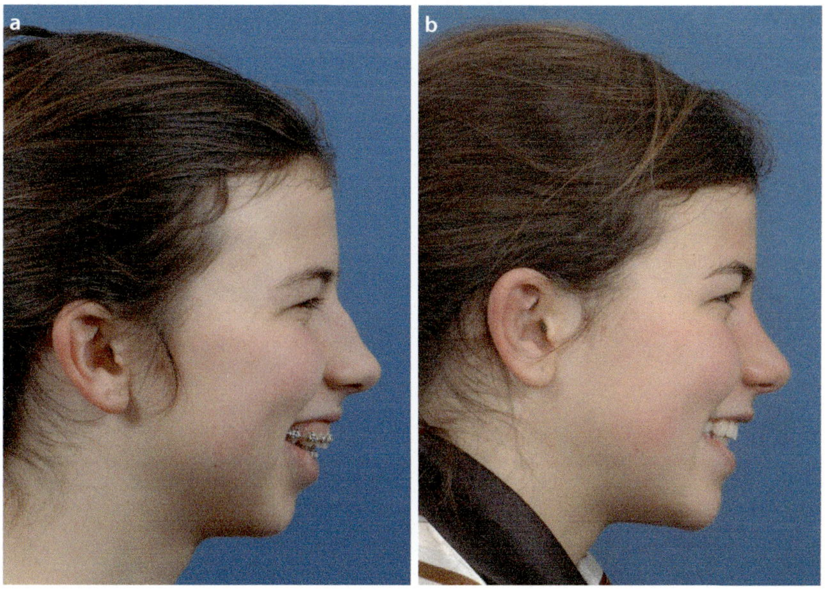

Fig. 6.8 Right profile clinical views during smiling, pre-surgical (**a**) and 1 year after (**b**) combined orthodontic-surgical treatment and closed rhinoplasty of patient V.E.W.

Case 1: Class II, Long Face, Clinical Treatment Outcome

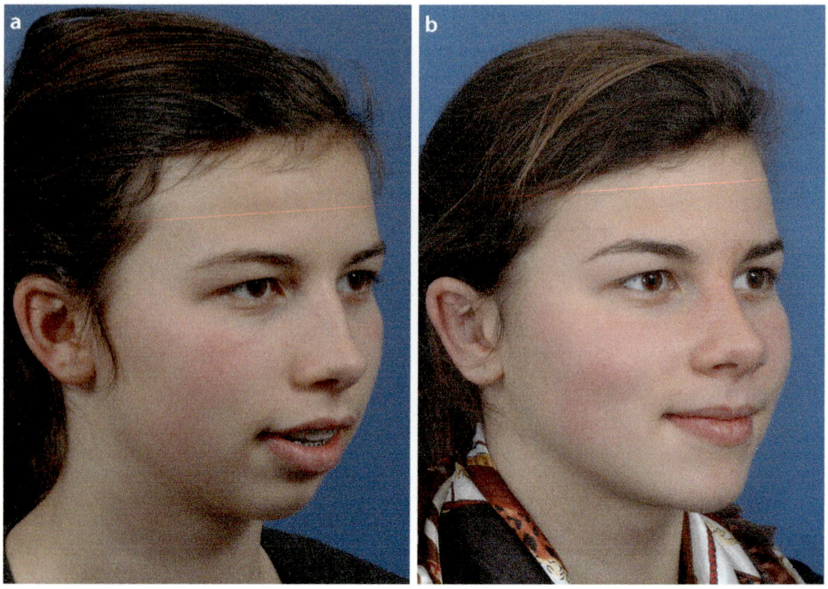

Fig. 6.9 2/3 right profile clinical views in rest, pre-surgical (**a**) and 1 year after (**b**) combined orthodontic-surgical treatment and closed rhinoplasty of patient V.E.W.

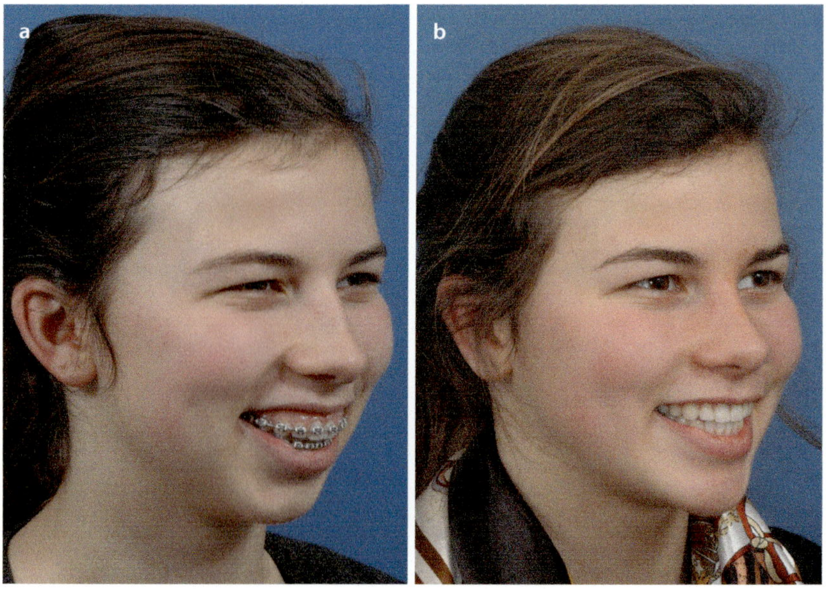

Fig. 6.10 2/3 right profile clinical views during smiling, pre-surgical (**a**) and 1 year after (**b**) combined orthodontic-surgical treatment and closed rhinoplasty of patient V.E.W.

Case 1: Class II, Long Face, Clinical Treatment Outcome

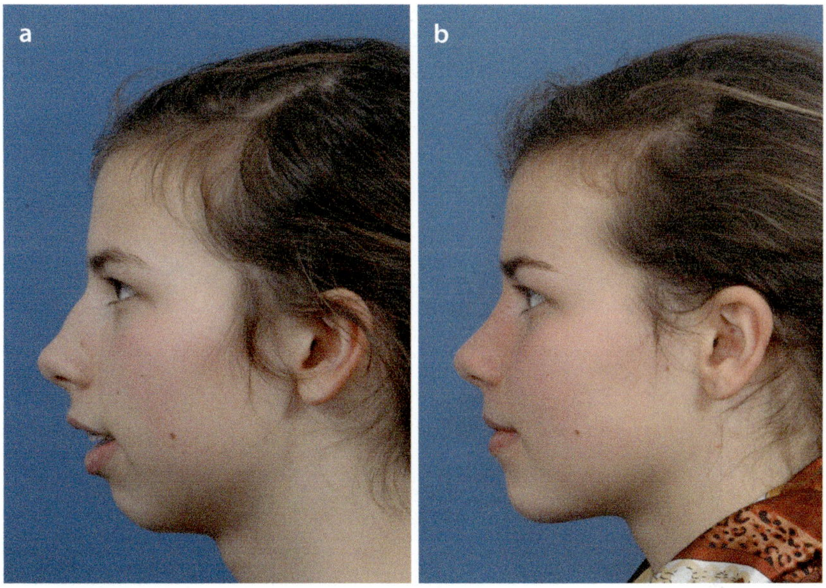

Fig. 6.11 Profile left clinical views in rest, pre-surgical (**a**) and 1 year after (**b**) combined orthodontic-surgical treatment and closed rhinoplasty of patient V.E.W.

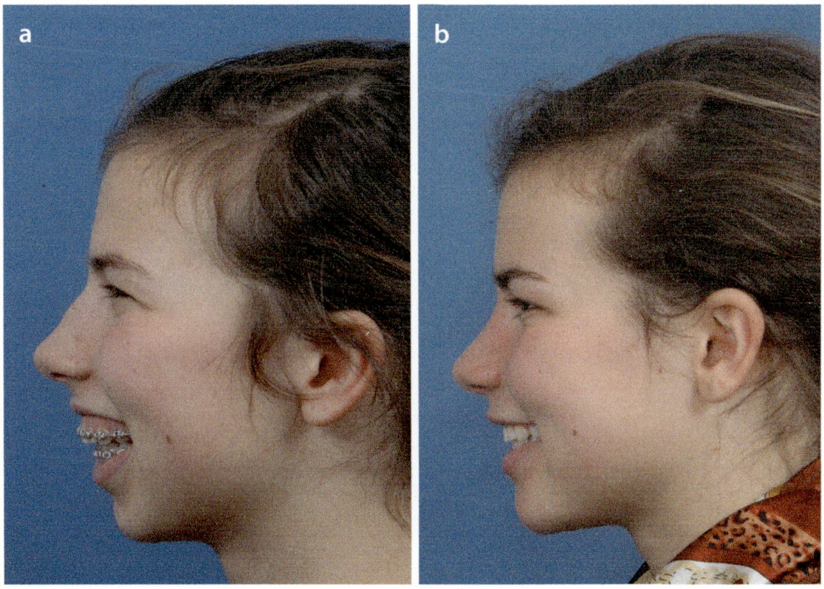

Fig. 6.12 Profile left clinical views during smiling, pre-surgical (**a**) and 1 year after (**b**) combined orthodontic-surgical treatment and closed rhinoplasty of patient V.E.W.

Case 1: Class II, Long Face, Clinical Treatment Outcome

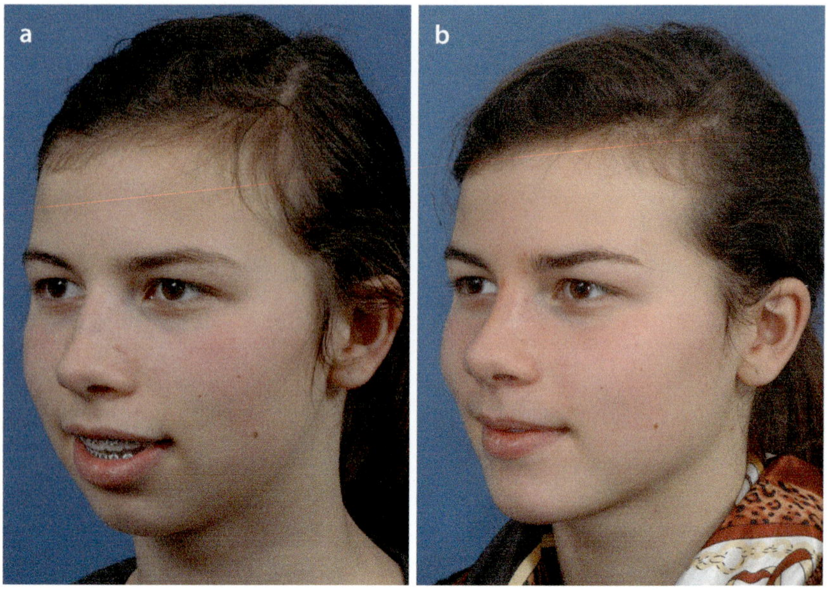

Fig. 6.13 2/3 profile left clinical views in rest, pre-surgical (**a**) and 1 year after (**b**) combined orthodontic-surgical treatment and closed rhinoplasty of patient V.E.W.

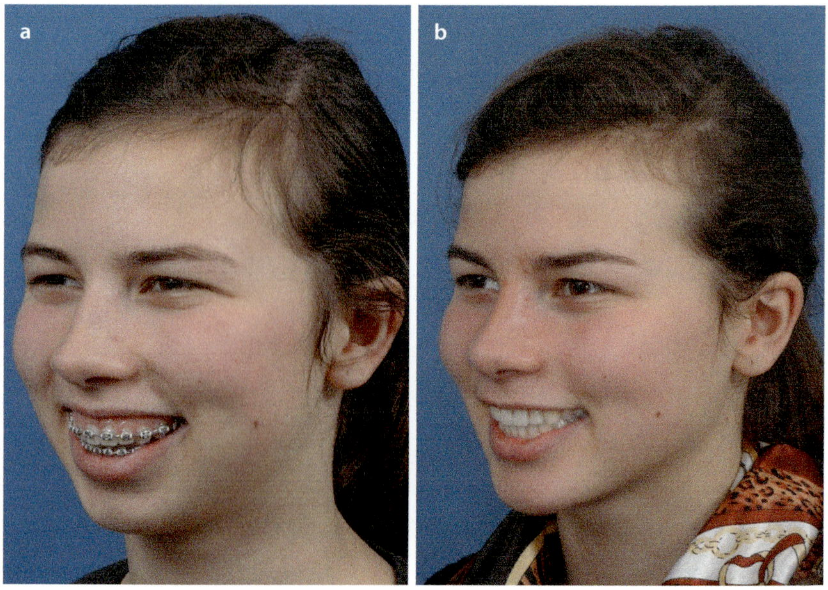

Fig. 6.14 2/3 profile left clinical views during smiling, pre-surgical (**a**) and 1 year after (**b**) combined orthodontic-surgical treatment and closed rhinoplasty of patient V.E.W.

Case 1: Class II, Long Face, Clinical Treatment Outcome

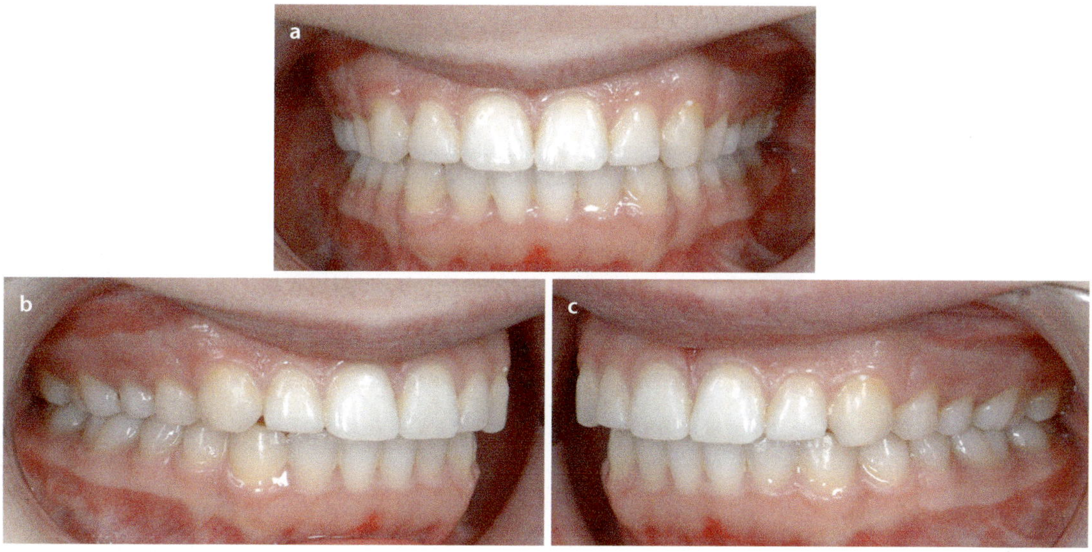

Fig. 6.15 Frontal (**a**), right (**b**) and left (**c**) intra-oral views of patient's V.E.W. occlusion 1 year after combined orthodontic-surgical treatment. The author acknowledges Toon Billiet for the orthodontic treatment

Fig. 6.16 Long-term clinical frontal (**a**) and 2/3 right profile (**b**) smiling views 2.5 years after combined orthodontic-surgical treatment and closed rhinoplasty of patient V.E.W.

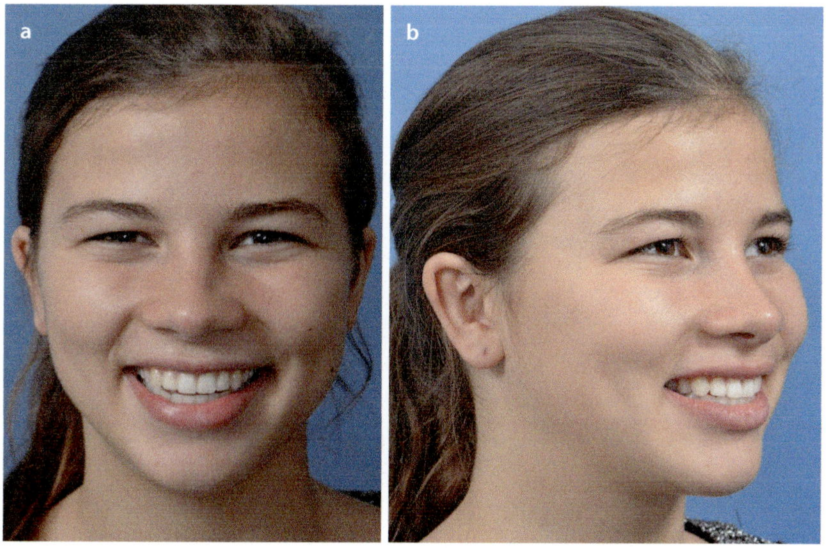

Case 2: Class II, Short Face

Patient D.C.M. is a 16-year-old girl with a Class II/2 short-face maxillofacial deformity due to vertical maxillary hypoplasia and mandibular retrusion. In the frontal view, she is clinically not presenting any obvious facial asymmetries although she has a slight chin deviation to the right. In rest, she has an upper incisal display of only 1 mm. During spontaneous smiling she has only 8 mm upper incisal exposure with an upper incisal crown length of 10 mm. In the profile view, she already presents with an adequate profile, although the mandible is retruded. She has an Angle Class II malocclusion with adequate transversal relationship. She has no history of TMJ dysfunction neither pain.

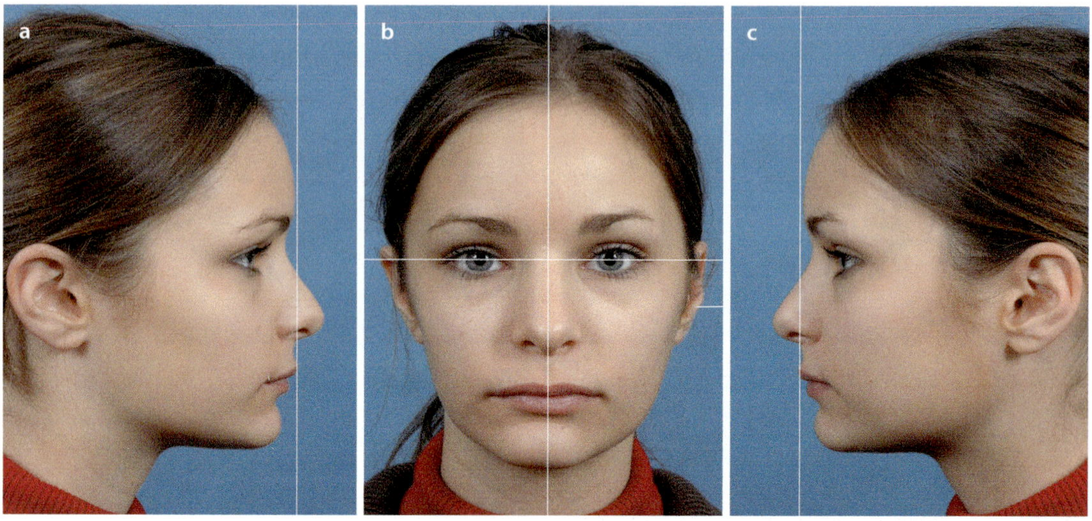

Fig. 6.17 Pre-surgical clinical right profile (**a**), frontal (**b**) and left profile (**c**) views of patient D.C.M. in her *c*-NHP in rest, at the time of the workup, approximately 3 weeks prior to surgery. Note the chin deviation to the right

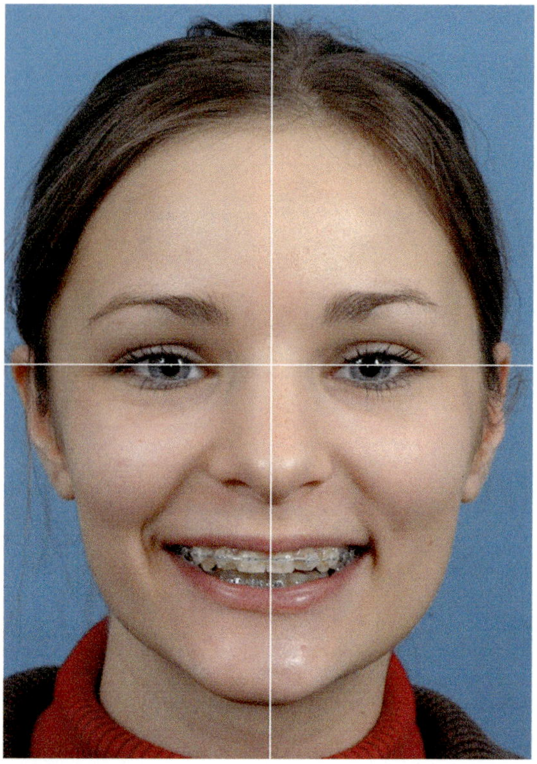

Fig. 6.18 Pre-surgical clinical frontal smiling view of patient D.C.M. at the time of the workup, approximately 3 weeks prior to surgery. Note the 1 mm upper dental midline deviation to the right. Note that the chin deviation to the right is more striking during smiling

Case 2: Class II, Short Face, v-NHP and PHP

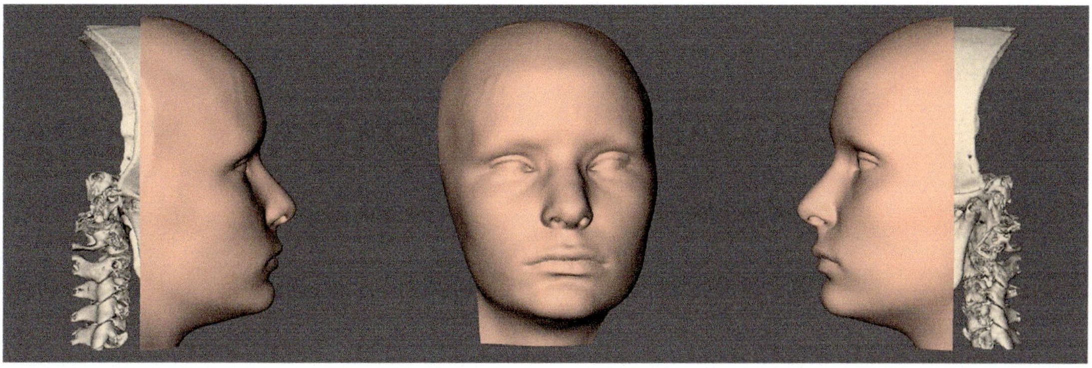

Fig. 6.19 Pre-surgical 3D "surface-rendered" right profile, frontal and left profile soft and hard tissue representations of the head of patient D.C.M., as generated during standardised CBCT image acquisition, at the time of the workup of patient D.C.M. (Maxilim v. 2.3.0.3). Note the incorrect position and orientation of the virtual head compared to the clinical pictures of patient D.C.M. (Fig. 6.17), although it was attempted to scan the patient in her correct *c*-NHP in rest

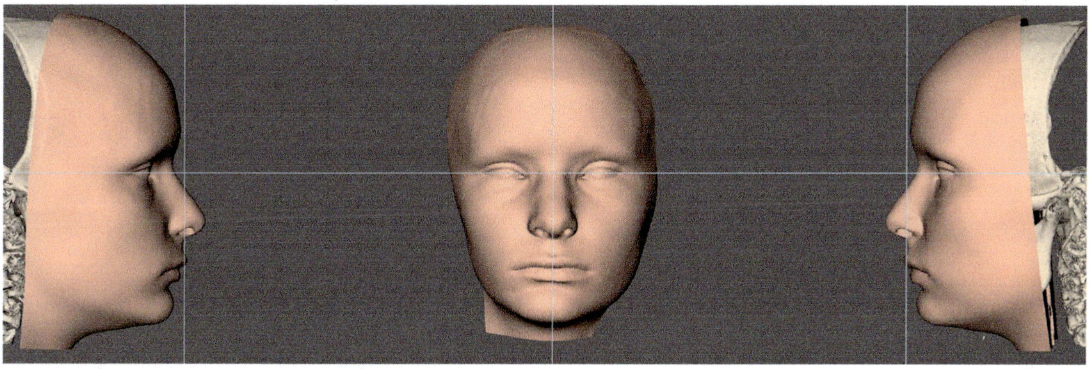

Fig. 6.20 Following a standardised "step-by-step" approach (▶ see Sect. 3.1), the scanned head position of patient D.C.M. (Fig. 6.19) was virtually modified towards her *c*-NHP (Fig. 6.17), which results in her *v*-NHP and corresponds to her individual "Planning Head Position (PHP)" (3D "surface-rendered" representations, patient D.C.M., Maxilim v. 2.3.0.3)

Case 2: Class II, Short Face, v-NHP and PHP

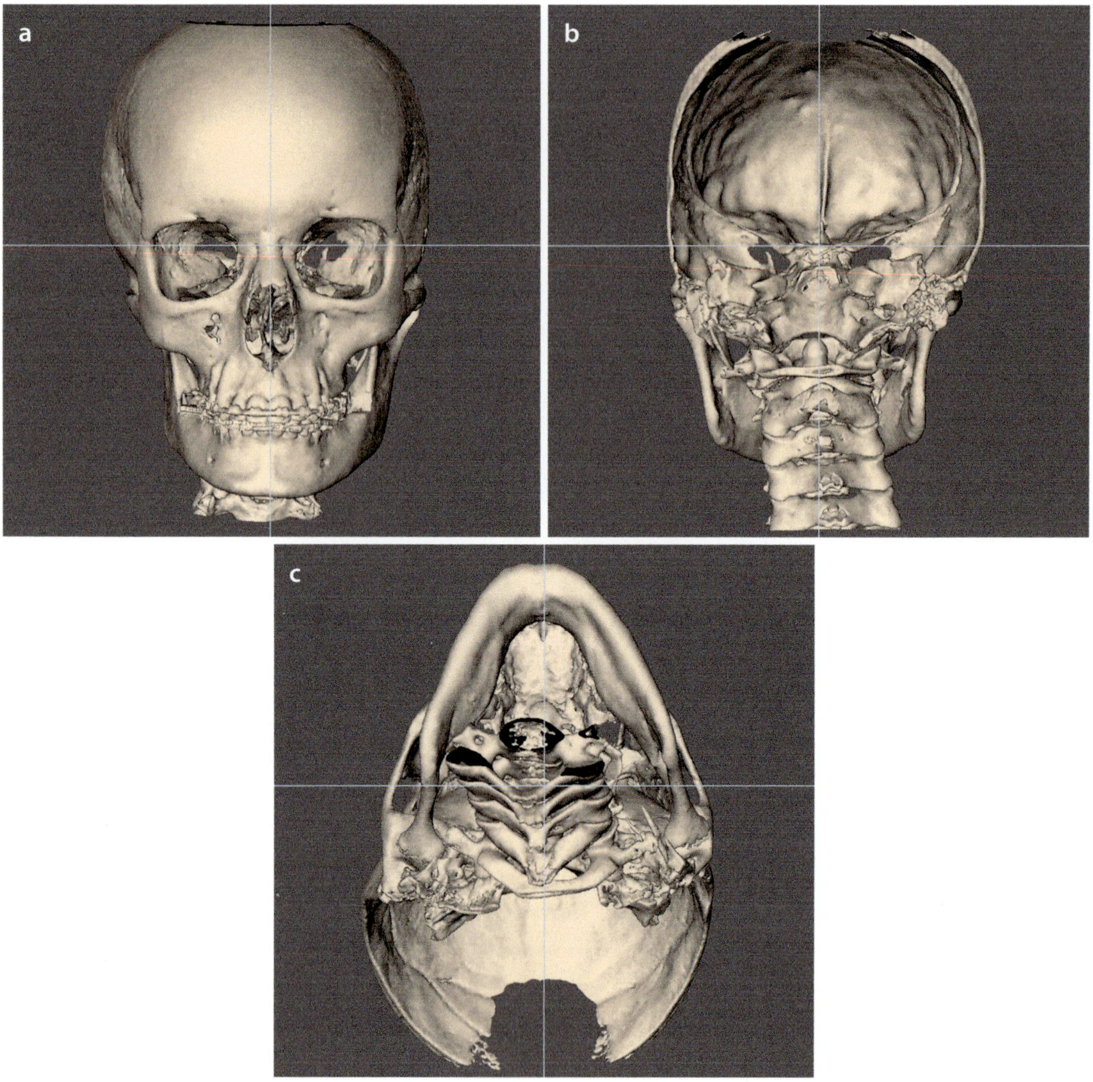

Fig. 6.21 The pre-surgical 3D "surface-rendered" frontal (**a**), posterior (**b**) and base (**c**) hard tissue representations of the virtual head of patient D.C.M., in her individual "Planning Head Position (PHP)" illustrate an important asymmetry of the cranial base and cervical torticollis

Case 2: Class II, Short Face

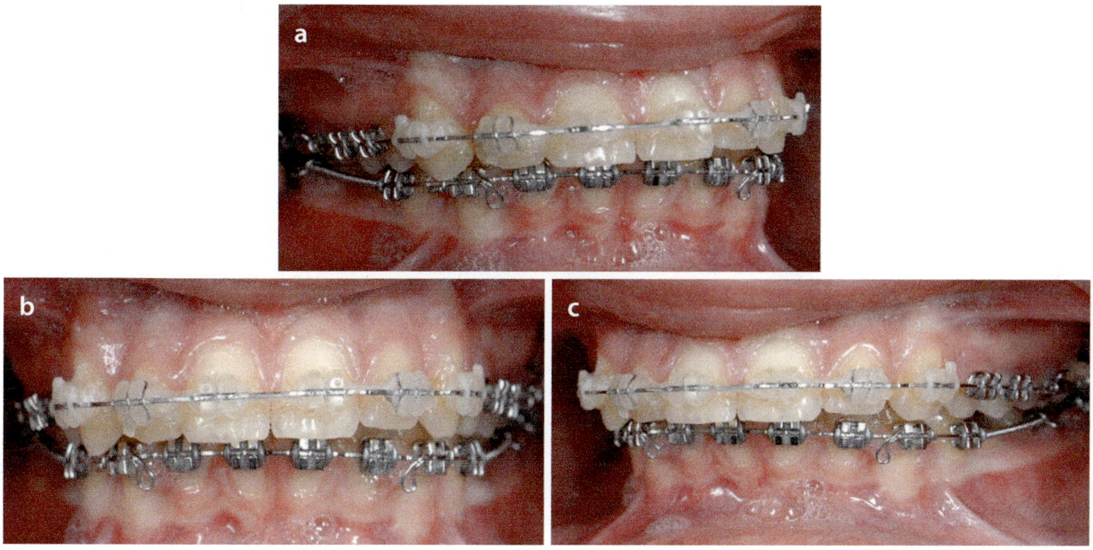

Fig. 6.22 Pre-surgical frontal (**a**), right (**b**) and left (**c**) intra-oral views of patient's D.C.M. occlusion at the time of the workup, approximately 3 weeks prior to surgery

■ Case 2: 3D-VPS$_5$ Step 1 Maxillary Occlusal Cant Evaluation/Correction ("Roll")

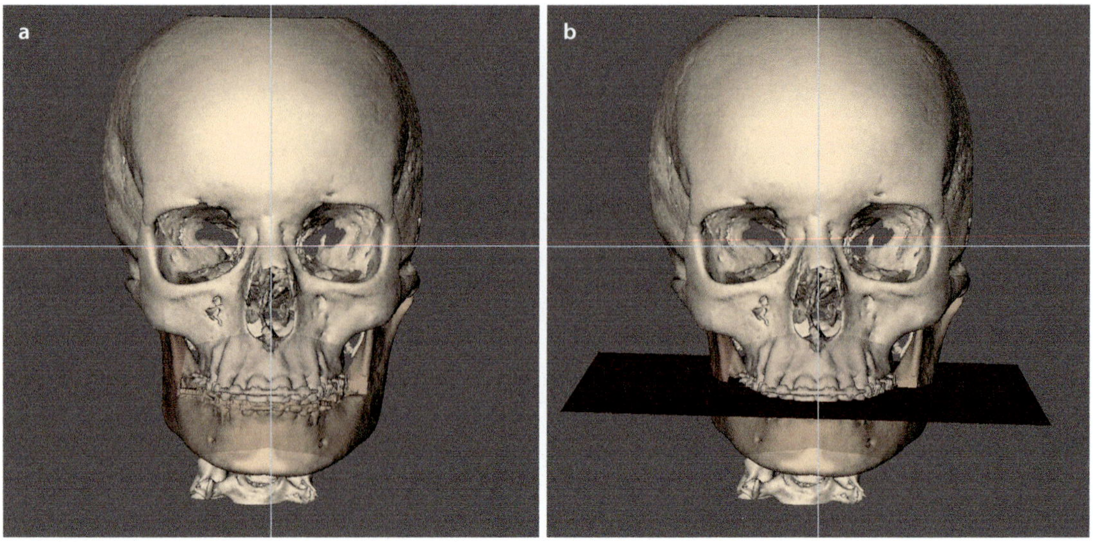

Fig. 6.23 The maxillary occlusal plane is evaluated both clinically (Fig. 6.18) and virtually (**a**) towards the horizontal 3D PHP reference plane in patient D.C.M. and shows virtually a clear cant (**b**) (3D "surface-rendered" representations, patient D.C.M., Maxilim v. 2.3.0.3). Note that this cant is clinically (Fig. 6.18) not so obvious

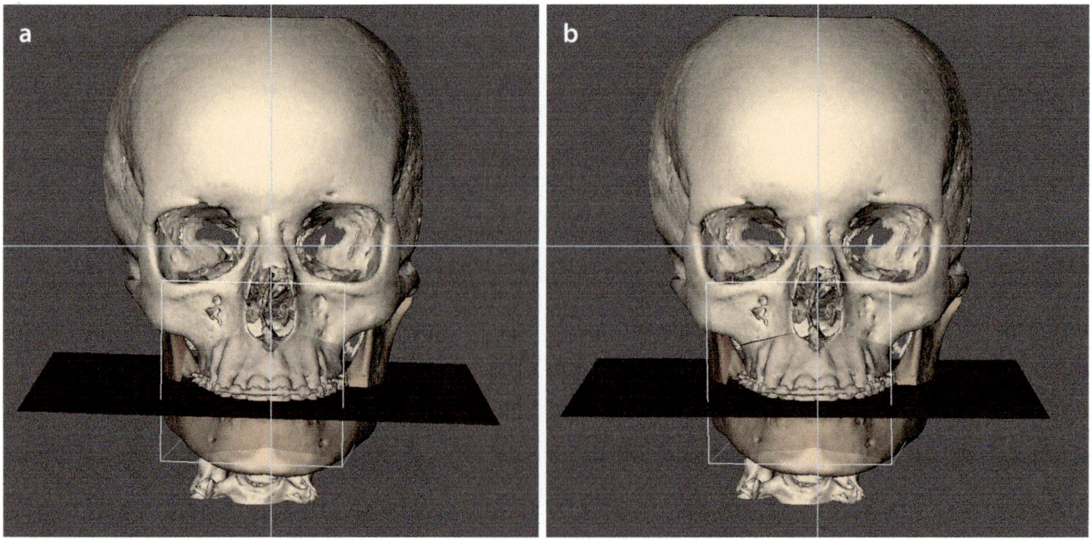

Fig. 6.24 The maxillary cant (**a**) in patient D.C.M. is corrected towards the horizontal 3D PHP reference plane by a CCW "Roll" rotational movement (**b**) (3D "surface-rendered" representations, Maxilim v. 2.3.0.3)

Case 2: 3D-VPS$_5$ Step 2 Upper Dental Midline Evaluation/Correction

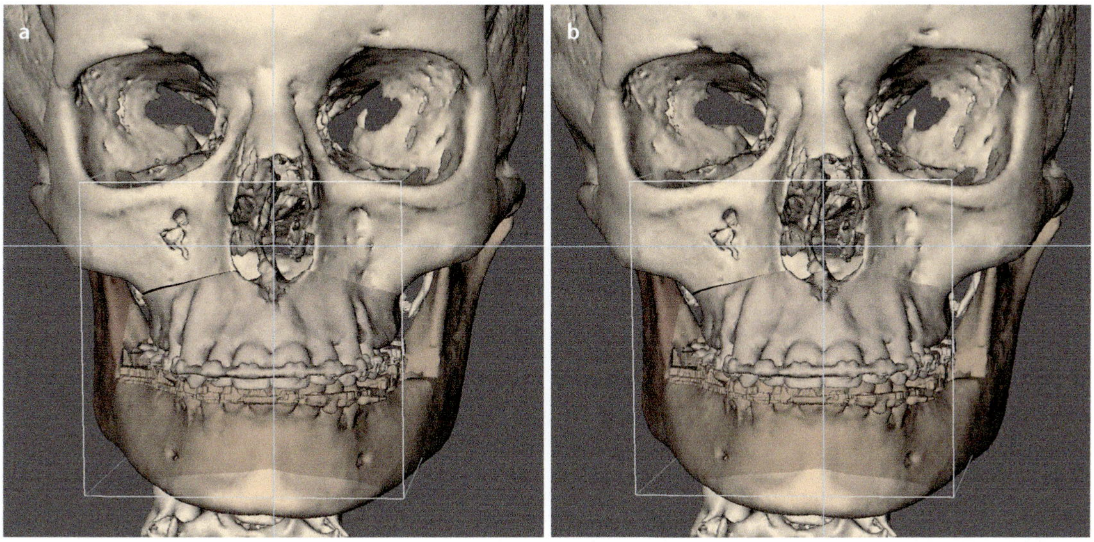

Fig. 6.25 The 1 mm deviation of the upper dental midline to the right (**a**) is corrected towards the facial midline 3D PHP reference plane, by a pure translational movement to the left in patient D.C.M. (**b**) (3D "surface-rendered" representations, Maxilim v. 2.3.0.3)

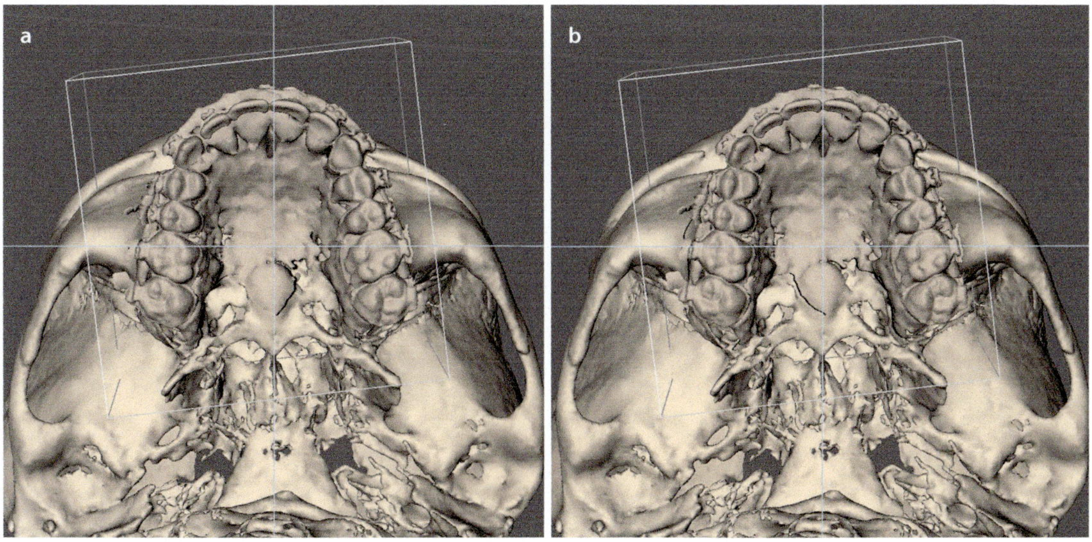

Fig. 6.26 The base views illustrate that the 1 mm deviation of the upper dental midline to the right (**a**) is corrected towards the facial midline 3D PHP reference plane, by a pure translational movement to the left (**b**) in patient D.C.M. (3D "surface-rendered" representations, Maxilim v. 2.3.0.3)

■ Case 2: 3D-VPS$_5$ Step 3 Overall Evaluation of Facial Asymmetry After Virtual Occlusal Definition

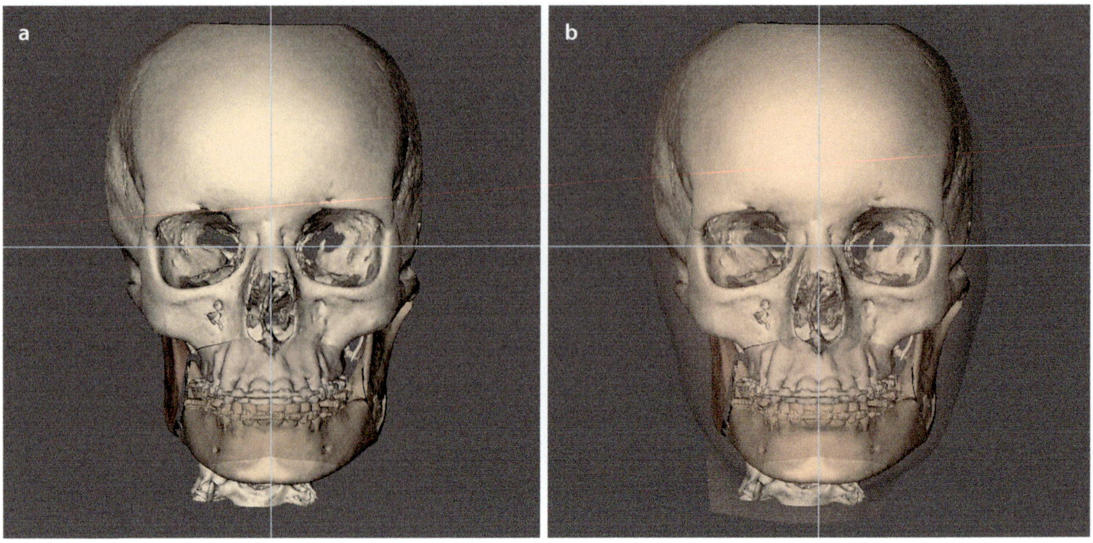

Fig. 6.27 Overall facial asymmetry of the head of patient D.C.M. (**a**) with transparent soft tissues (**b**) is assessed after virtual occlusal definition in the frontal view towards both the horizontal and facial midline 3D PHP reference planes. (3D "surface-rendered" representations, Maxilim v. 2.3.0.3). Note the flaring of the mandibular body to the left

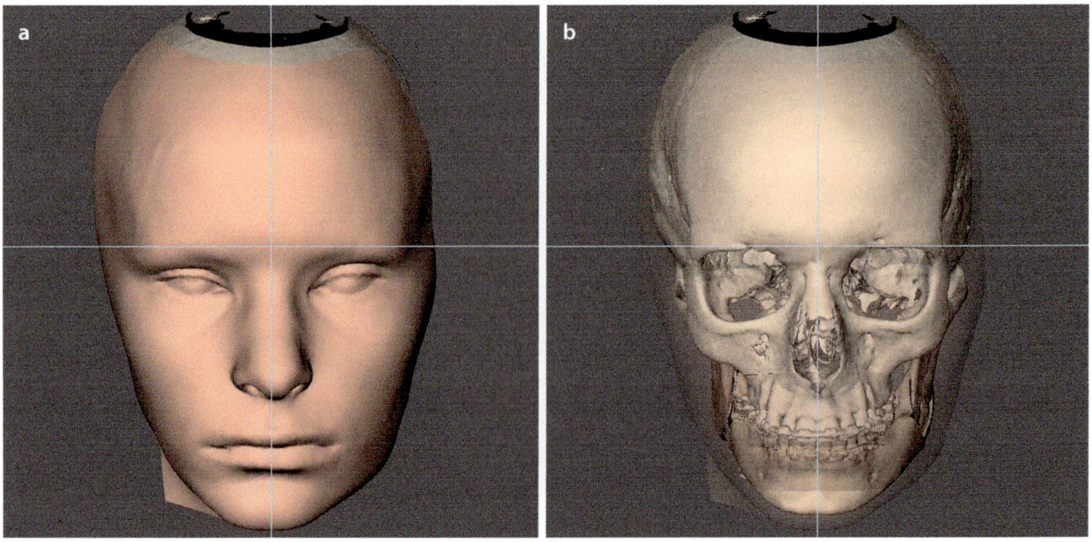

Fig. 6.28 To evaluate the overall facial asymmetry after virtual occlusal definition, the mandibular contour is evaluated both virtually on the soft tissues (**a**) and at the bony level towards the contour of the zygomatic bones and arches with soft tissues in transparency (**b**) (3D "surface-rendered" representations, patient D.C.M., Maxilim v. 2.3.0.3). Note the flaring of the mandibular body to the left

Case 2: 3D-VPS$_5$ Step 4 Evaluation/Correction of Flaring ("Yaw")

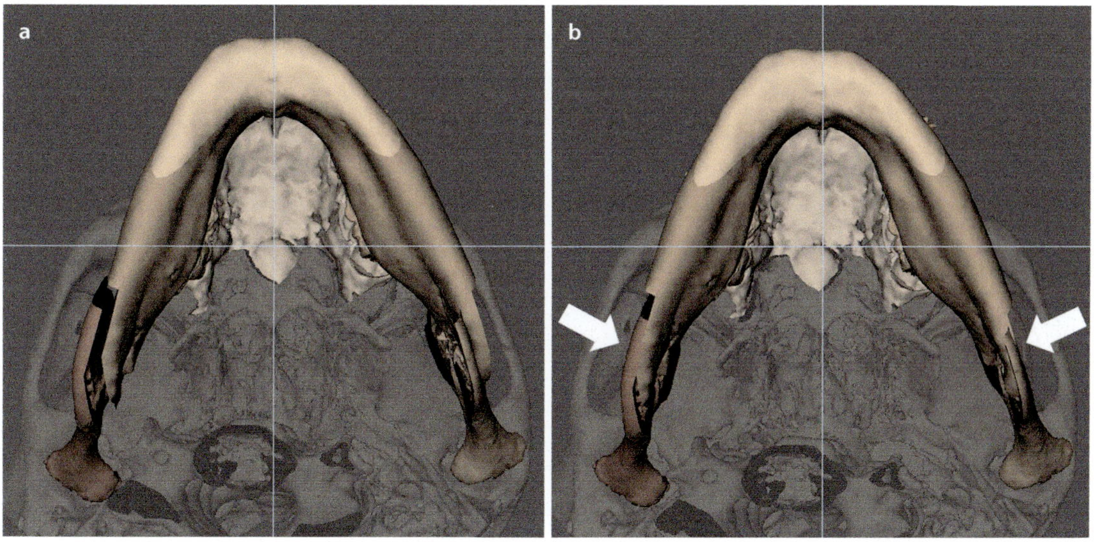

Fig. 6.29 The base views show that the flaring of the mandibular body to the left (**a**) is corrected by a CW "Yaw" rotational movement to the right (**b**) in patient D.C.M. (3D "surface-rendered" representations, Maxilim v. 2.3.0.3). Note the virtual bony overlap between the distal and proximal mandibular fragments at the left side

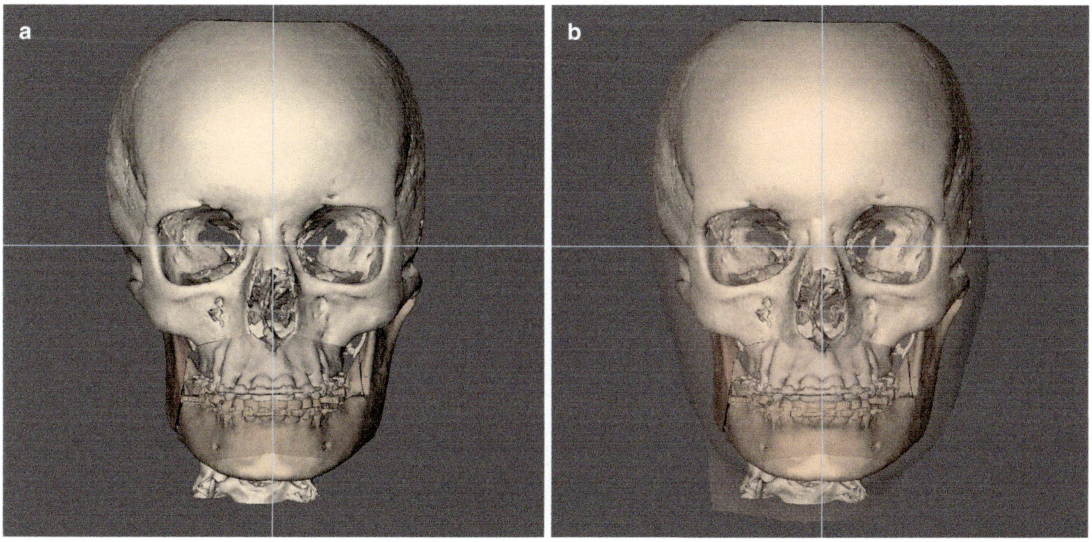

Fig. 6.30 Overall assessment of facial bony contour (**a**) with transparent soft tissues (**b**) after correction of flaring to the left by a "Yaw" rotational movement of the maxillo-mandibular complex to the right (3D "surface-rendered" representations, patient D.C.M., Maxilim v. 2.3.0.3)

Case 2: 3D-VPS$_5$ Step 5 Upper Vertical Incisal Position Evaluation/Correction

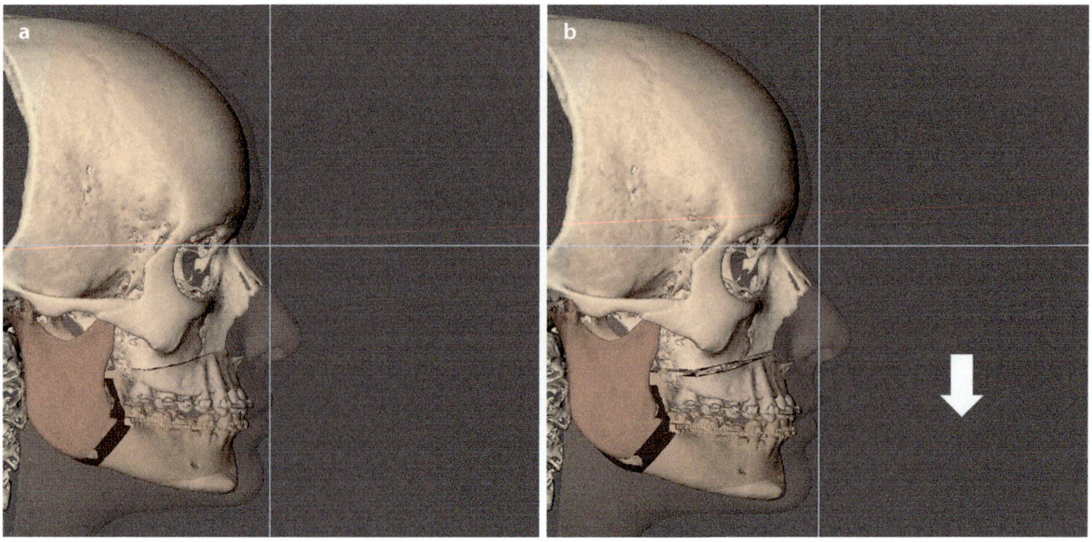

Fig. 6.31 Since patient D.C.M. has in rest only 1 mm and during spontaneous smiling only 8 mm upper incisal exposure (Fig. 6.18), it was decided clinically at this stage in "step 5" to virtually extrude the maxilla 2 mm at the upper incisal level (3D "surface-rendered" representations, patient D.C.M., Maxilim v. 2.3.0.3): before (**a**) and after (**b**) correction

Case 2: 3D-VPS$_5$ Step 6 Sagittal Upper Incisal Position Evaluation/Correction

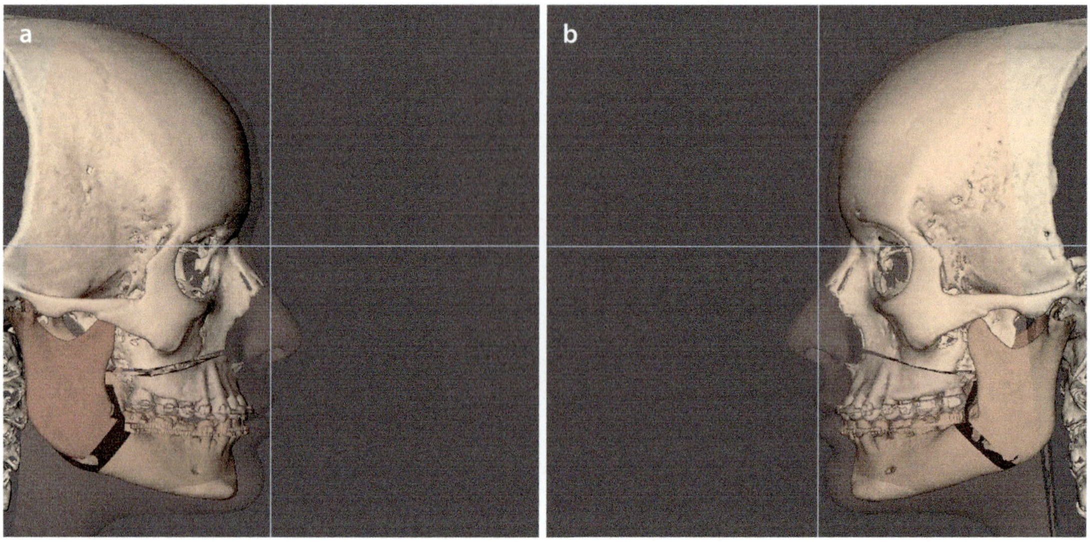

Fig. 6.32 From clinical examination but also 3D cephalometric analysis, it was decided not to advance the "maxillo-mandibular complex in final occlusion" in patient D.C.M. (3D "surface-rendered" representations, Maxilim v. 2.3.0.3). Profile views right (**a**) and left (**b**)

Case 2: 3D-VPS$_5$ Step 7 Profile Evaluation/Occlusal Plane Correction ("Pitch")

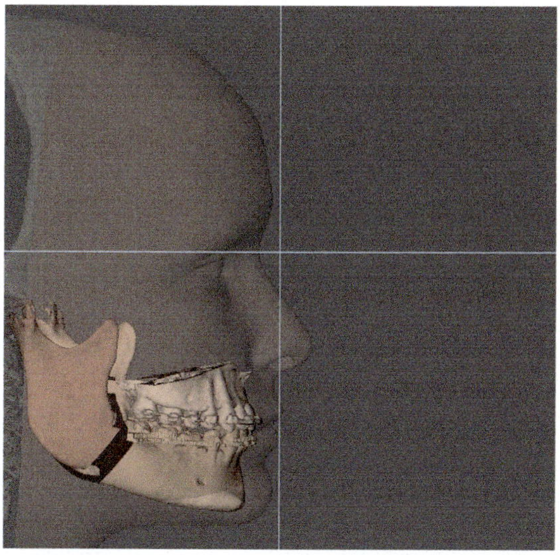

Fig. 6.33 At this stage in "step 7", the profile and dento-alveolar support of the upper lip are evaluated (3D "surface-rendered" representations, patient D.C.M., Maxilim v. 2.3.0.3)

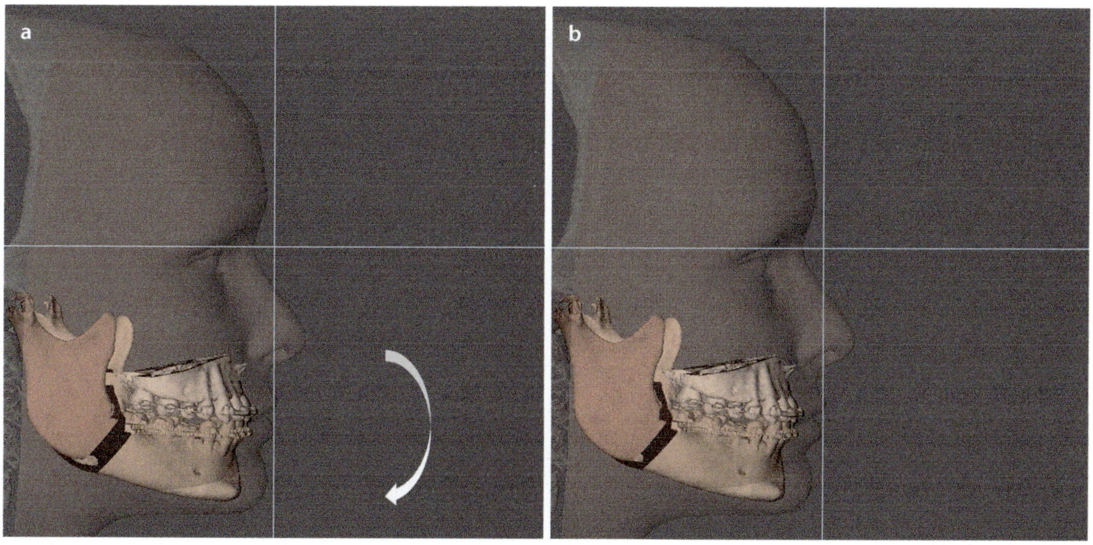

Fig. 6.34 Based on clinical and 3D cephalometric analysis, it was decided to perform a 2° CW occlusal plane rotation with the centre of rotation at the incisal level by a "Pitch" rotational movement (3D "surface-rendered" representations, patient D.C.M., Maxilim v. 2.3.0.3): before (**a**) and after (**b**) correction

Case 2: 3D-VPS$_5$ Step 8 3D Chin Position Evaluation/Correction

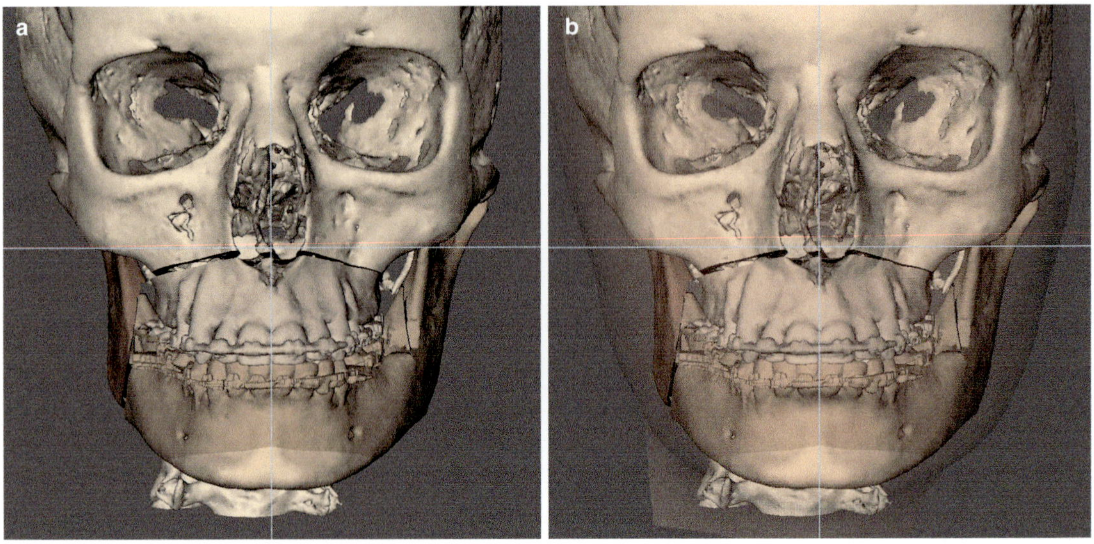

Fig. 6.35 Evaluation of the bony chin position in the frontal plane without (**a**) and with (**b**) the patient's 3D facial soft tissue mask in transparency (3D "surface-rendered" representations, patient D.C.M., Maxilim v. 2.3.0.3) does not show an obvious skeletal chin deviation neither asymmetry

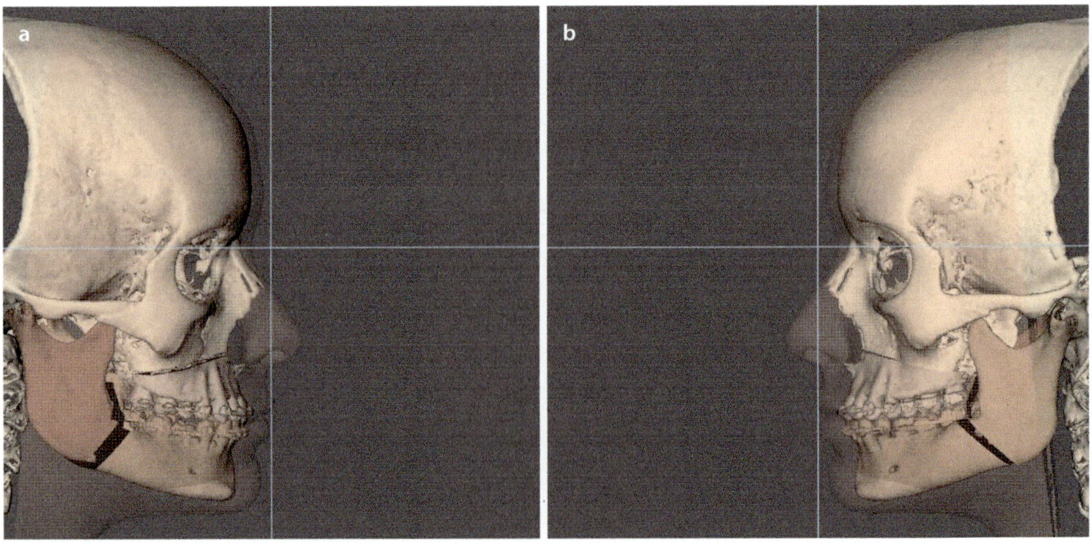

Fig. 6.36 Evaluation of the right (**a**) and left profile (**b**) views shows an adequate sagittal position of the chin in the face with a well-defined plica labio-mentalis. (3D "surface-rendered" representations, patient D.C.M., Maxilim v. 2.3.0.3). Note the nice 3D virtual soft tissue simulation at the level of the lips

Case 2: 3D-VPS$_5$ Step 9 Patient Communication of the Individualised Treatment Plan

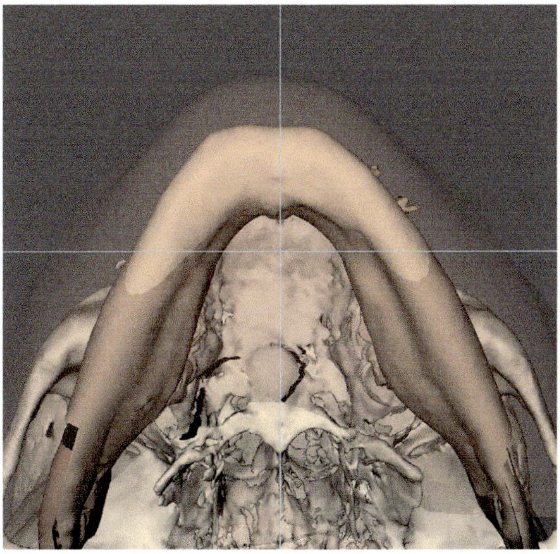

Fig. 6.37 Evaluation of the bony and soft tissue chin position in the base view however still shows a slight chin deviation to the right with asymmetric contour in patient D.C.M. (3D "surface-rendered" representations, Maxilim v. 2.3.0.3)

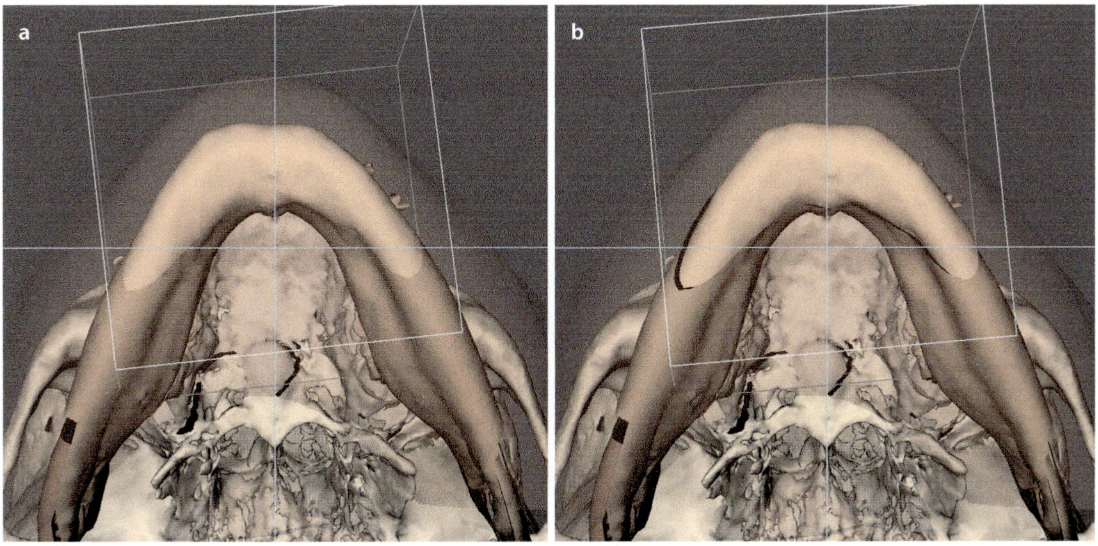

Fig. 6.38 At this stage, in "step 9", it is shown to the patient that the slight chin deviation and asymmetry can be additionally corrected by a 1.5 mm translation to the left with a subtile CCW "Yaw" rotational movement (3D "surface-rendered" representations, Maxilim v. 2.3.0.3). Before (**a**) and after (**b**) additional correction

▪ Case 2: 3D-VPS$_5$ Step 10 Final Adjustments of the 3D Virtual Treatment Plan

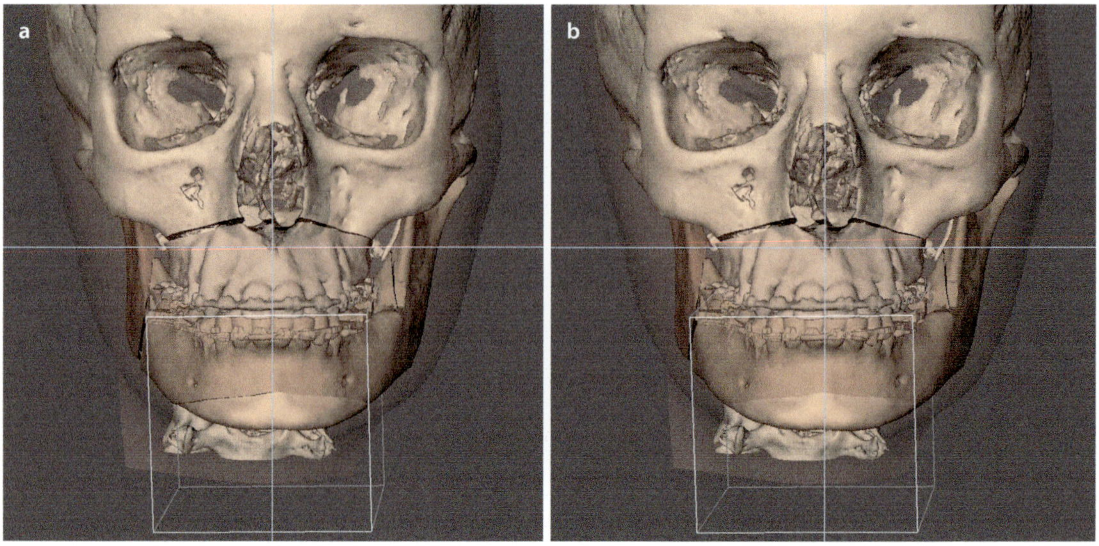

Fig. 6.39 In "step 10", after the final communication with patient D.C.M., it was decided not to perform final adjustments of the 3D virtual treatment plan anymore (3D "surface-rendered" representations, patient D.C.M., Maxilim v. 2.3.0.3). Frontal view with (**a**) and without (**b**) additional chin correction

Case 2: 3D-VPS$_5$ – Final Integrated "Individualised 3D Virtual Treatment Plan"

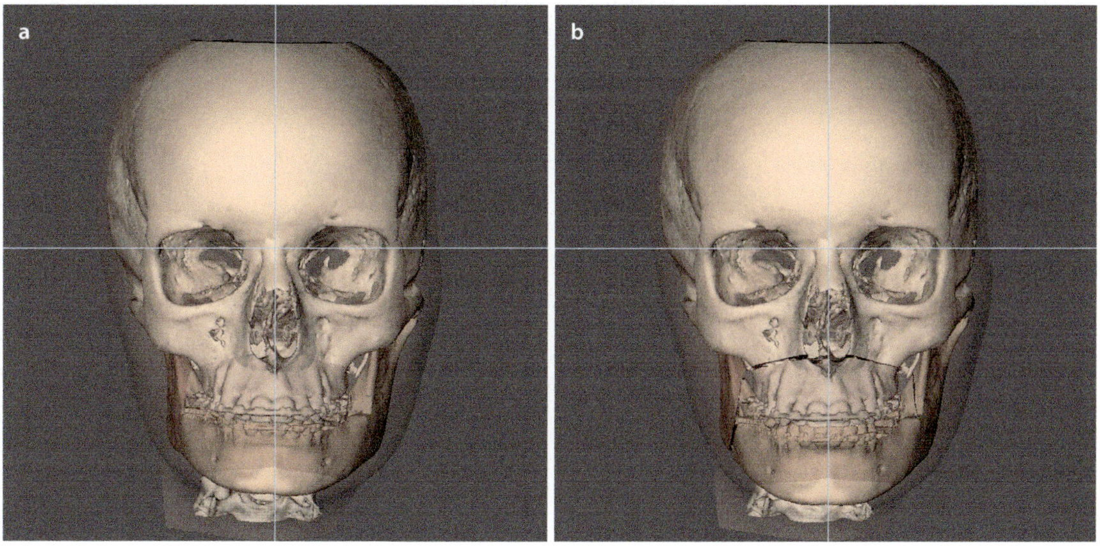

Fig. 6.40 Initial situation (**a**), and final "Individualised 3D Virtual Treatment Plan" (**b**), in the frontal plane (3D "surface-rendered" representations, patient D.C.M., Maxilim v. 2.3.0.3)

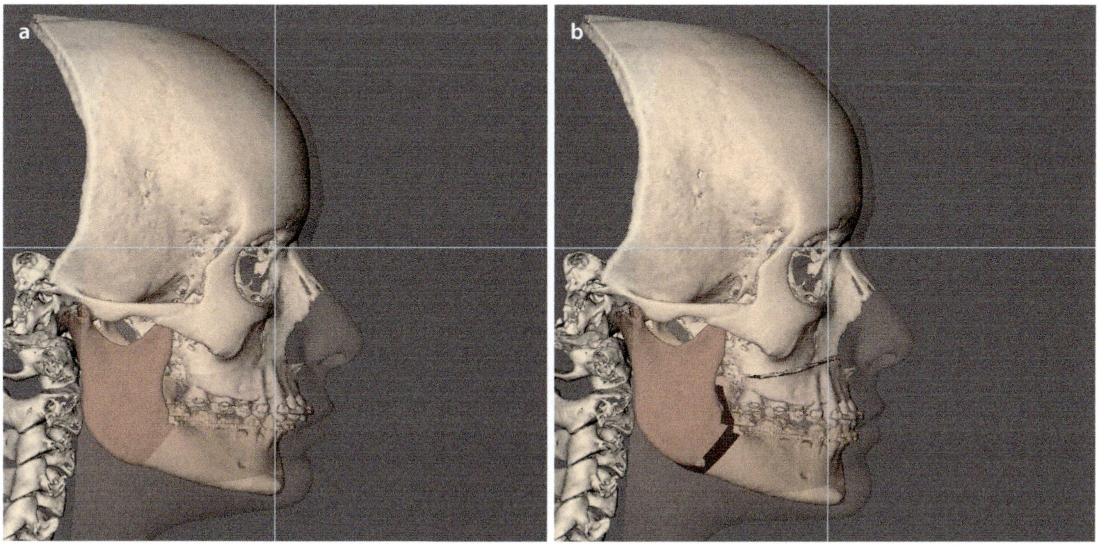

Fig. 6.41 Initial situation (**a**), and final "Individualised 3D Virtual Treatment Plan" (**b**), in the right profile plane (3D "surface-rendered" representations, patient D.C.M., Maxilim v. 2.3.0.3). Note the nice 3D virtual soft tissue simulation

Case 2: 3D-VPS$_5$- Final Integrated "Individualised 3D Virtual Treatment Plan"

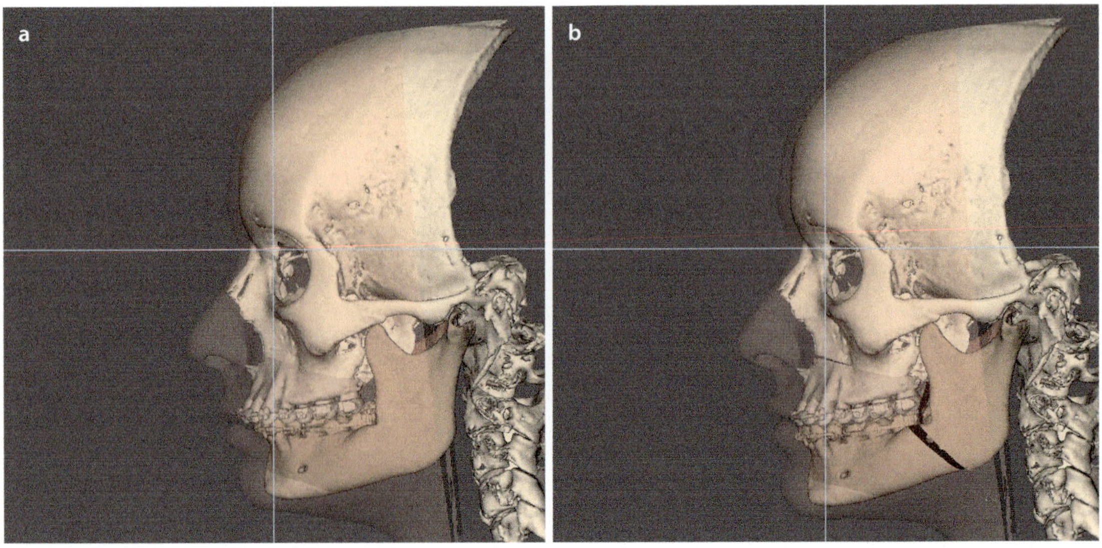

Fig. 6.42 Initial situation (**a**), and final "Individualised 3D Virtual Treatment Plan" (**b**), in the left profile plane (3D "surface-rendered" representations, patient D.C.M., Maxilim v. 2.3.0.3). Note the nice 3D virtual soft tissue simulation

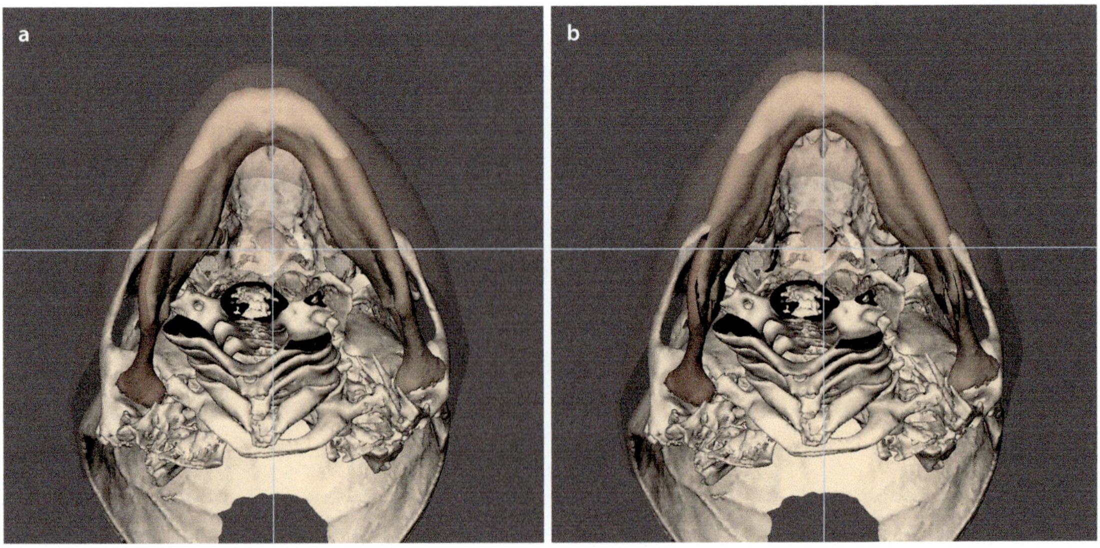

Fig. 6.43 Initial situation (**a**), and final "Individualised 3D Virtual Treatment Plan" (**b**), in the base plane (3D "surface-rendered" representations, patient D.C.M., Maxilim v. 2.3.0.3)

Case 2: "3D Virtual Treatment Planning, OR" Template

Maxillary osteotomy

- [x] Le Fort: [x] I [ ] II [ ] III
- [x] One-piece
- [ ] Segmental:
  - Pieces: ....
  - Interdental: ....
- [x] Advancement: 0.0 mm
- [ ] Set-back: ....
- [x] Midline: 1.0 mm [ ] R [x] L
- [x] Midline after Le Fort 1: inbetween 31/41
- [x] Vertical: (→)
- [x] "Yaw" correction: CW to the right
- [ ] Other: ....

Mandibular osteotomy

- [x] SSO [x] R [x] L
- [ ] Inverted-L [ ] R [ ] L
- [ ] VRO [ ] R [ ] L
- [x] Advancement: R 7.0 mm L 5.0 mm
- [ ] Set-back: R .... L ....
- [x] CW "Pitch" rotation
- [ ] CCW "Pitch" rotation
- [ ] Midline split
- [x] IAN course: R lingual L lingual
- [ ] Midline after BSSO: ....
- [ ] Other: ....

Chin osteotomy

- [ ] Advancement: ....
- [ ] Set-back: ....
- [ ] Midline: .... [ ] R [ ] L
- [ ] Intrusion:
  - [ ] Anterior: ....
  - [ ] Posterior: R ...... L ......
- [ ] Extrusion:
  - [ ] Anterior: ....
  - [ ] Posterior: R ...... L ......
- [ ] "Shield" osteotomy
- [ ] "Chin wing" osteotomy
  - *Mental Foramen level:*
    - [ ] Symmetric
    - [ ] Asymmetric
- [ ] Other: ....

Planning Requirements

- [x] Maxilla first
- [ ] Mandible first
- [ ] Minimally Invasive Le Fort I
- [ ] IO-CBCT
- [ ] Kobayashi wires: ....
- [ ] Skeletal anchorage: ....
- [ ] Orthodontic buttons: ....
- [ ] Occlusal grinding: ....
- [ ] Other: ....

1.5 mm	2.0 mm	2.0 mm	1.0 mm	0.0 mm
16	13	11	23	26

"Roll" correction: [ ] CW [x] CCW

Miscellaneous

- [x] Para-nasal cross sutures
- [ ] Alar cinch
- [ ] Septoplasty
- [ ] Inferior turbinectomy
- [ ] ANS: [ ] Shortening [ ] Midline
- [ ] Nasal base plasty [ ] R [ ] L
- [ ] Lateral nasal wall plasty [ ] R [ ] L
- [ ] Bone graft(s): ....
- [ ] Extraction(s): ....
- [ ] Other: ....

Adjuvant Cosmetic Procedures

- [ ] Bichatectomy [ ] R [ ] L
- [ ] Zygoma osteotomies [ ] R [ ] L
  - *Infraorbital Foramen level:*
    - [ ] Symmetric
    - [ ] Asymmetric
- [ ] Otoplasty: [ ] R [ ] L
- [ ] Rhinoplasty: ....
- [ ] Browlift: ....
- [ ] Blepharoplasty: ....
  - [ ] Upper [ ] Lower
- [ ] Facelift: ....
- [ ] Necklift: ....
- [ ] Liposuction: ....
- [ ] Lipofilling: ....
- [ ] Other: ....

Case 2: Class II, Short Face, 3D Virtual Treatment Outcome

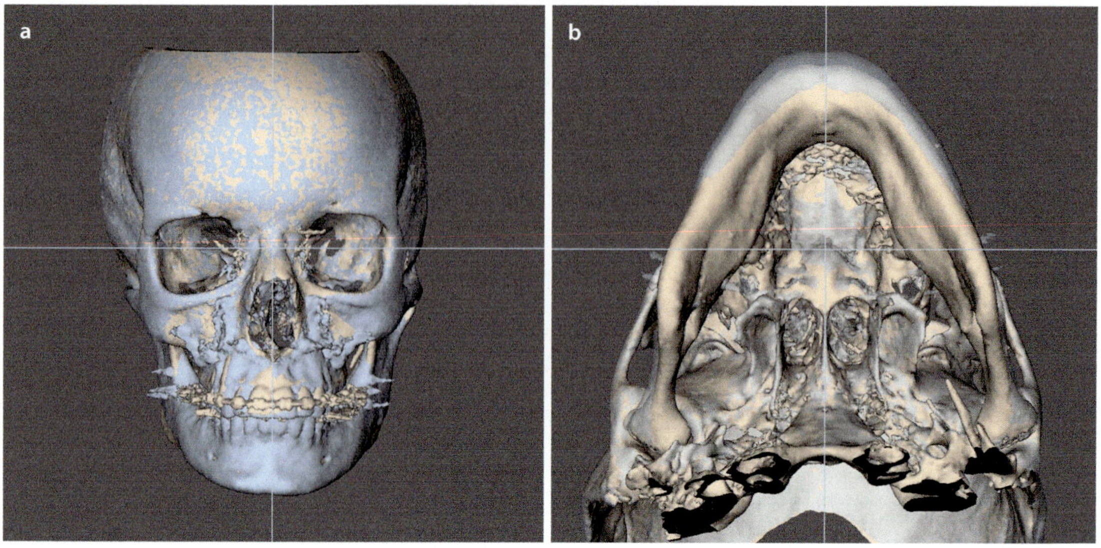

Fig. 6.44 Voxel-based superimposition on the cranial base of the pre-surgical and 10 months post-surgical (*blue*) 3D "surface-rendered" hard tissue representations. Frontal (**a**) and base (**b**) views (i-CAT, Imaging Sciences International Inc., Maxilim v. 2.3.0.3) (patient D.C.M.)

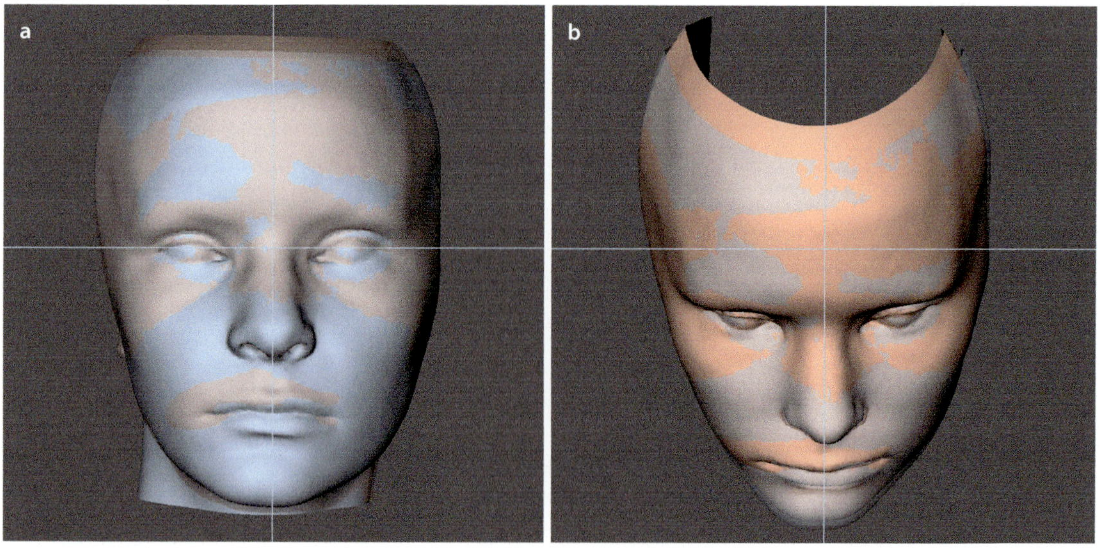

Fig. 6.45 Voxel-based superimposition on the cranial base of the pre-surgical and 10 months post-surgical (*blue*) 3D "surface-rendered" soft tissue representations. Frontal (**a**) and downward inclined (**b**) views (i-CAT, Imaging Sciences International Inc., Maxilim v. 2.3.0.3) (patient D.C.M.). Note the persistent post-surgical (*blue*) slight chin asymmetry and deviation to the right which was decided pre-surgically not to additionally correct

Case 2: Class II, Short Face, 3D Virtual Treatment Outcome

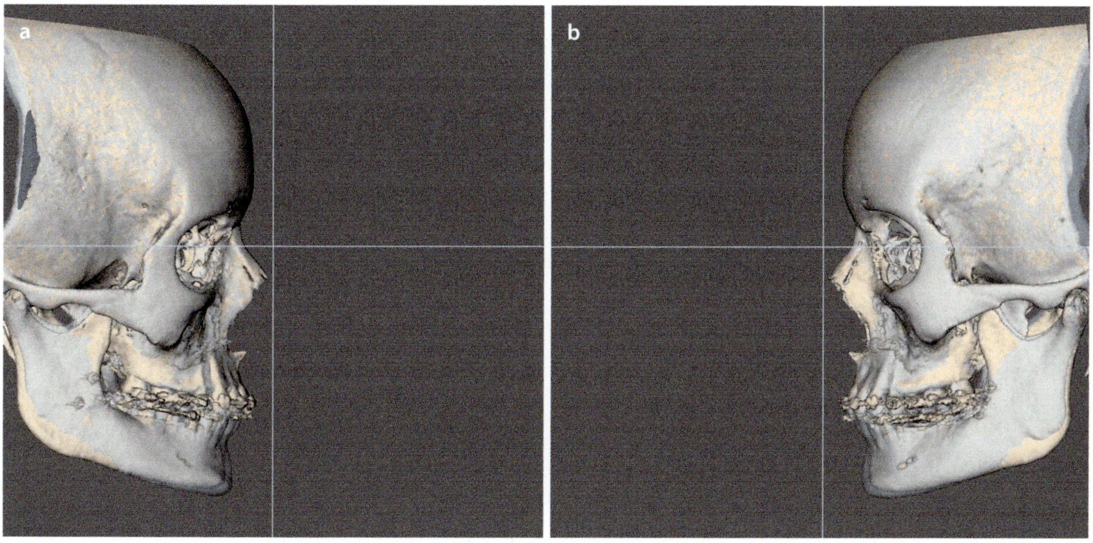

Fig. 6.46 Voxel-based superimposition on the cranial base of the pre-surgical and 10 months post-surgical (*blue*) 3D "surface-rendered" hard tissue representations. Right (**a**) and left (**b**) profile views (i-CAT, Imaging Sciences International Inc., Maxilim v. 2.3.0.3) (patient D.C.M.). Note the CW rotation of the bimaxillary complex

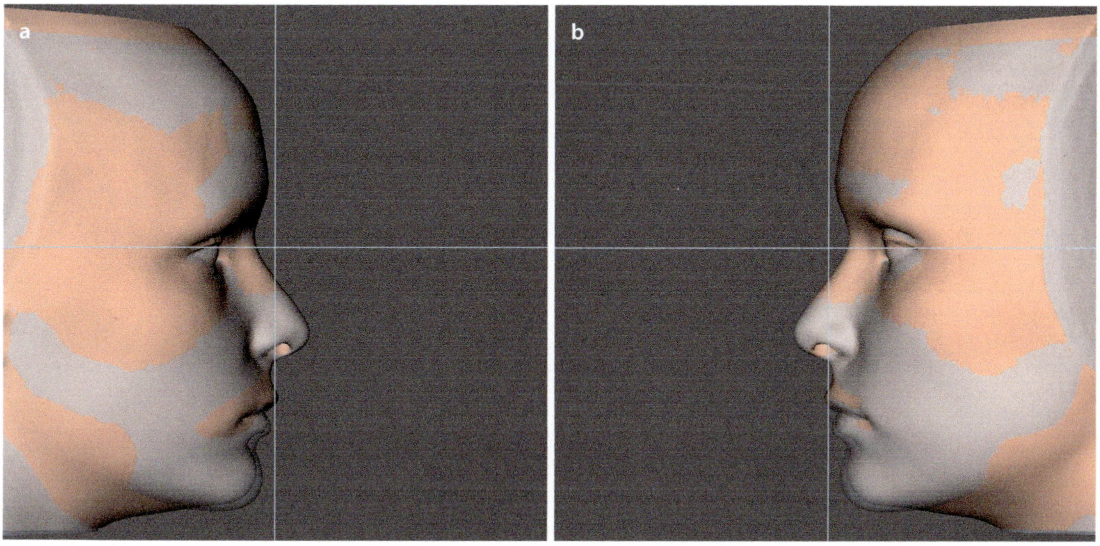

Fig. 6.47 Voxel-based superimposition on the cranial base of the pre-surgical and 10 months post-surgical (*blue*) 3D "surface-rendered" soft tissue representations. Right (**a**) and left (**b**) profile views (i-CAT, Imaging Sciences International Inc., Maxilim v. 2.3.0.3) (patient D.C.M.). Note the changes at the lower lip/chin aesthetic unit. Also note that there are no postural changes of the nose/upper lip aesthetic unit

Case 2: Class II, Short Face, Clinical Treatment Outcome

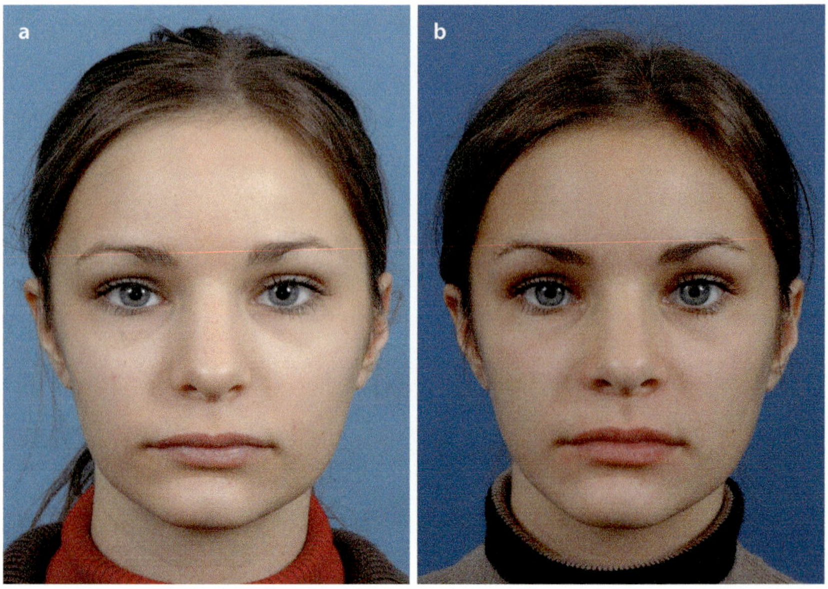

Fig. 6.48 Frontal views in rest, pre-surgical (**a**) and 6 months after (**b**) combined orthodontic-surgical treatment (patient D.C.M.)

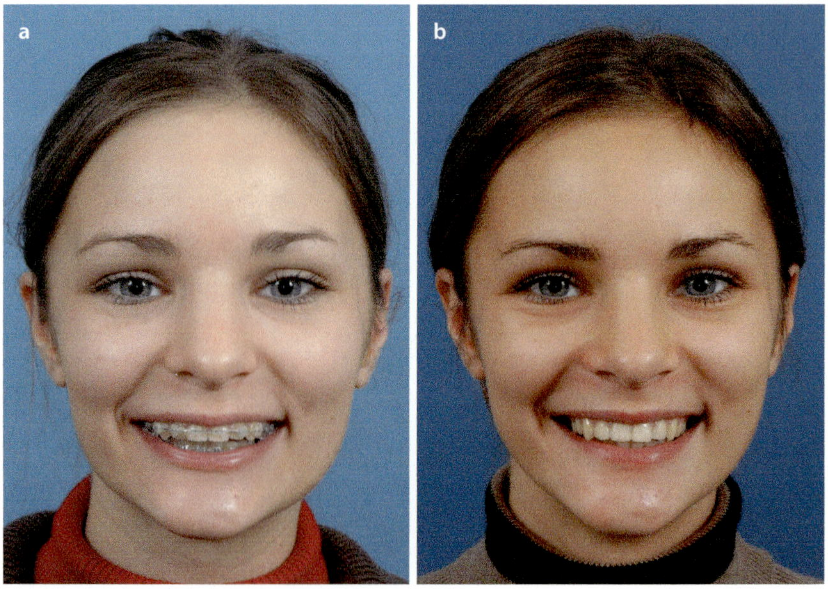

Fig. 6.49 Frontal views during smiling, pre-surgical (**a**) and 6 months after (**b**) combined orthodontic-surgical treatment (patient D.C.M.). Note the jaw movement of the patient's head during clinical photographing in the post-surgical photograph at 6 months which is not present in the 2 years post-surgical clinical photograph (Fig. 6.59b)

Case 2: Class II, Short Face, Clinical Treatment Outcome

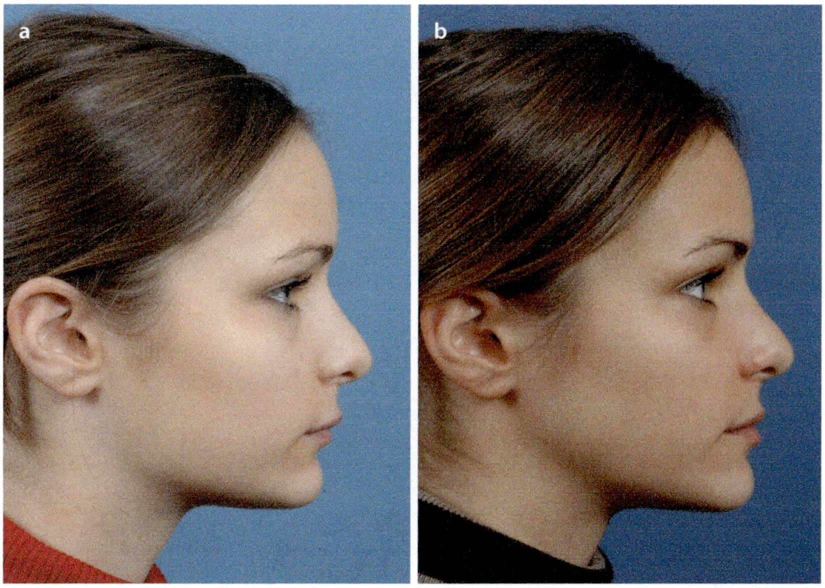

Fig. 6.50 Right profile views in rest, pre-surgical (**a**) and 6 months after (**b**) combined orthodontic-surgical treatment (patient D.C.M.)

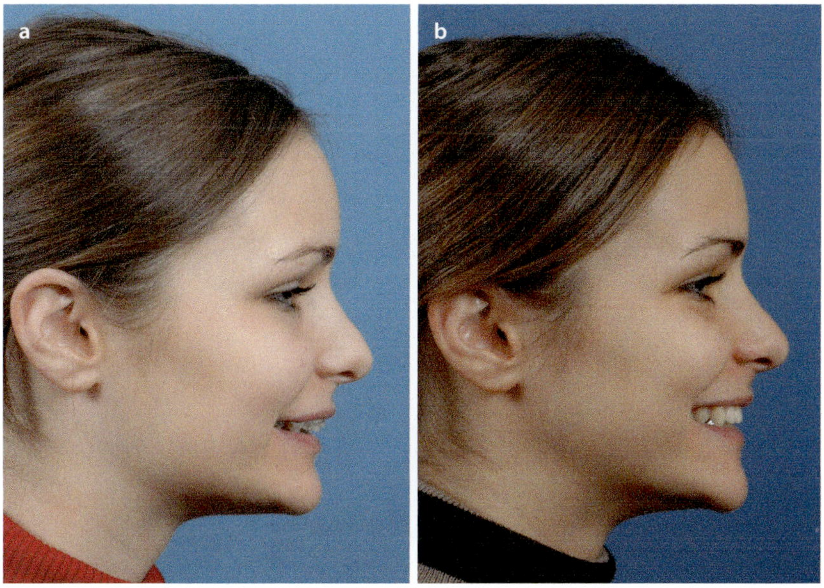

Fig. 6.51 Right profile views during smiling, pre-surgical (**a**) and 6 months after (**b**) combined orthodontic-surgical treatment (patient D.C.M.)

Case 2: Class II, Short Face, Clinical Treatment Outcome

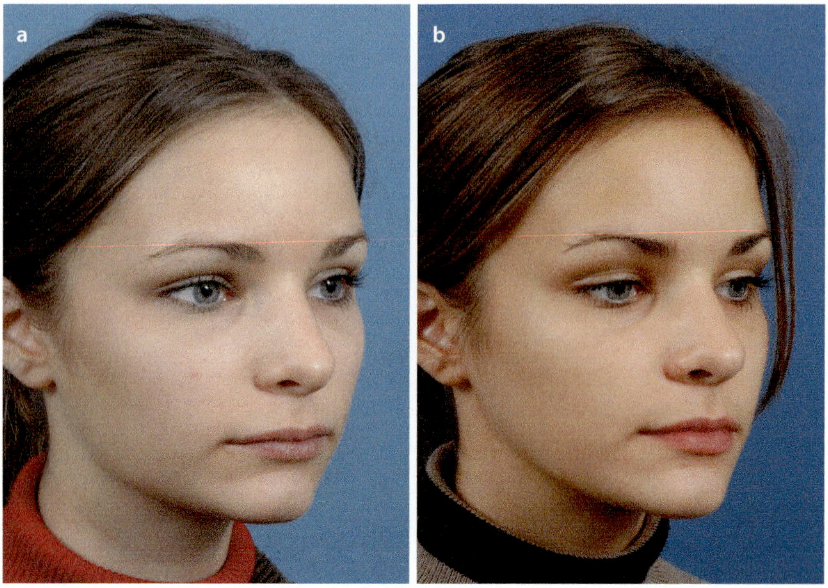

Fig. 6.52 2/3 right profile views in rest, pre-surgical (**a**) and 6 months after (**b**) combined orthodontic-surgical treatment (patient D.C.M.)

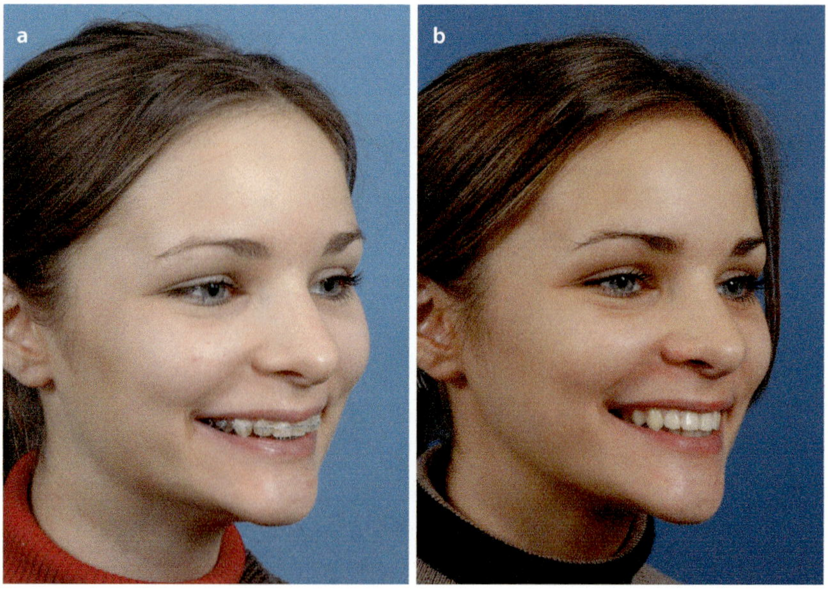

Fig. 6.53 2/3 right profile views during smiling, pre-surgical (**a**) and 6 months after (**b**) combined orthodontic-surgical treatment (patient D.C.M.)

Case 2: Class II, Short Face, Clinical Treatment Outcome

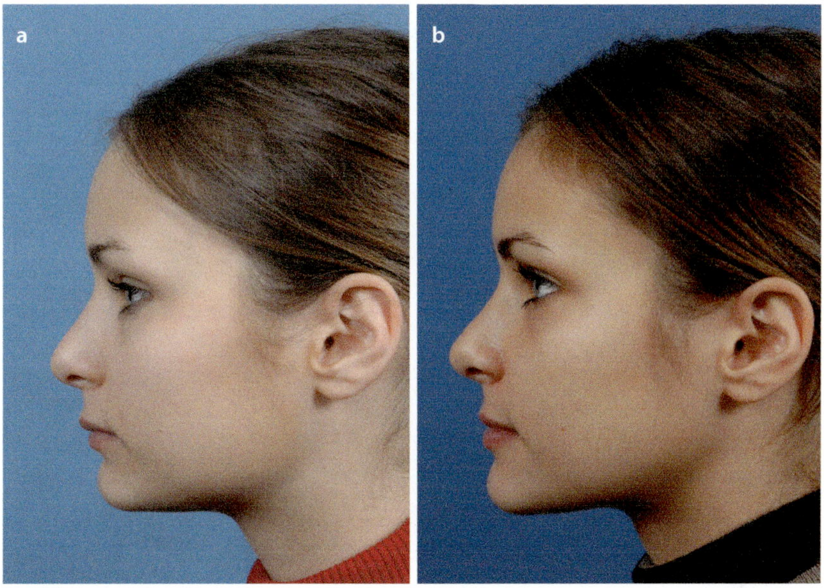

Fig. 6.54 Left profile views in rest, pre-surgical (**a**) and 6 months after (**b**) combined orthodontic-surgical treatment (patient D.C.M.)

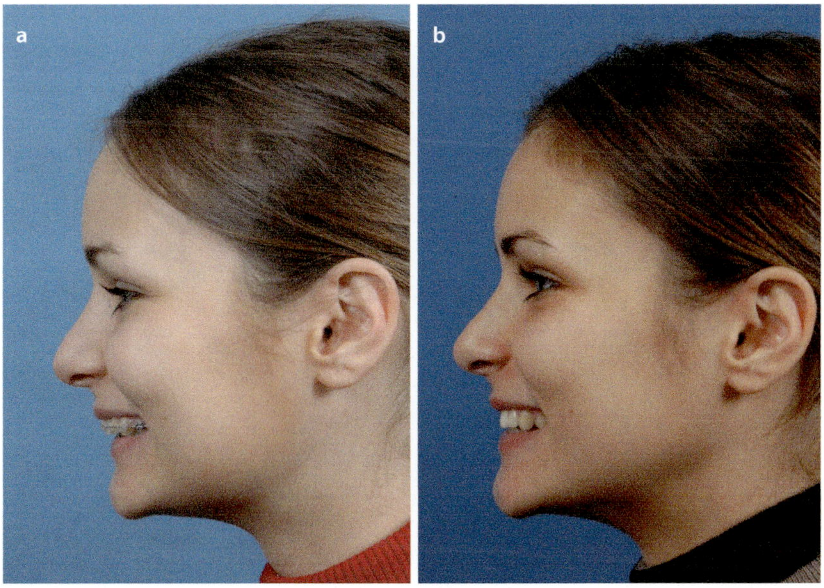

Fig. 6.55 Left profile views during smiling, pre-surgical (**a**) and 6 months after (**b**) combined orthodontic-surgical treatment (patient D.C.M.)

Case 2: Class II, Short Face, Clinical Treatment Outcome

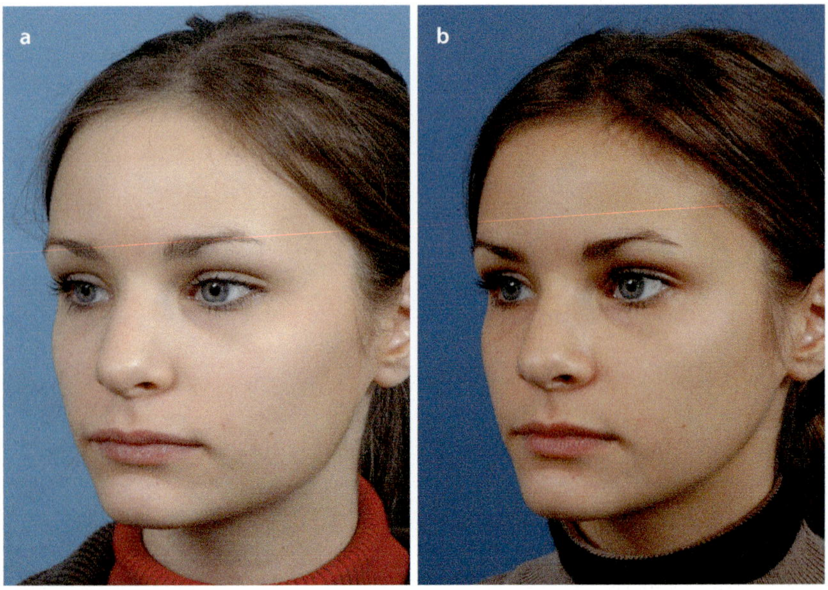

Fig. 6.56 2/3 left profile views in rest, pre-surgical (**a**) and 6 months after (**b**) combined orthodontic-surgical treatment (patient D.C.M.)

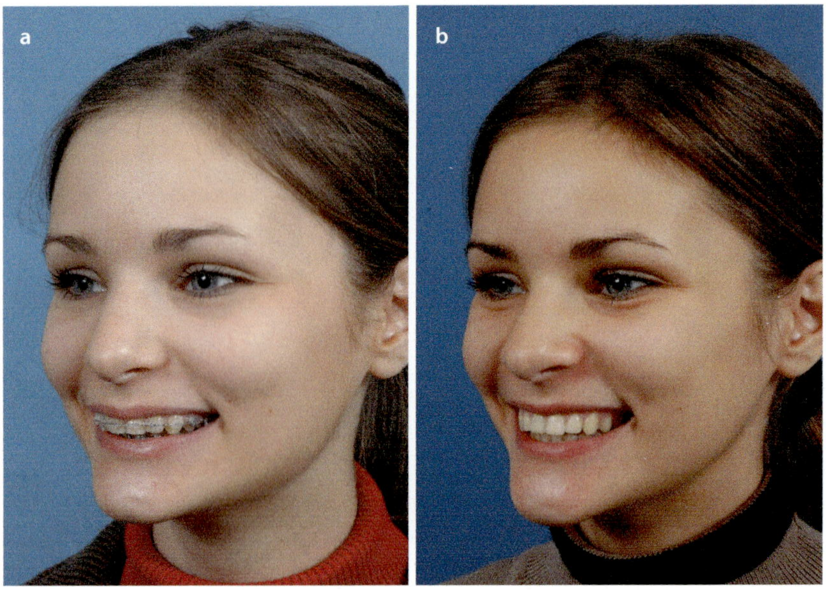

Fig. 6.57 2/3 left profile views during smiling, pre-surgical (**a**) and 6 months after (**b**) combined orthodontic-surgical treatment (patient D.C.M.)

Case 2: Class II, Short Face, Clinical Treatment Outcome

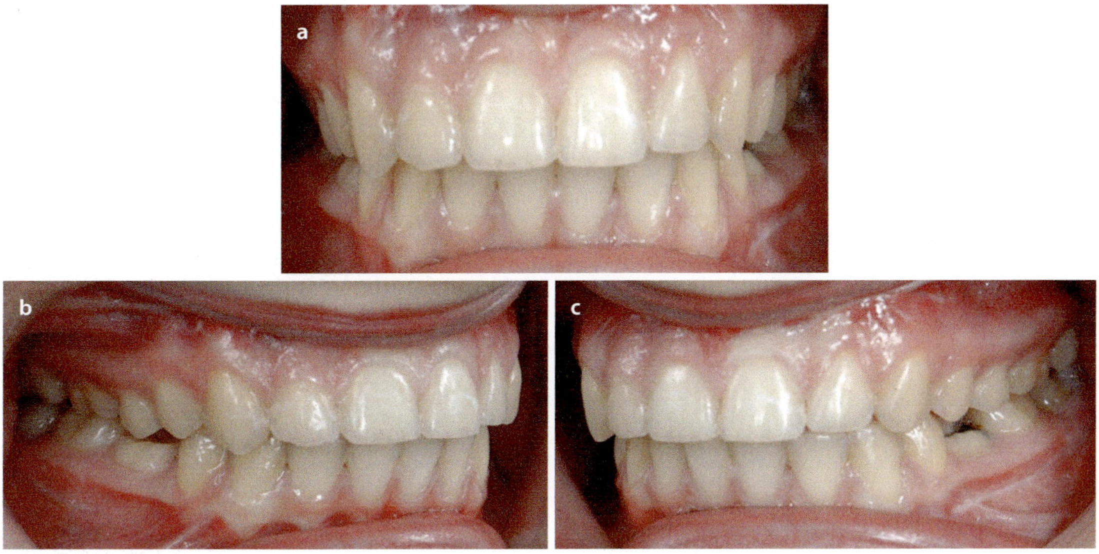

Fig. 6.58 Frontal (**a**), right (**b**) and left (**c**) intra-oral views of the patient's occlusion 6 months after combined orthodontic-surgical treatment (patient D.C.M.). Note the presence of the deciduous second molars in the lower jaw which are kept in place until the age of 19 years to preserve the bone prior to implant-prosthodontic treatment. The author acknowledges Prof. Hugo De Clerck for the orthodontic treatment

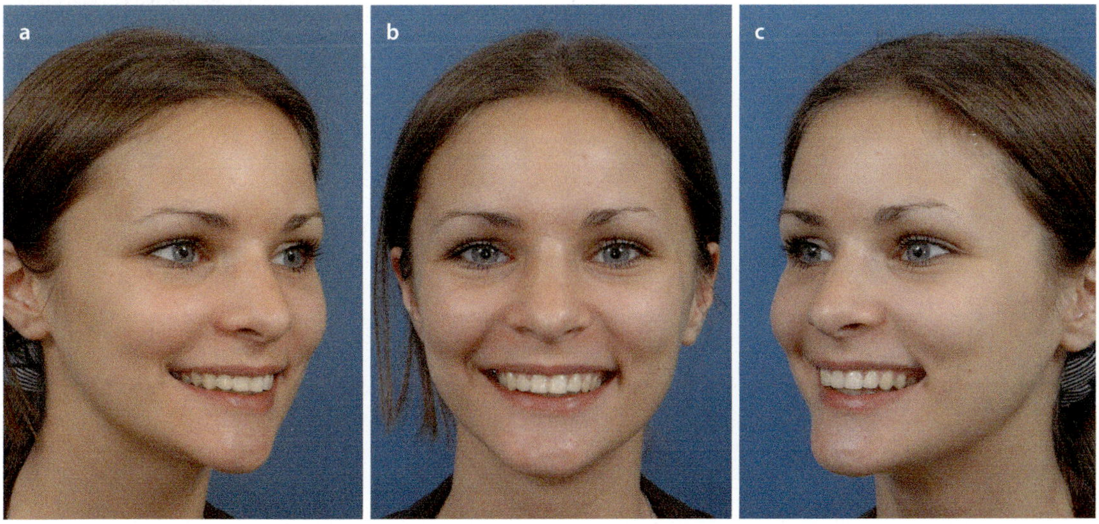

Fig. 6.59 Long-term clinical 2/3 right profile (**a**), frontal (**b**) and 2/3 left profile (**c**) smiling views 2 years after combined orthodontic-surgical treatment (patient D.C.M.)

Case 3: Class II, Anterior Open Bite (AOB), Orthofacial, Clinical Treatment Outcome

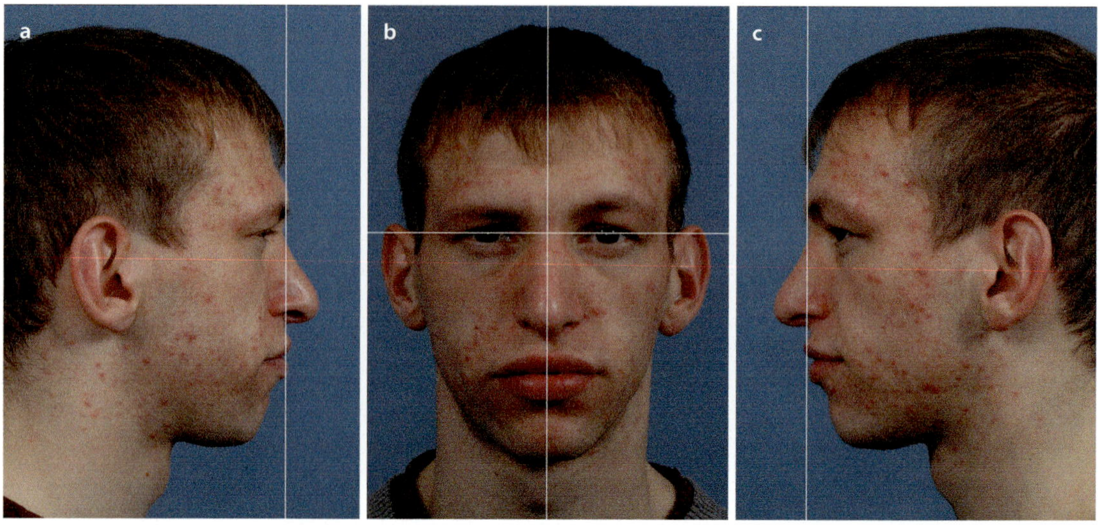

Fig. 6.60 Pre-surgical clinical right profile (**a**), frontal (**b**) and left profile (**c**) views of patient B.J. in his *c*-NHP in rest, at the time of the workup, approximately 3 weeks prior to surgery. Note the "V"-shaped face and retruded chin. Also note the discrete ear asymmetry with a prominent left ear

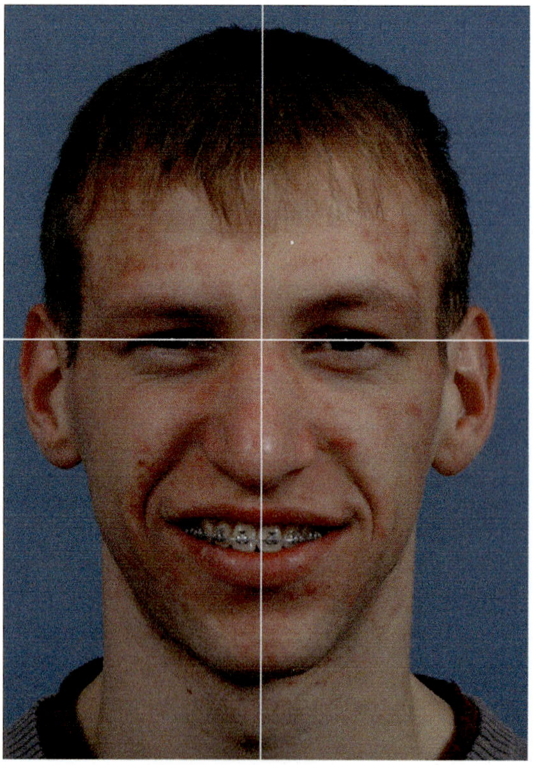

Fig. 6.61 Pre-surgical clinical frontal smiling view of patient B.J. at the time of the workup, approximately 3 weeks prior to surgery. Note the upper dental midline deviation to the right

Patient B.J. is a 22-year-old male with a Class II, anterior open bite (AOB) maxillofacial deformity due to combined posterior vertical maxillary excess (VME) and mandibular hypoplasia. In the frontal view, he is clinically presenting with a "V"-shaped face with poor bilateral zygoma and gonial angle definition, a prominent nasal tip with hanging columella and slight chin deviation to the left. In rest, he has clinically an incisal display of 2 mm, while during spontaneous smiling, he has almost (-1 mm) full incisal exposure. In the profile view, he presents with an acute nasolabial angle with short upper lip and a retruded mandible with poor chin definition. He has an Angle Class II malocclusion with an anterior open bite (AOB), adequate transversal relationship and a 1 mm lower dental midline deviation to the right. He has no history of TMJ dysfunction neither pain.

Case 3: Class II, Anterior Open Bite (AOB), Orthofacial, *v*-NHP and PHP

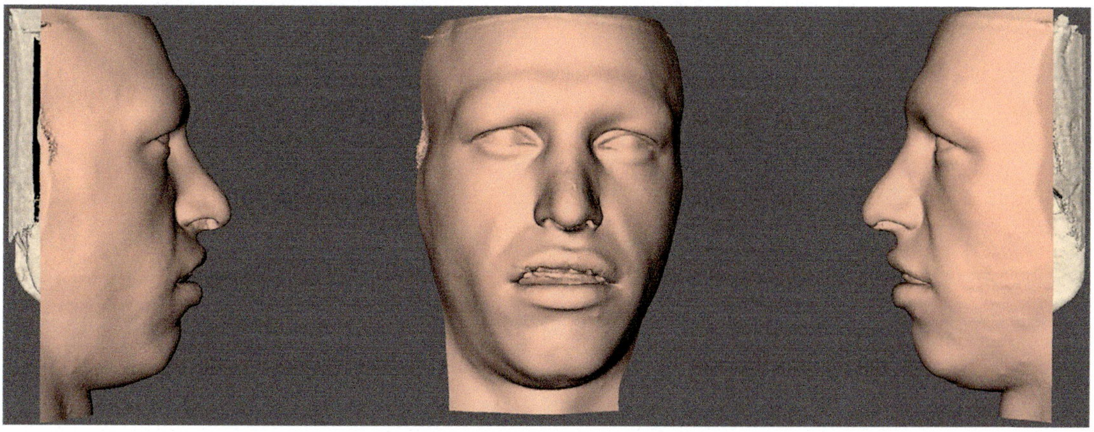

Fig. 6.62 Pre-surgical 3D "surface-rendered" right profile, frontal and left profile soft and hard tissue representations of the head of patient B.J., as generated during standardised CBCT image acquisition, at the time of the workup (Maxilim v. 2.3.0.3). Note the incorrect position and orientation of the virtual head compared to the clinical pictures of patient B.J. (Fig. 6.60), although it was attempted to scan the patient in his correct *c*-NHP in rest

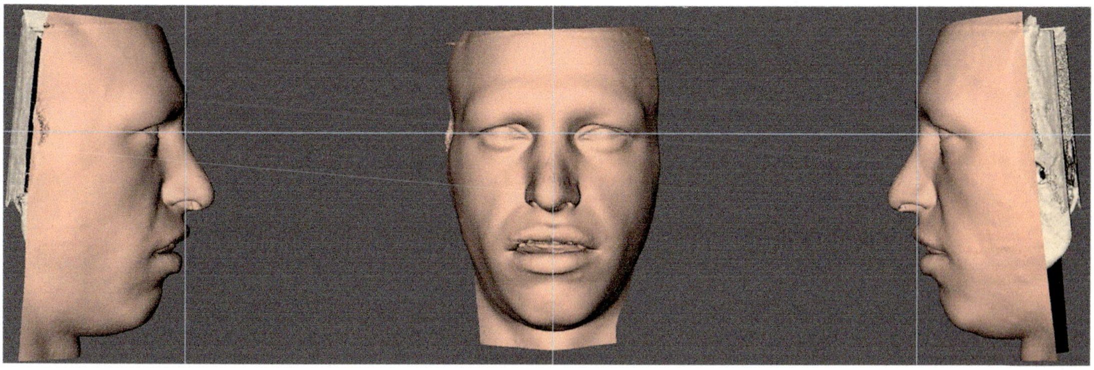

Fig. 6.63 Following a standardised "step-by-step" approach (see Sect. 3.1), the scanned head position of patient B.J. (Fig. 6.62) was virtually modified towards his *c*-NHP (Fig. 6.60), which results in his *v*-NHP and corresponds to his individual "Planning Head Position (PHP)" (3D "surface-rendered" representations, Maxilim v. 2.3.0.3)

Patient B.J. is used to illustrate the potential of colour surface distance maps (see Sect. 5.3.1) in 3D virtual evaluation of treatment outcome of orthofacial surgery (Fig. 6.92)

Case 3: Class II, Anterior Open Bite (AOB), Orthofacial, Clinical Treatment Outcome

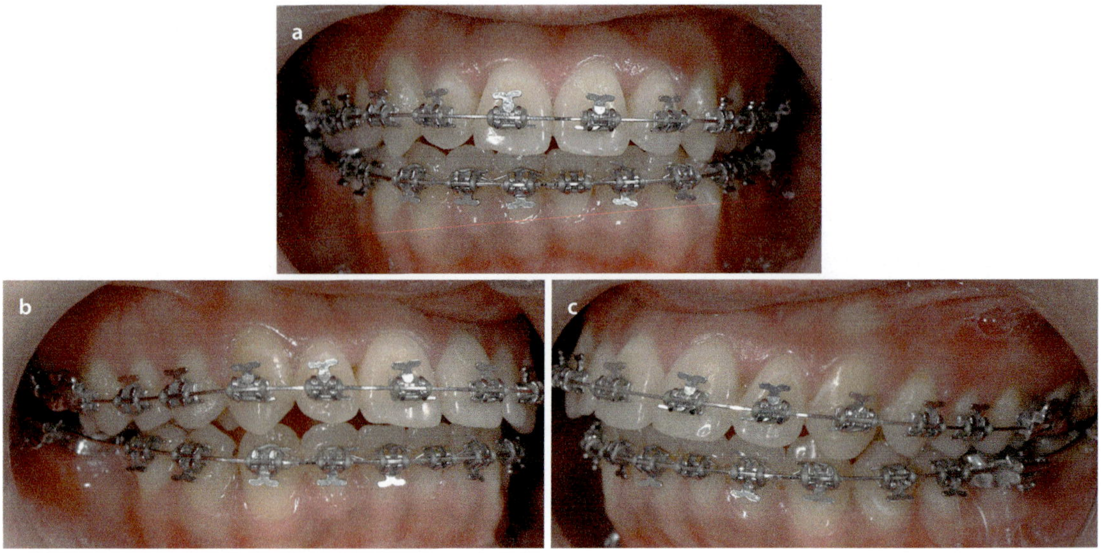

Fig. 6.64 Pre-surgical frontal (**a**), right (**b**) and left (**c**) intra-oral views of the occlusion of patient B.J. at the time of the workup, approximately 3 weeks prior to surgery. Note the 2 mm lower dental midline deviation to the right

Case 3: 3D-VPS$_5$ Step 1 Maxillary Occlusal Cant Evaluation/Correction ("Roll")

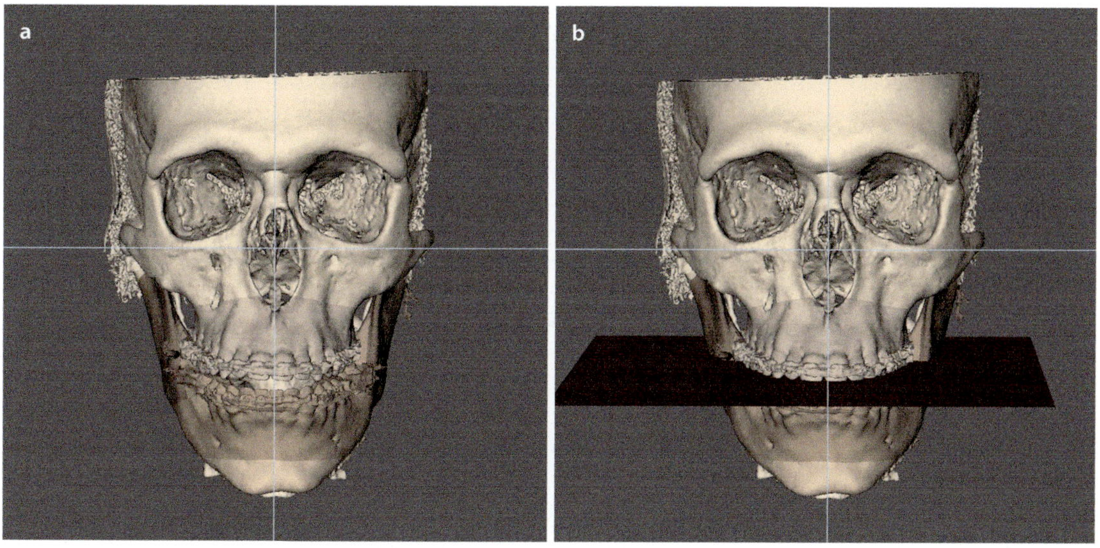

Fig. 6.65 The maxillary occlusal plane is evaluated both clinically (Fig. 6.61) and virtually (**a**) towards the horizontal 3D PHP reference plane and does not need to be corrected in patient B.J. (**b**) (3D "surface-rendered" representations, Maxilim v. 2.3.0.3). Note the presence of "halo" artefacts on the hard tissue surface representation of patient B.J.

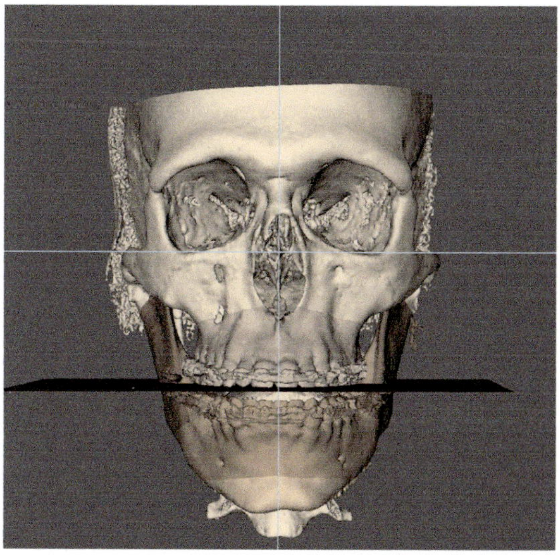

Fig. 6.66 Slight virtual rotation of the patient's skull to the back more clearly shows virtually that the maxillary occlusal plane is parallel to the horizontal 3D PHP reference plane and does not need to be modified (3D "surface-rendered" representations, patient B.J., Maxilim v. 2.3.0.3)

▪ Case 3: 3D-VPS$_5$ Step 2 Upper Dental Midline Evaluation/Correction

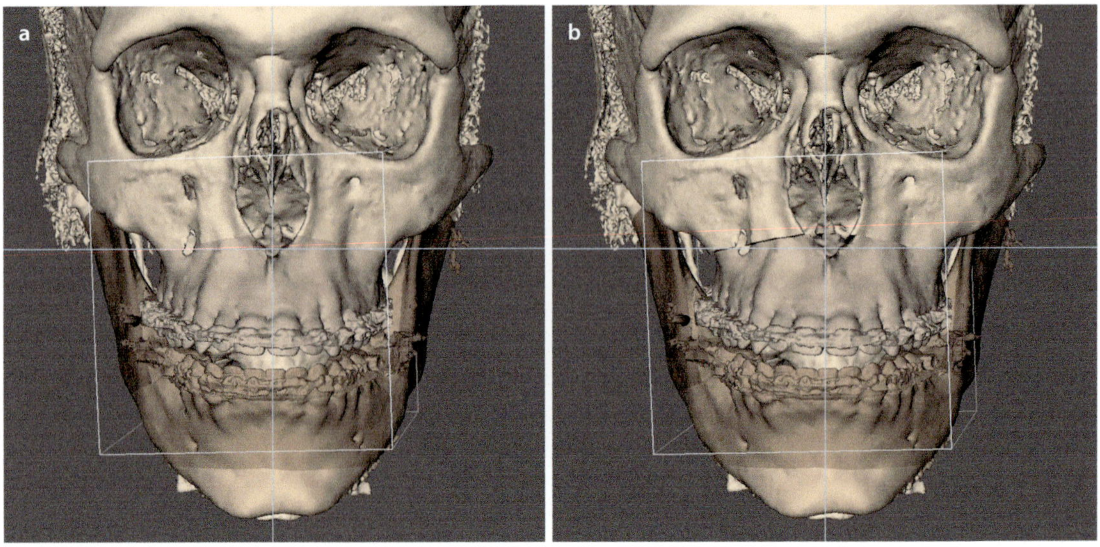

Fig. 6.67 The 1.5 mm deviation of the upper dental midline to the right (**a**) is corrected towards the facial midline 3D PHP reference plane, by a pure translational movement to the left (**b**) in patient B.J. (3D "surface-rendered" representations, Maxilim v. 2.3.0.3)

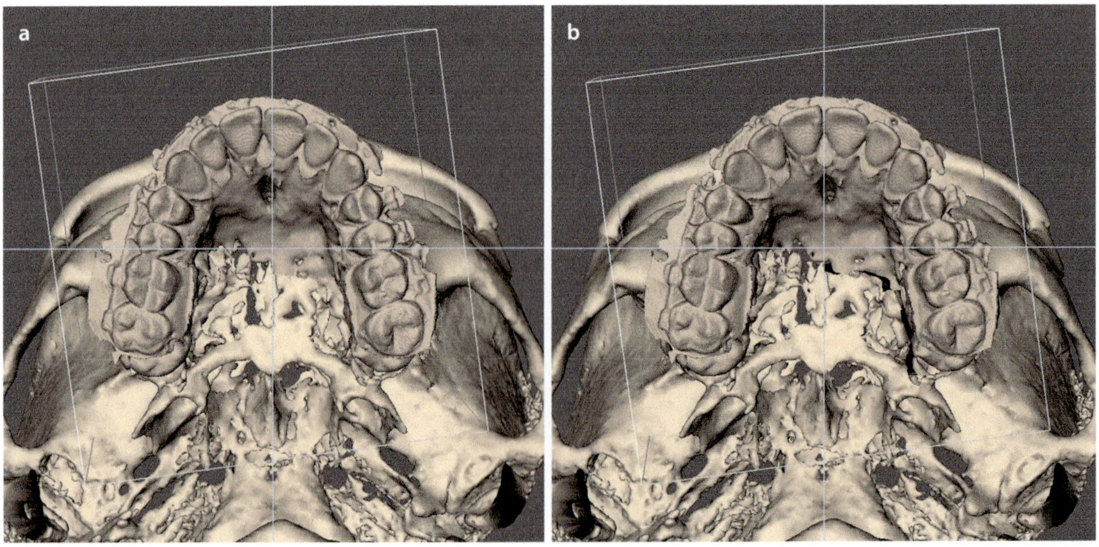

Fig. 6.68 The base views illustrate that the 1.5 mm deviation of the upper dental midline to the right (**a**) is corrected towards the facial midline 3D PHP reference plane, by a pure translational movement to the left (**b**) (3D "surface-rendered" representations, patient B.J., Maxilim v. 2.3.0.3)

Case 3: 3D-VPS$_5$ Step 3 Overall Evaluation of Facial Asymmetry After Virtual Occlusal Definition

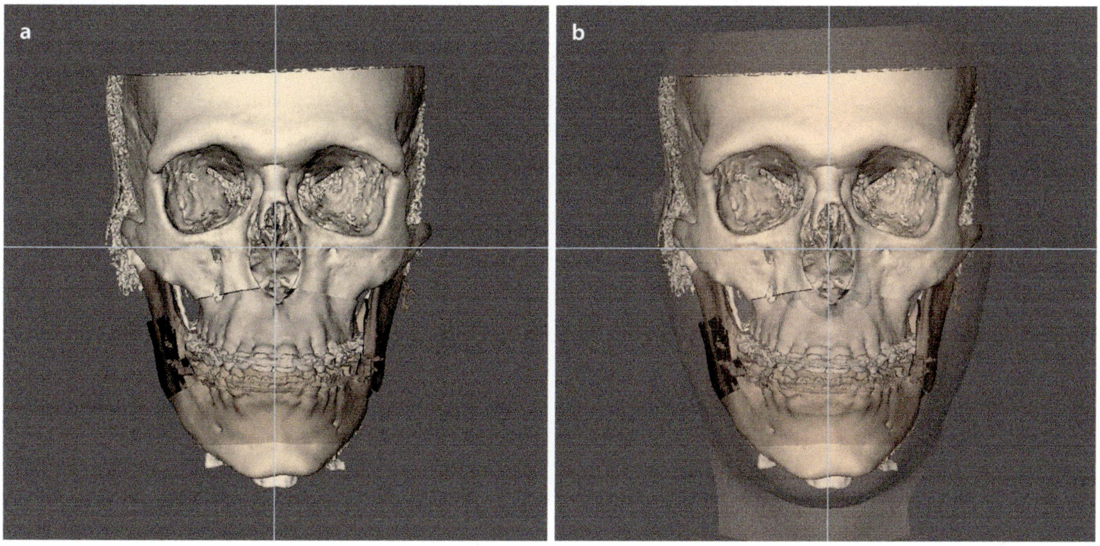

Fig. 6.69 Overall facial asymmetry of the skull of patient B.J. (**a**) with transparent soft tissues (**b**) is assessed after virtual occlusal definition in the frontal view towards both the horizontal and facial midline 3D PHP reference planes (3D "surface-rendered" representations, Maxilim v. 2.3.0.3). Note the important flaring of the mandibular body to the right and the chin deviation to the left

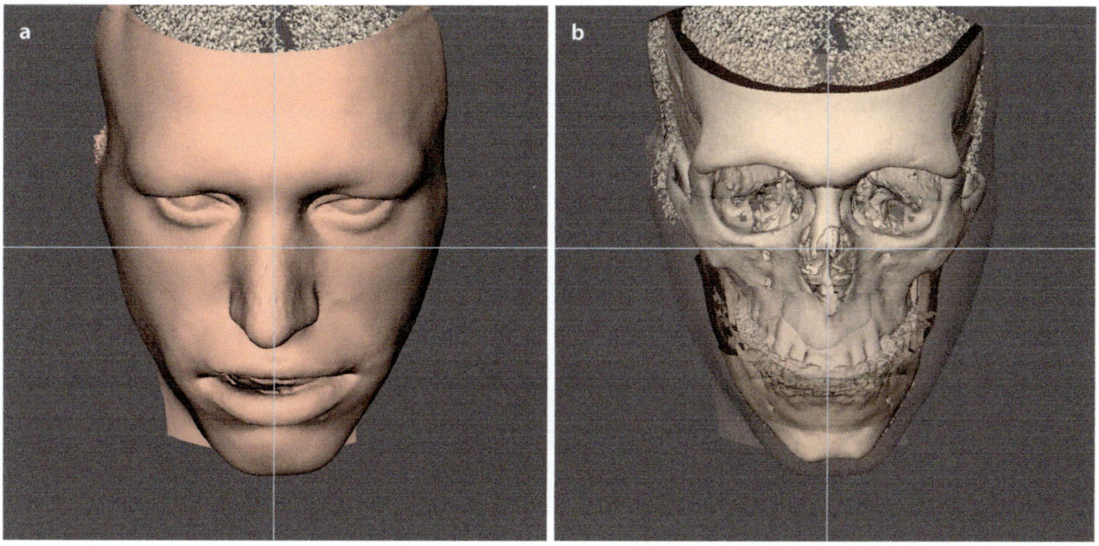

Fig. 6.70 To evaluate the overall facial asymmetry after virtual occlusal definition, the mandibular contour is evaluated both virtually on the soft tissues (**a**) and at the bony level towards the contour of the zygomatic bones and arches with soft tissues in transparency (**b**) (3D "surface-rendered" representations, patient B.J., Maxilim v. 2.3.0.3). Note the deviation of the nasal tip to the right although the bony nasal pyramid is straight

■ Case 3: 3D-VPS$_5$ Step 4 Evaluation/Correction of Flaring ("Yaw")

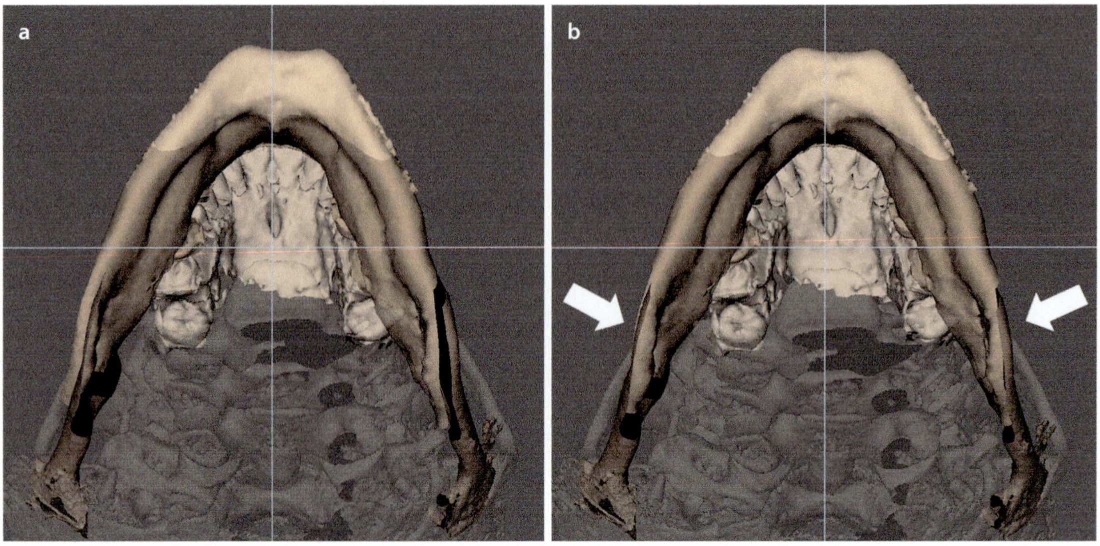

Fig. 6.71 The base views show that the flaring of the mandibular body to the right (**a**) is corrected by a CCW "Yaw" rotational movement to the left (**b**) (3D "surface-rendered" representations, patient B.J., Maxilim v. 2.3.0.3)

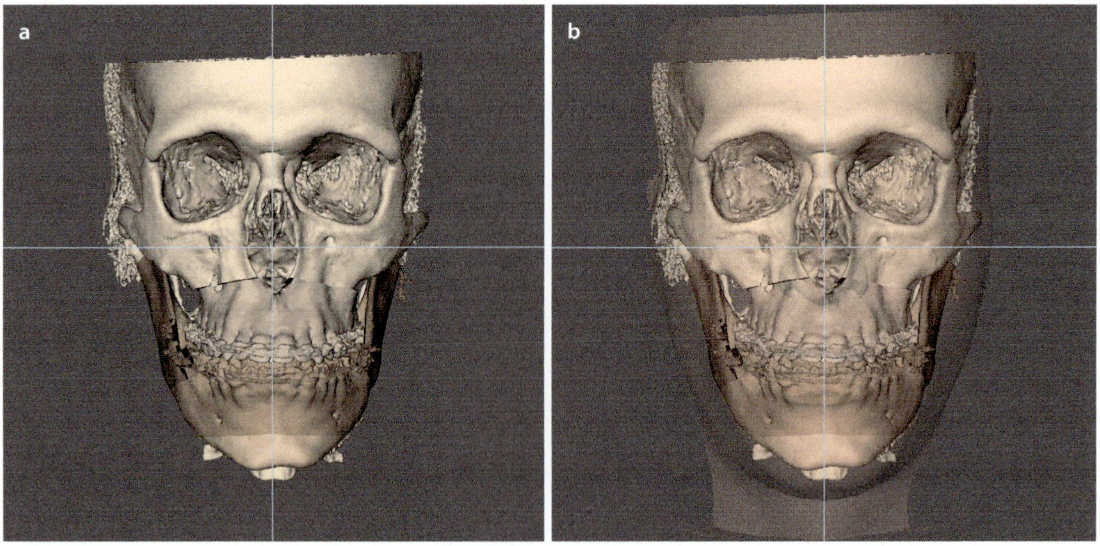

Fig. 6.72 Overall assessment of facial bony contour of patient B.J. (**a**) with transparent soft tissues (**b**) after correction of flaring to the right by a "Yaw" rotational movement of the maxillo-mandibular complex to the left (3D "surface-rendered" representations, Maxilim v. 2.3.0.3)

Case 3: 3D-VPS$_5$ Step 5 Upper Vertical Incisal Position Evaluation/Correction

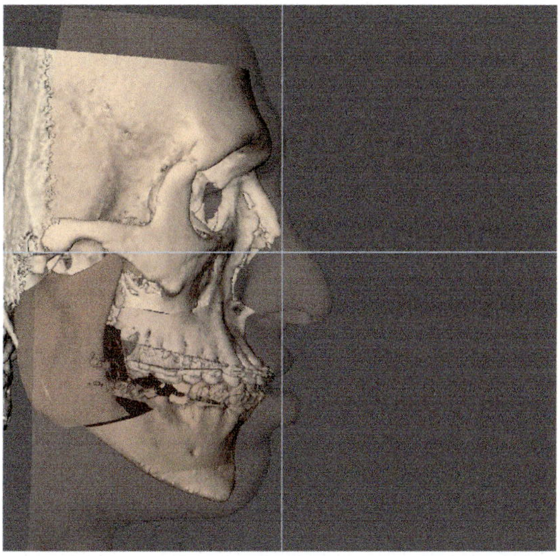

Fig. 6.73 Since patient B.J. has clinically in rest 2 mm and during spontaneous smiling almost full (−1 mm) upper incisal exposure, it was decided at this stage to keep the upper incisal vertical level at "0" anticipating already the maxillary advancement in "step 6" (3D "surface-rendered" representations, Maxilim v. 2.3.0.3)

Case 3: 3D-VPS$_5$ Step 6 Sagittal Upper Incisal Position Evaluation/Correction

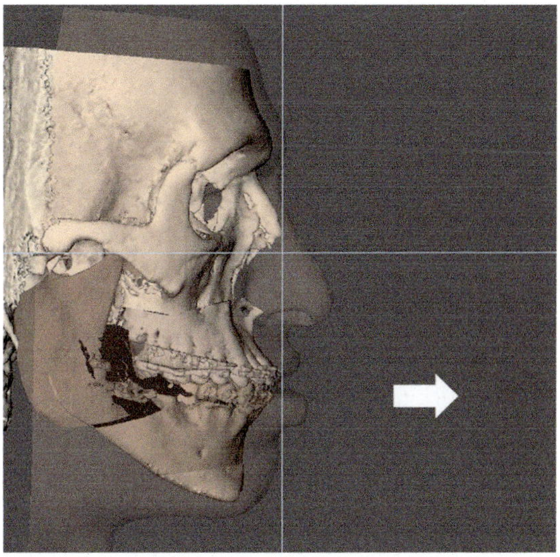

Fig. 6.74 From 3D cephalometric analysis and clinically, it was decided to advance the "maxillo-mandibular complex in final occlusion" 3 mm at the upper incisal level in patient B.J. which results according to the authors' experience in 1 mm additional incisal exposure (3D "surface-rendered" representations, Maxilim v. 2.3.0.3)

■ Case 3: 3D-VPS$_5$ Step 7 Profile Evaluation/Occlusal Plane Correction ("Pitch")

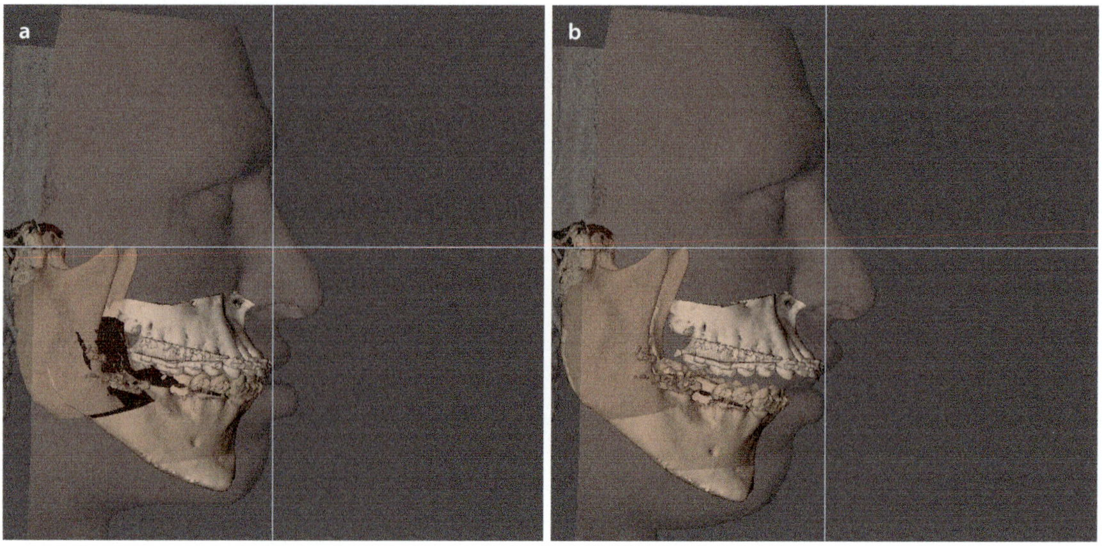

Fig. 6.75 At this stage in "step 7", the profile and dento-alveolar support of the upper lip are evaluated (**a**) (3D "surface-rendered" representations, patient B.J., Maxilim v. 2.3.0.3). Note that the labioversion of the upper incisors (**b**) that was prepared orthodontically to anticipate the posterior maxillary impaction for AOB closure results in an acute nasolabial angle, on the soft tissue simulation

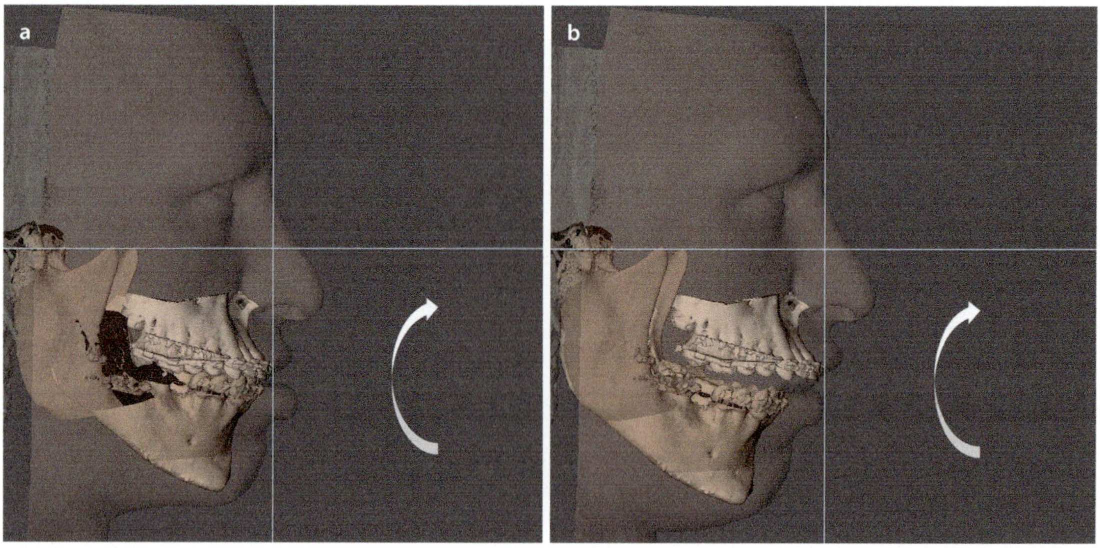

Fig. 6.76 At this stage in "step 7", a 3° CW rotation of the "maxillo-mandibular complex" (**a**) is virtually performed (3D "surface-rendered" representations, patient B.J., Maxilim v. 2.3.0.3) which results in a 2 mm posterior impaction at the mesial cusps of the first upper molars and partial correction of the AOB (**b**)

Case 3-3D-VPS$_5$ Step 8 3D Chin Position Evaluation/Correction

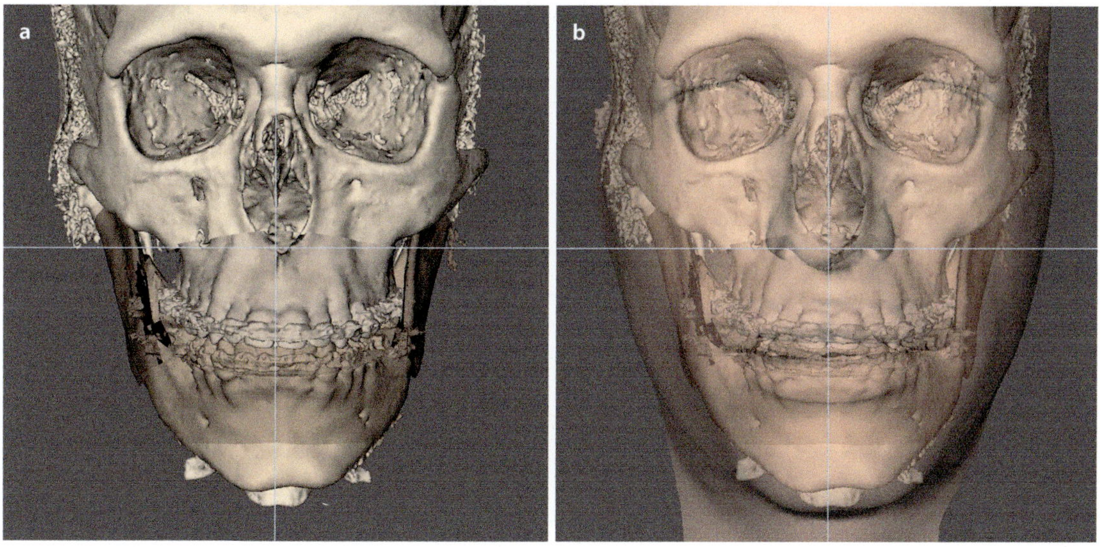

Fig. 6.77 Evaluation of the chin position in the frontal plane without (**a**) and with (**b**) the patient's 3D facial soft tissue mask in transparency (3D "surface-rendered" representations, Maxilim v. 2.3.0.3). Note that at this stage, there is still a significant chin deviation to the left with a slight cant in patient B.J.

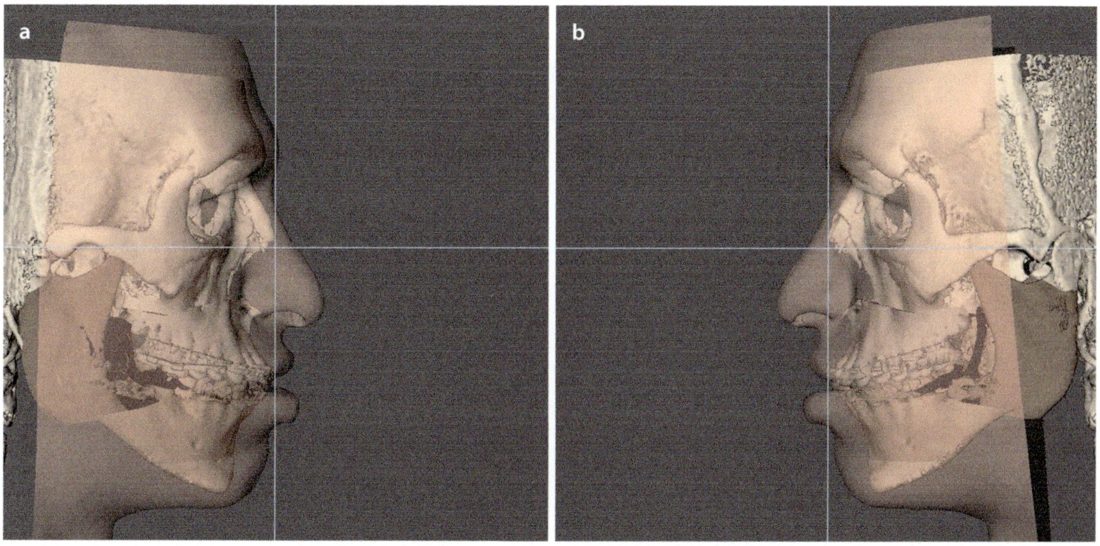

Fig. 6.78 Evaluation of the sagittal chin position in the right (**a**) and left profile (**b**) views needs to be individually assessed (3D "surface-rendered" representations, Maxilim v. 2.3.0.3). Note that the chin is still retruded in the face with the absence of a well-defined plica labio-mentalis in patient B.J. Note also the limits of the actual 3D virtual soft tissue simulation at the level of the lower lip

Case 3: 3D-VPS$_5$ Step 8 3D Chin Position Evaluation/Correction

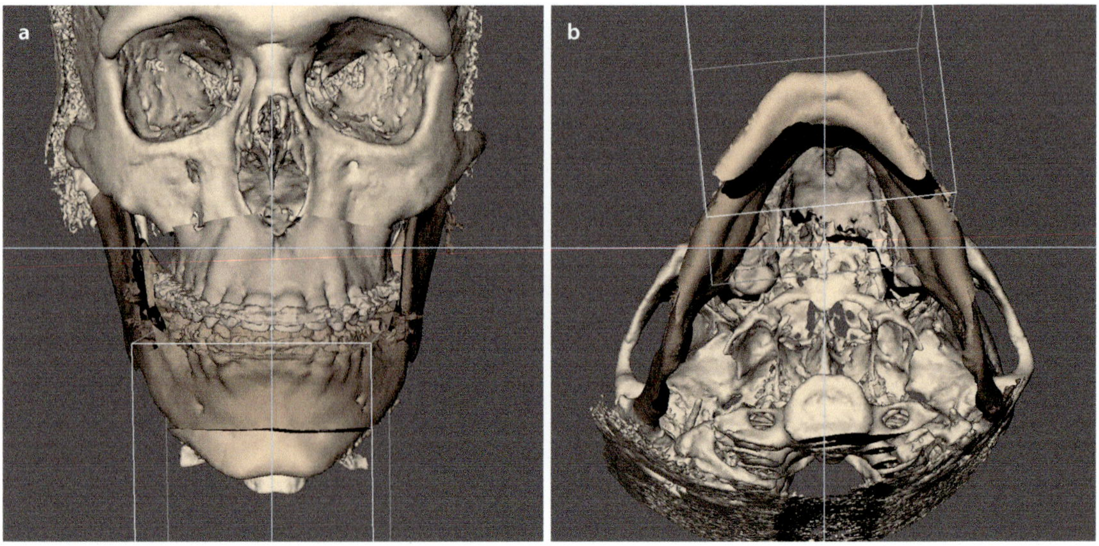

Fig. 6.79 In the frontal plane (**a**), a 1 mm translation to the right with a CW "Roll" movement of the chin with 1 mm posterior extrusion at the left was virtually planned in patient B.J. to correct the midline deviation and the cant (Fig. 6.77). The base view (**b**) shows no flaring of the chin after 6 mm advancement (3D "surface-rendered" representations, Maxilim v. 2.3.0.3). Note that the chin needs to be recontoured at the right lateral side during actual surgery

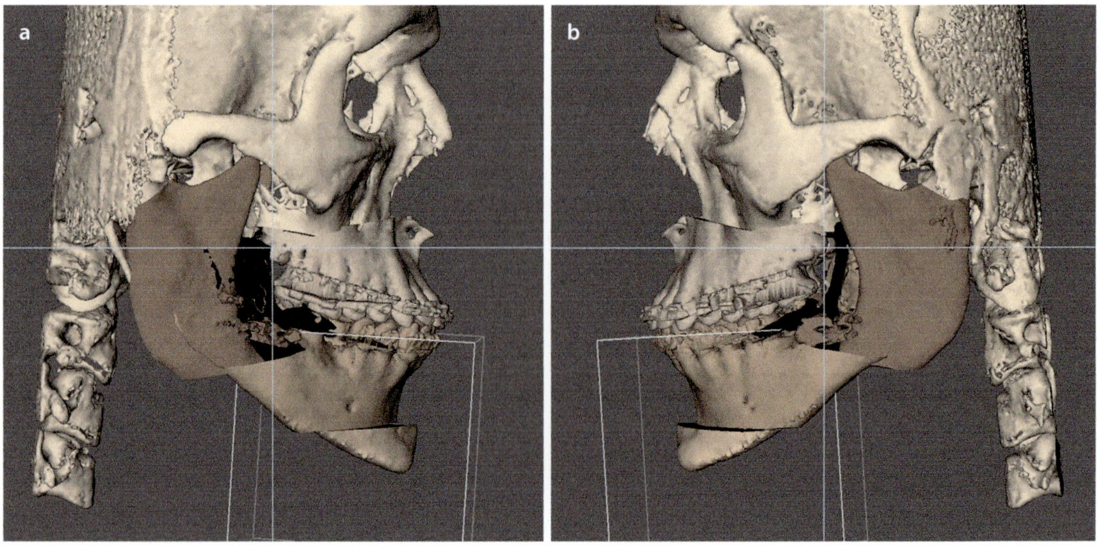

Fig. 6.80 The right (**a**) and left (**b**) profile views show that a chin advancement of 6 mm with a posterior extrusion of 1 mm at the left was virtually planned in patient B.J. (3D "surface-rendered" representations, Maxilim v. 2.3.0.3)

Case 3: 3D-VPS$_5$ Step 9 Patient Communication of the Individualised Treatment Plan

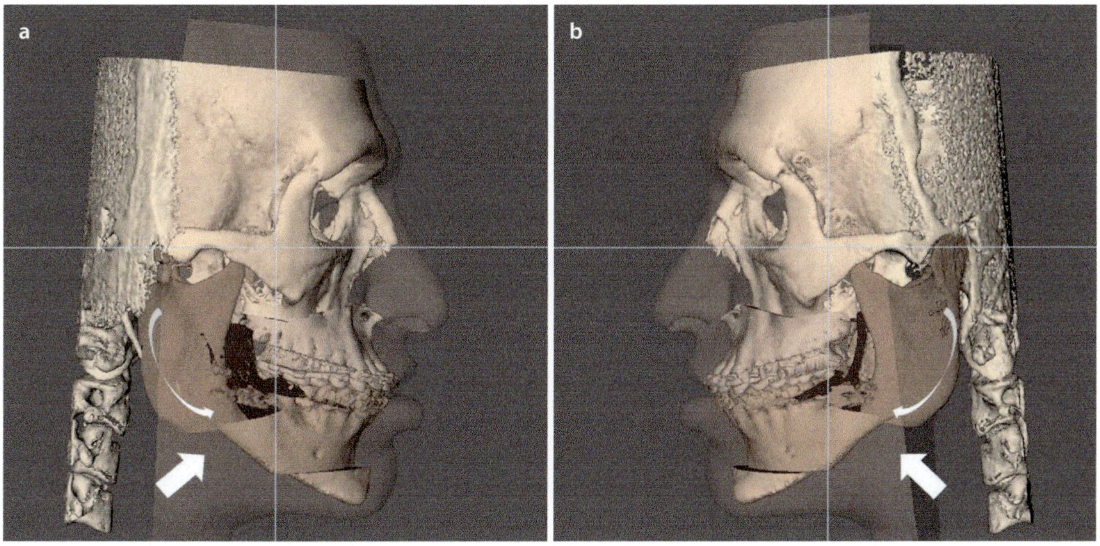

Fig. 6.81 Right (**a**) and left (**b**) profile views of the "Individualised 3D Virtual Treatment Plan" show that a gentle CCW rotation of both proximal fragments would be beneficial to decrease the step at the antegonial notch (3D "surface-rendered" representations, Maxilim v. 2.3.0.3). Note the limits of the actual 3D virtual soft tissue simulation at the level of the lips

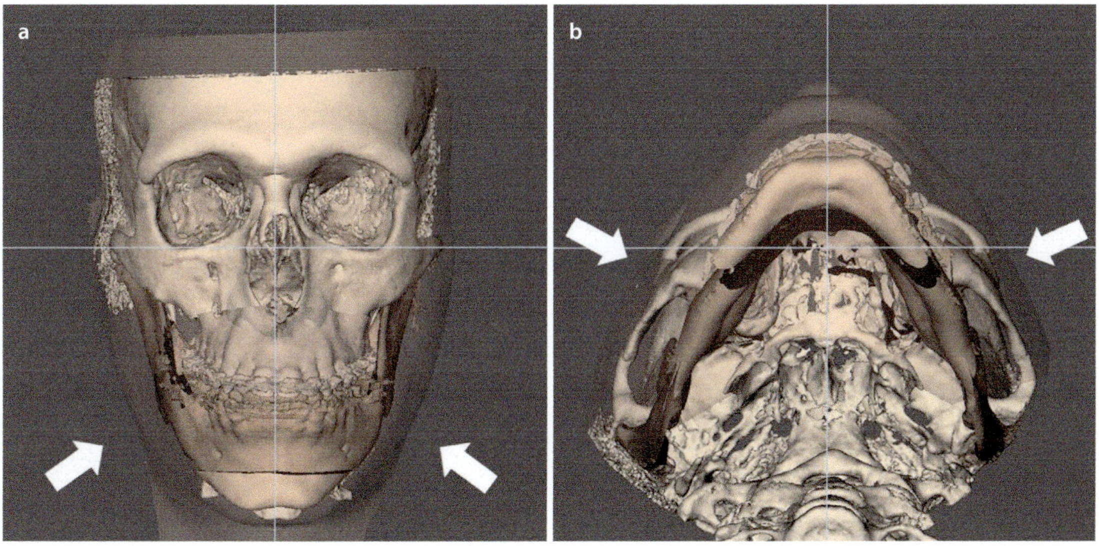

Fig. 6.82 Frontal (**a**) and base (**b**) views of the "Individualised 3D Virtual Treatment Plan", as presented to patient B.J., before the actual surgery (3D "surface-rendered" representations, Maxilim v. 2.3.0.3). Patient B.J. is complaining of the "V"-shaped appearance of his face and the poor definition of his zygomatic bones

■ Case 3: 3D-VPS$_5$ Step 10 Final Adjustments of the 3D Virtual Treatment Plan

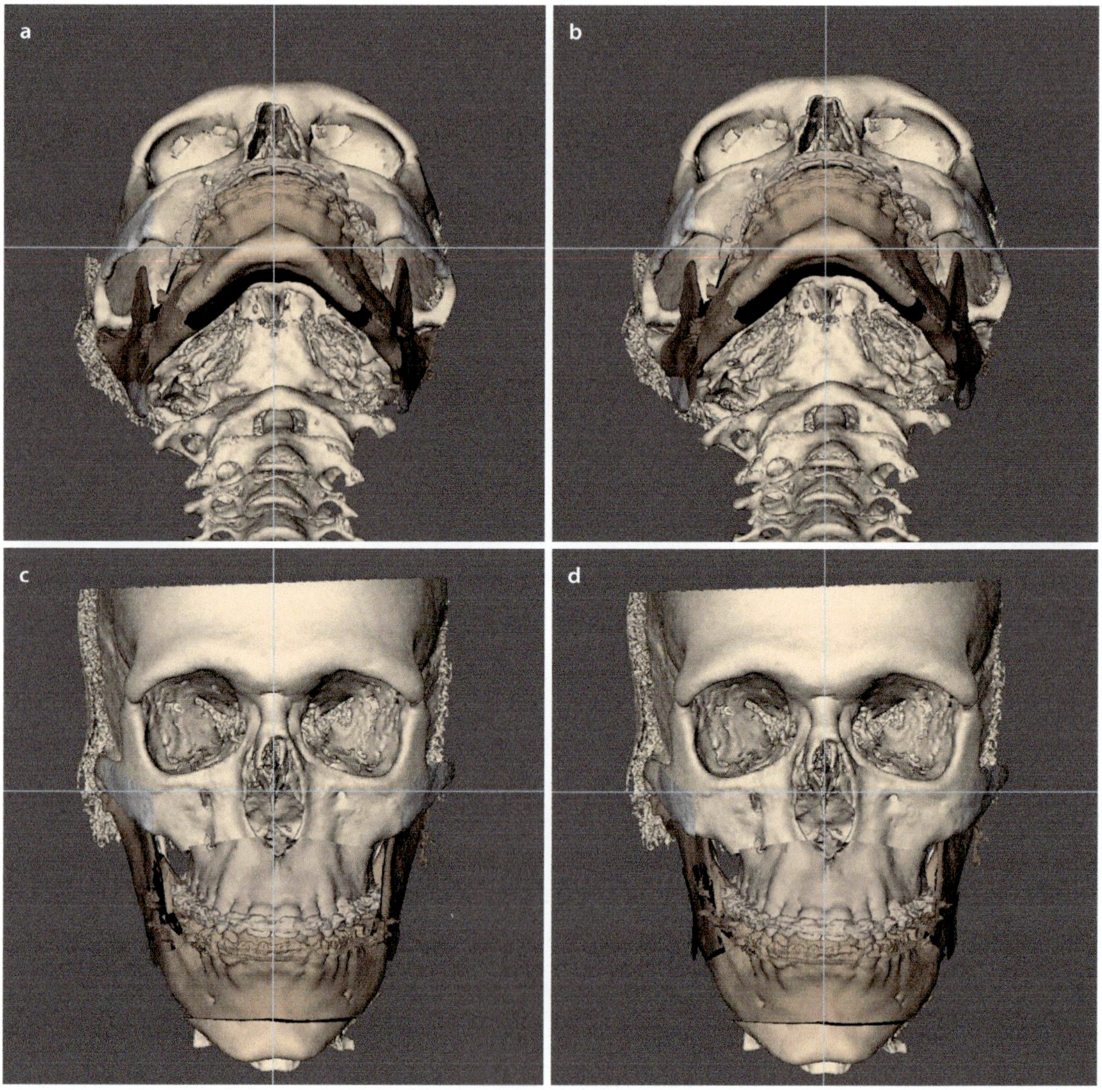

◘ **Fig. 6.83** Final adjustments of the "Individualised 3D Virtual Treatment Plan" after communication with patient B.J. consisted of additional zygomatic sandwich osteotomies to correct the flattened infraorbital contour of the midface and bilateral gonial angle augmentation (3D "surface-rendered" representations, Maxilim v. 2.3.0.3): before (**a**) and after (**b**) frontal upward inclined and before (**c**) and after (**d**) frontal views

▪ Case 3: 3D-VPS$_5$- Final Integrated "Individualised 3D Virtual Treatment Plan"

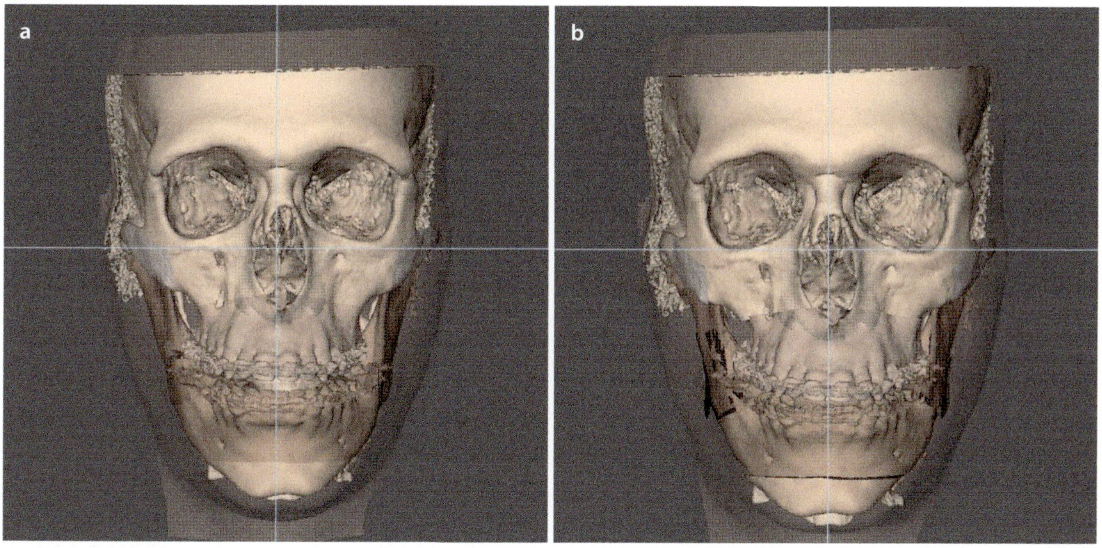

Fig. 6.84 Initial situation (**a**), and final "Individualised 3D Virtual Treatment Plan" (**b**), of patient B.J. in the frontal plane (3D "surface-rendered" representations, Maxilim v. 2.3.0.3)

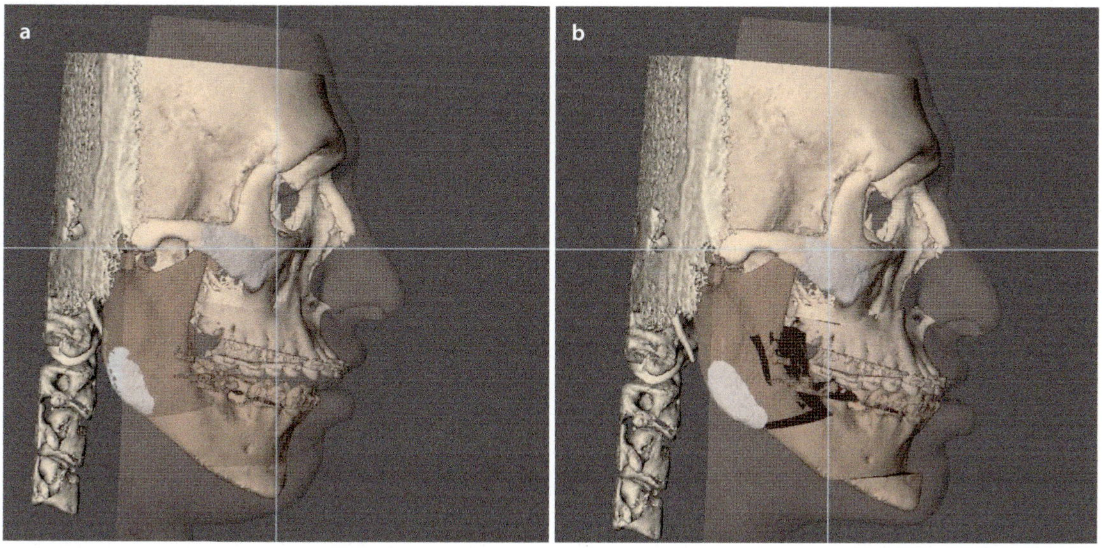

Fig. 6.85 Initial situation (**a**), and final "Individualised 3D Virtual Treatment Plan" (**b**), of patient B.J. in the right profile plane (3D "surface-rendered" representations, Maxilim v. 2.3.0.3). Note the limits of the actual 3D virtual soft tissue simulation at the level of the lips

■ Case 3: 3D-VPS$_5$- Final Integrated "Individualised 3D Virtual Treatment Plan"

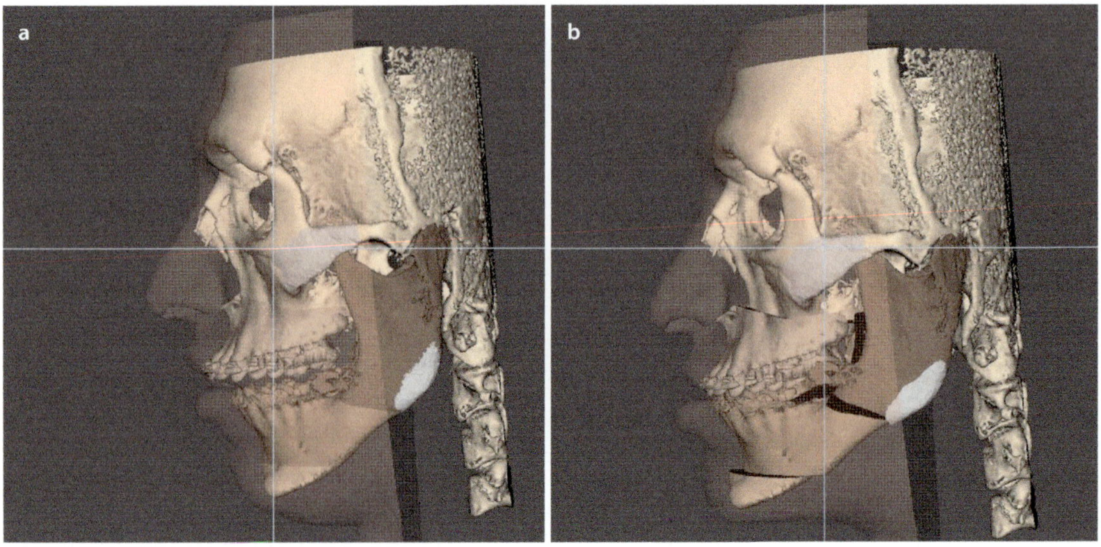

Fig. 6.86 Initial situation (**a**), and final "Individualised 3D Virtual Treatment Plan" (**b**), of patient B.J. in the left profile plane (3D "surface-rendered" representations, Maxilim v. 2.3.0.3). Note the limits of the actual 3D virtual soft tissue simulation at the level of the lips

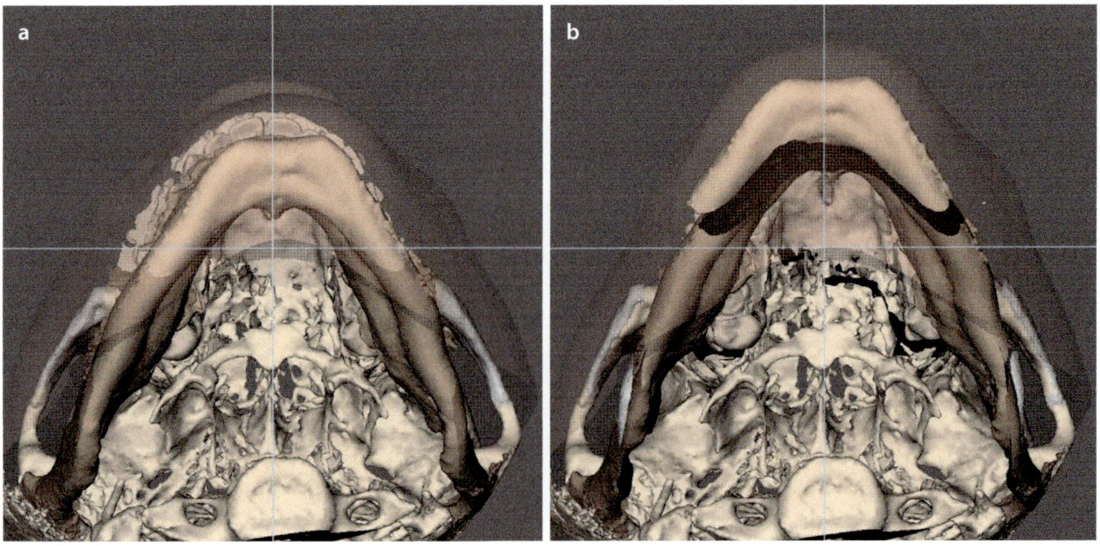

Fig. 6.87 Initial situation (**a**), and final "Individualised 3D Virtual Treatment Plan" (**b**), of patient B.J. in the base plane (3D "surface-rendered" representations, patient B.J., Maxilim v. 2.3.0.3). Note the virtual bilateral zygomatic and gonial angle expansion

■ Case 3: "3D Virtual Treatment Planning, OR" Template

Maxillary osteotomy

- ■ Le Fort: ■I □II □III
- ■ One-piece
- □ Segmental:
  - Pieces: ....
  - Interdental: ....
- ■ Advancement: 3.0 mm
- □ Set-back: ....
- ■ Midline: 1.5 mm □R ■L
- ■ Midline after Le Fort 1: mesial 31
- ■ Vertical: (➔)
- ■ "Yaw" correction: CCW to the left
- ■ Other: CW "Pitch" rotation

Mandibular osteotomy

- ■ SSO ■R ■L
- □ Inverted-L □R □L
- □ VRO □R □L
- ■ Advancement: R 9.0 mm L 8.0 mm
- □ Set-back: R .... L ....
- ■ CW "Pitch" rotation the distal fragment
- ■ CCW "Pitch" rotation the proximal fragments
- □ Midline split
- ■ IAN course: R lingual L lingual
- □ Midline after BSSO: ....
- □ Other: ....

Chin osteotomy

- ■ Advancement: 6.0 mm
- □ Set-back: ....
- ■ Midline: 1.0 mm ■R □L
- □ Intrusion:
  - □Anterior: ....
  - □Posterior: R ...... L ......
- ■ Extrusion:
  - □Anterior: ....
  - ■Posterior: R ...... L 2.0 mm
- □ "Shield" osteotomy
- □ "Chin wing" osteotomy
  - *Mental Foramen level:*
  - □ Symmetric
  - ■ Asymmetric
- ■ Other: duplicated foramen mentale left

Planning Requirements

- ■ Maxilla first
- □ Mandible first
- □ Minimally Invasive Le Fort I
- □ IO-CBCT
- □ Kobayashi wires : ....
- ■ Skeletal anchorage : frontal
- □ Orthodontic buttons : ....
- ■ Occlusal grinding : ....
- □ Other : ....

2.5 mm	1.0 mm	0.0 mm	1.0 mm	2.5 mm
16	13	11	23	26

"Roll" correction: □CW □CCW

Miscellaneous

- ■ Para-nasal cross sutures
- □ Alar cinch
- □ Septoplasty
- □ Inferior turbinectomy
- ■ ANS: □Shortening ■Midline
- ■ Nasal base plasty ■R ■L
- ■ Lateral nasal wall plasty ■R ■L
- □ Bone graft(s): ....
- □ Extraction(s): ....
- □ Other: ....

Adjuvant Cosmetic Procedures

- □ Bichatectomy □R □L
- ■ Zygoma osteotomies ■R ■L
  - *Infraorbital Foramen level:*
  - ■ Symmetric
  - □ Asymmetric
- ■ Otoplasty: □R ■L
- ■ Rhinoplasty: Closed
- □ Browlift: ....
- □ Blepharoplasty: ....
  - □Upper □Lower
- □ Facelift: ....
- □ Necklift: ....
- □ Liposuction: ....
- ■ Lipofilling: midfacial
- ■ Other: bilateral gonial angle augmentation with rib cartilage

In patient B.J. the bilateral gonial angle augmentation was performed with rib cartilage grafts. The current alternative would be the use of patient-specific implants (PSIs) in PEEK or titanium.

■ Case 3: Class II, Anterior Open Bite (AOB), Orthofacial, 3D Virtual Treatment Outcome

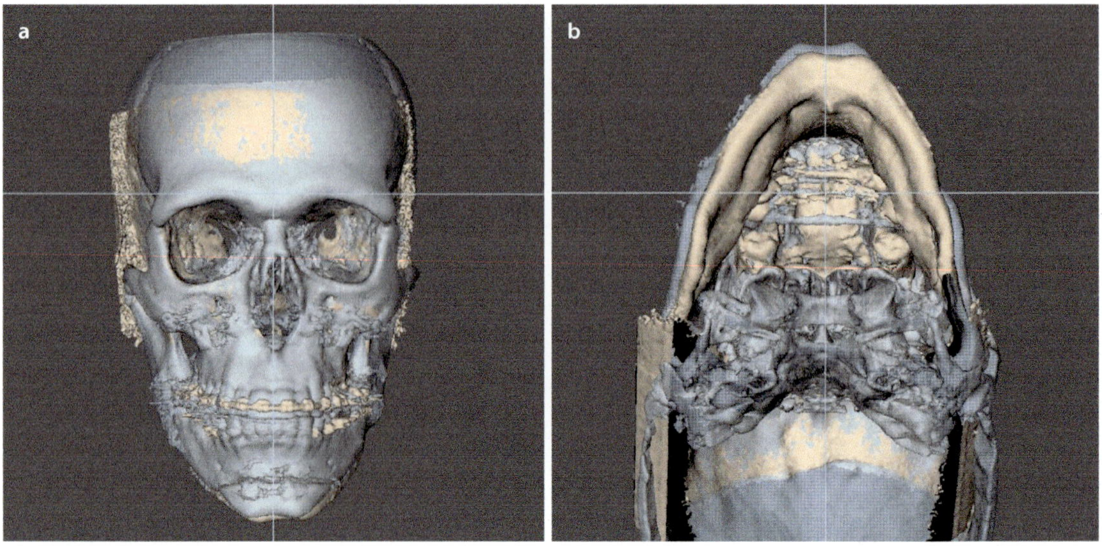

Fig. 6.88 Voxel-based superimposition on the cranial base of the pre-surgical and 6 months post-surgical (*blue*) 3D "surface-rendered" hard tissue representations. Frontal (**a**) and base (**b**) views (i-CAT, Imaging Sciences International Inc., Maxilim v. 2.3.0.3) (patient B.J.). Note the correction of the chin deviation

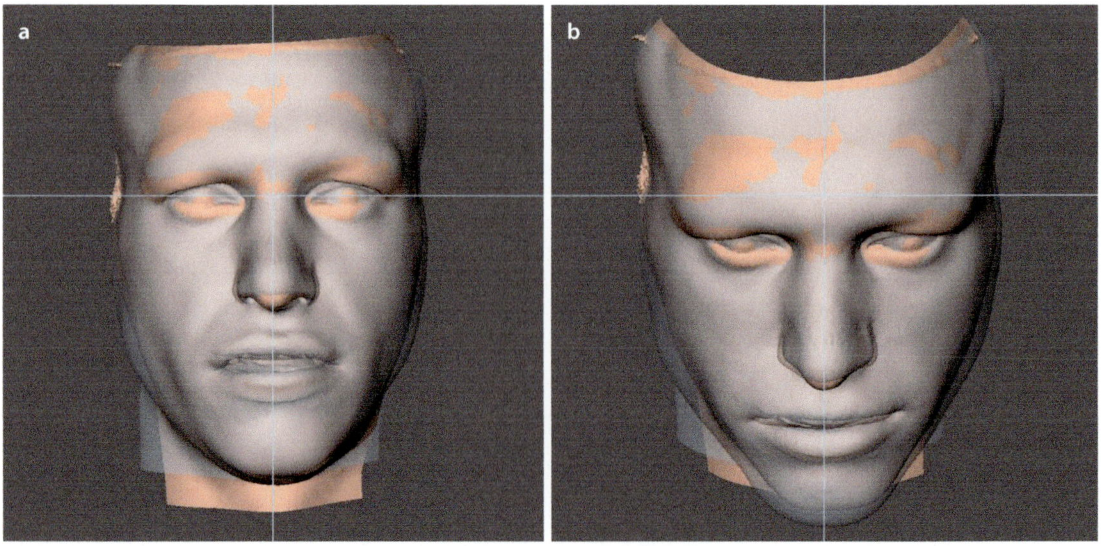

Fig. 6.89 Voxel-based superimposition on the cranial base of the pre-surgical and 6 months post-surgical (*blue*) 3D "surface-rendered" soft tissue representations. Frontal (**a**) and downward inclined (**b**) views (i-CAT, Imaging Sciences International Inc., Maxilim v. 2.3.0.3) (patient B.J.). Note the post-surgical (*blue*) widening of the upper and lower face width

Case 3: Class II, Anterior Open Bite (AOB), Orthofacial, 3D Virtual Treatment Outcome

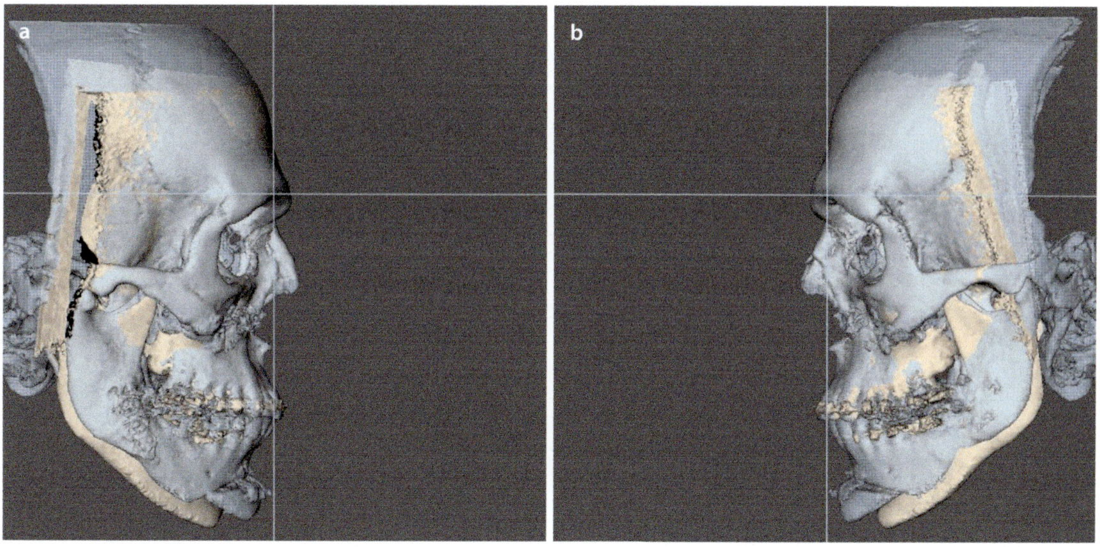

Fig. 6.90 Voxel-based superimposition on the cranial base of the pre-surgical and 6 months post-surgical (*blue*) 3D "surface-rendered" hard tissue representations. Right (**a**) and left (**b**) profile views (i-CAT, Imaging Sciences International Inc, Maxilim v. 2.3.0.3) (patient B.J.). Note the CCW rotation of the bimaxillary complex

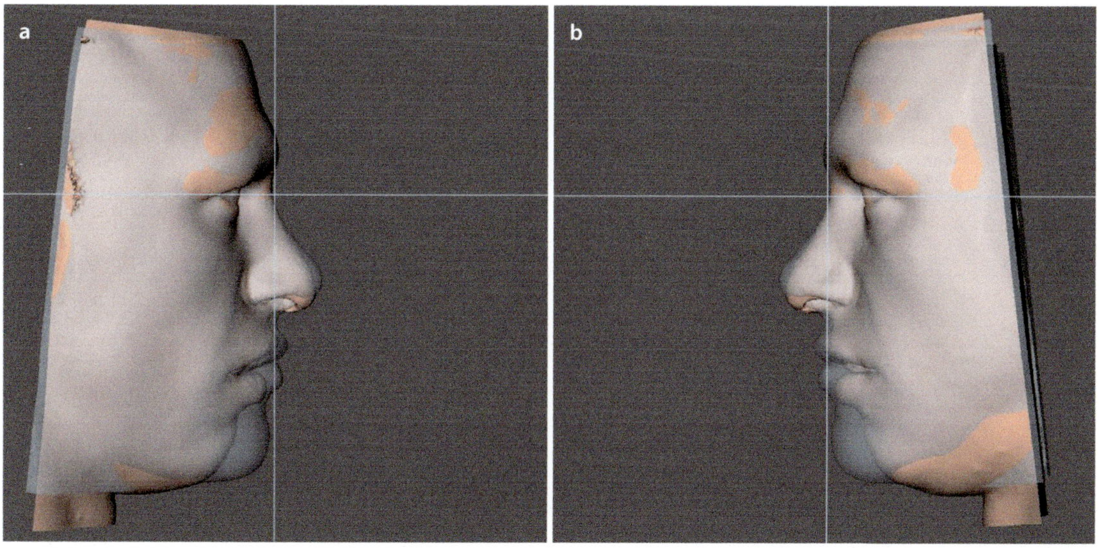

Fig. 6.91 Voxel-based superimposition on the cranial base of the pre-surgical and 6 months post-surgical (*blue*) 3D "surface-rendered" soft tissue representations. Right (**a**) and left (**b**) profile views (i-CAT, Imaging Sciences International Inc., Maxilim v. 2.3.0.3) (patient B.J.). Note the post-surgical changes at the nasolabial aesthetic unit (cranial nasal tip rotation with opening of the nasolabial angle and nasal dorsum correction), post-surgical changes of lip posture with lip competence and well-defined chin position and morphology

Case 3: Class II, Anterior Open Bite (AOB), Orthofacial, 3D Virtual Treatment Outcome

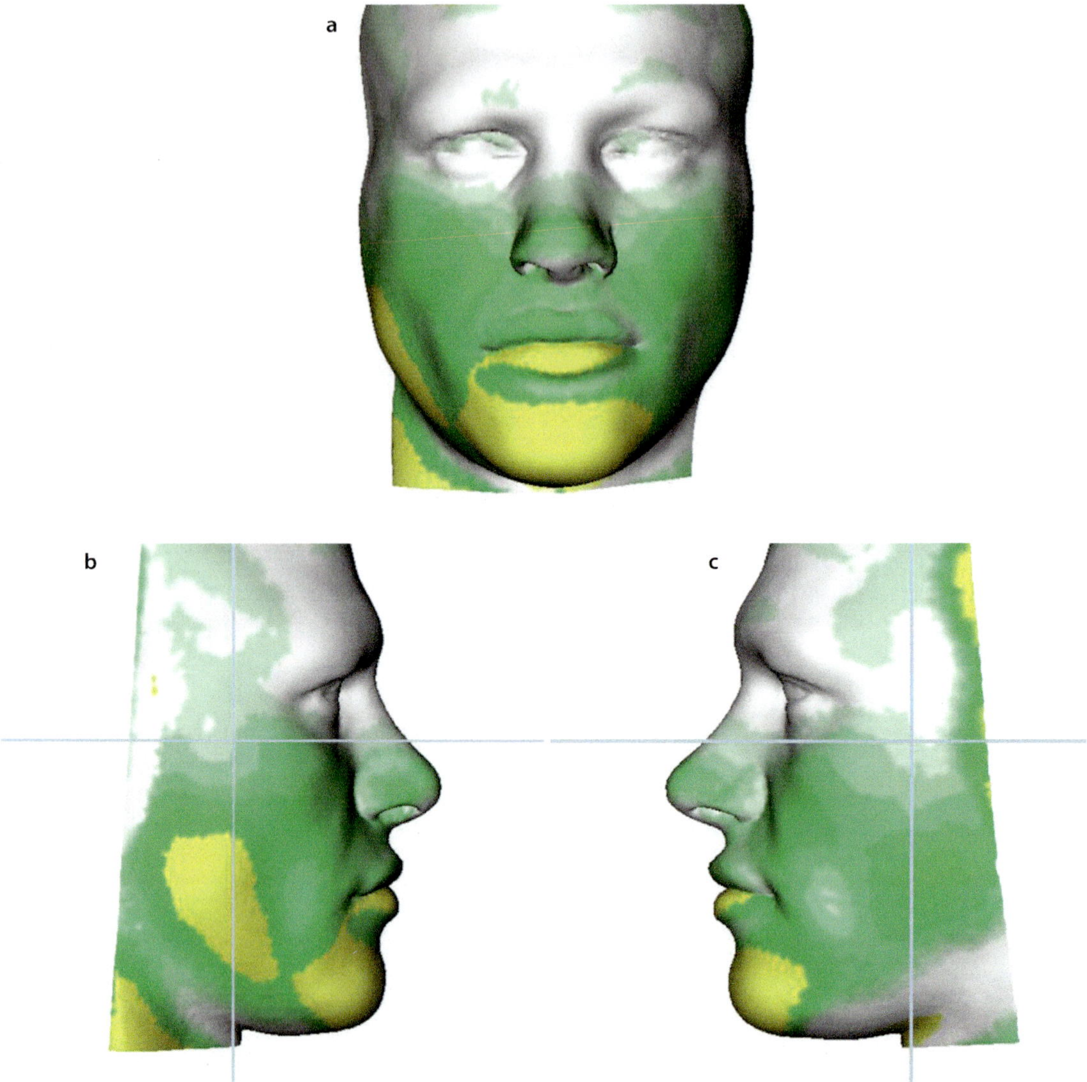

Fig. 6.92 Colour surface distance maps visualising the inter-surface distance between the "pre-surgical" and "6 months post-surgical" "surface-rendered" soft tissue representations of the patient's head after voxel-based superimposition on the cranial base and cranial bones (▶ see Sect. 5.3.1): frontal (**a**), right profile (**b**) and left profile (**c**) views (i-CAT, Imaging Sciences International Inc., Maxilim v. 2.3.0.3, patient B.J.). The *yellow* colour implies an inter-surface distance of more than 10 mm. Note the increased right gonial augmentation compared to the left side

Case 3: Class II, Anterior Open Bite (AOB), Orthofacial, Clinical Treatment Outcome

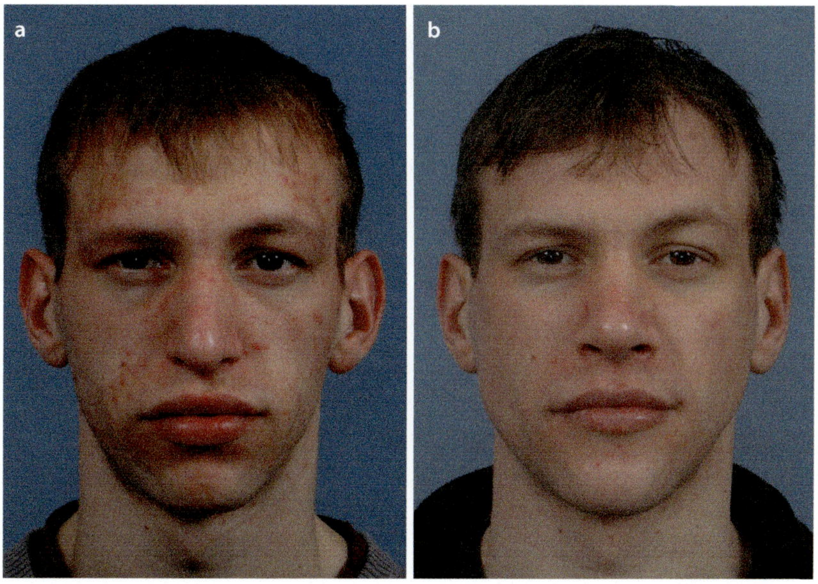

Fig. 6.93 Frontal views in rest, pre-surgical (**a**) and 1 year after (**b**) combined orthodontic-surgical treatment with bilateral zygomatic osteotomies, bilateral gonial augmentation, closed rhinoplasty, left otoplasty and midfacial liposculpture (patient B.J.)

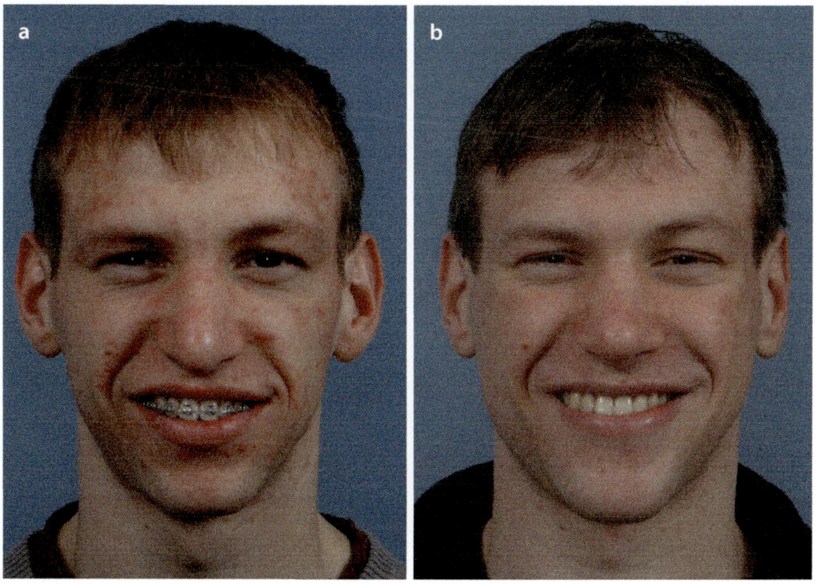

Fig. 6.94 Frontal views during smiling, pre-surgical (**a**) and 1 year after (**b**) combined orthodontic-surgical treatment with bilateral zygomatic osteotomies, bilateral gonial augmentation, closed rhinoplasty, left otoplasty and midfacial liposculpture (patient B.J.)

Case 3: Class II, Anterior Open Bite (AOB), Orthofacial, Clinical Treatment Outcome

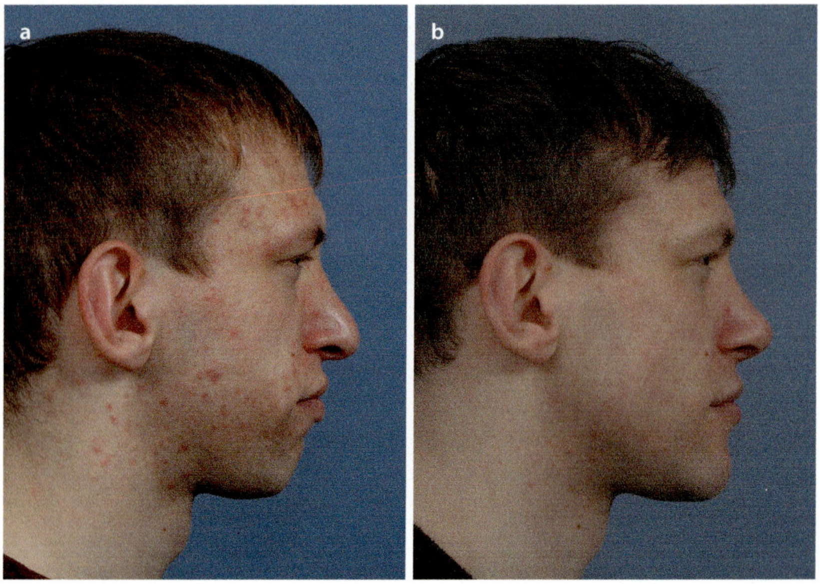

Fig. 6.95 Right profile views in rest, pre-surgical (**a**) and 1 year after (**b**) combined orthodontic-surgical treatment with bilateral zygomatic osteotomies, bilateral gonial augmentation, closed rhinoplasty, left otoplasty and midfacial liposculpture (patient B.J.)

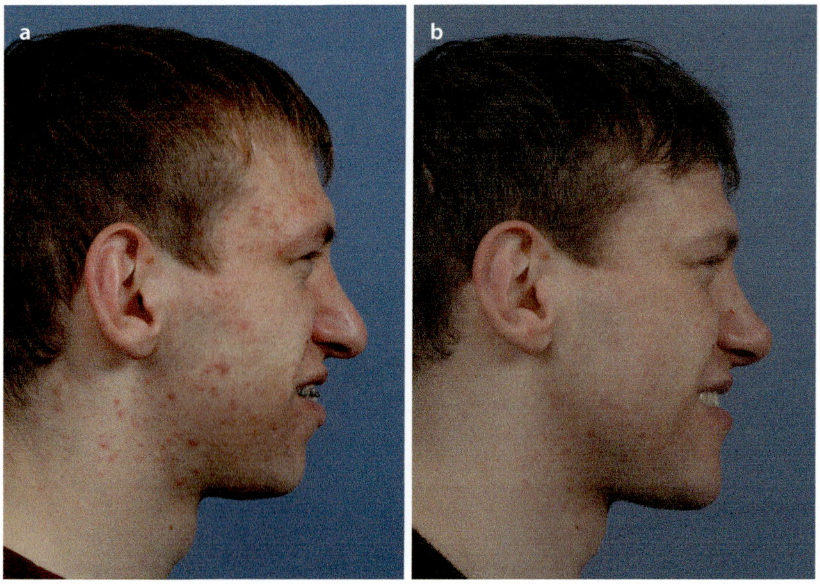

Fig. 6.96 Right profile views during smiling, pre-surgical (**a**) and 1 year after (**b**) combined orthodontic-surgical treatment with bilateral zygomatic osteotomies, bilateral gonial augmentation, closed rhinoplasty, left otoplasty and midfacial liposculpture (patient B.J.)

Case 3: Class II, Anterior Open Bite (AOB), Orthofacial, Clinical Treatment Outcome

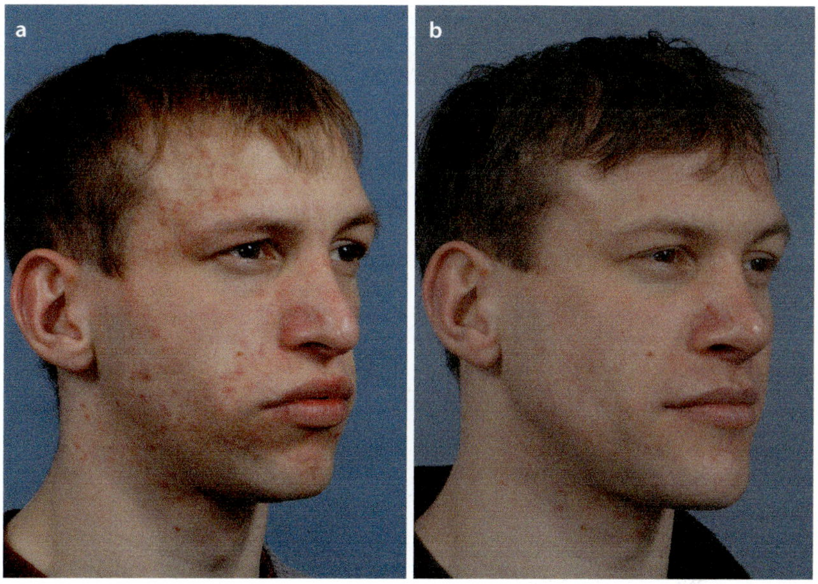

Fig. 6.97 2/3 right profile views in rest, pre-surgical (**a**) and 1 year after (**b**) combined orthodontic-surgical treatment with bilateral zygomatic osteotomies, bilateral gonial augmentation, closed rhinoplasty, left otoplasty and midfacial liposculpture (patient B.J.)

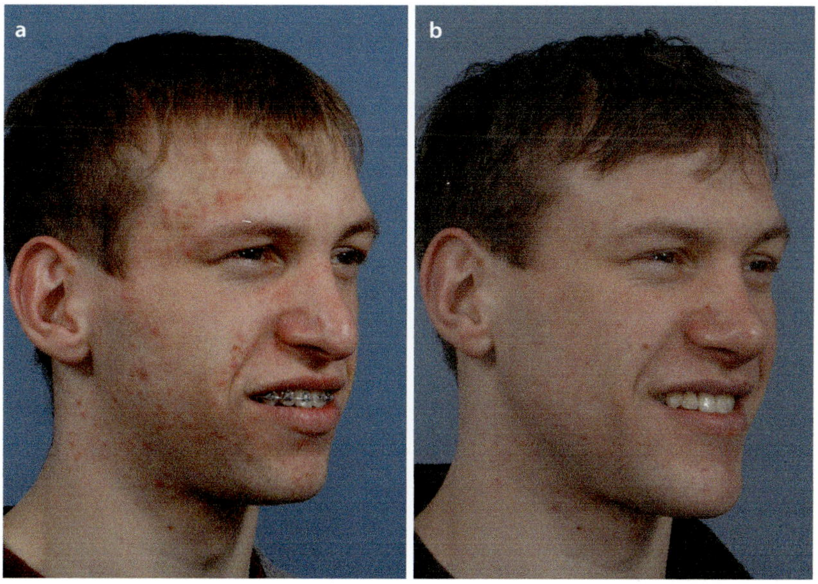

Fig. 6.98 2/3 right profile views during smiling, pre-surgical (**a**) and 1 year after (**b**) combined orthodontic-surgical treatment with bilateral zygomatic osteotomies, bilateral gonial augmentation, closed rhinoplasty, left otoplasty and midfacial liposculpture (patient B.J.)

Case 3: Class II, Anterior Open Bite (AOB), Orthofacial, Clinical Treatment Outcome

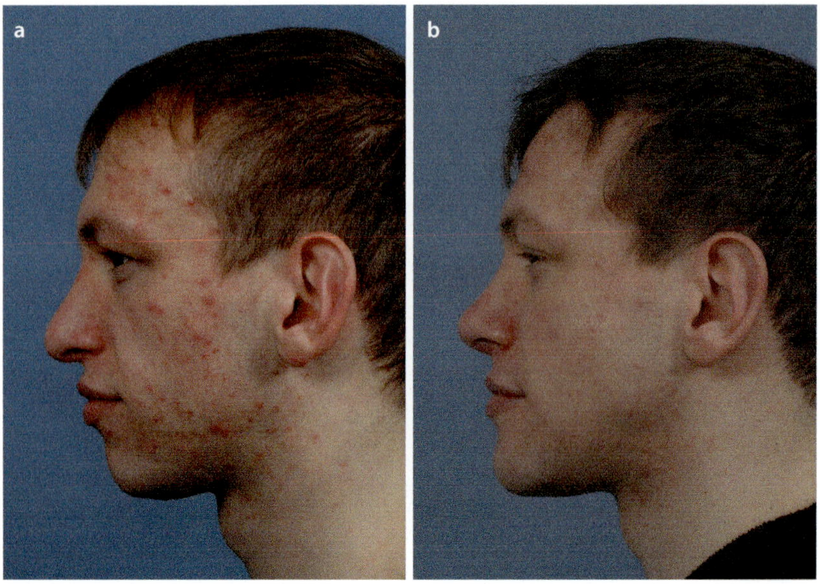

Fig. 6.99 Left profile views in rest, pre-surgical (**a**) and 1 year after (**b**) combined orthodontic-surgical treatment with bilateral zygomatic osteotomies, bilateral gonial augmentation, closed rhinoplasty, left otoplasty and midfacial liposculpture (patient B.J.)

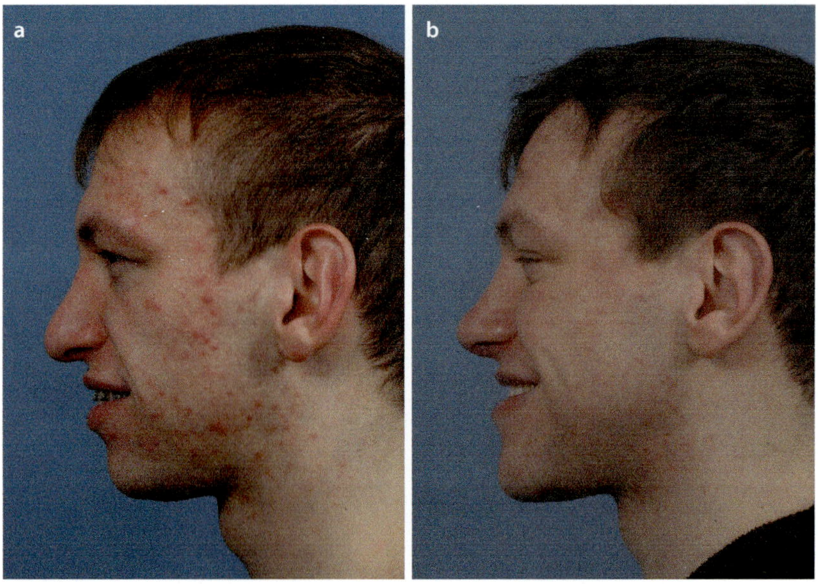

Fig. 6.100 Left profile views during smiling, pre-surgical (**a**) and 1 year after (**b**) combined orthodontic-surgical treatment with bilateral zygomatic osteotomies, bilateral gonial augmentation, closed rhinoplasty, left otoplasty and midfacial liposculpture (patient B.J.)

Case 3: Class II, Anterior Open Bite (AOB), Orthofacial, Clinical Treatment Outcome

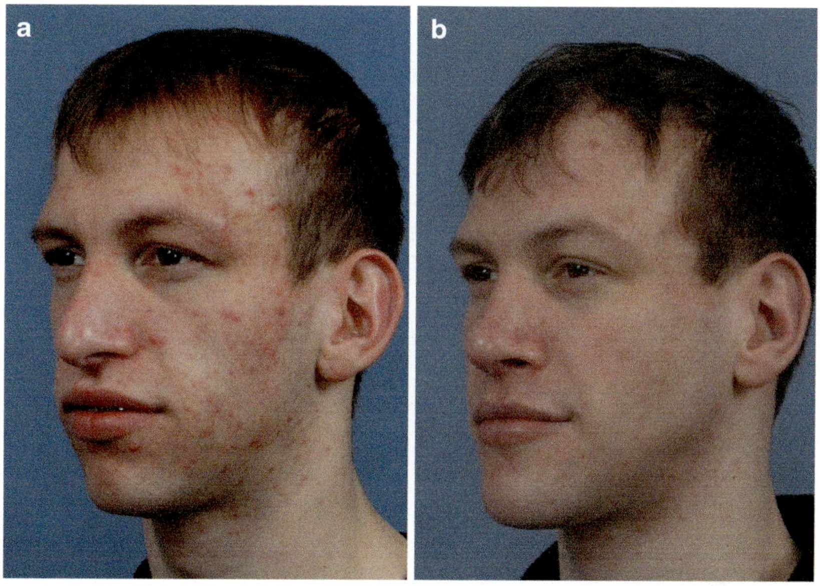

Fig. 6.101 2/3 left profile views in rest, pre-surgical (**a**) and 1 year after (**b**) combined orthodontic-surgical treatment with bilateral zygomatic osteotomies, bilateral gonial augmentation, closed rhinoplasty, left otoplasty and midfacial liposculpture (patient B.J.)

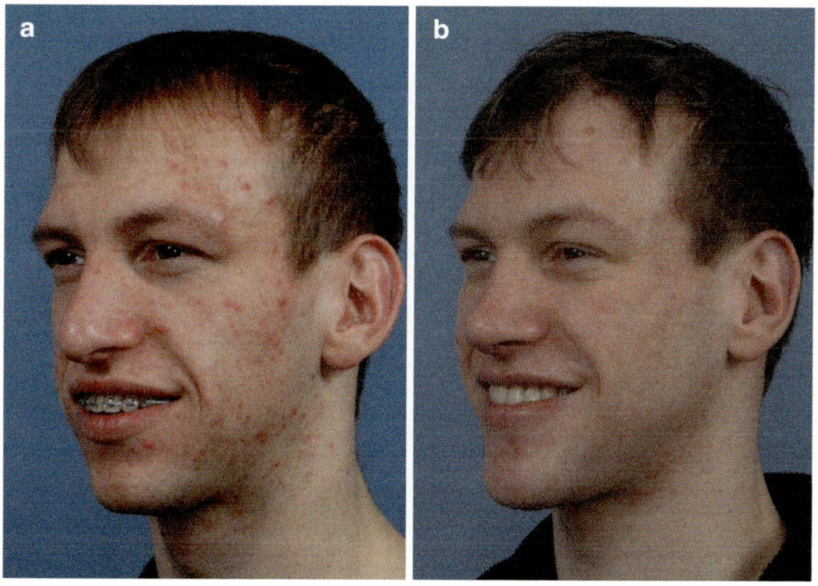

Fig. 6.102 2/3 left profile views during smiling, pre-surgical (**a**) and 1 year after (**b**) combined orthodontic-surgical treatment with bilateral zygomatic osteotomies, bilateral gonial augmentation, closed rhinoplasty, left otoplasty and midfacial liposculpture (patient B.J.)

Case 3: Class II, Anterior Open Bite (AOB), Orthofacial, Clinical Treatment Outcome

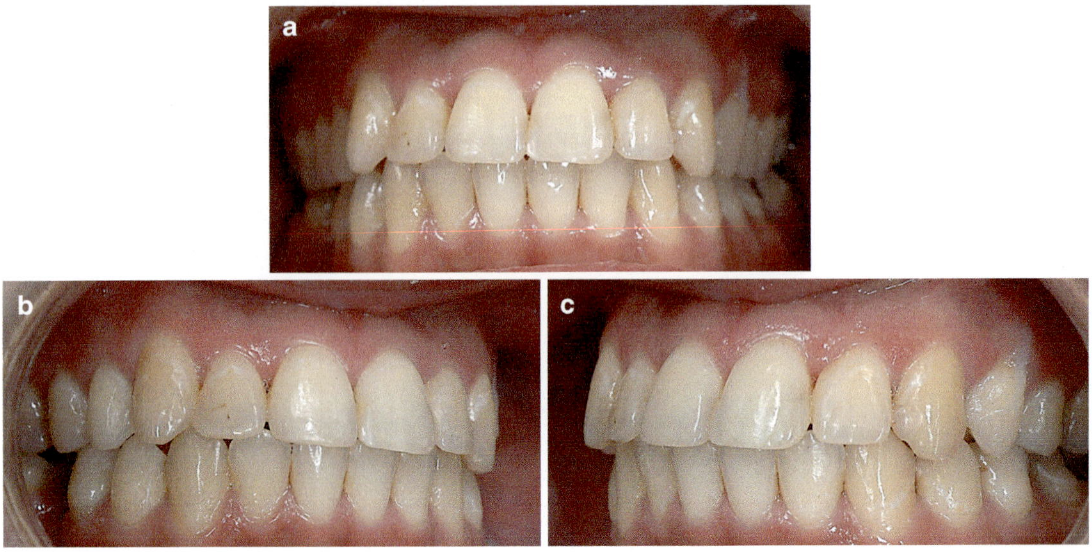

Fig. 6.103 Frontal (**a**), right (**b**) and left (**c**) intra-oral views of the patient's occlusion 1 year after combined orthodontic-surgical treatment (patient B.J.). The author acknowledges Prof. Bart Vande Vannet for the orthodontic treatment

Case 4: Class III, Midfacial Hypoplasia, Anterior Open Bite (AOB)

Patient B.B. is an 18.5-year-old male with a Class III, anterior open bite (AOB) maxillofacial deformity due to midfacial hypoplasia. Prior to the surgical workup, a bone scintigraphy was performed which did not show any residual condylar growth. In the frontal view, he is clinically presenting with a flattened midface, a slight deviation of the nasal tip to the right and no clinical obvious mandibular asymmetry. In rest, he has an incisal display of 2 mm, while during spontaneous smiling, he has almost (−1 mm at 11) full incisal exposure and presents with a slightly canted maxillary occlusal plane. In the profile view, he presents with a flattened midface with poor bilateral zygoma definition, a subtile nasal hump, a lip incompetence and an atonic lower lip. He has a Class II profile with an Angle Class III malocclusion with adequate transversal relationship, an anterior open bite (AOB) and a 1 mm upper dental midline deviation to the left. There is no history of TMJ dysfunction neither pain.

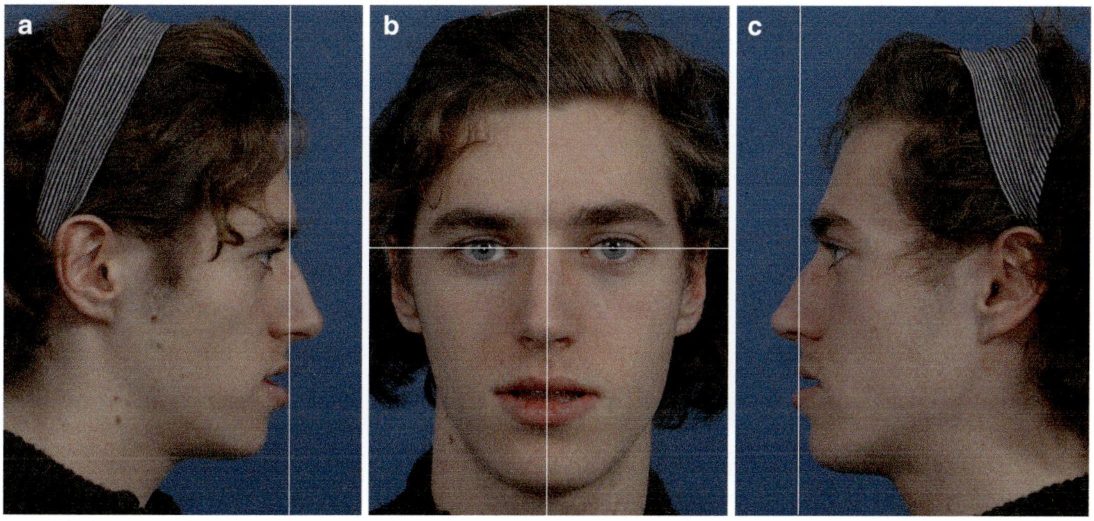

Fig. 6.104 Pre-surgical clinical right profile (**a**), frontal (**b**) and left profile (**c**) views of patient B.B. in his *c*-NHP in rest, at the time of the workup, approximately 3 weeks prior to surgery (patient B.B.)

Case 4: Class III, Midfacial Hypoplasia, Anterior Open Bite (AOB)

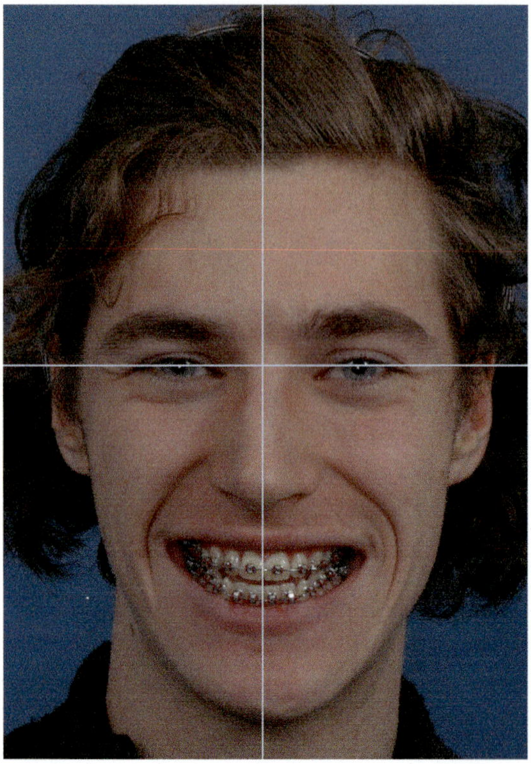

Fig. 6.105 Pre-surgical clinical frontal smiling view of patient B.B. at the time of the workup, approximately 3 weeks prior to surgery

Case 4: Class III, Midfacial Hypoplasia, Anterior Open Bite (AOB), v-NHP and PHP

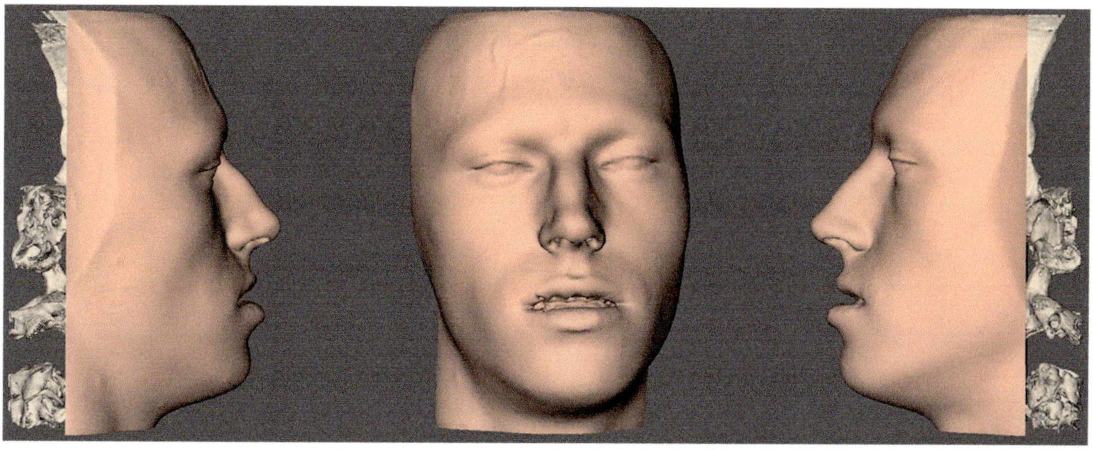

Fig. 6.106 Pre-surgical 3D "surface-rendered" right profile, frontal and left profile soft and hard tissue representations of the head of patient B.B., as generated during standardised CBCT image acquisition, at the time of the workup (Maxilim v. 2.3.0.3). Note the incorrect position and orientation of the virtual head compared to the clinical pictures of patient B.B. (Fig. 6.104), although it was attempted to scan patient B.B. in his correct *c*-NHP in rest

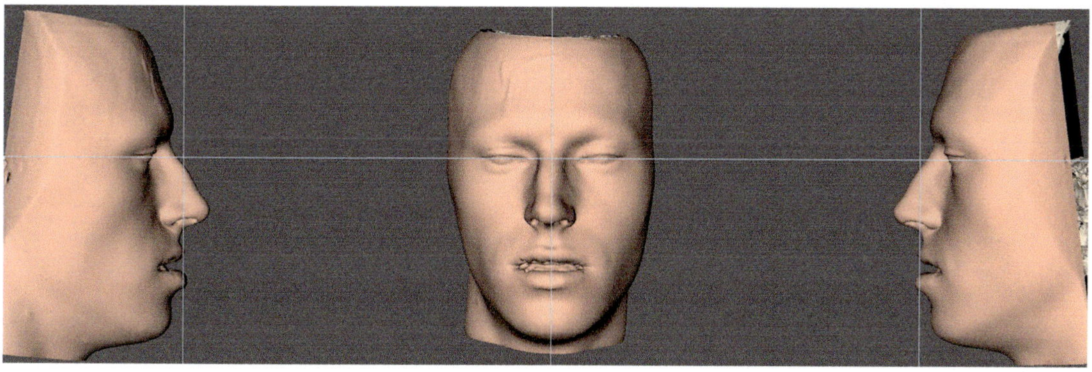

Fig. 6.107 Following a standardised "step-by-step" approach (▶ see Sect. 3.1), the scanned head position of patient B.B. (Fig. 6.106) was virtually modified towards his *c*-NHP (Fig. 6.104), which results in his *v*-NHP and corresponds to his individual "Planning Head Position (PHP)" (3D "surface-rendered" representations, Maxilim v. 2.3.0.3). Note that since both clinical profile photographs (Fig. 6.104a, c) showed a different *c*-NHP, it was clinically decided to virtually modify to a *v*-NHP in between

■ Case 4: Class III, Midfacial Hypoplasia, Anterior Open Bite (AOB)

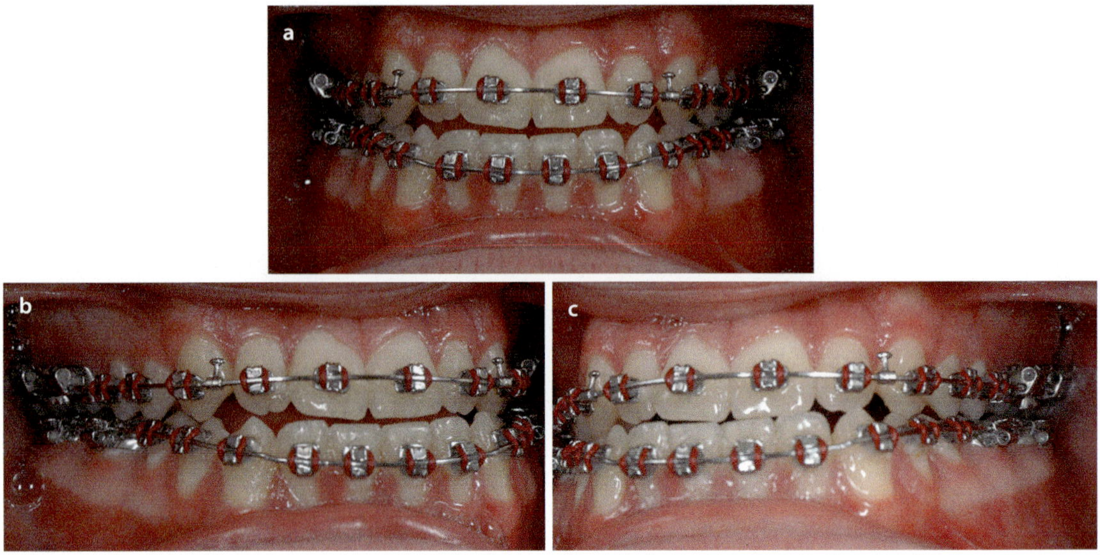

Fig. 6.108 Pre-surgical frontal (**a**), right (**b**) and left (**c**) intra-oral views of the occlusion of patient B.B. at the time of the workup, approximately 3 weeks prior to surgery

Patient B.B. illustrates clinically the potential of 3D virtual mandibular autorotation (▶ see also Sect. 1.3) in 3D virtual treatment planning of orthognathic surgery.

Case 4: 3D-VPS$_5$ Step 1 Maxillary Occlusal Cant Evaluation/Correction ("Roll")

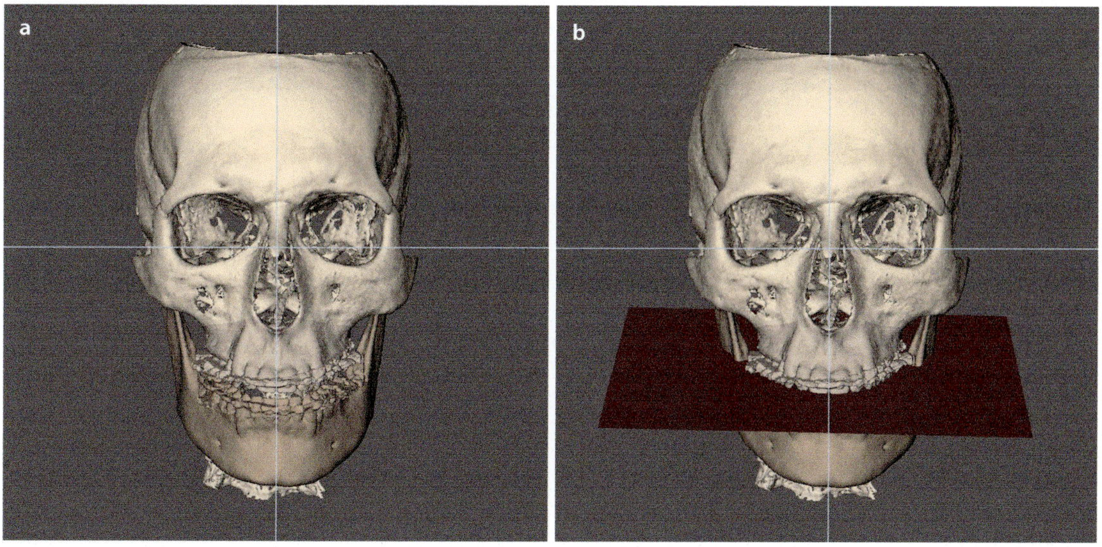

Fig. 6.109 The maxillary occlusal plane is evaluated both clinically (Fig. 6.105) and virtually (**a**) towards the horizontal 3D PHP reference plane and is slightly canted (**b**) in patient B.B. (3D "surface-rendered" representations, patient B.B., Maxilim v. 2.3.0.3)

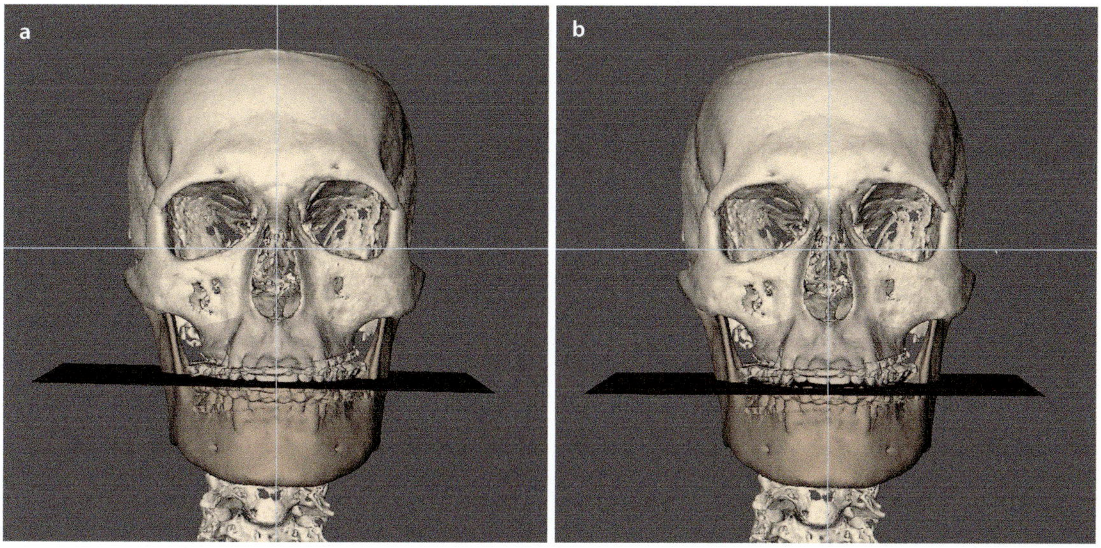

Fig. 6.110 Virtual rotation of the patient's skull to the back more clearly shows the slightly canted maxillary occlusal plane (**a**), whereas the mandibular occlusal plane (**b**) is parallel to the horizontal 3D PHP reference plane and does not need to be modified (3D "surface-rendered" representations, patient B.B., Maxilim v. 2.3.0.3)

Case 4: 3D-VPS$_5$ Step 2 Upper Dental Midline Evaluation/Correction

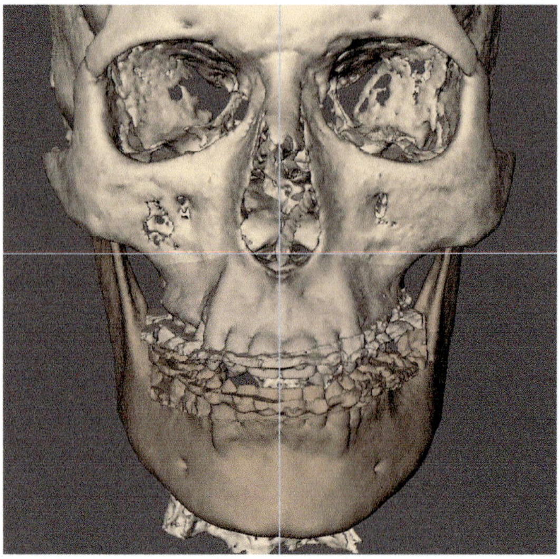

Fig. 6.111 The upper dental midline is 1 mm deviated to the left towards the facial midline 3D PHP reference plane in patient B.B., whereas the lower dental midline is centred (3D "surface-rendered" representations, Maxilim v. 2.3.0.3)

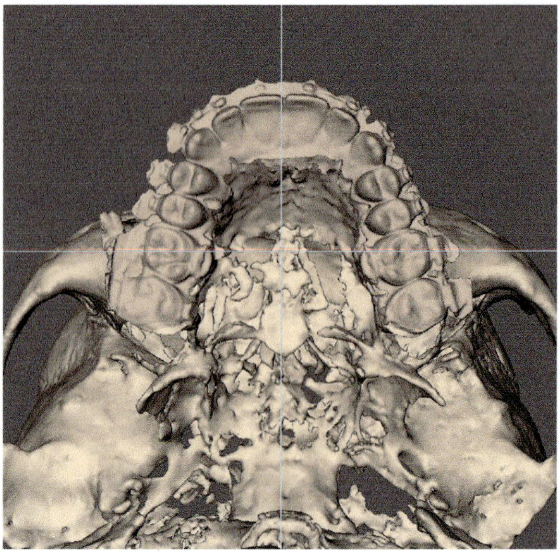

Fig. 6.112 The base views illustrate a 1 mm deviation of the upper dental midline to the left towards the facial midline 3D PHP reference plane in patient B.B. (3D "surface-rendered" representations, Maxilim v. 2.3.0.3)

Case 4: 3D-VPS$_5$ Step 3 Overall Evaluation of Facial Asymmetry After Virtual Occlusal Definition

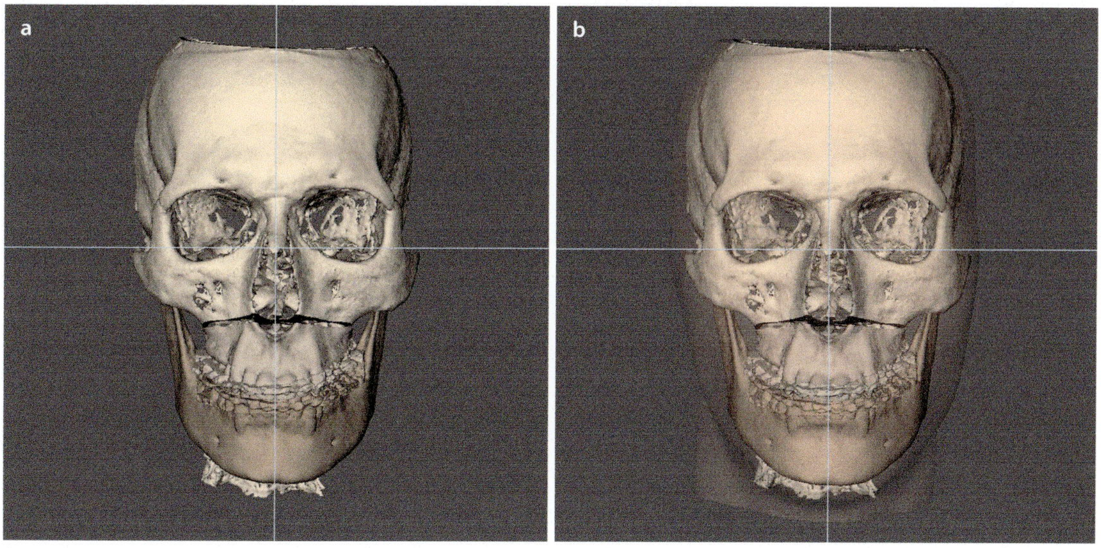

Fig. 6.113 Overall facial asymmetry of the patient's skull (**a**) with transparent soft tissues (**b**) is assessed after virtual occlusal definition in the frontal view towards both the horizontal and facial midline 3D PHP reference planes in patient B.B. (3D "surface-rendered" representations, Maxilim v. 2.3.0.3). Note the overall adequate symmetry of the mandibular contour

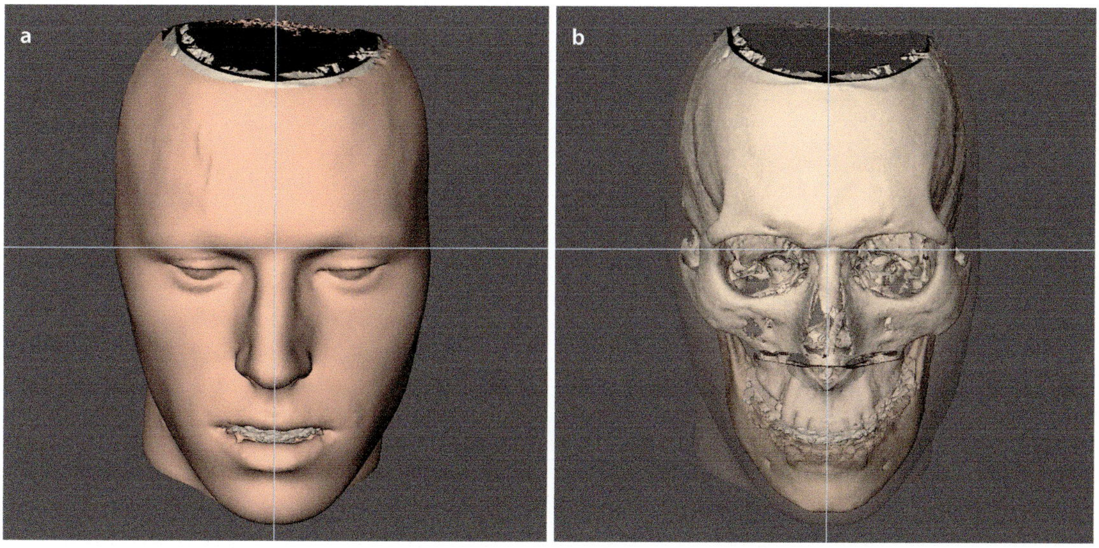

Fig. 6.114 To evaluate the overall facial asymmetry after virtual occlusal definition, the mandibular contour is evaluated both virtually on the soft tissues (**a**) and at the bony level towards the contour of the zygomatic bones and arches with soft tissues in transparency (**b**) in patient B.B. (3D "surface-rendered" representations, Maxilim v. 2.3.0.3). Note the overall symmetry of the midfacial and mandibular contour and a slight deviation of the nasal tip to the right although the bony nasal pyramid is straight

■ Case 4: 3D-VPS$_5$ Step 4 Evaluation/Correction of Flaring ("Yaw")

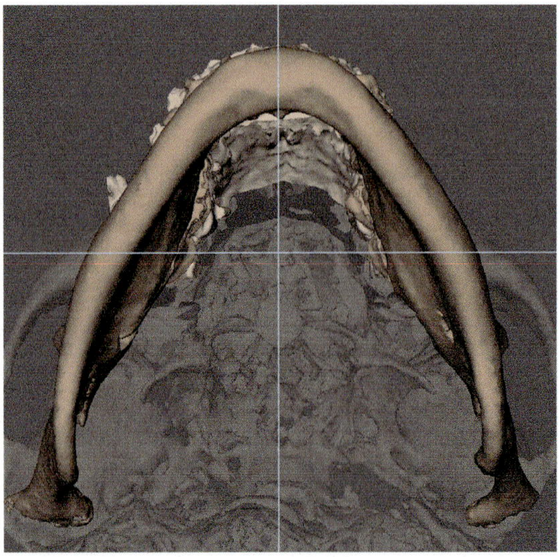

Fig. 6.115 The base view shows good overall mandibular symmetry in patient B.B. (3D "surface-rendered" representations, Maxilim v. 2.3.0.3)

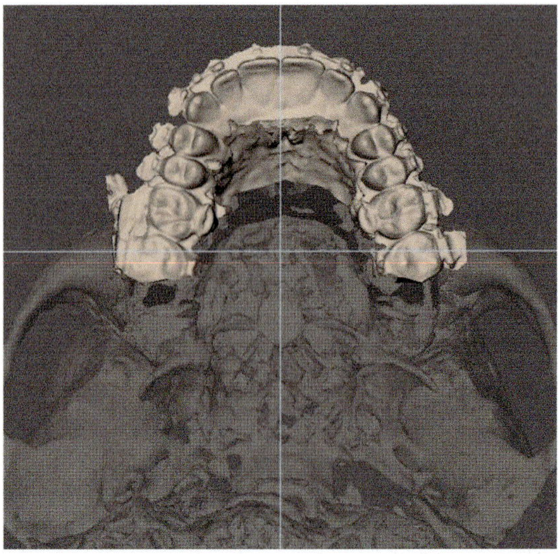

Fig. 6.116 The base view shows no flaring of the maxilla after 3D virtual occlusal definition in patient B.B. (3D "surface-rendered" representations, Maxilim v. 2.3.0.3)

■ Case 4: 3D-VPS$_5$ Step 5 Upper Vertical Incisal Position Evaluation/Correction

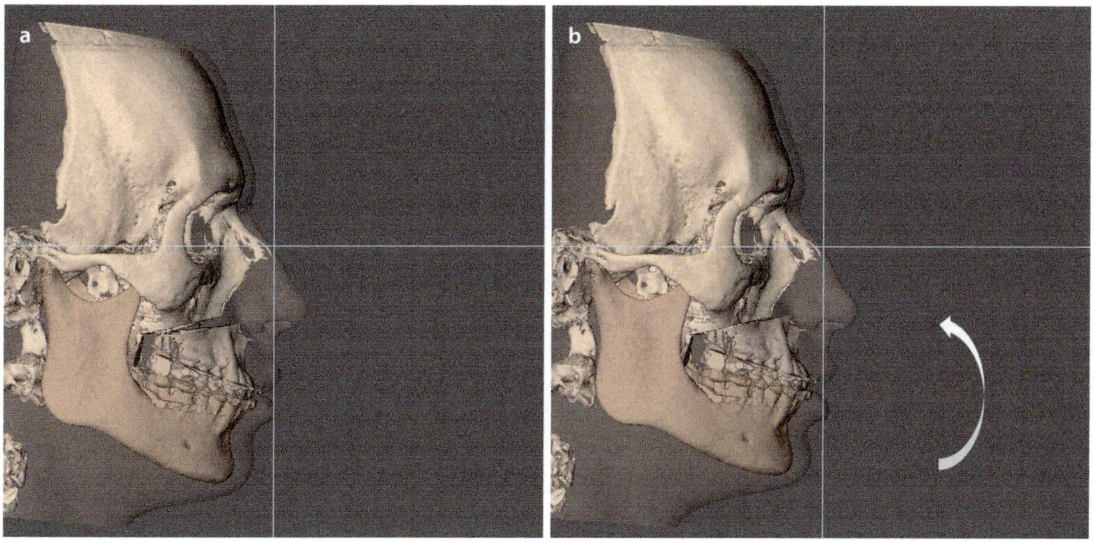

Fig. 6.117 After 3D virtual occlusal definition without mandibular autorotation (**a**), the upper incisal level is 4.5 mm extruded, while a 3° CCW autorotation of the mandible (**b**) keeps the upper incisal level on "0" (3D "surface-rendered" representations, patient B.B., Maxilim v. 2.3.0.3)

▪ Case 4: 3D-VPS$_5$ Step 6 Sagittal Upper Incisal Position Evaluation/Correction

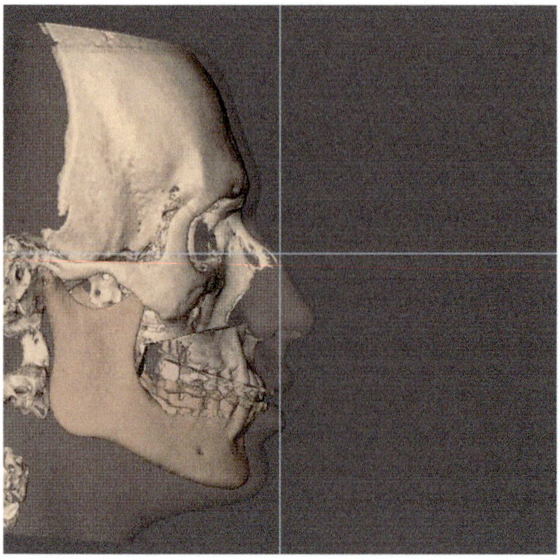

Fig. 6.118 A 3° CCW autorotation of the mandible (Fig. 6.117) advances the upper incisal level for 8.5 mm which is clinically assessed as exaggerated in patient B.B. (3D "surface-rendered" representations, Maxilim v. 2.3.0.3)

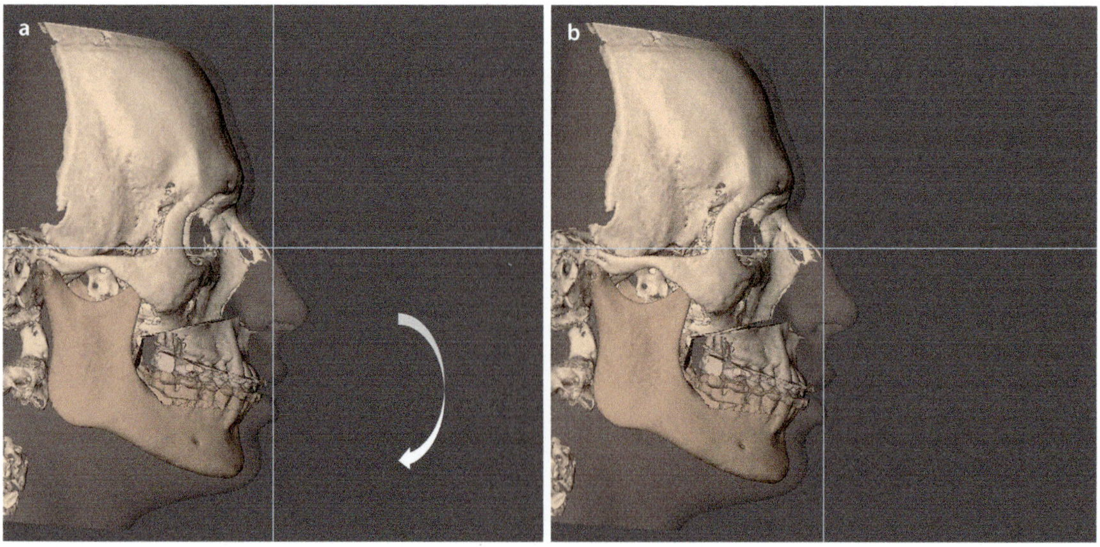

Fig. 6.119 The mandible is therefore again virtually autorotated 1.5° CW (**a**) which results in a 1.5 mm extrusion at the upper incisal level in patient B.B. and clinically acceptable advancement of 6 mm (**b**) (3D "surface-rendered" representations, patient B.B., Maxilim v. 2.3.0.3)

▪ Case 4: 3D-VPS$_5$ Step 7 Profile Evaluation/Occlusal Plane Correction ("Pitch")

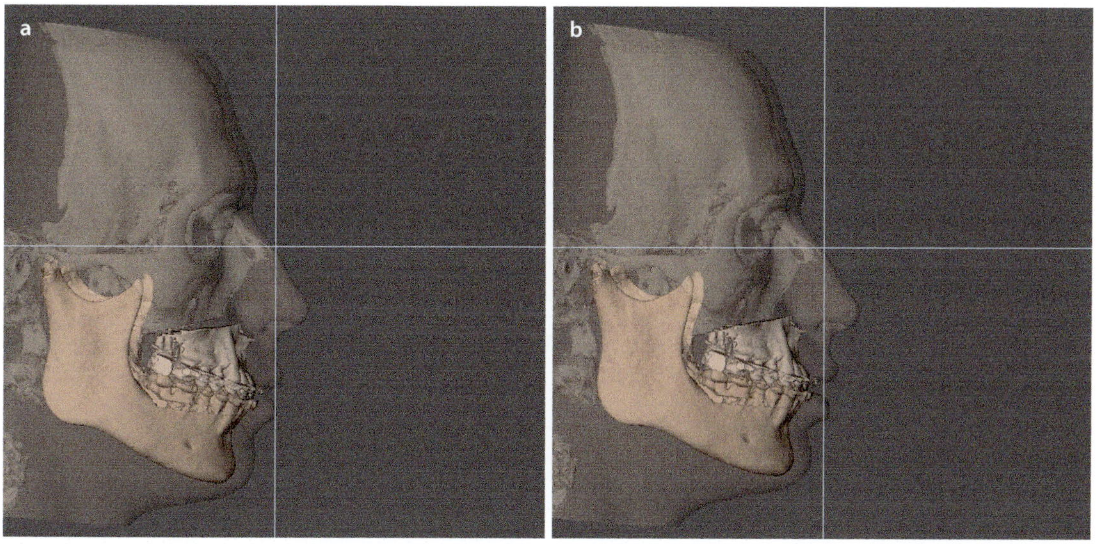

Fig. 6.120 At this stage in "step 7", the profile is evaluated without mandibular autorotation (**a**) and after 3° CCW autorotation of the mandible (**b**) (3D "surface-rendered" representations, patient B.B., Maxilim v. 2.3.0.3)

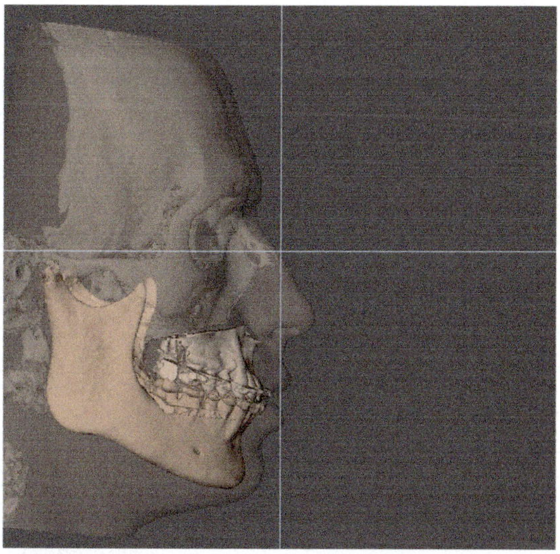

Fig. 6.121 Clinically it was decided to perform a 1.5° CCW virtual mandibular autorotation which results in an advancement of 6 mm and an extrusion of 1.5 mm, at the upper incisal level (Fig. 6.119b) (3D "surface-rendered" representations, patient B.B., Maxilim v. 2.3.0.3)

■ Case 4: 3D-VPS$_5$ Step 8 3D Chin Position Evaluation/Correction

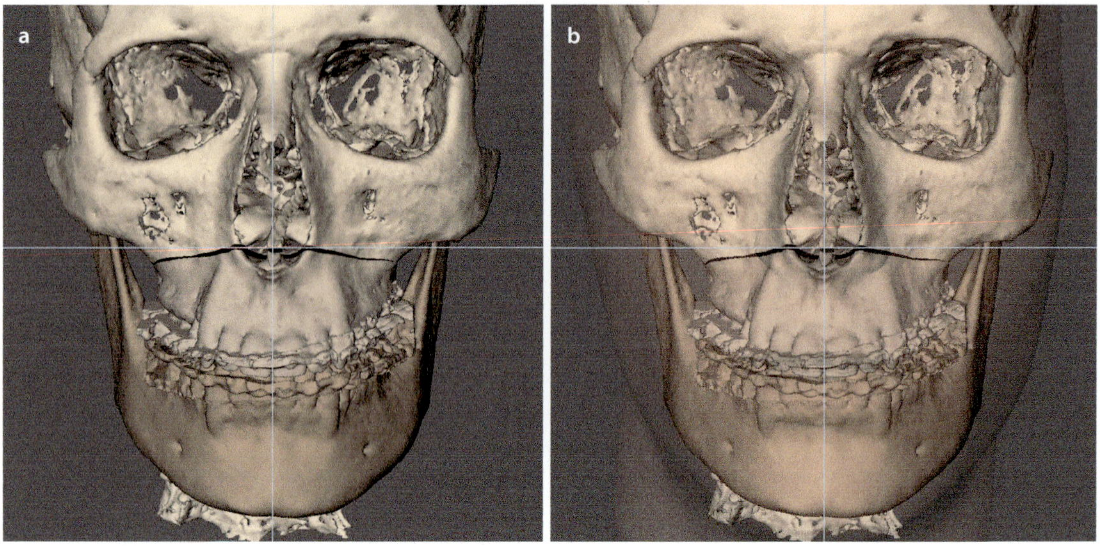

Fig. 6.122 Evaluation of the chin position in the frontal plane after isolated virtual Le Fort I osteotomy with 1.5° CCW virtual mandibular autorotation without (**a**) and with (**b**) the patient's 3D facial soft tissue mask in transparency (3D "surface-rendered" representations, patient B.B., Maxilim v. 2.3.0.3). Note the adequate overall symmetry of the chin

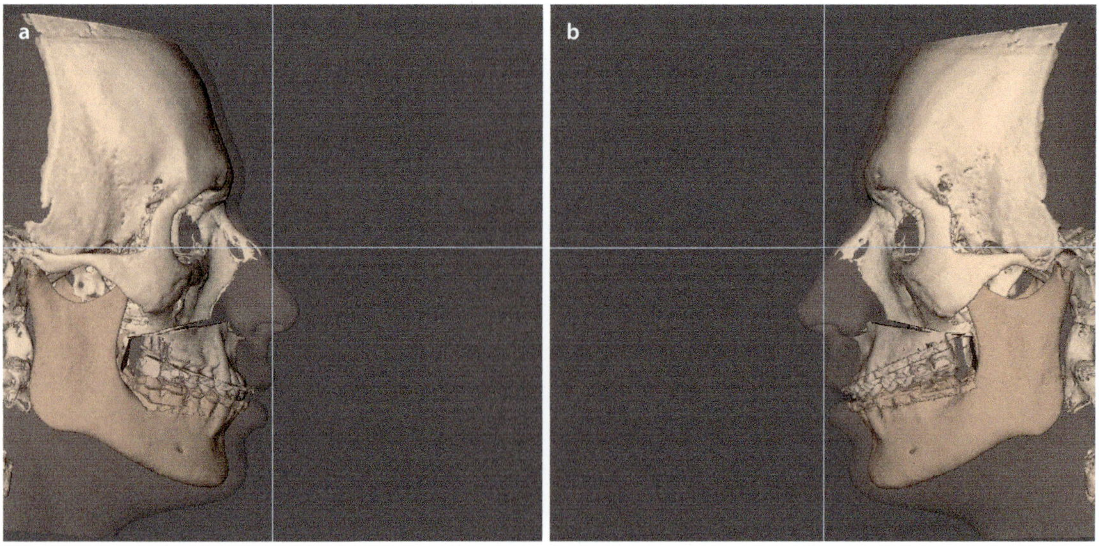

Fig. 6.123 Evaluation of the sagittal chin position after isolated virtual Le Fort I osteotomy with 1.5° CCW virtual mandibular autorotation needs to be individually assessed in the right (**a**) and left profile (**b**) views (3D "surface-rendered" representations, patient B.B., Maxilim v. 2.3.0.3)

Case 4: 3D-VPS$_5$ Step 8 3D Chin Position Evaluation/Correction

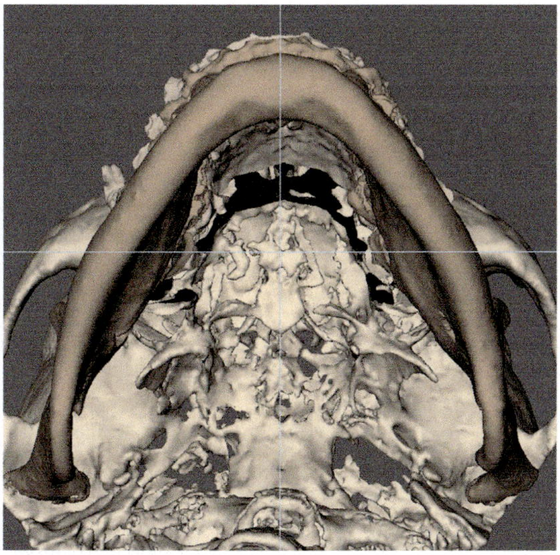

Fig. 6.124 Evaluation of the chin position in the base view after isolated virtual Le Fort I osteotomy with 1.5° CCW virtual mandibular autorotation shows overall symmetric mandibular contour in patient B.B. (3D "surface-rendered" representations, patient B.B., Maxilim v. 2.3.0.3)

Case 4: 3D-VPS$_5$ Step 9 Patient Communication of the Individualised Treatment Plan

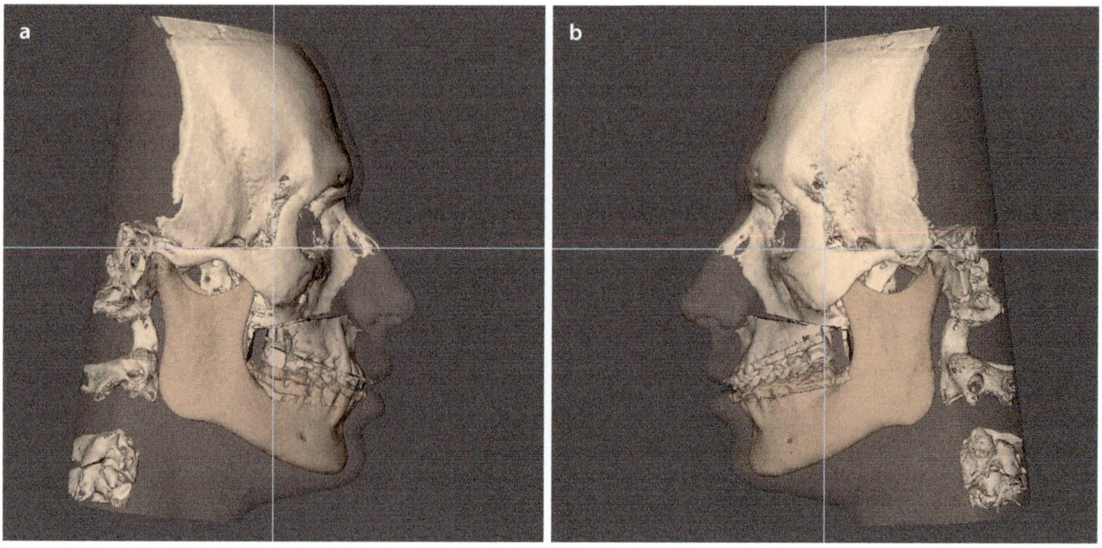

Fig. 6.125 Right (**a**) and left (**b**) profile views of the "Individualised 3D Virtual Treatment Plan", as presented to patient B.B., before the actual surgery (3D "surface-rendered" representations, Maxilim v. 2.3.0.3)

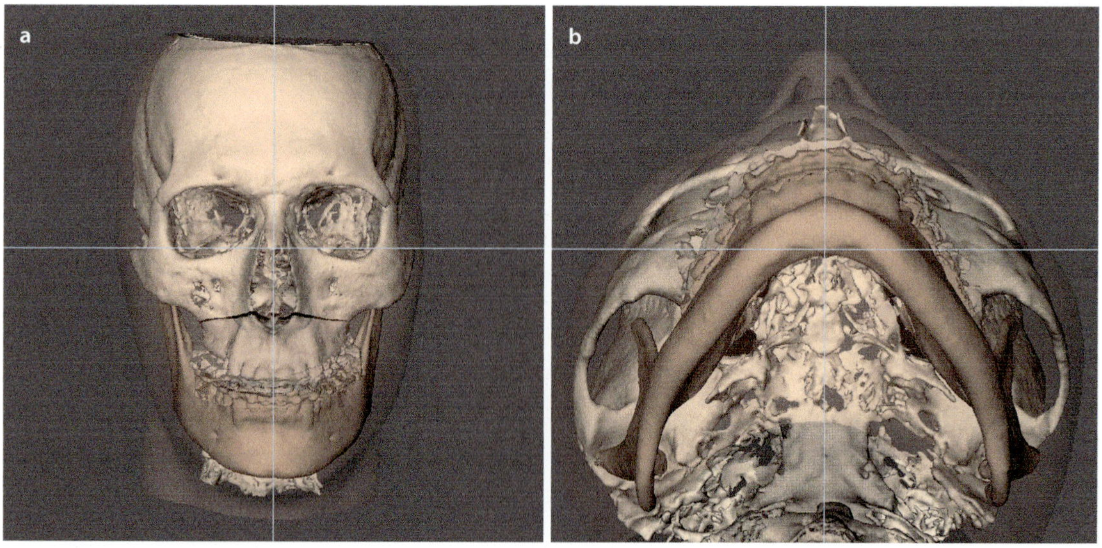

Fig. 6.126 Frontal (**a**) and base (**b**) views of the "Individualised 3D Virtual Treatment Plan", as presented to patient B.B., before the actual surgery (3D "surface-rendered" representations, Maxilim v. 2.3.0.3). Note the slight deviation of the nasal tip to the right although the bony nasal pyramid is straight. Also note the flattened zygomatic bones

Case 4: 3D-VPS$_5$ Step 9 Patient Communication of the Individualised Treatment Plan

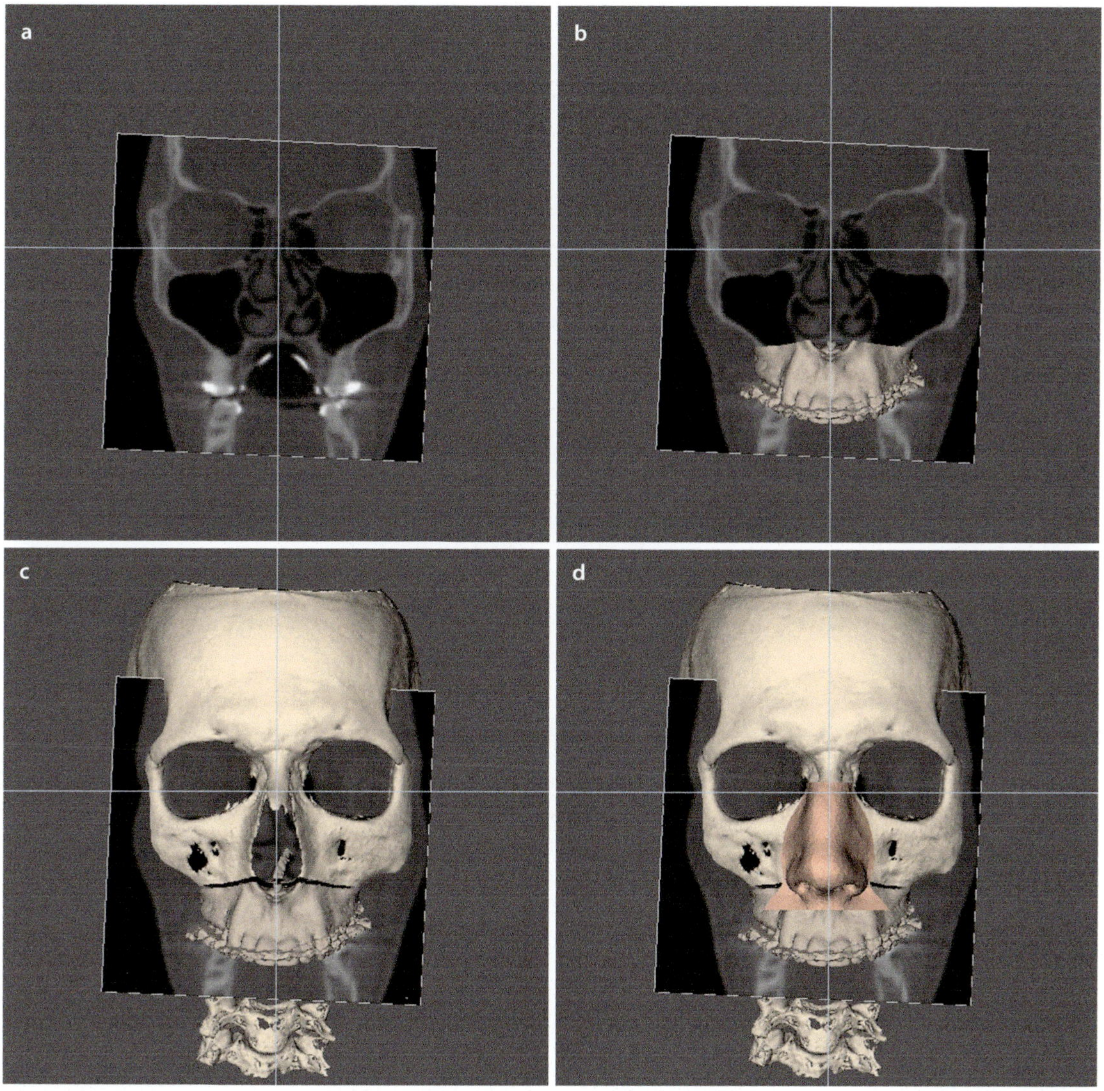

Fig. 6.127 The combination of 3D virtual evaluation of the underlying coronal slices (**a**), the segmented maxilla (**b**), the bony skull (**c**) and the soft tissue of the nose (**d**) shows that the anterior nasal spine (ANS) is centred and the nasal floor is symmetric, but an important septal deviation which pushes the nasal tip to the right in patient B.B. (3D "surface-rendered" representations, Maxilim v. 2.3.0.3)

■ Case 4: 3D-VPS$_5$ Step 10 Final Adjustments of the 3D Virtual Treatment Plan

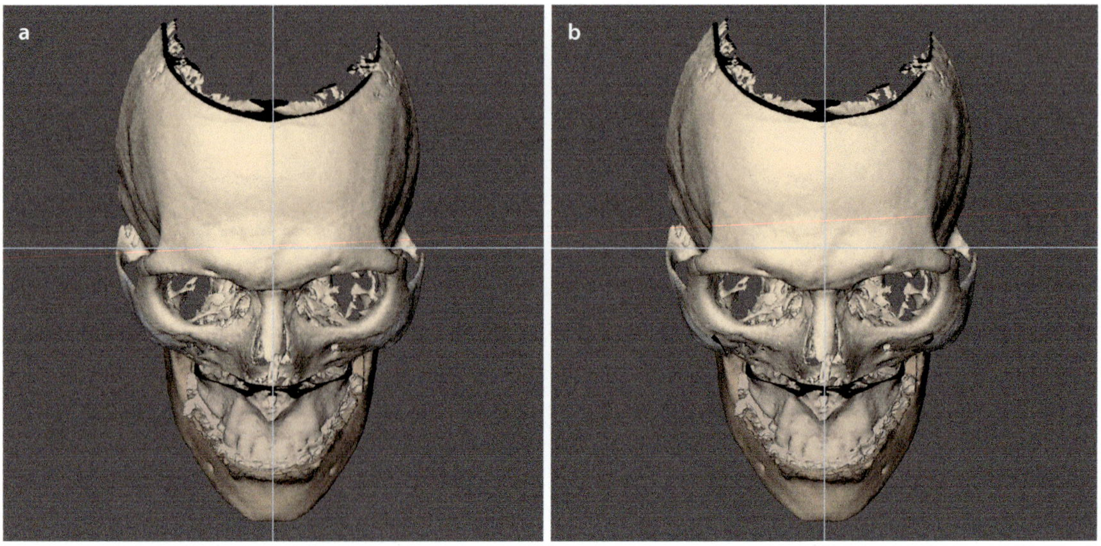

Fig. 6.128 Final adjustments of the "Individualised 3D Virtual Treatment Plan" after communication with patient B.B. consisted of additional zygomatic sandwich osteotomies to correct the flattened infraorbital contour of the midface and comprehensive septoplasty to correct the right nasal tip deviation and the left nasal obstruction (3D "surface-rendered" representations, Maxilim v. 2.3.0.3): before (**a**) and after (**b**) frontal downward inclined views

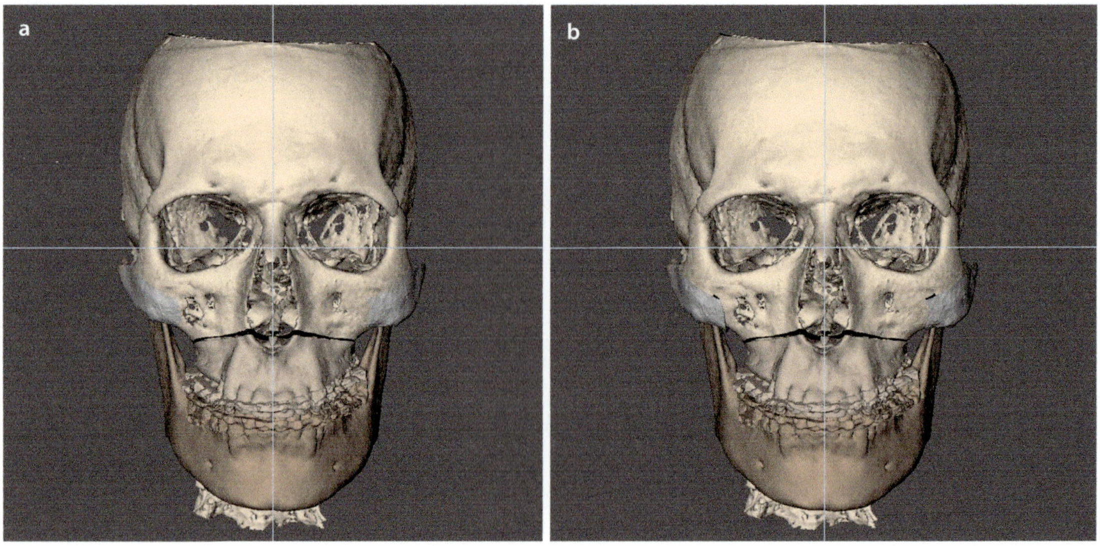

Fig. 6.129 Final adjustments of the "Individualised 3D Virtual Treatment Plan" after communication with patient B.B. consisted of additional zygomatic sandwich osteotomies to correct the flattened infraorbital contour of the midface and comprehensive septoplasty to correct the right nasal tip deviation and the left nasal obstruction (3D "surface-rendered" representations, Maxilim v. 2.3.0.3): before (**a**) and after (**b**) frontal views

Case 4: 3D-VPS$_5$- Final Integrated "Individualised 3D Virtual Treatment Plan"

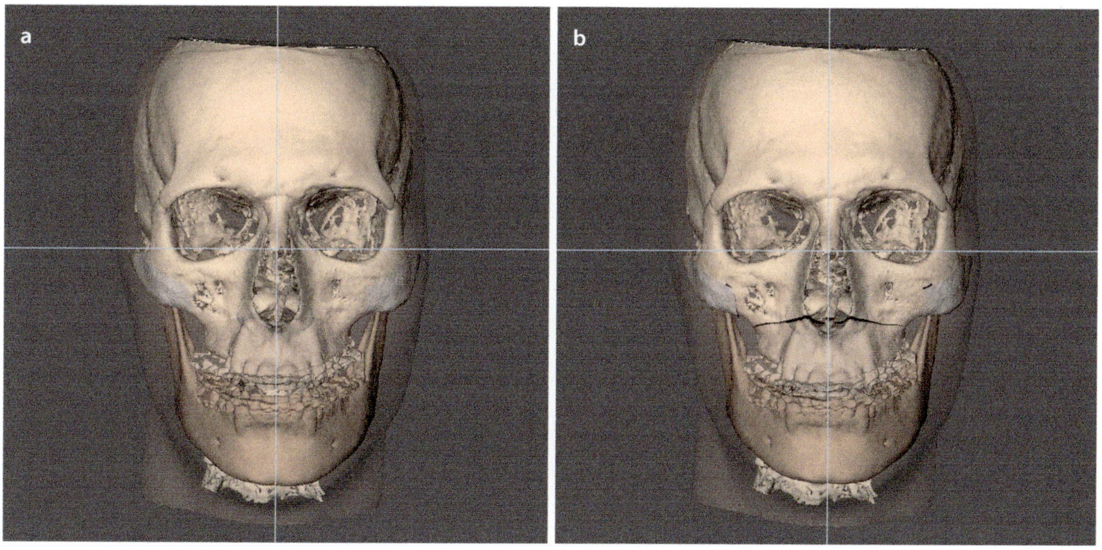

Fig. 6.130 Initial situation (**a**), and final "Individualised 3D Virtual Treatment Plan" (**b**), in the frontal plane (3D "surface-rendered" representations, patient B.B., Maxilim v. 2.3.0.3)

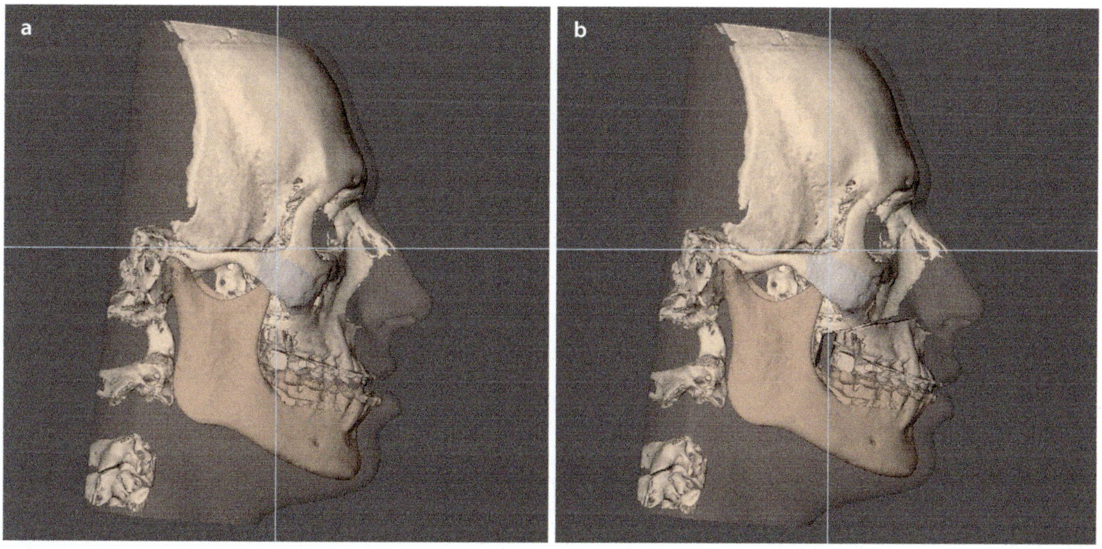

Fig. 6.131 Initial situation (**a**), and final "Individualised 3D Virtual Treatment Plan" (**b**), in the right profile plane (3D "surface-rendered" representations, patient B.B., Maxilim v. 2.3.0.3)

Case 4: 3D-VPS$_5$- Final Integrated "Individualised 3D Virtual Treatment Plan"

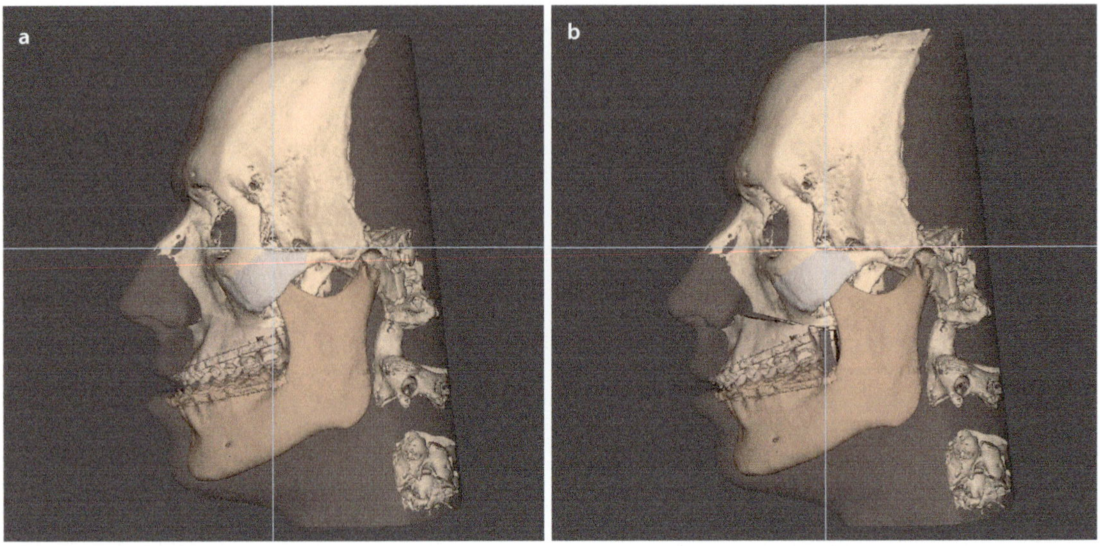

Fig. 6.132 Initial situation (**a**), and final "Individualised 3D Virtual Treatment Plan" (**b**), in the left profile plane (3D "surface-rendered" representations, patient B.B., Maxilim v. 2.3.0.3)

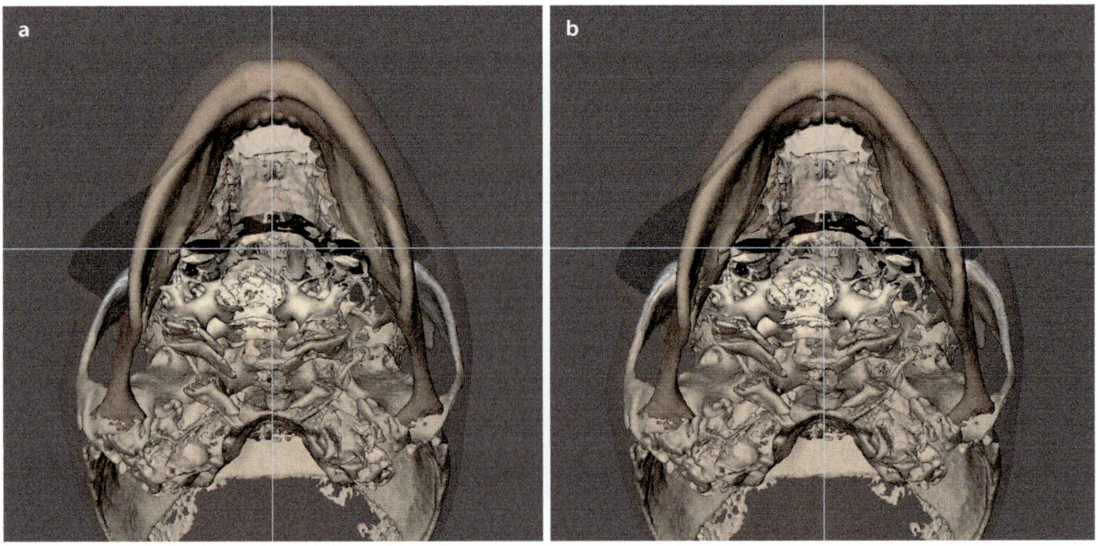

Fig. 6.133 Initial situation (**a**), and final "Individualised 3D Virtual Treatment Plan" (**b**), in the base plane (3D "surface-rendered" representations, patient B.B., Maxilim v. 2.3.0.3). Note the bilateral zygomatic expansion

Case 4: "3D Virtual Treatment Planning, OR" Template

Maxillary osteotomy

- ■ Le Fort: ■I ☐II ☐III
- ■ One-piece
- ☐ Segmental:
  - Pieces: ....
  - Interdental: ....
- ■ Advancement: 6.0 mm..........................
- ☐ Set-back : ....
- ■ Midline: 1 mm.................. ■R ☐L
- ■ Midline after Le Fort 1: inbetween 31/41
- ■ Vertical: (➔)
- ☐ "Yaw" correction: ....
- ☐ Other: ....

Mandibular osteotomy

- ☐ SSO ☐R ☐L
- ☐ Inverted-L ☐R ☐L
- ☐ VRO ☐R ☐L
- ☐ Advancement: R .... L ....
- ☐ Set-back: R .... L ....
- ☐ CW "Pitch" rotation
- ☐ CCW "Pitch" rotation
- ☐ Midline split
- ☐ IAN course: R .... L ....
- ☐ Midline after BSSO: ....
- ☐ Other: ....

Chin osteotomy

- ☐ Advancement: ....
- ☐ Set-back: ....
- ☐ Midline: .... ☐R ☐L
- ☐ Intrusion:
  - ☐ Anterior: ....
  - ☐ Posterior: R ...... L ......
- ☐ Extrusion:
  - ☐ Anterior: ....
  - ☐ Posterior: R ...... L ......
- ☐ "Shield" osteotomy
- ☐ "Chin wing" osteotomy
  - *Mental Foramen level:*
    - ☐ Symmetric
    - ☐ Asymmetric
- ☐ Other: ....

Planning Requirements

- ■ Maxilla first
- ☐ Mandible first
- ☐ Minimally Invasive Le Fort I
- ☐ IO-CBCT
- ☐ Kobayashi wires : ....
- ■ Skeletal anchorage : frontal..............
- ☐ Orthodontic buttons : ....
- ☐ Occlusal grinding : ....
- ☐ Other : ....

0.5 mm	1.5 mm	1.5 mm	1.0 mm	0.0 mm
16	13	11	23	26

"Roll" correction: ☐ CW ■ CCW

Miscellaneous

- ■ Para-nasal cross sutures
- ■ Alar cinch
- ■ Septoplasty
- ☐ Inferior turbinectomy
- ☐ ANS: ☐Shortening ☐Midline
- ☐ Nasal base plasty ☐R ☐L
- ■ Lateral nasal wall plasty ■R ■L
- ☐ Bone graft(s): ....
- ☐ Extraction(s): ....
- ☐ Other: ....

Adjuvant Cosmetic Procedures

- ☐ Bichatectomy ☐R ☐L
- ■ Zygoma osteotomies ■R ■L
  - *Infraorbital Foramen level:*
    - ☐ Symmetric
    - ■ Asymmetric
- ☐ Otoplasty: ☐R ☐L
- ☐ Rhinoplasty: ....
- ☐ Browlift: ....
- ☐ Blepharoplasty: ....
  - ☐Upper ☐Lower
- ☐ Facelift: ....
- ☐ Necklift: ....
- ☐ Liposuction: ....
- ☐ Lipofilling: ....
- ☐ Other: ....

■ Case 4: Class III, Midfacial Hypoplasia, Anterior Open Bite (AOB), 3D Virtual Treatment Outcome

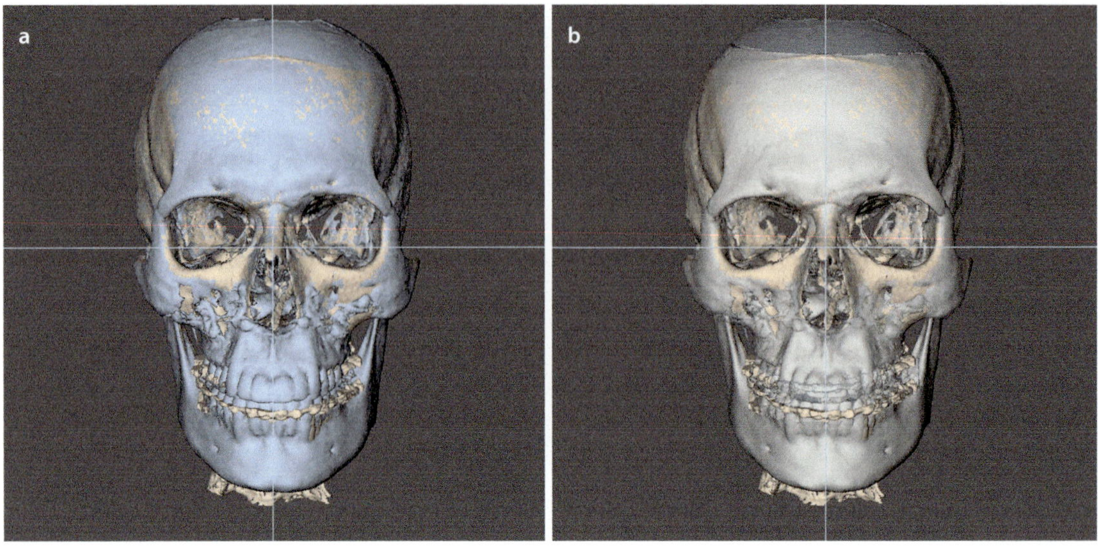

Fig. 6.134 Voxel-based superimposition on the cranial base of the pre-surgical and 6 months post-surgical (*blue*) frontal "surface-rendered" hard tissue representations (i-CAT, Imaging Sciences International Inc., Maxilim v. 2.3.0.3) (patient B.B.): post-surgical without (**a**) and with transparency (**b**)

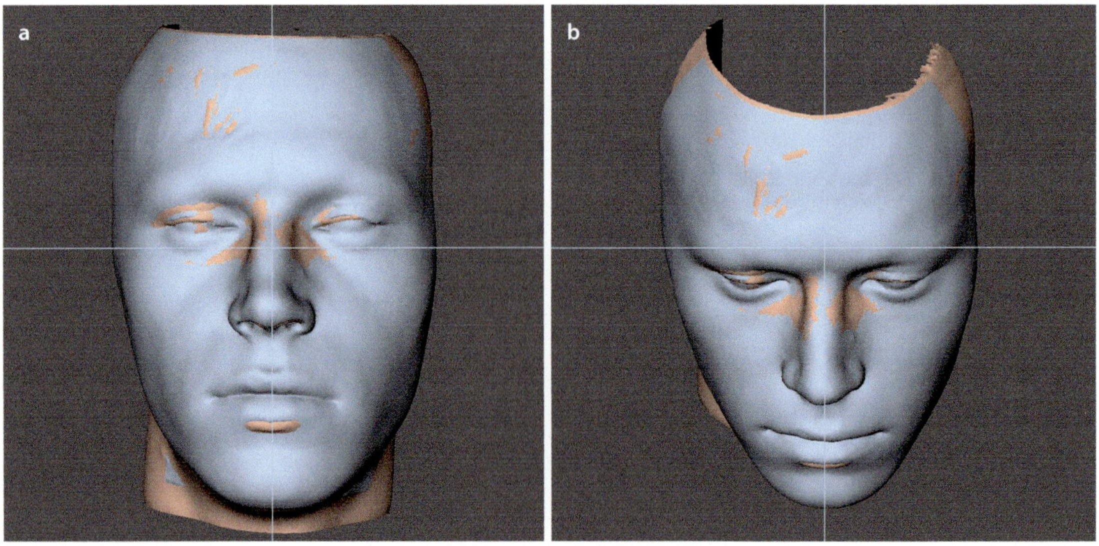

Fig. 6.135 Voxel-based superimposition on the cranial base of the pre-surgical and 6 months post-surgical (*blue*) 3D "surface-rendered" soft tissue representations. Frontal (**a**) and downward inclined (**b**) views (i-CAT, Imaging Sciences International Inc., Maxilim v. 2.3.0.3) (patient B.B.). Note the post-surgical (*blue*) facial symmetry and harmony. Note that the nasal tip deviation is almost completely corrected by the septoplasty

Case 4: Class III, Midfacial Hypoplasia, Anterior Open Bite (AOB), 3D Virtual Treatment Outcome

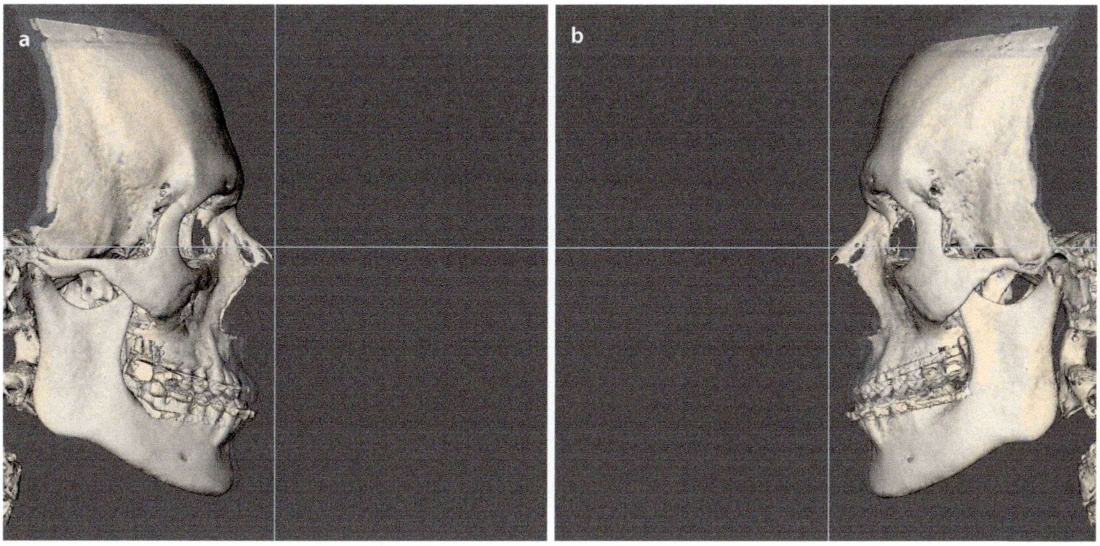

Fig. 6.136 Voxel-based superimposition on the cranial base of the pre-surgical and 6 months post-surgical (*blue*) 3D "surface-rendered" hard tissue representations. Right (**a**) and left profile (**b**) views (i-CAT, Imaging Sciences International Inc., Maxilim v. 2.3.0.3) (patient B.B.)

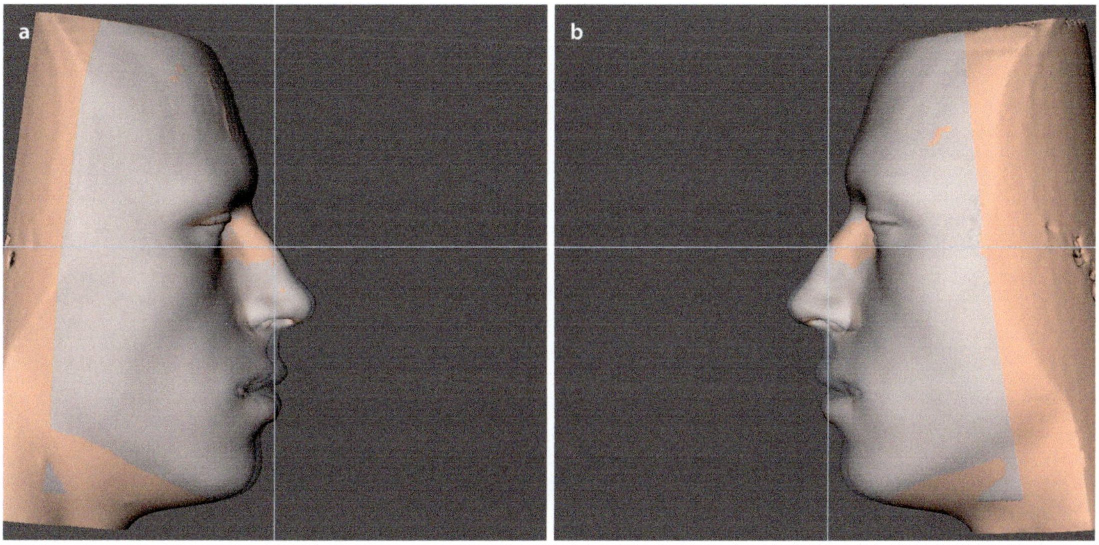

Fig. 6.137 Voxel-based superimposition on the cranial base of the pre-surgical and 6 months post-surgical (*blue*) 3D "surface-rendered" soft tissue representations. Right (**a**) and left (**b**) profile views (i-CAT, Imaging Sciences International Inc., Maxilim v. 2.3.0.3) (patient B.B.). Note the post-surgical lip competence and the changes at the nasolabial aesthetic unit with enhanced nasal tip projection since the ANS was deliberately not shortened

Case 4: Class III, Midfacial Hypoplasia, Anterior Open Bite (AOB), Clinical Treatment Outcome

Fig. 6.138 Frontal views in rest, pre-surgical (**a**) and 6 months after (**b**) combined orthodontic-surgical treatment and bilateral zygomatic osteotomies (patient B.B.)

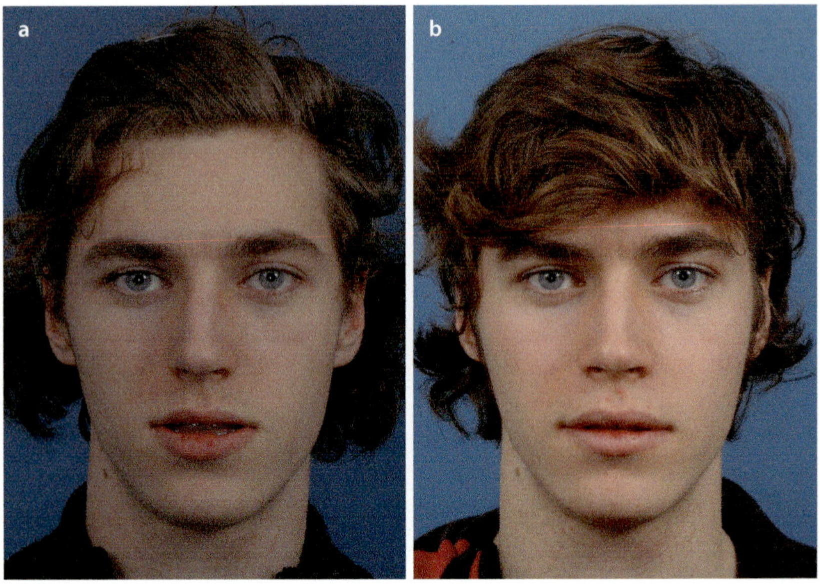

Fig. 6.139 Frontal views during smiling, pre-surgical (**a**) and 6 months after (**b**) combined orthodontic-surgical treatment and bilateral zygomatic osteotomies (patient B.B.)

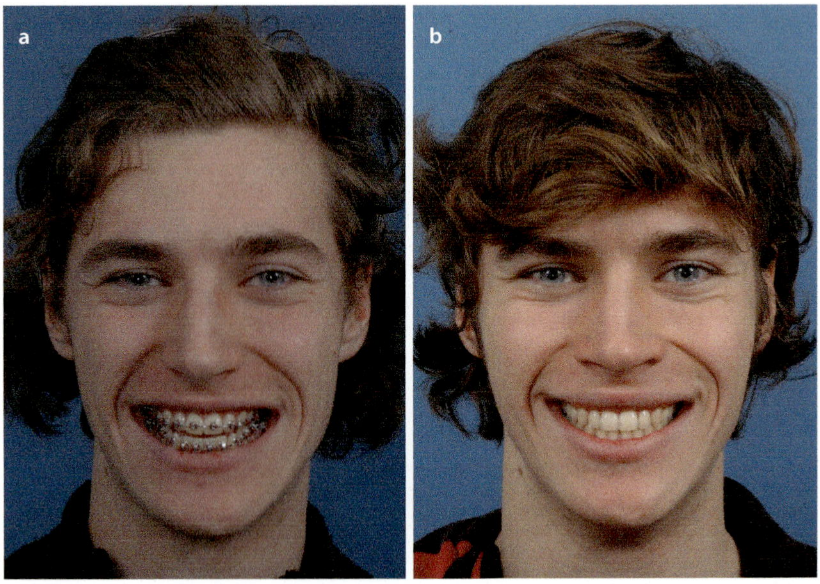

Case 4: Class III, Midfacial Hypoplasia, Anterior Open Bite (AOB), Clinical Treatment Outcome

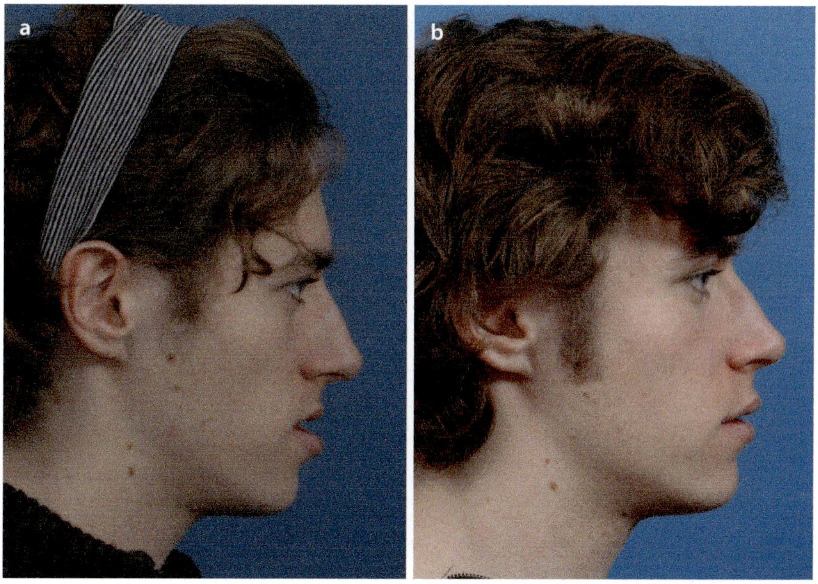

Fig. 6.140 Right profile views in rest, pre-surgical (**a**) and 6 months after (**b**) combined orthodontic-surgical treatment and bilateral zygomatic osteotomies (patient B.B.)

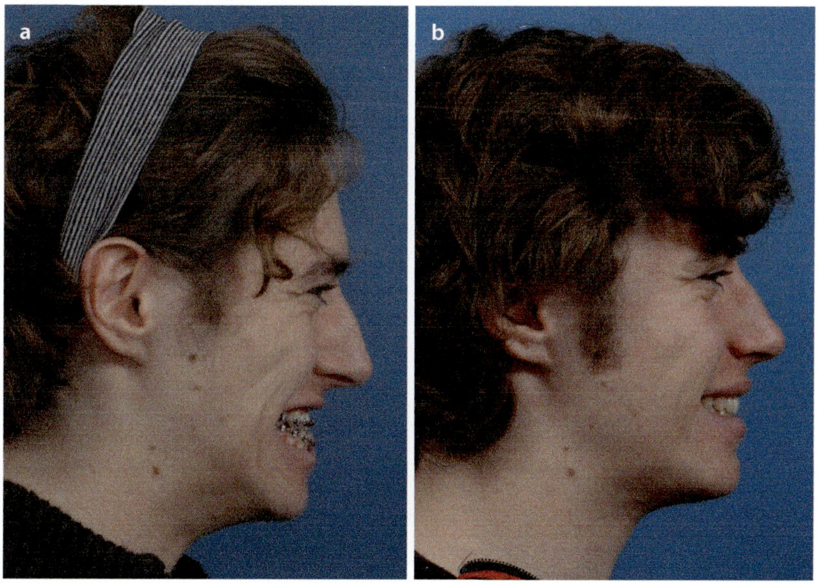

Fig. 6.141 Right profile views during smiling, pre-surgical (**a**) and 6 months after (**b**) combined orthodontic-surgical treatment and bilateral zygomatic osteotomies (patient B.B.)

Case 4: Class III, Midfacial Hypoplasia, Anterior Open Bite (AOB), Clinical Treatment Outcome

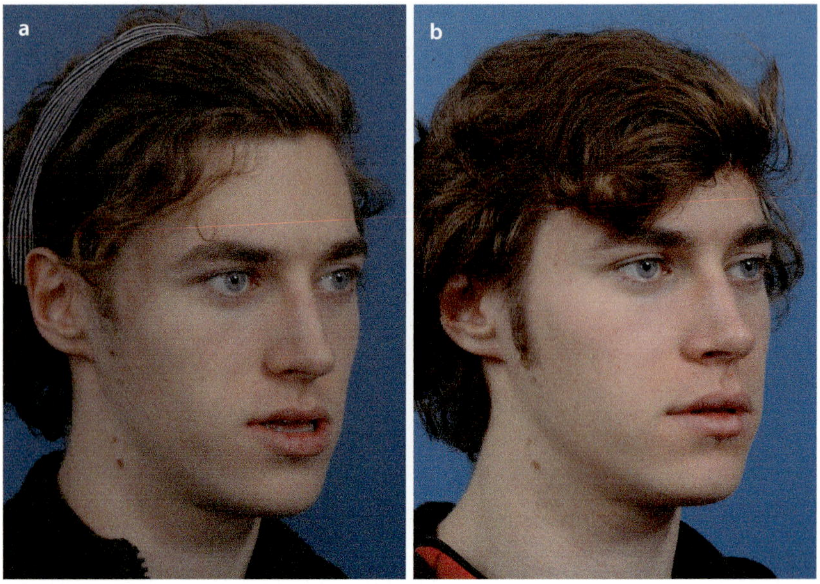

Fig. 6.142 2/3 right profile views in rest, pre-surgical (**a**) and 6 months after (**b**) combined orthodontic-surgical treatment and bilateral zygomatic osteotomies (patient B.B.)

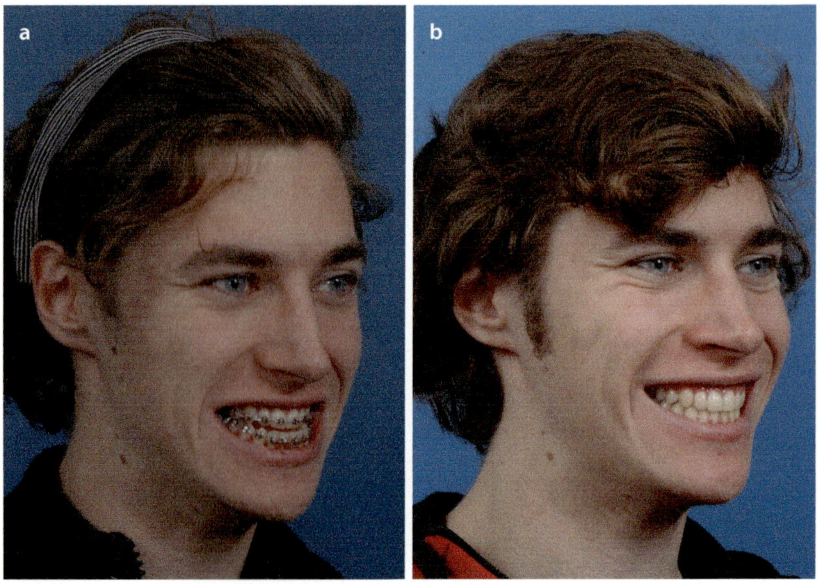

Fig. 6.143 2/3 right profile views during smiling, pre-surgical (**a**) and 6 months after (**b**) combined orthodontic-surgical treatment and bilateral zygomatic osteotomies (patient B.B.)

Case 4: Class III, Midfacial Hypoplasia, Anterior Open Bite (AOB), Clinical Treatment Outcome

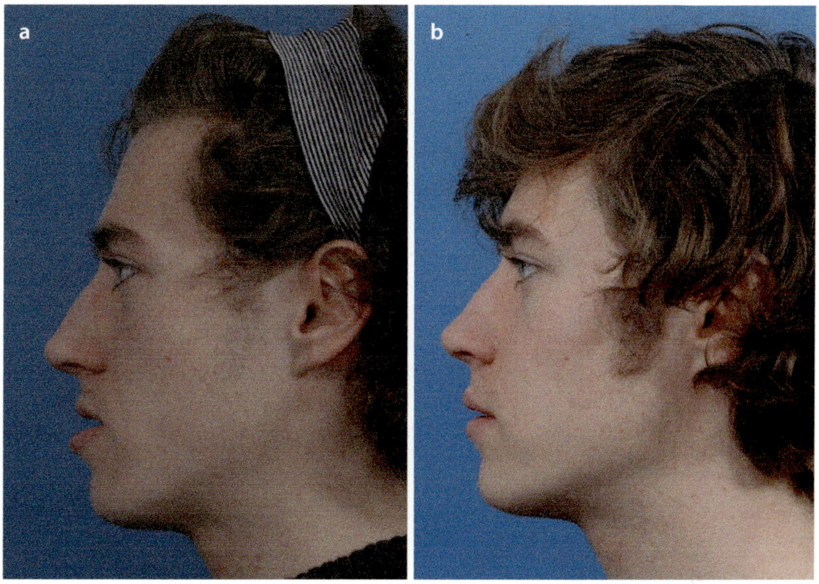

Fig. 6.144 Left profile views in rest, pre-surgical (**a**) and 6 months after (**b**) combined orthodontic-surgical treatment and bilateral zygomatic osteotomies (patient B.B.)

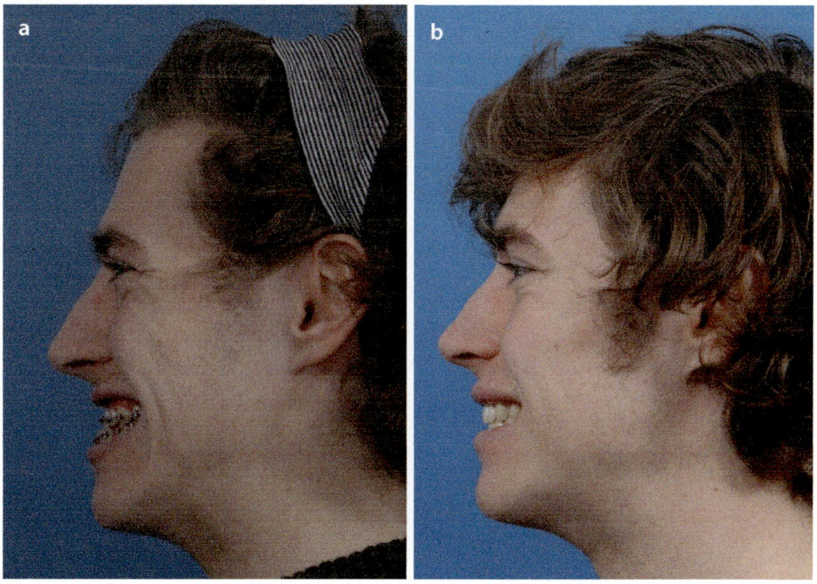

Fig. 6.145 Left profile views during smiling, pre-surgical (**a**) and 6 months after (**b**) combined orthodontic-surgical treatment and bilateral zygomatic osteotomies (patient B.B.)

Case 4: Class III, Midfacial Hypoplasia, Anterior Open Bite (AOB), Clinical Treatment Outcome

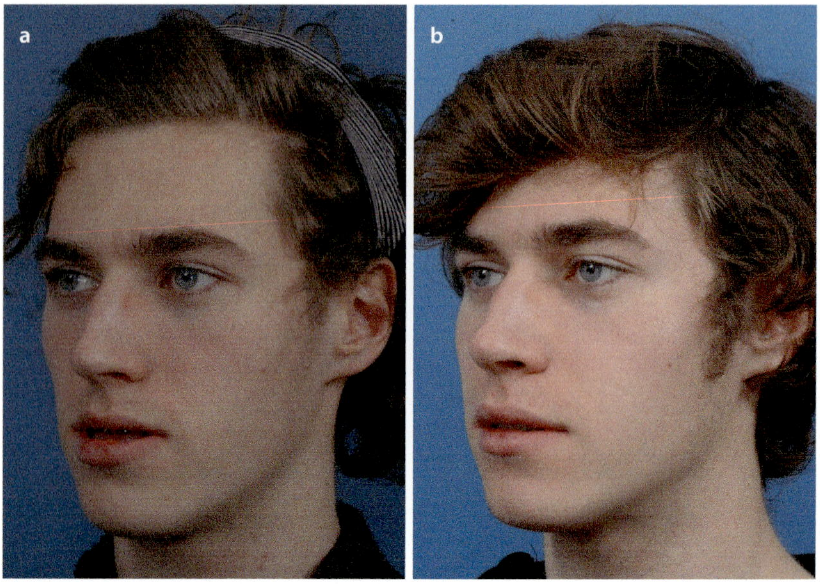

Fig. 6.146 2/3 left profile views in rest, pre-surgical (**a**) and 6 months after (**b**) combined orthodontic-surgical treatment and bilateral zygomatic osteotomies (patient B.B.)

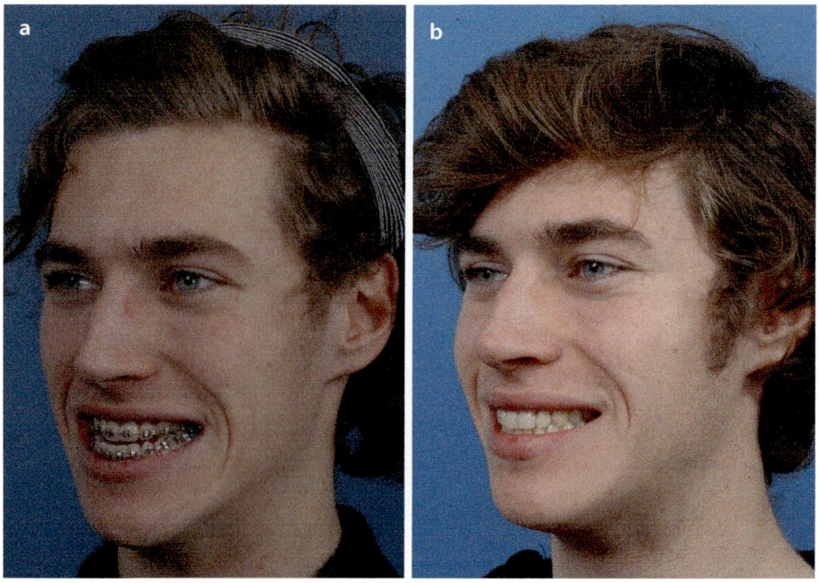

Fig. 6.147 2/3 left profile views during smiling, pre-surgical (**a**) and 6 months after (**b**) combined orthodontic-surgical treatment and bilateral zygomatic osteotomies (patient B.B.)

Case 4: Class III, Midfacial Hypoplasia, Anterior Open Bite (AOB), Clinical Treatment Outcome

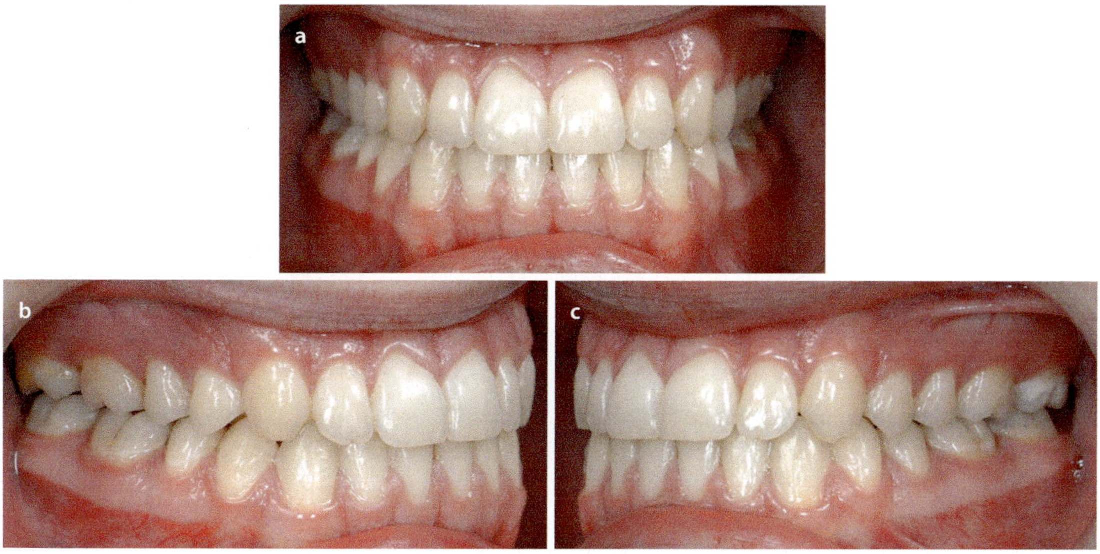

Fig. 6.148 Frontal (**a**), right (**b**) and left (**c**) intra-oral views of the patient's occlusion 6 months after combined orthodontic-surgical treatment (patient B.B.). The author acknowledges Annelies Müller and Prof. Guy De Pauw for the orthodontic treatment

Case 5: Class III, Midfacial Hypoplasia, Mandibular Hyperplasia

Patient L.E. is a 16-year-old girl with a Class III maxillofacial deformity due to combined midfacial hypoplasia and mandibular hyperplasia. A bone scintigraphy was performed prior to the surgical workup and did not show any condylar growth anymore. In the frontal view, she is clinically presenting with a flattened midface, a nasal root asymmetry and a chin deviation to the left. In rest, she has an incisal display of 5 mm, while during spontaneous smiling, she has full incisal exposure with 2 mm gingival display at incisal level. In the profile view, she presents with a retruded midface with poor bilateral zygoma definition, a prominent nose, a limited vermilion exposure, a negative lip trap, and a rather strong mandible with poor chin definition. She has an Angle Class III malocclusion with adequate transversal relationship and a 1 mm lower dental midline deviation to the left. She has no history of TMJ dysfunction neither pain.

6

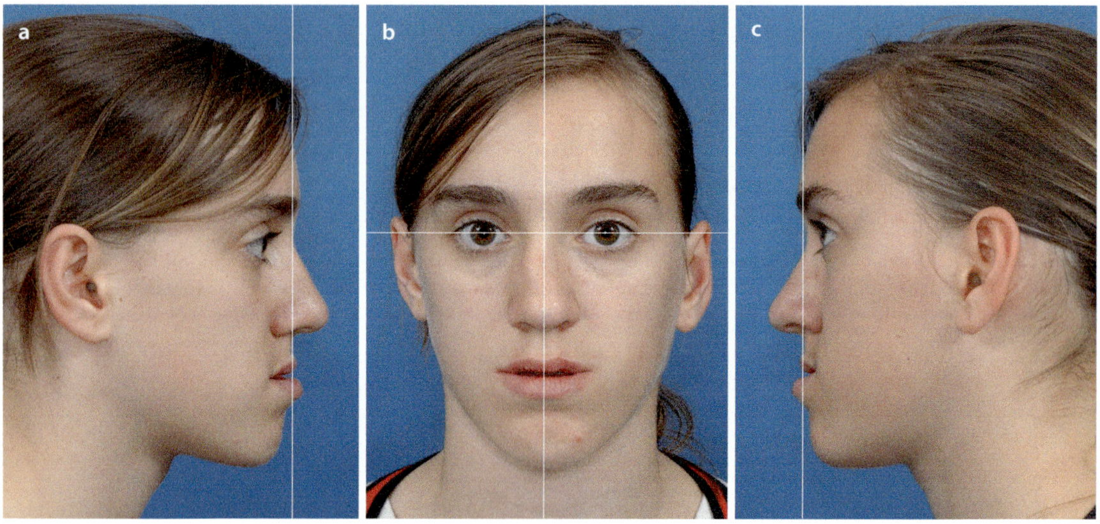

Fig. 6.149 Pre-surgical clinical right profile (**a**), frontal (**b**) and left profile (**c**) views of patient L.E. in her *c*-NHP in rest, at the time of the workup, approximately 3 weeks prior to surgery. Note the flattened midface, nasal root asymmetry and chin deviation to the left

Case 5: Class III, Midfacial Hypoplasia, Mandibular Hyperplasia

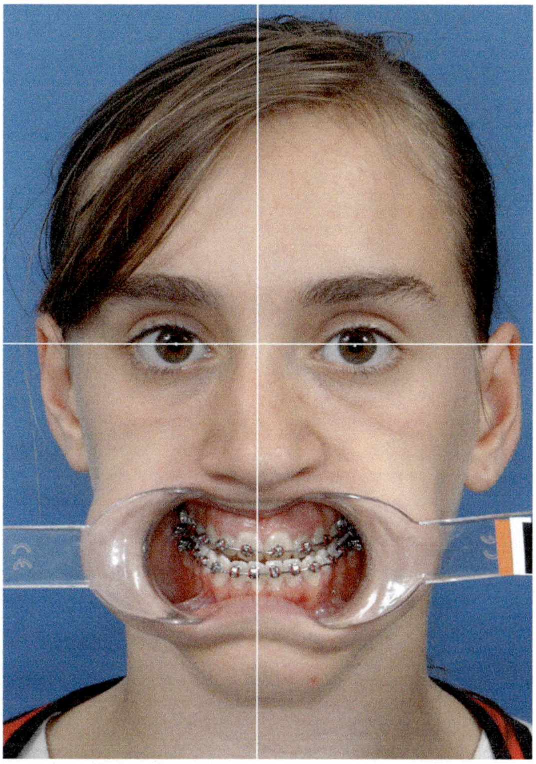

Fig. 6.150 Pre-surgical clinical frontal view of patient L.E. with cheek retractors at the time of the workup, approximately 3 weeks prior to surgery. Note the 2 mm upper dental midline deviation to the left

■ Case 5: Class III, Midfacial Hypoplasia, Mandibular Hyperplasia, *v*-NHP and PHP

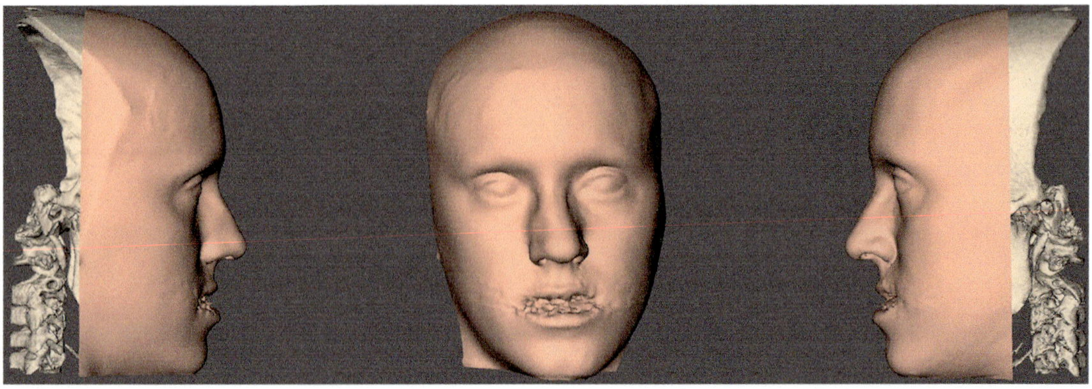

Fig. 6.151 Pre-surgical 3D "surface-rendered" right profile, frontal and left profile soft and hard tissue representations of the head of patient L.E., as generated during standardised CBCT image acquisition, at the time of the workup (Maxilim v. 2.3.0.3). Note the incorrect position and orientation of the virtual head compared to the clinical pictures of patient L.E. (Fig. 6.149), although it was attempted to scan the patient in her correct *c*-NHP in rest

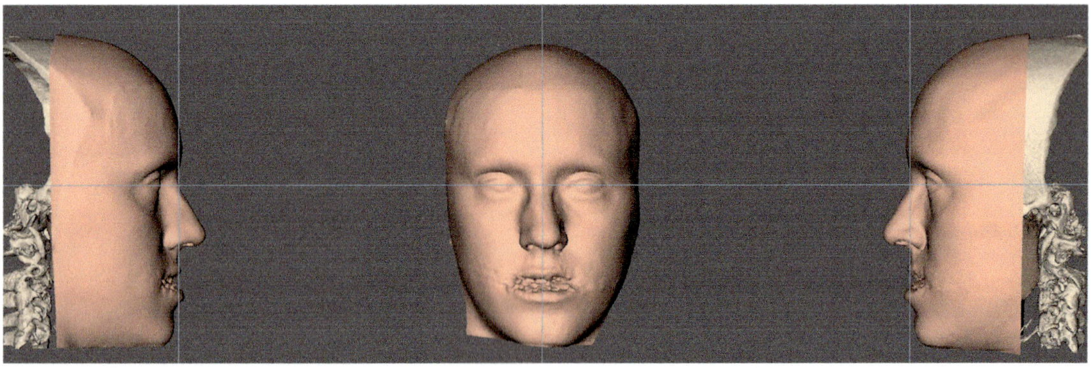

Fig. 6.152 Following a standardised "step-by-step" approach (▶ see Sect. 3.1), the scanned head position of patient L.E. (Fig. 6.151) was virtually modified towards her *c*-NHP (Fig. 6.149), which results in her *v*-NHP and corresponds to her individual "Planning Head Position (PHP)" (3D "surface-rendered" representations, Maxilim v. 2.3.0.3)

Case 5: Class III, Midfacial Hypoplasia, Mandibular Hyperplasia

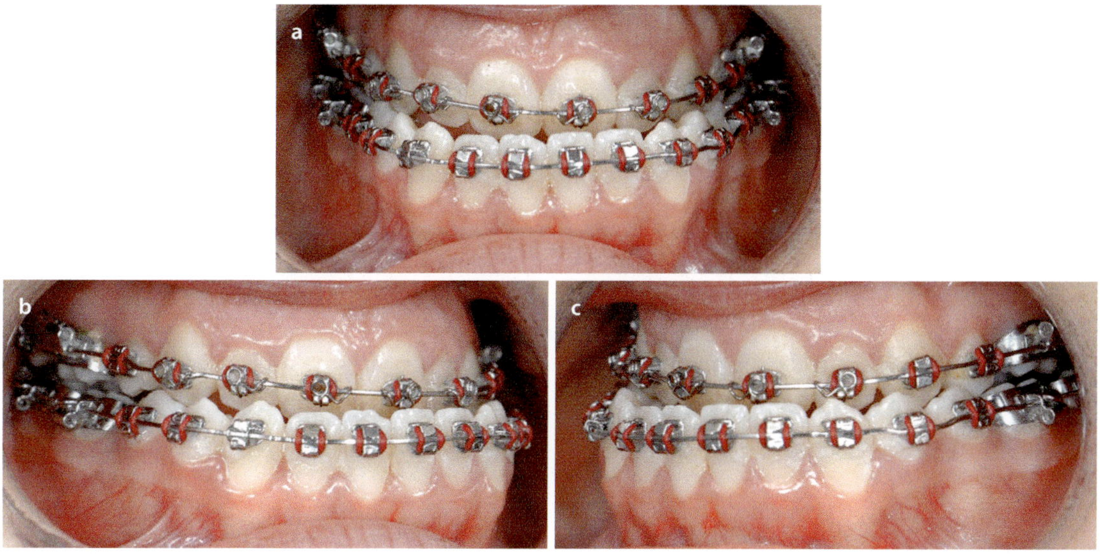

Fig. 6.153 Pre-surgical frontal (**a**), right (**b**) and left (**c**) intra-oral views of the occlusion of patient L.E. at the time of the workup, approximately 3 weeks prior to surgery. Note the slight 1 mm lower dental midline deviation to the left

Fig. 6.154 Pre-surgical frontal clinical view of patient L.E. with a full spontaneous smile approximately 3 months prior to the workup. Note that the patient's smile at the time of the workup (Fig. 6.186a) is not fully spontaneous

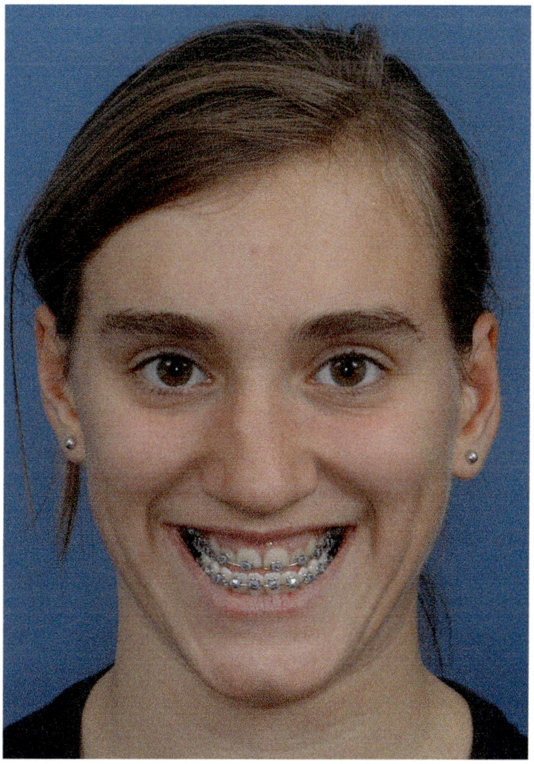

Case 5: 3D-VPS$_5$ Step 1 Maxillary Occlusal Cant Evaluation/Correction ("Roll")

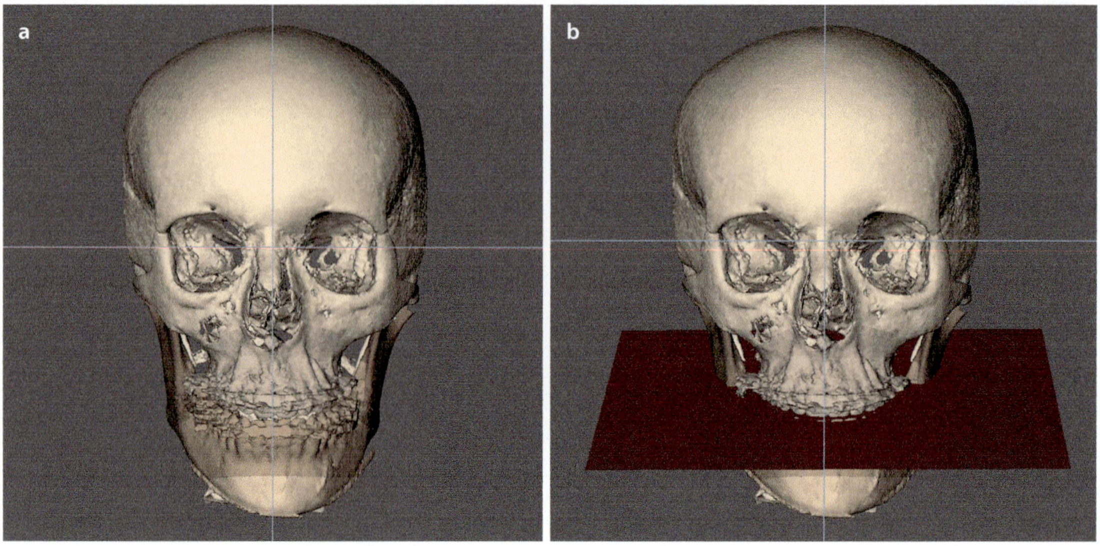

Fig. 6.155 The maxillary occlusal plane is evaluated both clinically (Fig. 6.154) and virtually (**a**) towards the horizontal 3D PHP reference plane and does not need to be corrected (**b**) in patient L.E. (3D "surface-rendered" representations, Maxilim v. 2.3.0.3)

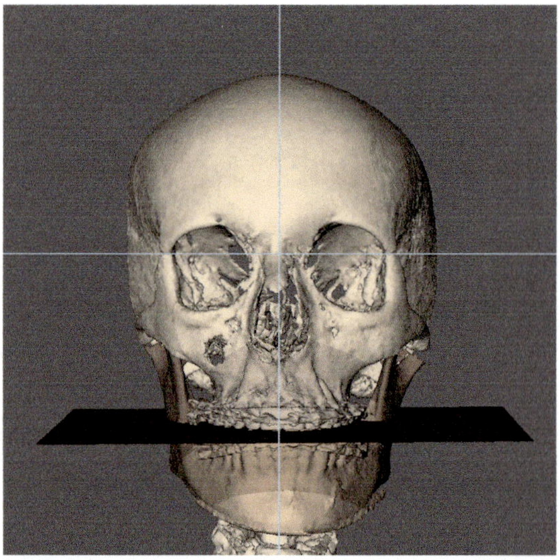

Fig. 6.156 Slight virtual rotation of the patient's skull to the back more clearly shows virtually that the maxillary occlusal plane is parallel to the horizontal 3D PHP reference plane and does not need to be modified (3D "surface-rendered" representations, patient L.E., Maxilim v. 2.3.0.3)

Case 5: 3D-VPS$_5$ Step 2 Upper Dental Midline Evaluation/Correction

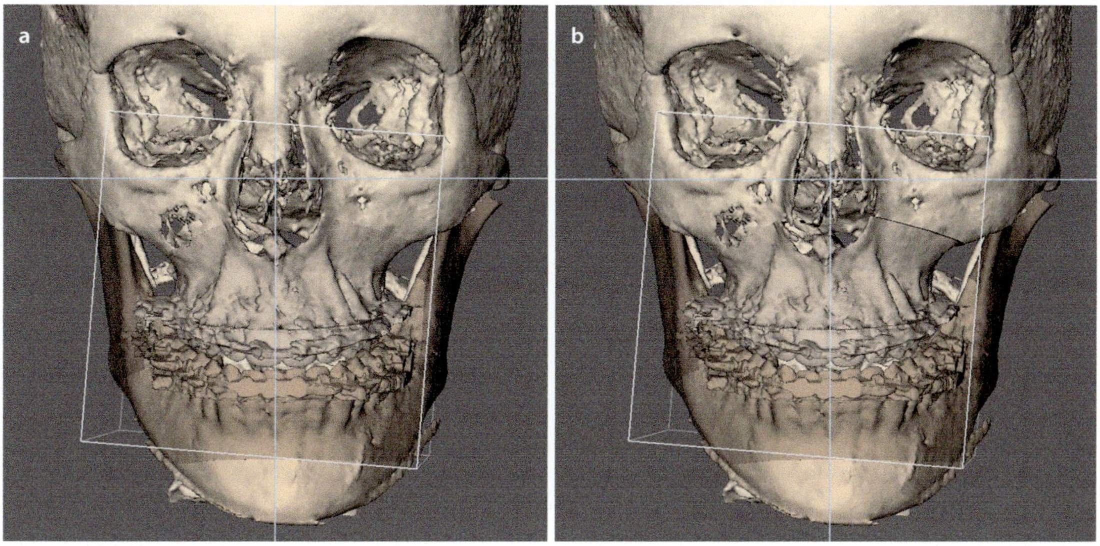

Fig. 6.157 The 2 mm deviation of the upper dental midline to the left (**a**) is corrected towards the facial midline 3D PHP reference plane, by a pure translational movement to the right (**b**) in patient L.E. (3D "surface-rendered" representations, Maxilim v. 2.3.0.3)

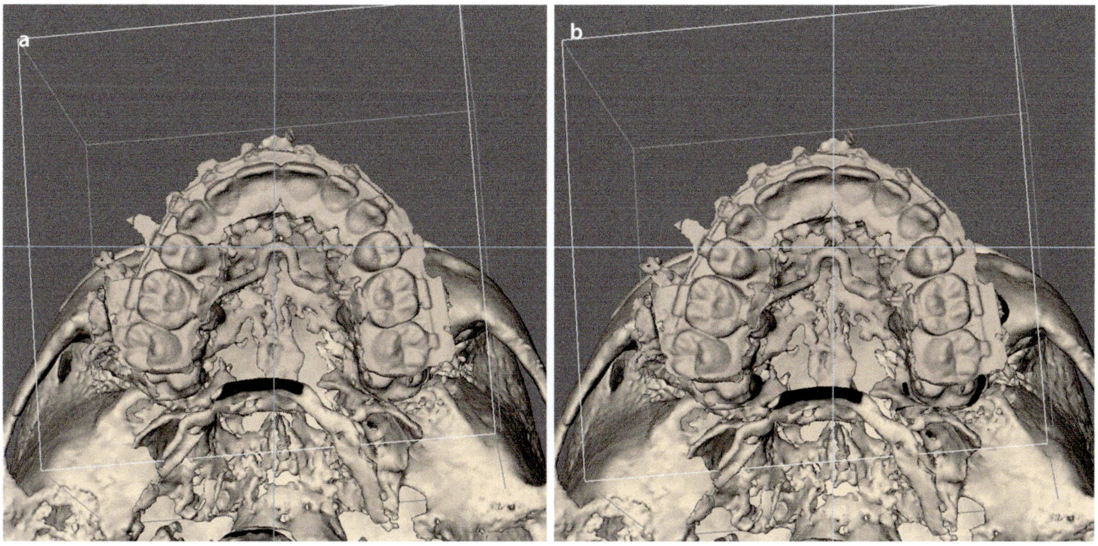

Fig. 6.158 The base views illustrate that the 2 mm deviation of the upper dental midline to the left (**a**) is corrected towards the facial midline 3D PHP reference plane, by a pure translational movement to the right (**b**) (3D "surface-rendered" representations, patient L.E., Maxilim v. 2.3.0.3)

Case 5: 3D-VPS$_5$ Step 3 Overall Evaluation of Facial Asymmetry After Virtual Occlusal Definition

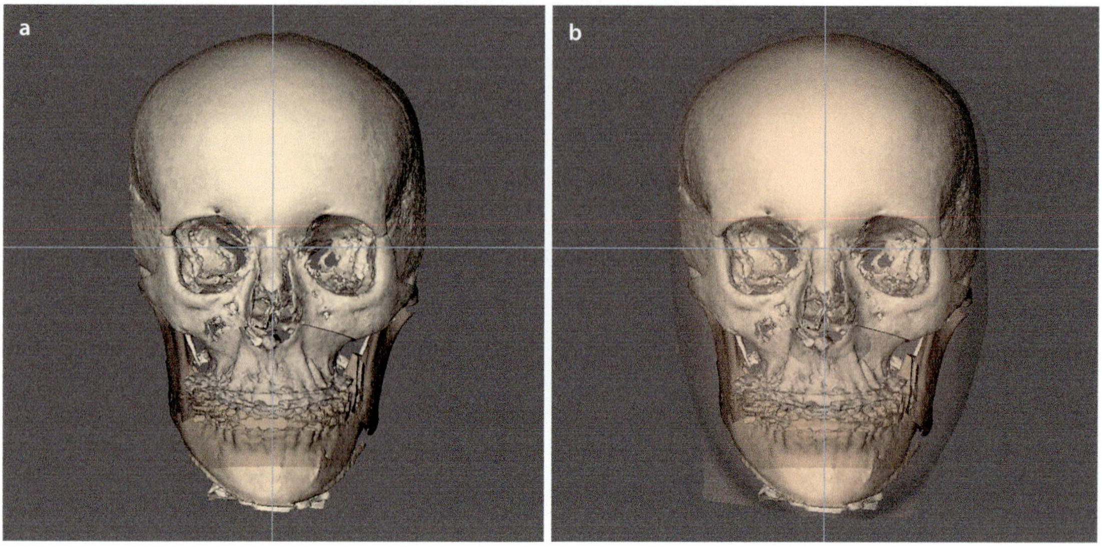

Fig. 6.159 Overall facial asymmetry of the skull of patient L.E. (**a**) with transparent soft tissues (**b**) is assessed after virtual occlusal definition in the frontal view towards both the horizontal and facial midline 3D PHP reference planes. Note the flaring of the mandibular body to the right (3D "surface-rendered" representations, Maxilim v. 2.3.0.3)

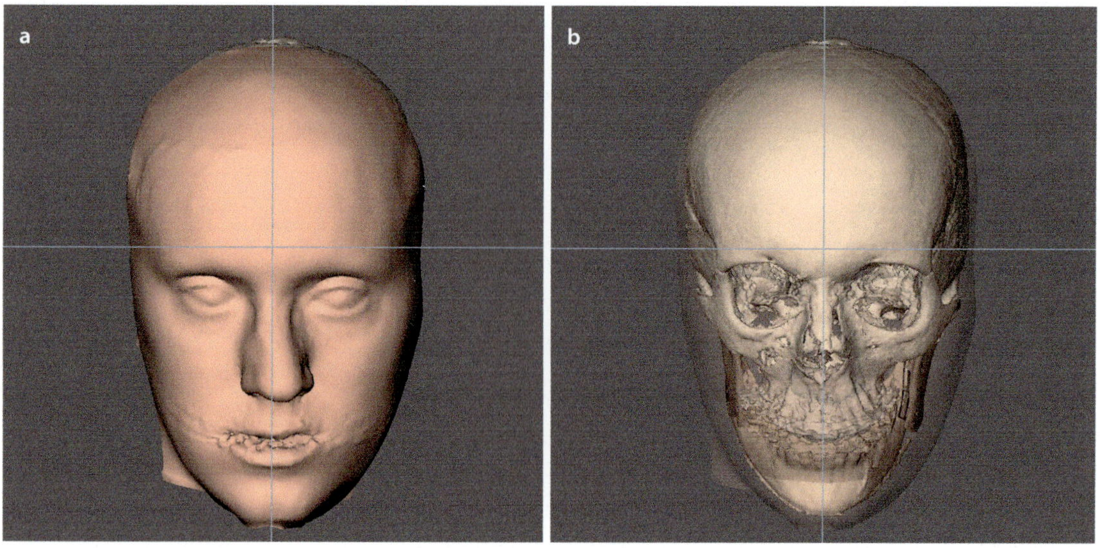

Fig. 6.160 To evaluate the overall facial asymmetry after virtual occlusal definition, the mandibular contour is evaluated both virtually on the soft tissues (**a**) and at the bony level towards the contour of the zygomatic bones and arches with soft tissues in transparency (**b**) (3D "surface-rendered" representations, patient L.E., Maxilim v. 2.3.0.3). Note the important deviation of the nasal tip although the bony nasal pyramid is straight

Case 5: 3D-VPS$_5$ Step 4 Evaluation/Correction of Flaring ("Yaw")

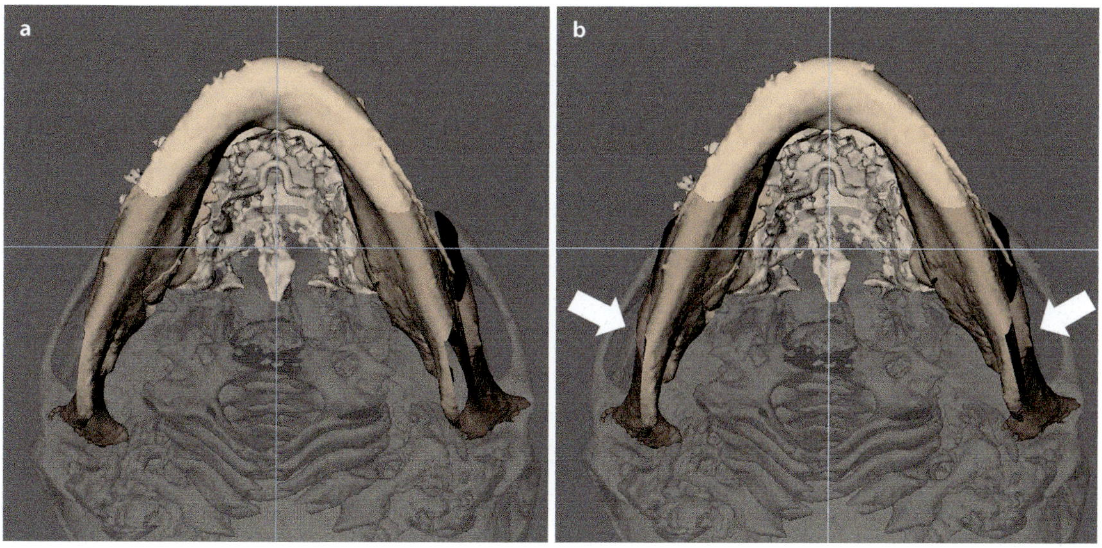

Fig. 6.161 The base views show that the flaring of the mandibular body to the right (**a**) is corrected by a CCW "Yaw" rotational movement to the left (**b**) (3D "surface-rendered" representations, patient L.E., Maxilim v. 2.3.0.3). Note the asymmetric bony overlap between the distal and both proximal mandibular fragments

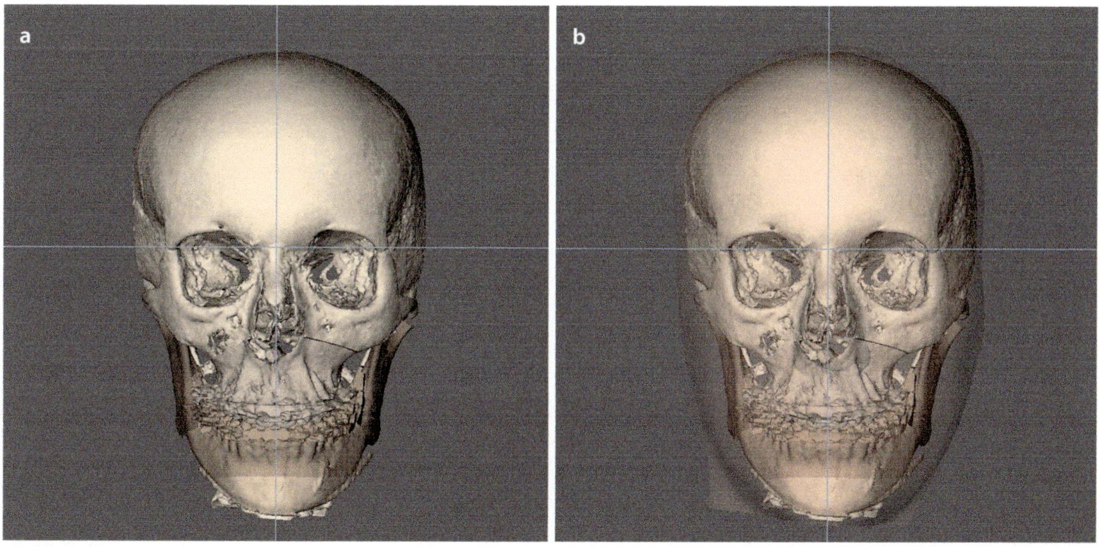

Fig. 6.162 Overall assessment of facial bony contour of patient L.E. (**a**) with transparent soft tissues (**b**) after correction of flaring to the right by a "Yaw" rotational movement of the maxillo-mandibular complex to the left (3D "surface-rendered" representations, Maxilim v. 2.3.0.3)

Case 5: 3D-VPS$_5$ Step 5 Upper Vertical Incisal Position Evaluation/Correction

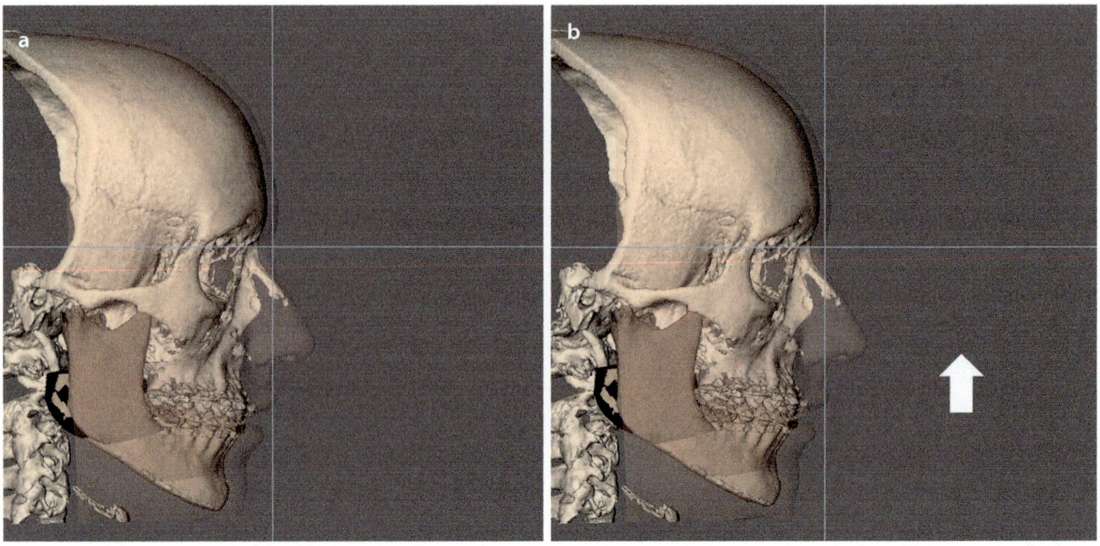

Fig. 6.163 Since the patient has an upper incisal exposure in rest of 5 mm and a gingival exposure of 2 mm, it was decided clinically at this stage in "step 5" to virtually intrude the maxilla of patient L.E. 2 mm at the upper incisal level (3D "surface-rendered" representations, Maxilim v. 2.3.0.3): before (**a**) and after (**b**) correction

Case 5: 3D-VPS$_5$ Step 6 Sagittal Upper Incisal Position Evaluation/Correction

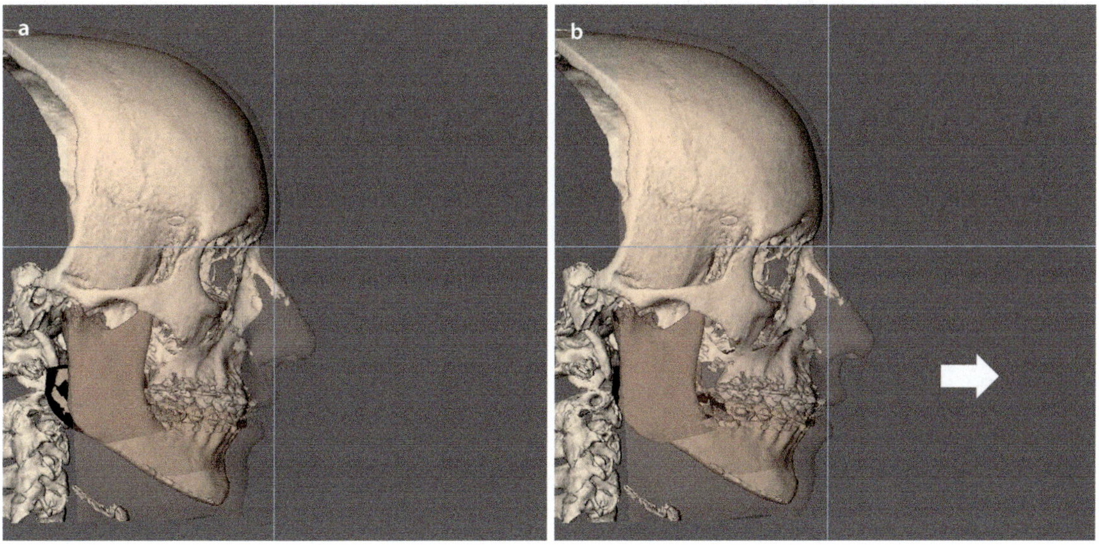

Fig. 6.164 From especially clinical examination but also 3D cephalometric analysis, it was decided to advance the "maxillo-mandibular complex in final occlusion" 7 mm at the upper incisal level in patient L.E. (3D "surface-rendered" representations, Maxilim v. 2.3.0.3): before (**a**) and after (**b**) correction

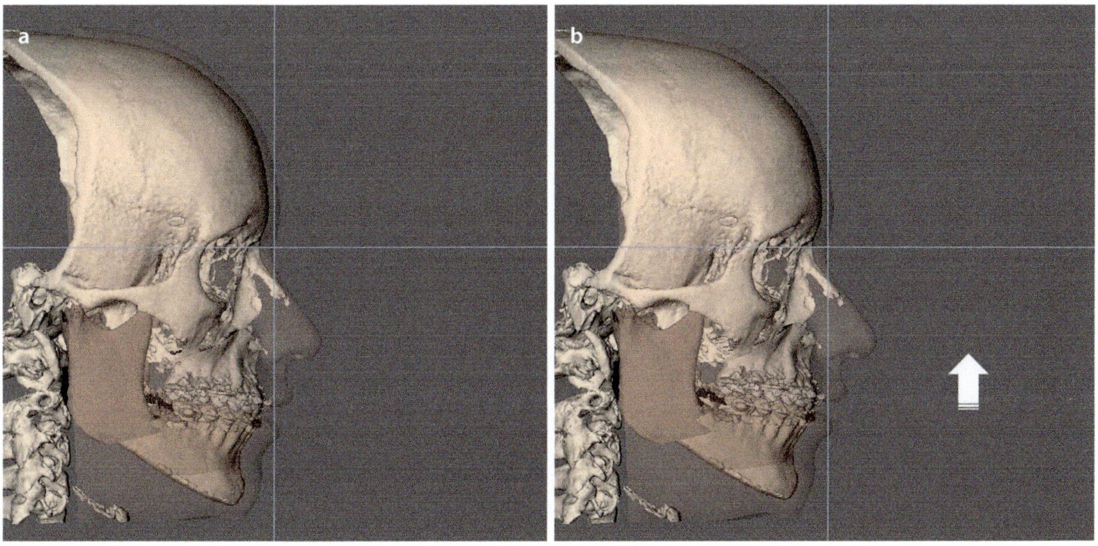

Fig. 6.165 Since it was clinically judged based on the authors' experience that the 7 mm maxillary advancement would result in approximately 2.5 mm additional incisal and gingival exposure, the "maxillo-mandibular complex in final occlusion" was virtually intruded for 2.5 mm extra at the upper incisal level in patient L.E. (3D "surface-rendered" representations, Maxilim v. 2.3.0.3): before (**a**) and after (**b**) correction

▪ Case 5: 3D-VPS$_5$ Step 7 Profile Evaluation/Occlusal Plane Correction ("Pitch")

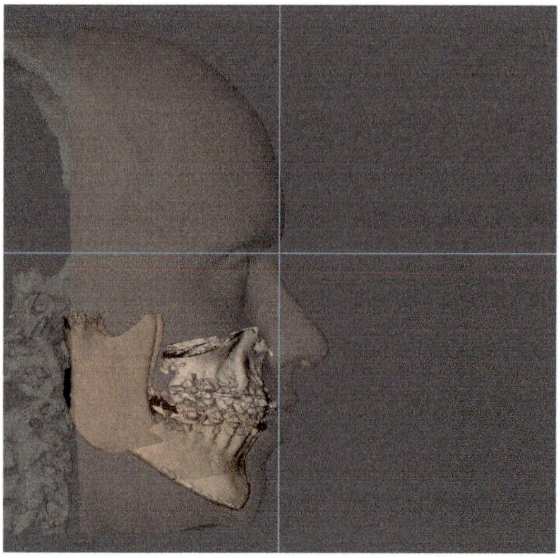

Fig. 6.166 At this stage in "step 7", the profile and dento-alveolar support of the upper lip are evaluated (3D "surface-rendered" representations, patient L.E., Maxilim v. 2.3.0.3). Note the retruded chin and antegonial step

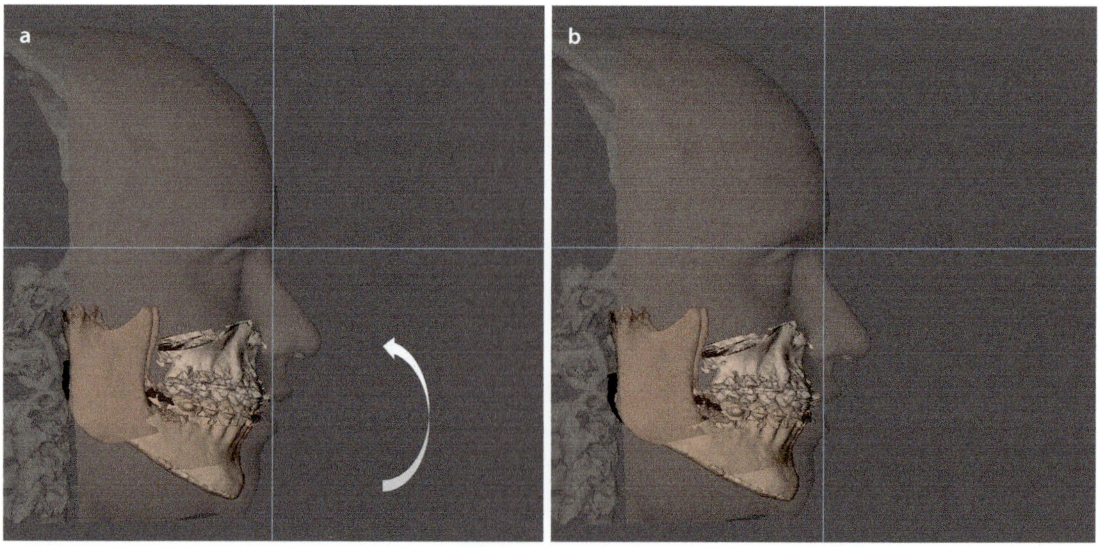

Fig. 6.167 Based on clinical and 3D cephalometric analysis, it was decided to perform a 4° CCW occlusal plane rotation with the centre of rotation at the incisal level by a "Pitch" rotational movement, which result in 1 mm differential impaction at the first molar (3D "surface-rendered" representations, patient L.E., Maxilim v. 2.3.0.3): before (**a**) and after (**b**) correction

Case 5: 3D-VPS$_5$ Step 8 3D Chin Position Evaluation/Correction

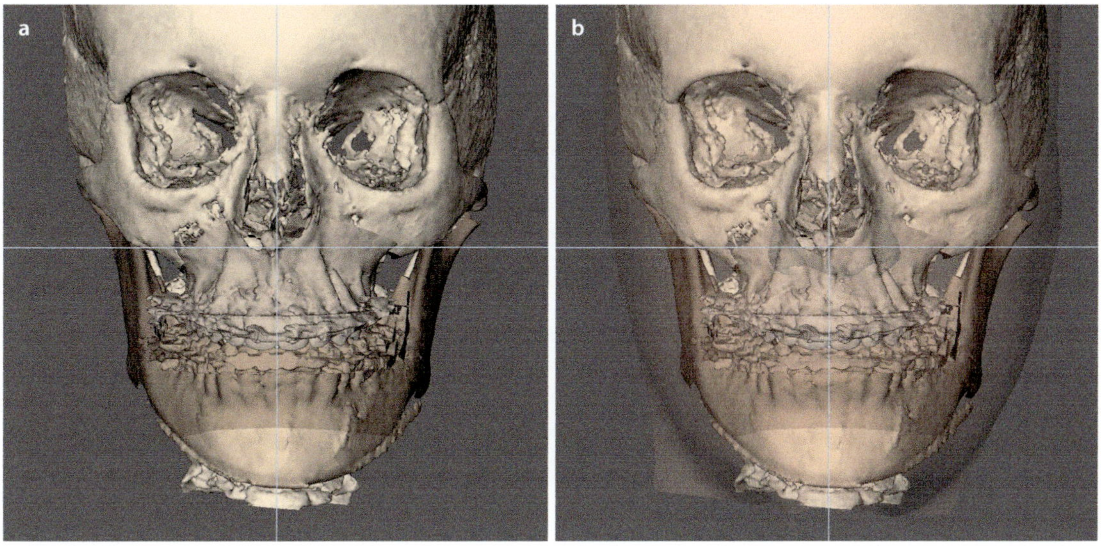

Fig. 6.168 Evaluation of the chin position in the frontal plane without (**a**) and with (**b**) the patient's 3D facial soft tissue mask in transparency (3D "surface-rendered" representations, Maxilim v. 2.3.0.3). Note that the initial chin deviation to the left in patient L.E. has already been corrected by the previous steps. Also note that there is still a slight cant of the chin

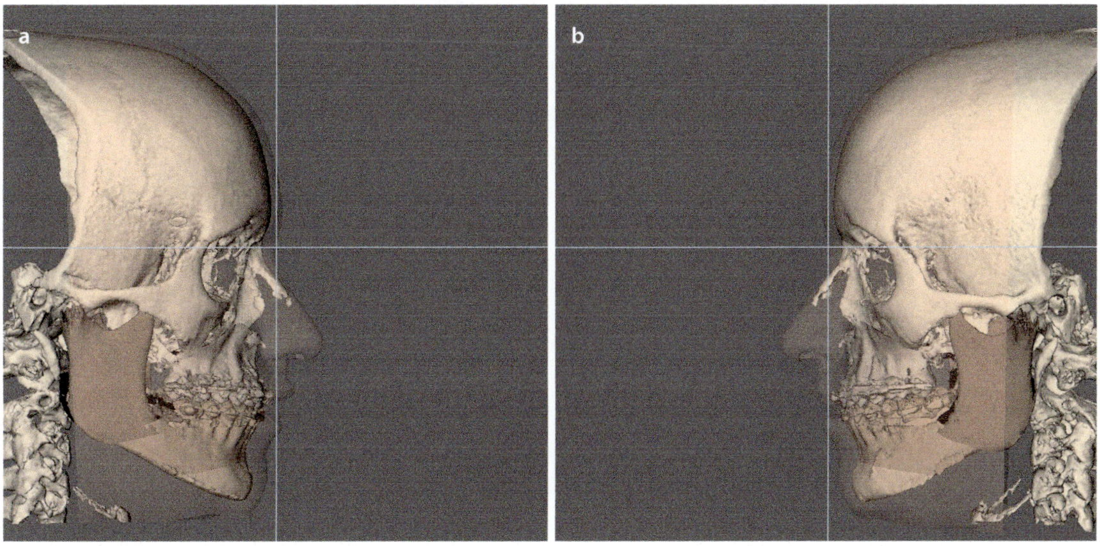

Fig. 6.169 Evaluation of the sagittal chin position in the right (**a**) and left profile (**b**) views needs to be individually assessed (3D "surface-rendered" representations, Maxilim v. 2.3.0.3). Note the discrepancy between the prominent bony chin and its overlying flattened soft tissue contour with the absence of a well-defined plica labio-mentalis in patient L.E.

Case 5: 3D-VPS$_5$ Step 8 3D Chin Position Evaluation/Correction

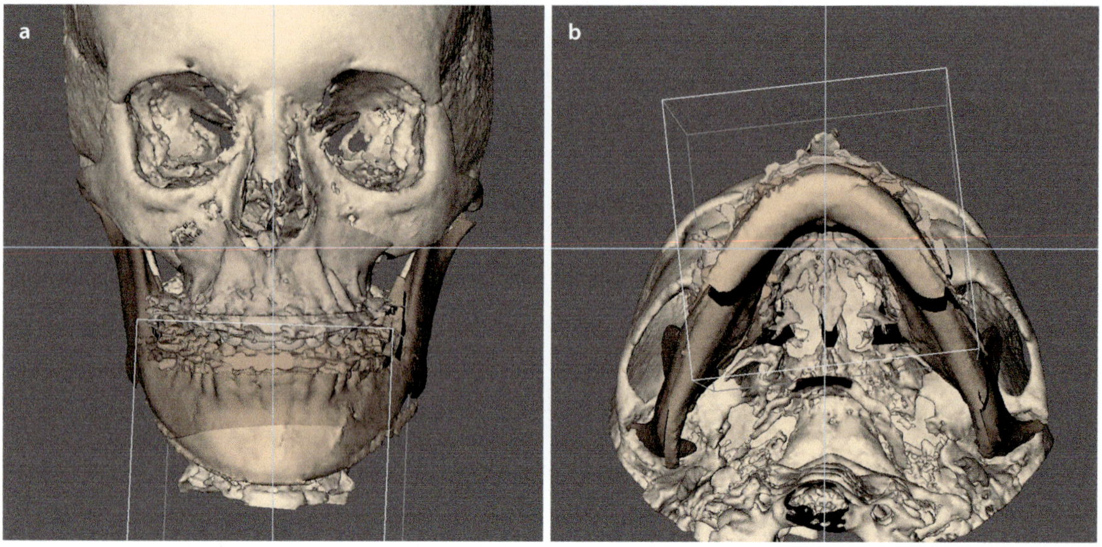

Fig. 6.170 In the frontal plane (**a**), a CCW "Roll" movement of the chin with 2 mm posterior intrusion at the left was virtually planned in patient L.E. to correct the cant (Fig. 6.168). The base view (**b**) shows no flaring of the chin after 4 mm advancement (3D "surface-rendered" representations, Maxilim v. 2.3.0.3)

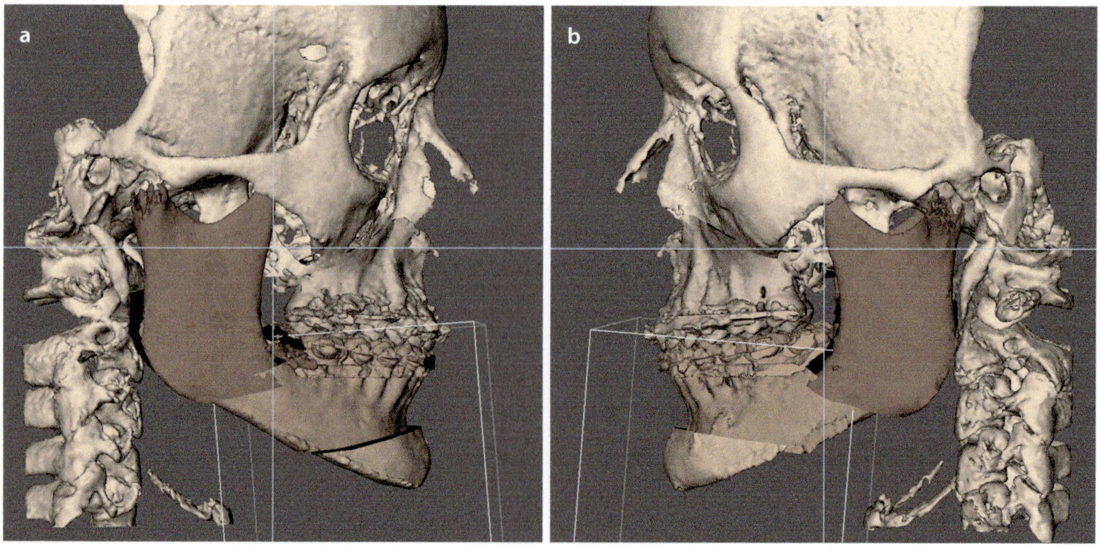

Fig. 6.171 The right (**a**) and left profile (**b**) views show that a chin advancement of 4 mm with a posterior intrusion of 2 mm at the left was virtually planned in patient L.E. (3D "surface-rendered" representations, Maxilim v. 2.3.0.3)

Case 5: 3D-VPS$_5$ Step 9 Patient Communication of the Individualised Treatment Plan

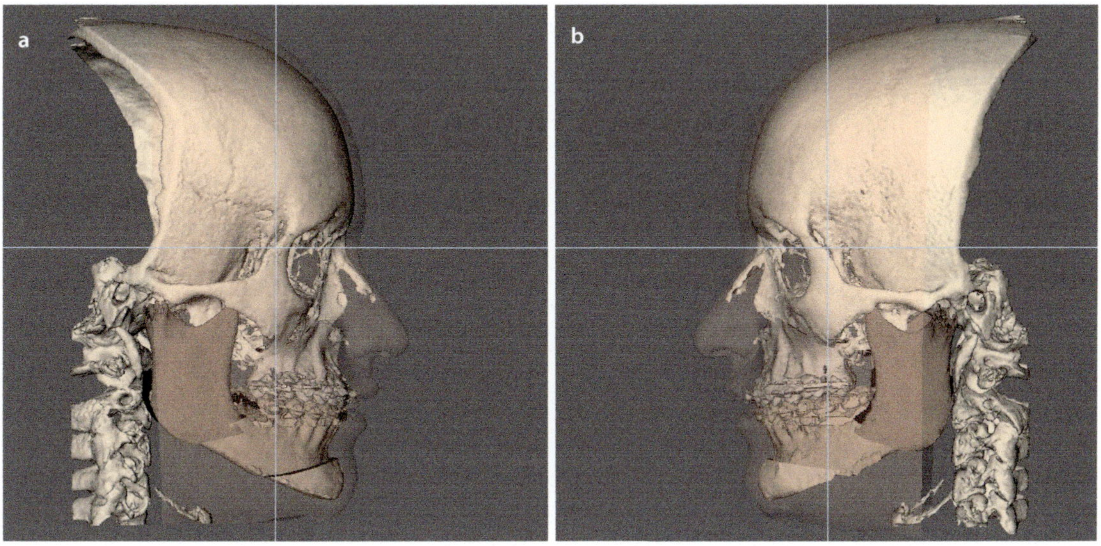

Fig. 6.172 Right (**a**) and left profile (**b**) views of the "Individualised 3D Virtual Treatment Plan", as presented to patient L.E., before the actual surgery (3D "surface-rendered" representations, Maxilim v. 2.3.0.3). Note the limits of the actual 3D virtual soft tissue simulation at the level of the lips

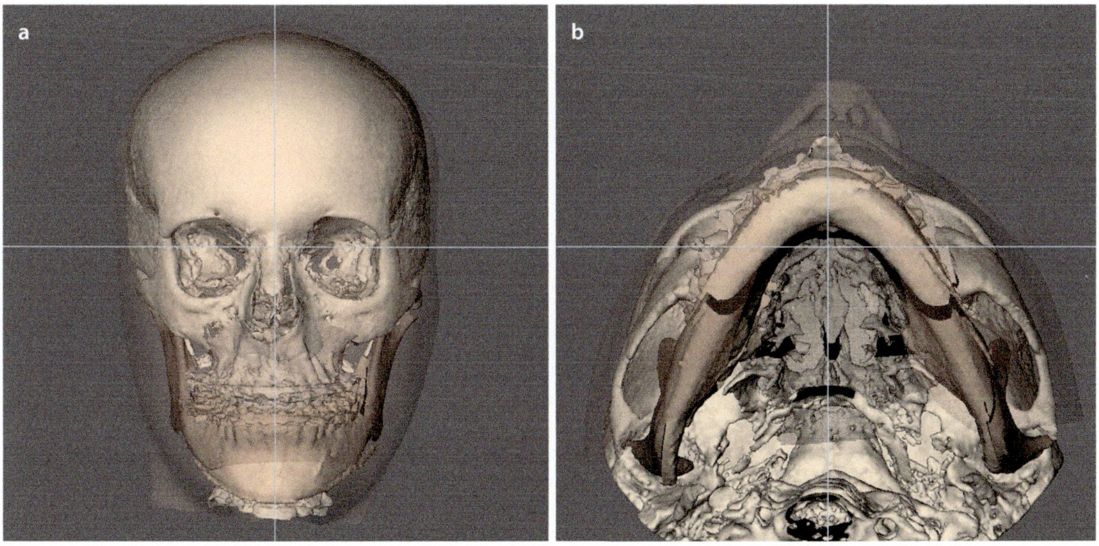

Fig. 6.173 Frontal (**a**) and base (**b**) views of the "Individualised 3D Virtual Treatment Plan", as presented to patient L.E., before the actual surgery (3D "surface-rendered" representations, Maxilim v. 2.3.0.3). Note the important deviation of the nasal tip to the left although the bony nasal pyramid is straight. Also note the flattened zygomatic bones

Case 5: 3D-VPS$_5$ Step 9 Patient Communication of the Individualised Treatment Plan

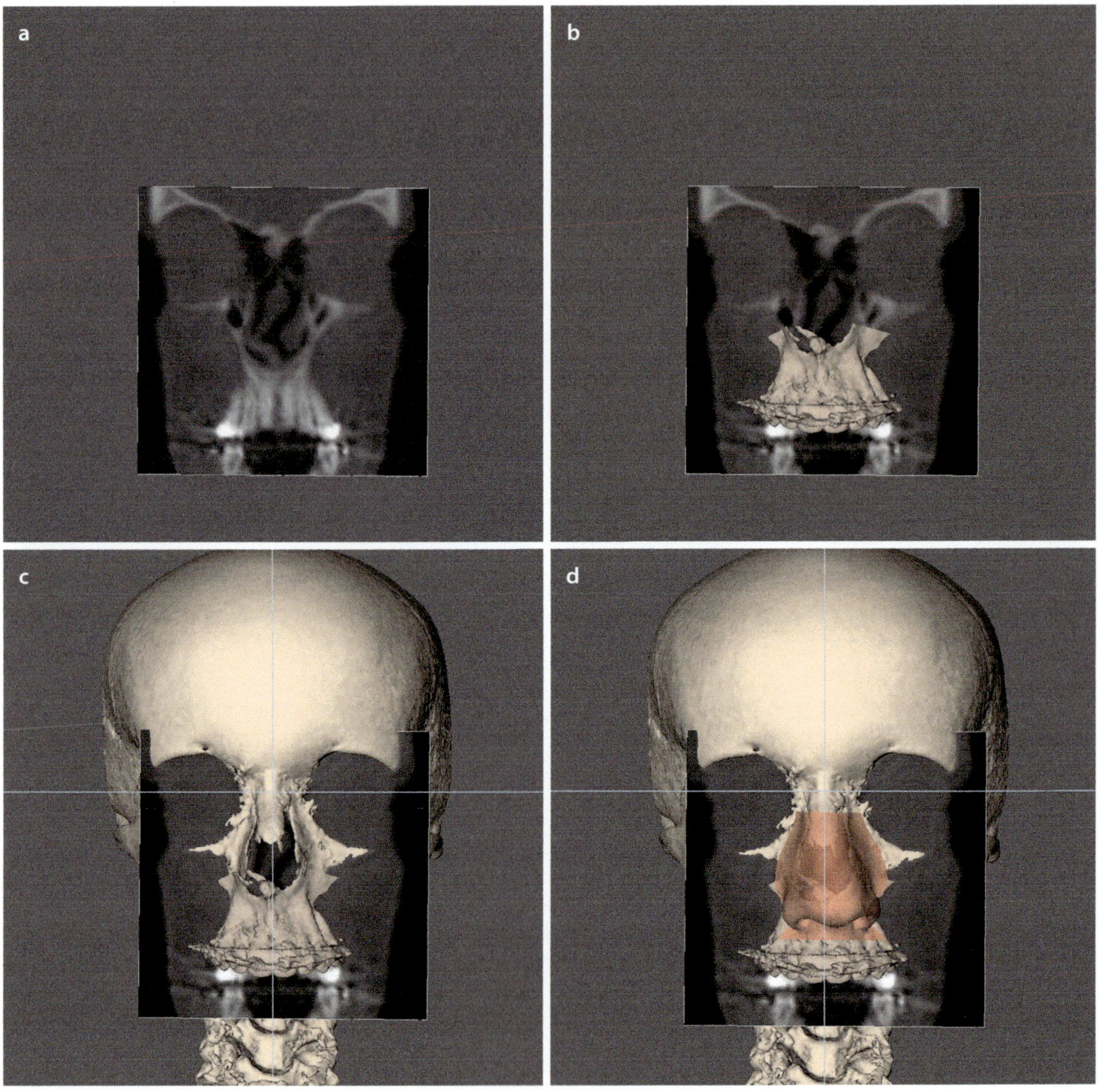

Fig. 6.174 The combination of 3D virtual evaluation of the underlying coronal slices (**a**), the segmented maxilla (**b**), the bony skull (**c**) and the soft tissue of the nose (**d**) shows a deviation of the anterior nasal spine (ANS) to the right, an important asymmetry of the left nasal floor and lateral wall and above an important septal deviation which pushes the nasal tip to the left in patient L.E. (3D "surface-rendered" representations, Maxilim v. 2.3.0.3)

Case 5: 3D-VPS$_5$ Step 10 Final Adjustments of the 3D Virtual Treatment Plan

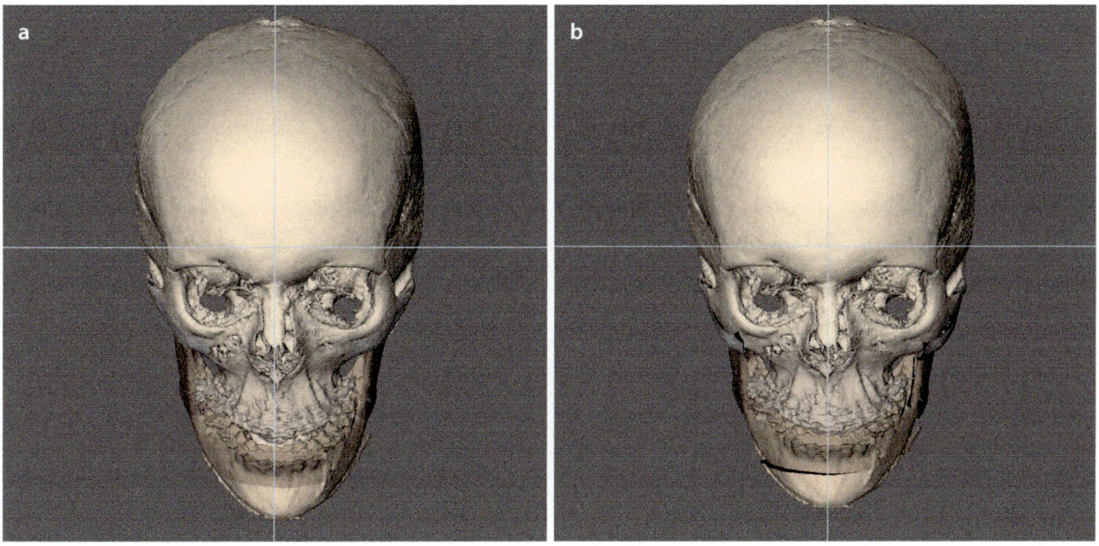

Fig. 6.175 Final adjustments of the "Individualised 3D Virtual Treatment Plan" after communication with patient L.E. consisted of additional zygomatic sandwich osteotomies to correct the flattened infraorbital contour of the midface (3D "surface-rendered" representations, Maxilim v. 2.3.0.3): before (**a**) and after (**b**) frontal downward inclined views

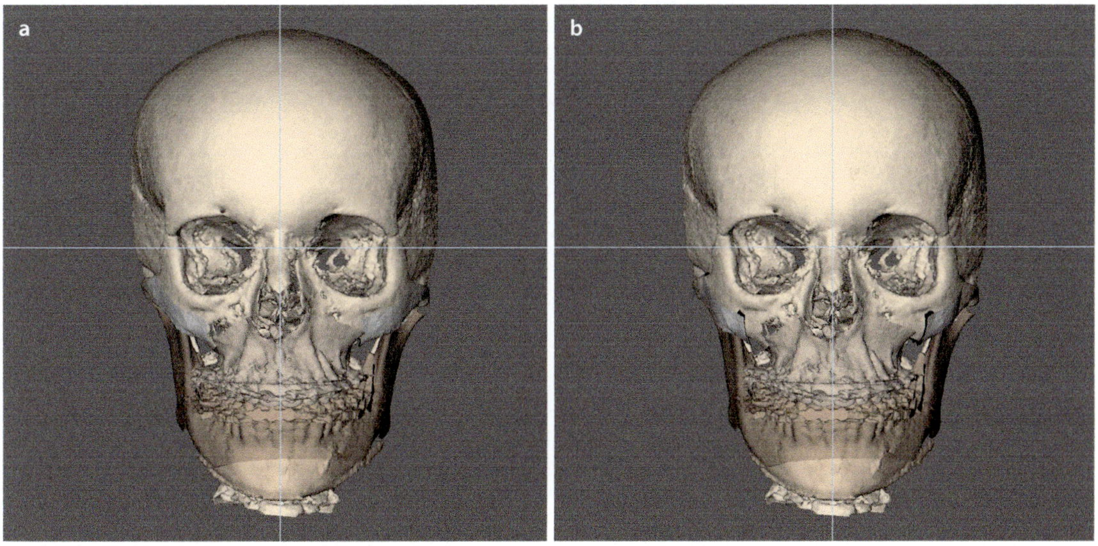

Fig. 6.176 Final adjustments of the "Individualised 3D Virtual Treatment Plan" after communication with patient L.E. consisted of additional zygomatic sandwich osteotomies to correct the flattened infraorbital contour of the midface (3D "surface-rendered" representations, Maxilim v. 2.3.0.3): before (**a**) and after (**b**) frontal views

Case 5: 3D-VPS$_5$- Final Integrated "Individualised 3D Virtual Treatment Plan"

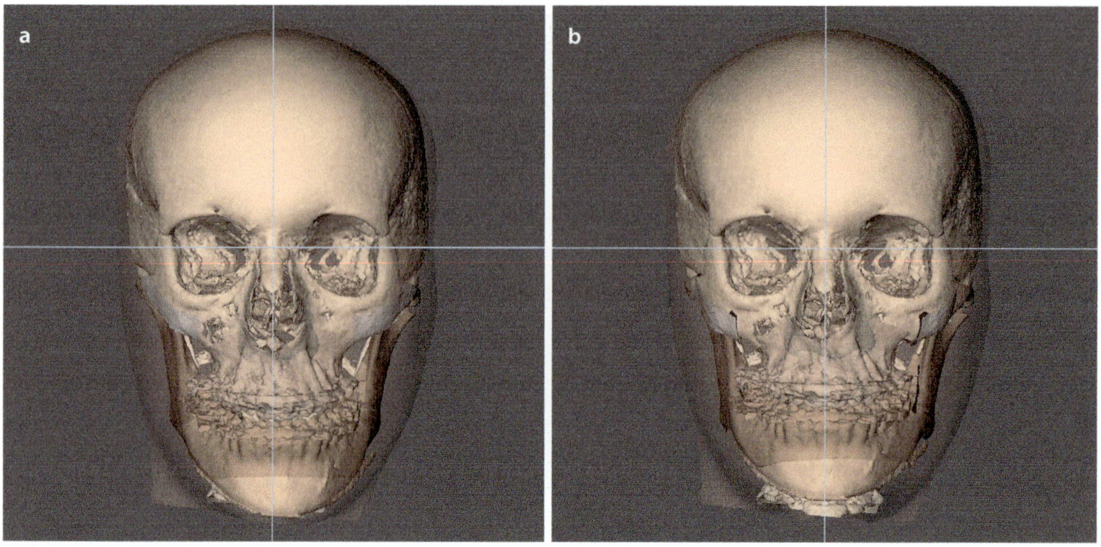

Fig. 6.177 Initial situation (**a**) and final "Individualised 3D Virtual Treatment Plan" (**b**) of patient L.E. in the frontal plane (3D "surface-rendered" representations, Maxilim v. 2.3.0.3)

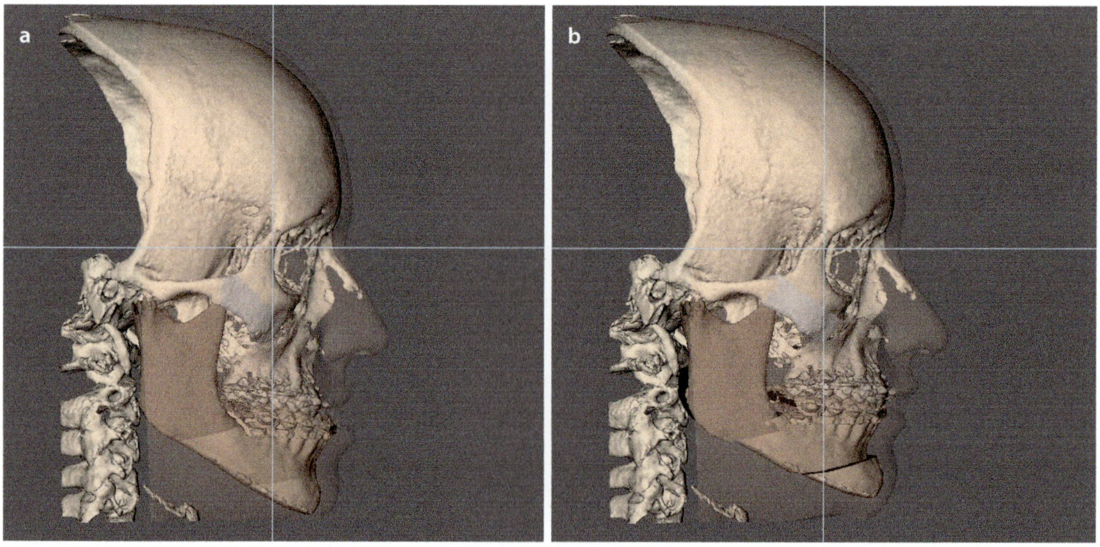

Fig. 6.178 Initial situation (**a**), and final "Individualised 3D Virtual Treatment Plan" (**b**), of patient L.E. in the right profile plane (3D "surface-rendered" representations, Maxilim v. 2.3.0.3). Note the limits of the actual 3D virtual soft tissue simulation at the level of the lips

Case 5: 3D-VPS$_5$- Final Integrated "Individualised 3D Virtual Treatment Plan"

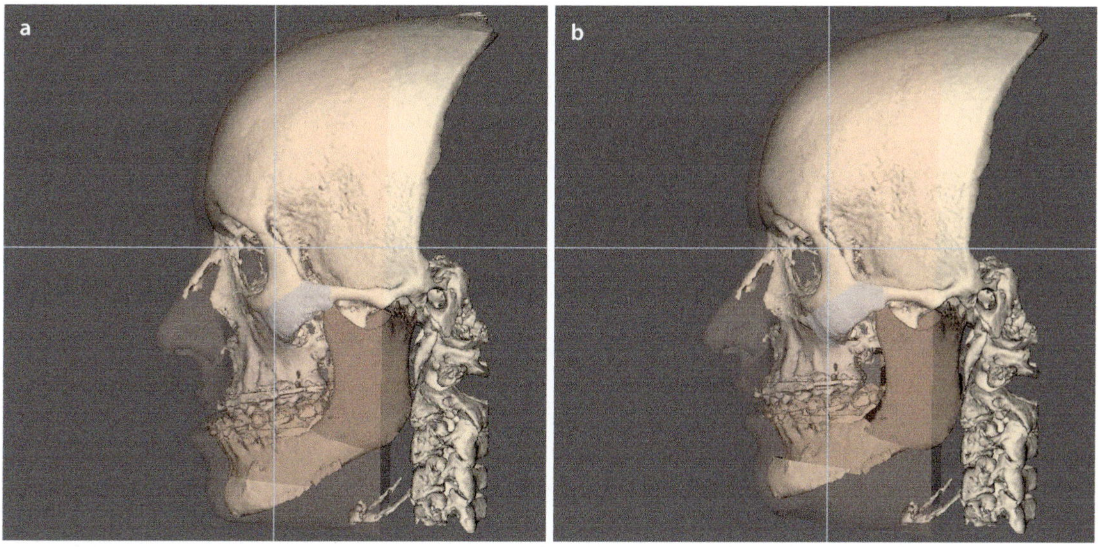

Fig. 6.179 Initial situation (**a**) and final "Individualised 3D Virtual Treatment Plan" (**b**) of patient L.E. in the left profile plane (3D "surface-rendered" representations, Maxilim v. 2.3.0.3). Note the limits of the actual 3D virtual soft tissue simulation at the level of the lips

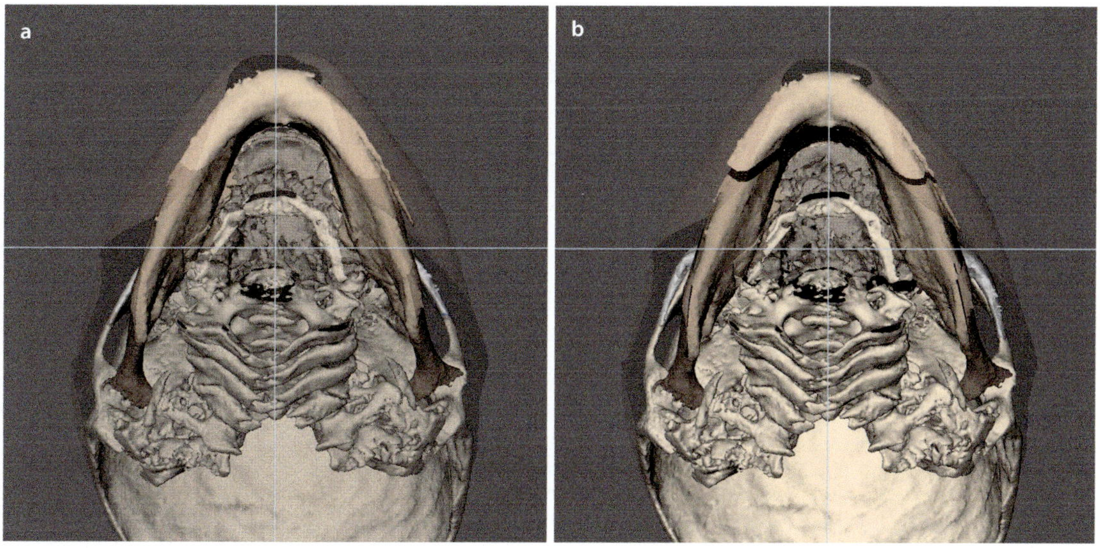

Fig. 6.180 Initial situation (**a**) and final "Individualised 3D Virtual Treatment Plan" (**b**) of patient L.E. in the base plane (3D "surface-rendered" representations, patient L.E., Maxilim v. 2.3.0.3). Note the bilateral zygomatic expansion

▪ Case 5: "3D Virtual Treatment Planning, OR" Template

Maxillary osteotomy

- ■ Le Fort: ■I □II □III
- ■ One-piece
- □ Segmental:
  - Pieces: ....
  - Interdental: ....
- ■ Advancement: 7.0 mm......................
- □ Set-back : ....
- ■ Midline: 2.0 mm.............. ■R □L
- ■ Midline after Le Fort 1: 1/3 mesial 41
- ■ Vertical: (➔)
- ■ "Yaw" correction: CCW to the left.....
- □ Other: ....

Mandibular osteotomy

- ■ SSO ■R ■L
- □ Inverted-L □R □L
- □ VRO □R □L
- □ Advancement: R .... L ....
- ■ Set-back: R 5.0 mm L 6.0 mm
- □ CW "Pitch" rotation
- ■ CCW "Pitch" rotation
- □ Midline split
- ■ IAN course: R lingual L lingual
- □ Midline after BSSO: ....
- □ Other: ....

Chin osteotomy

- ■ Advancement: 4.0 mm......................
- □ Set-back: ....
- □ Midline: .... □R □L
- ■ Intrusion:
  - □ Anterior: ....
  - ■ Posterior: R ...... L 2.0 mm
- □ Extrusion:
  - □ Anterior: ....
  - □ Posterior: R ...... L ......
- □ "Shield" osteotomy
- □ "Chin wing" osteotomy
  - *Mental Foramen level:*
    - □ Symmetric
    - ■ Asymmetric
- □ Other: ....

Planning Requirements

- ■ Maxilla first
- □ Mandible first
- □ Minimally Invasive Le Fort I
- □ IO-CBCT
- □ Kobayashi wires : ....
- □ Skeletal anchorage : ....
- □ Orthodontic buttons : ....
- □ Occlusal grinding : ....
- □ Other : ....

↑	↑	↑	↑	↑
3.5 mm	4.25 mm	4.5 mm	4.25 mm	3.5 mm
16	13	11	23	26

"Roll" correction: □CW □CCW

Miscellaneous

- ■ Para-nasal cross sutures
- ■ Alar cinch
- ■ Septoplasty
- ■ Inferior turbinectomy
- ■ ANS: ■Shortening ■Midline
- ■ Nasal base plasty ■R ■L
- ■ Lateral nasal wall plasty ■R □L
- □ Bone graft(s): ....
- □ Extraction(s): ....
- □ Other: ....

Adjuvant Cosmetic Procedures

- □ Bichatectomy □R □L
- ■ Zygoma osteotomies ■R ■L
  - *Infraorbital Foramen level:*
    - ■ Symmetric
    - □ Asymmetric
- □ Otoplasty: □R □L
- ■ Rhinoplasty: Closed.............................
- □ Browlift: ....
- □ Blepharoplasty: ....
  - □Upper □Lower
- □ Facelift: ....
- □ Necklift: ....
- □ Liposuction: ....
- □ Lipofilling: ....
- □ Other: ....

Case 5: Class III, Midfacial Hypoplasia, Mandibular Hyperplasia, 3D Virtual Treatment Outcome

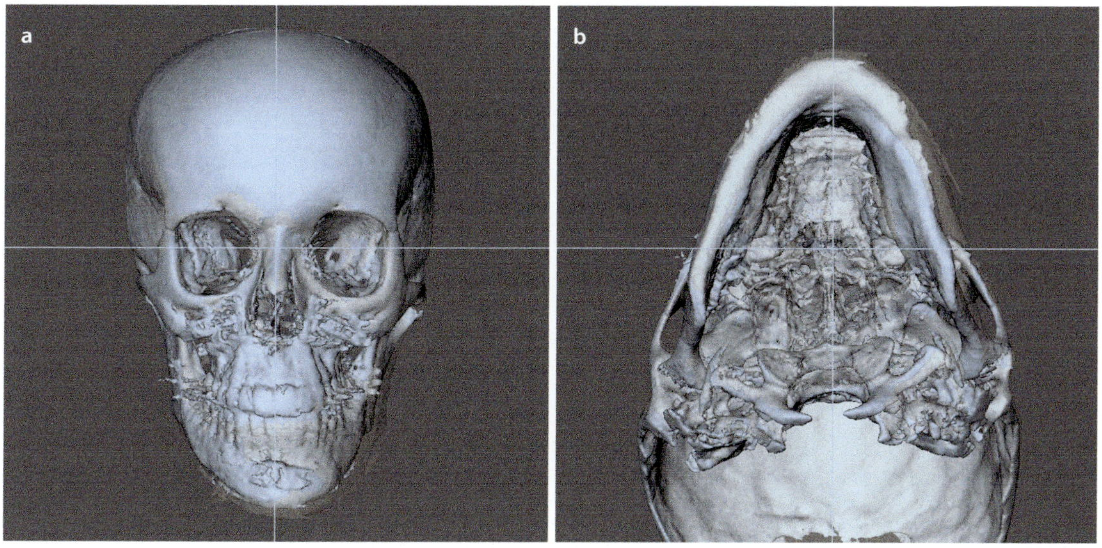

Fig. 6.181 Voxel-based superimposition on the cranial base of the pre-surgical and 10 months post-surgical (*blue*) 3D "surface-rendered" hard tissue representations. Frontal (**a**) and base (**b**) views (i-CAT, Imaging Sciences International Inc., Maxilim v. 2.3.0.3) (patient L.E.). Note the correction of the chin deviation

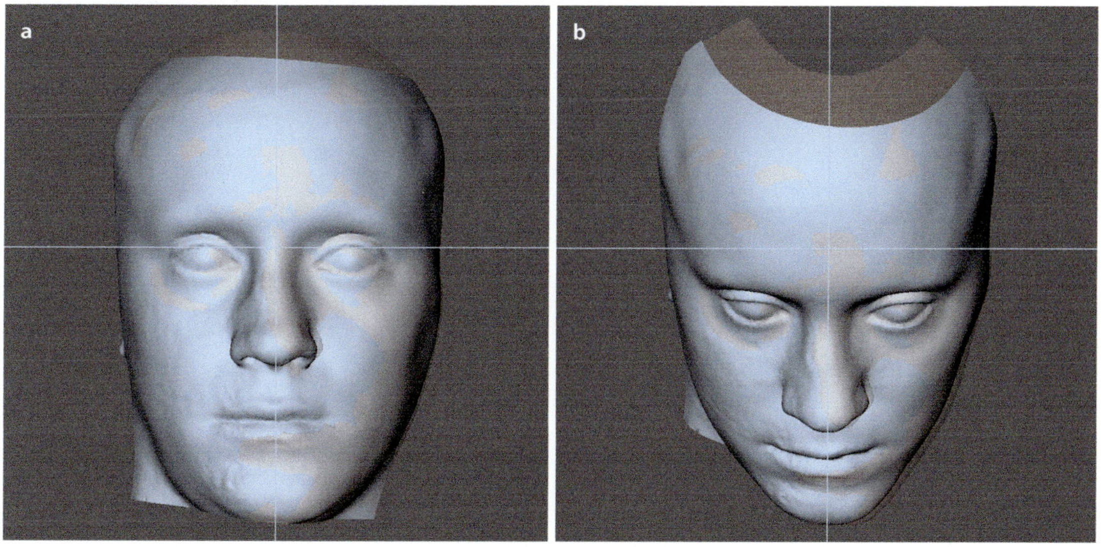

Fig. 6.182 Voxel-based superimposition on the cranial base of the pre-surgical and 10 months post-surgical (*blue*) 3D "surface-rendered" soft tissue representations. Frontal (**a**) and downward inclined (**b**) views (i-CAT, Imaging Sciences International Inc., Maxilim v. 2.3.0.3) (patient L.E.). Note the post-surgical (*blue*) facial symmetry and harmony

Case 5: Class III, Midfacial Hypoplasia, Mandibular Hyperplasia, 3D Virtual Treatment Outcome

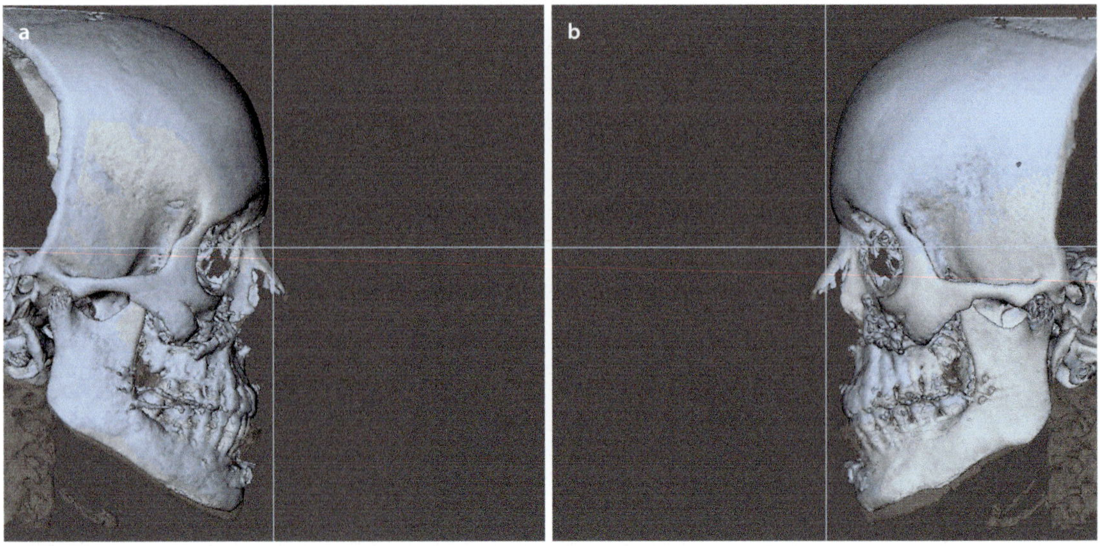

Fig. 6.183 Voxel-based superimposition on the cranial base of the pre-surgical and 10 months post-surgical (*blue*) 3D "surface-rendered" hard tissue representations. Right (**a**) and left profile (**b**) views (i-CAT, Imaging Sciences International Inc., Maxilim v. 2.3.0.3) (patient L.E.). Note the anterior impaction of the bimaxillary complex

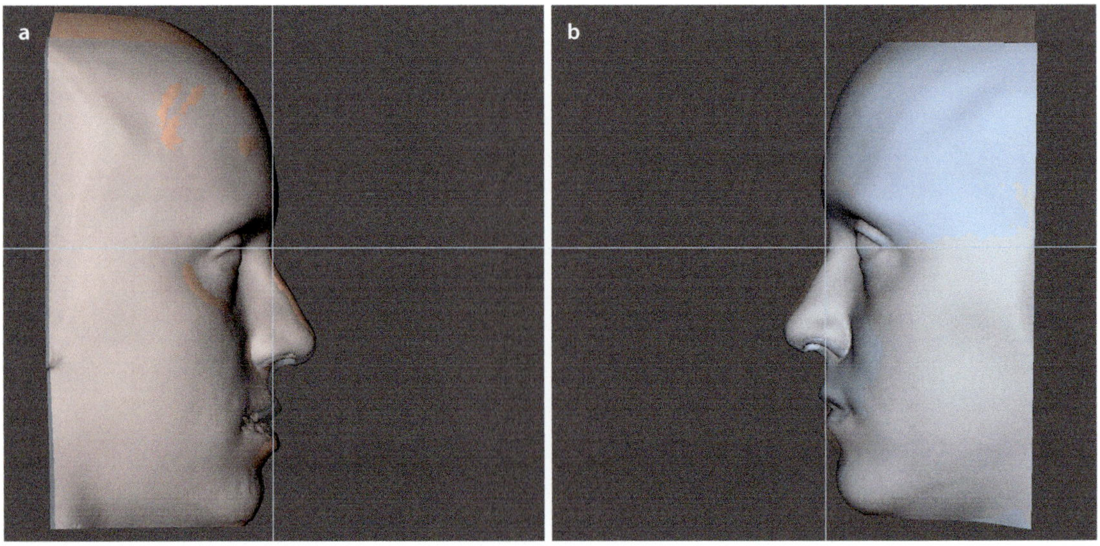

Fig. 6.184 Voxel-based superimposition on the cranial base of the pre-surgical and 10 months post-surgical (*blue*) 3D "surface-rendered" soft tissue representations. Right (**a**) and left profile (**b**) views (i-CAT, Imaging Sciences International Inc., Maxilim v. 2.3.0.3) (patient L.E.). Note the changes at the nasolabial aesthetic unit with nasal dorsum correction and post-surgical changes of lip posture

Case 5: Class III, Midfacial Hypoplasia, Mandibular Hyperplasia, Clinical Treatment Outcome

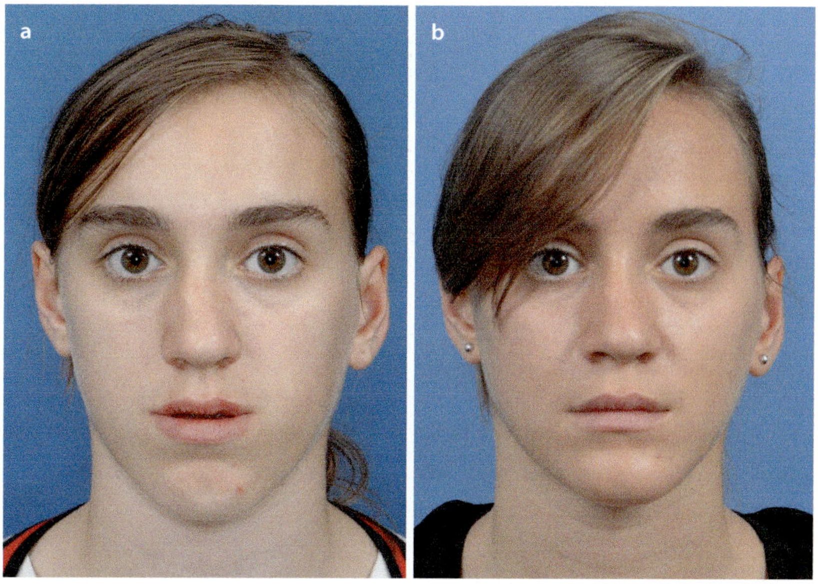

Fig. 6.185 Frontal views in rest, pre-surgical (**a**) and 10 months after (**b**) combined orthodontic-surgical treatment, bilateral zygomatic osteotomies and closed rhinoplasty (patient L.E.)

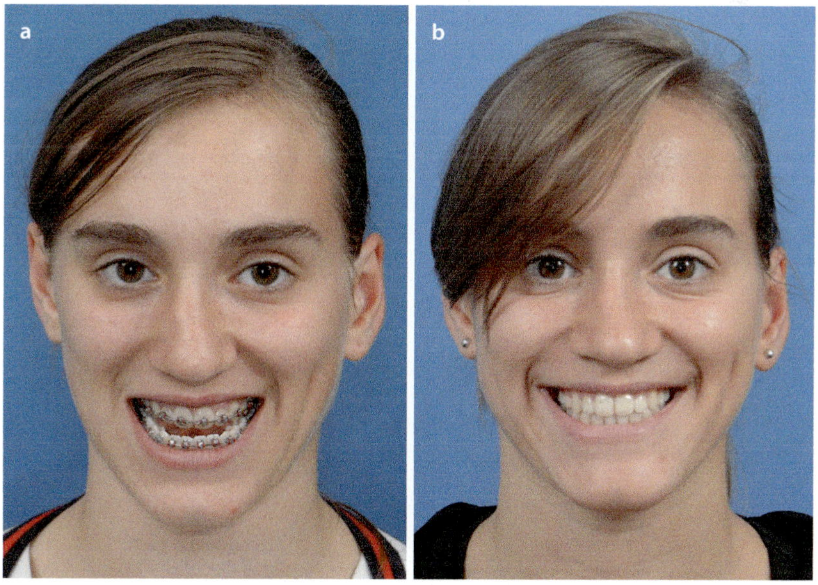

Fig. 6.186 Frontal views during smiling, pre-surgical (**a**) and 10 months after (**b**) combined orthodontic-surgical treatment, bilateral zygomatic osteotomies and closed rhinoplasty (patient L.E.)

Case 5: Class III, Midfacial Hypoplasia, Mandibular Hyperplasia, Clinical Treatment Outcome

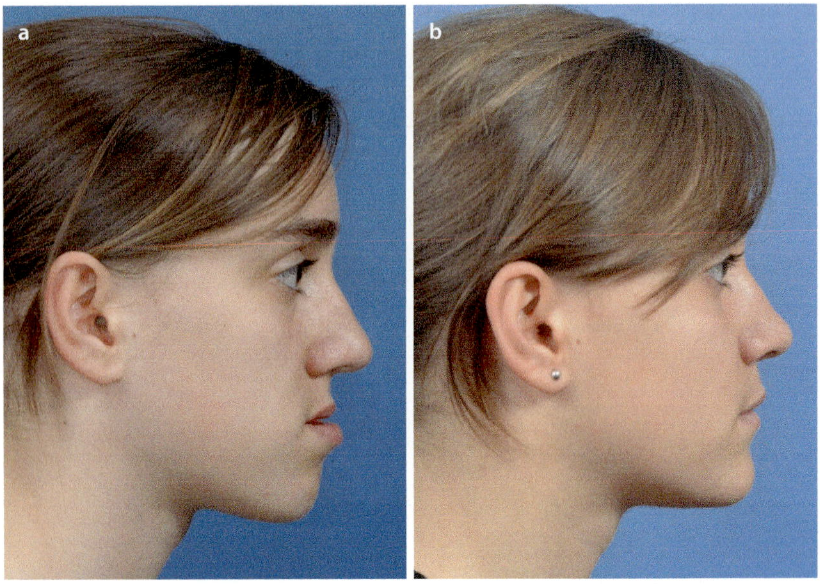

Fig. 6.187 Right profile views in rest, pre-surgical (**a**) and 10 months after (**b**) combined orthodontic-surgical treatment, bilateral zygomatic osteotomies and closed rhinoplasty (patient L.E.)

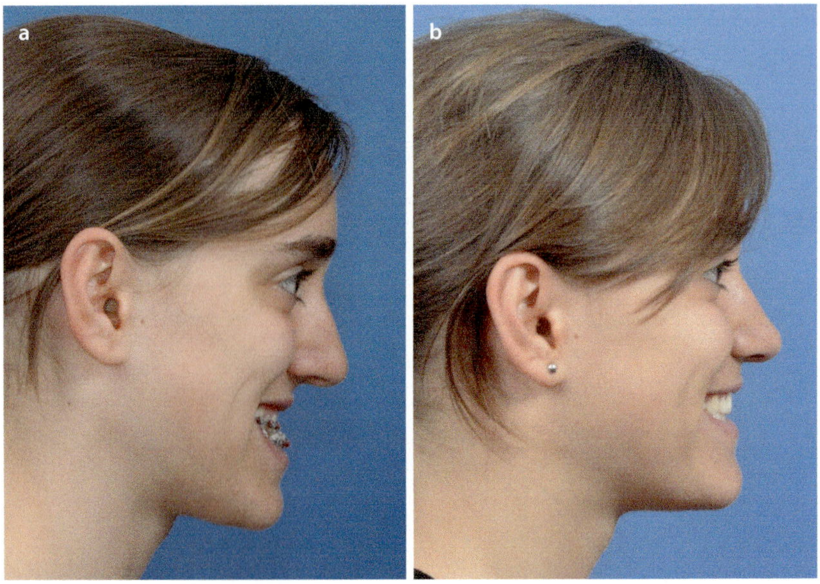

Fig. 6.188 Right profile views during smiling, pre-surgical (**a**) and 10 months after (**b**) combined orthodontic-surgical treatment, bilateral zygomatic osteotomies and closed rhinoplasty (patient L.E.)

Case 5: Class III, Midfacial Hypoplasia, Mandibular Hyperplasia, Clinical Treatment Outcome

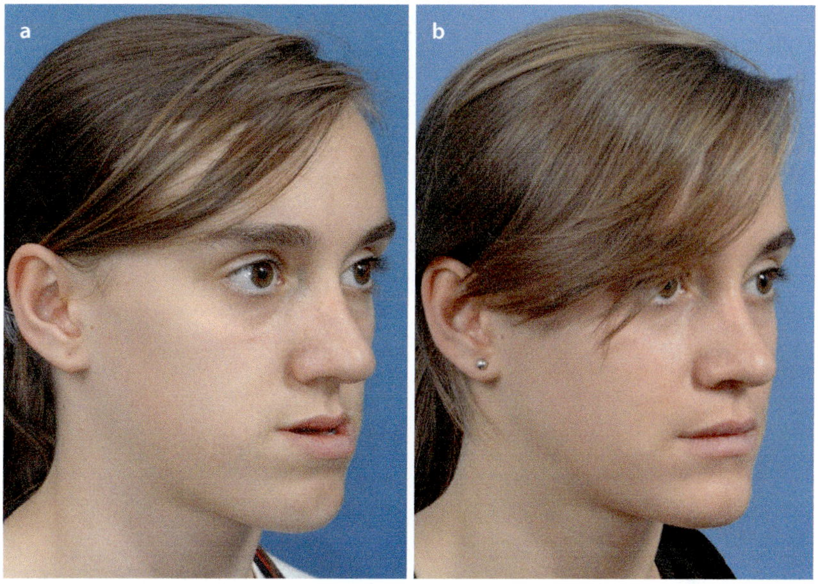

Fig. 6.189 2/3 right profile views in rest, pre-surgical (**a**) and 10 months after (**b**) combined orthodontic-surgical treatment, bilateral zygomatic osteotomies and closed rhinoplasty (patient L.E.)

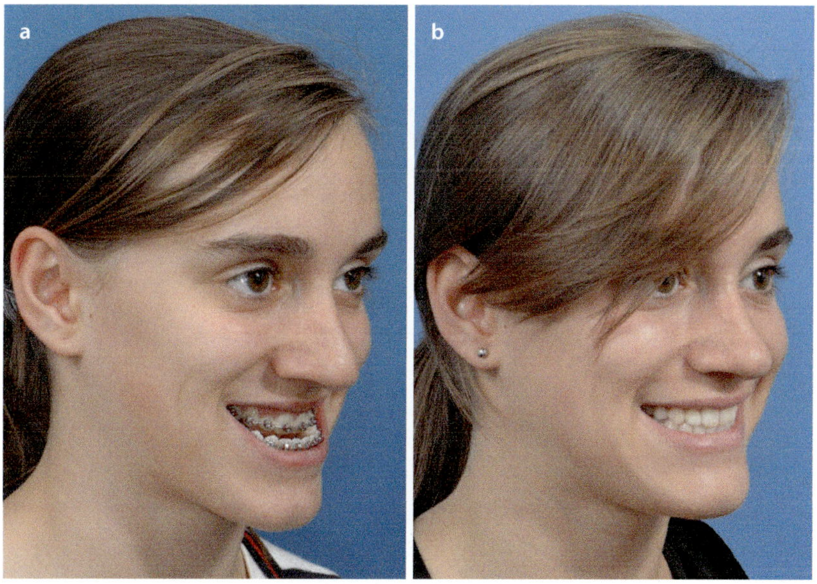

Fig. 6.190 2/3 right profile views during smiling, pre-surgical (**a**) and 10 months after (**b**) combined orthodontic-surgical treatment, bilateral zygomatic osteotomies and closed rhinoplasty (patient L.E.)

Case 5: Class III, Midfacial Hypoplasia, Mandibular Hyperplasia, Clinical Treatment Outcome

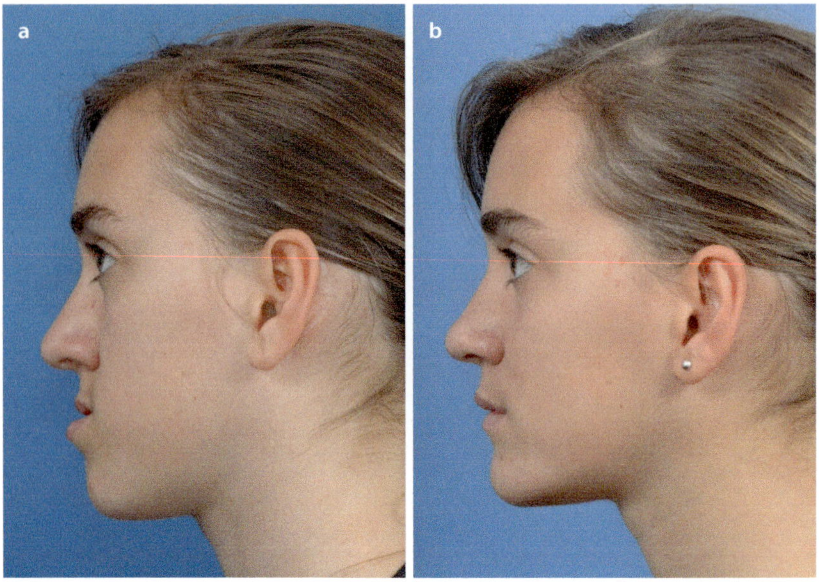

Fig. 6.191 Left profile views in rest, pre-surgical (**a**) and 10 months after (**b**) combined orthodontic-surgical treatment, bilateral zygomatic osteotomies and closed rhinoplasty (patient L.E.)

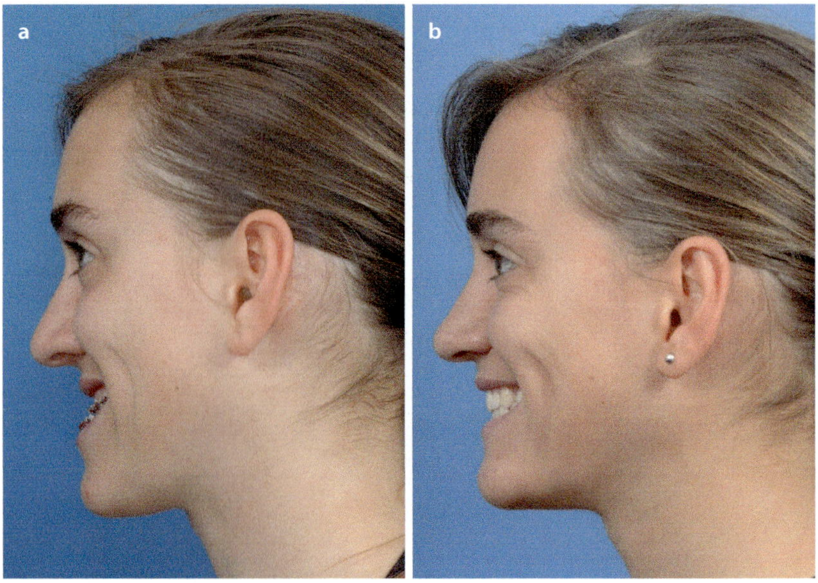

Fig. 6.192 Left profile views during smiling, pre-surgical (**a**) and 10 months after (**b**) combined orthodontic-surgical treatment, bilateral zygomatic osteotomies and closed rhinoplasty (patient L.E.)

Case 5: Class III, Midfacial Hypoplasia, Mandibular Hyperplasia, Clinical Treatment Outcome

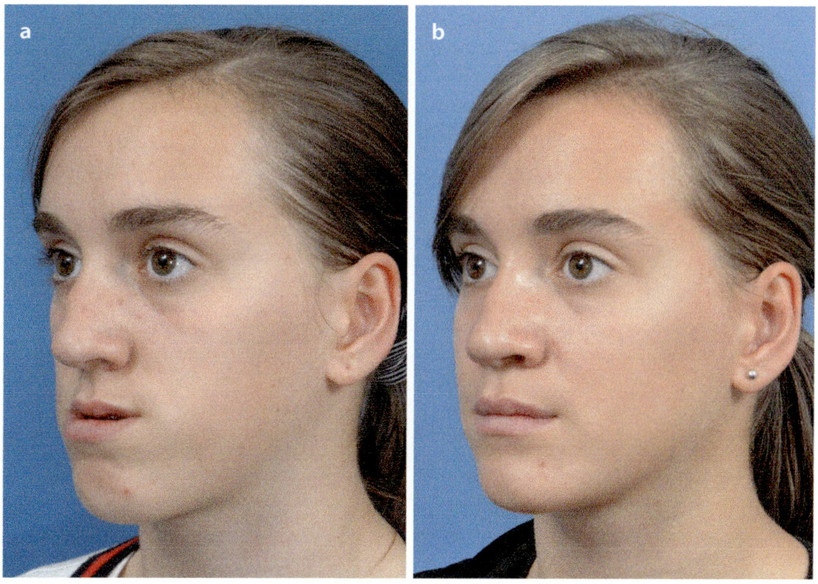

Fig. 6.193 2/3 left profile views in rest, pre-surgical (**a**) and 10 months after (**b**) combined orthodontic-surgical treatment, bilateral zygomatic osteotomies and closed rhinoplasty (patient L.E.)

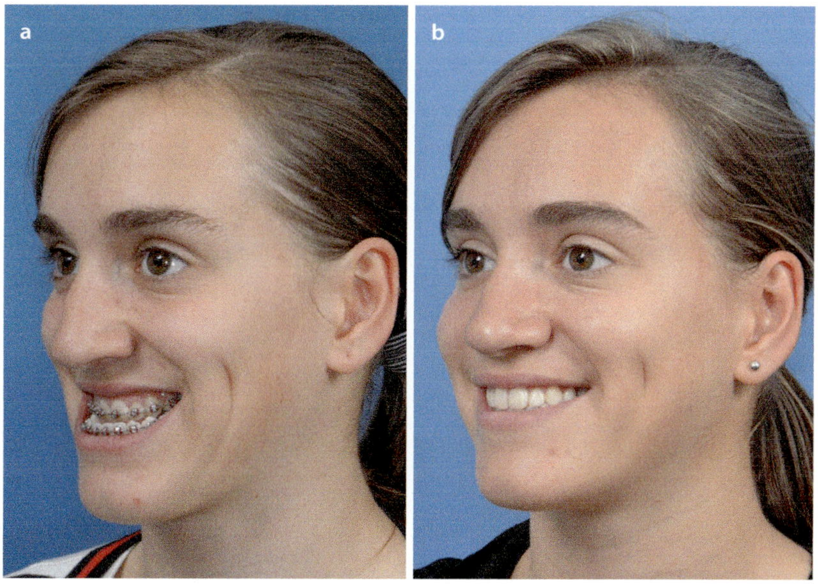

Fig. 6.194 2/3 left profile views during smiling, pre-surgical (**a**) and 10 months after (**b**) combined orthodontic-surgical treatment, bilateral zygomatic osteotomies and closed rhinoplasty (patient L.E.)

Case 5: Class III, Midfacial Hypoplasia, Mandibular Hyperplasia, Clinical Treatment Outcome

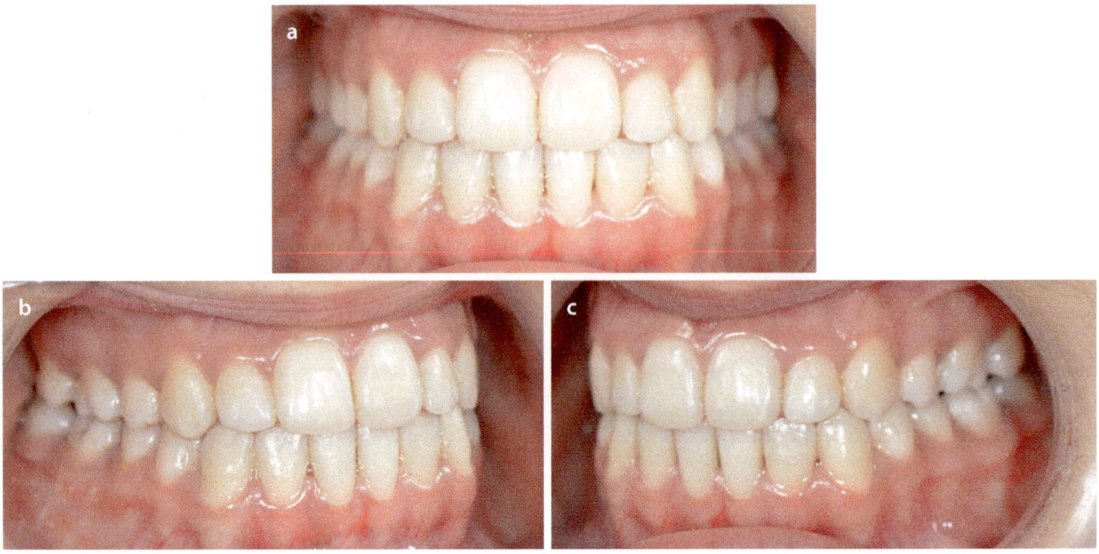

Fig. 6.195 Frontal (**a**), right (**b**) and left (**c**) intra-oral views of the patient's occlusion 10 months after combined orthodontic-surgical treatment (patient L.E.). The author acknowledges Charlotte Van Elst and Prof. Guy De Pauw for the orthodontic treatment

Case 6: Class III, Anterior Open Bite (AOB)

Patient D.B. is a 17-year-old boy with a Class III, anterior open bite (AOB) maxillofacial deformity due to Beckwith-Wiedemann syndrome. In the frontal view, he is clinically not presenting any obvious facial asymmetry. In rest, he has no incisal display and neither during spontaneous smiling. He has an upper incisal crown length of 11 mm. In the profile view, he presents with rather a Class I profile. He has an Angle Class III malocclusion, a severe anterior open bite and adequate transversal relationship. He has no history of TMJ dysfunction neither pain.

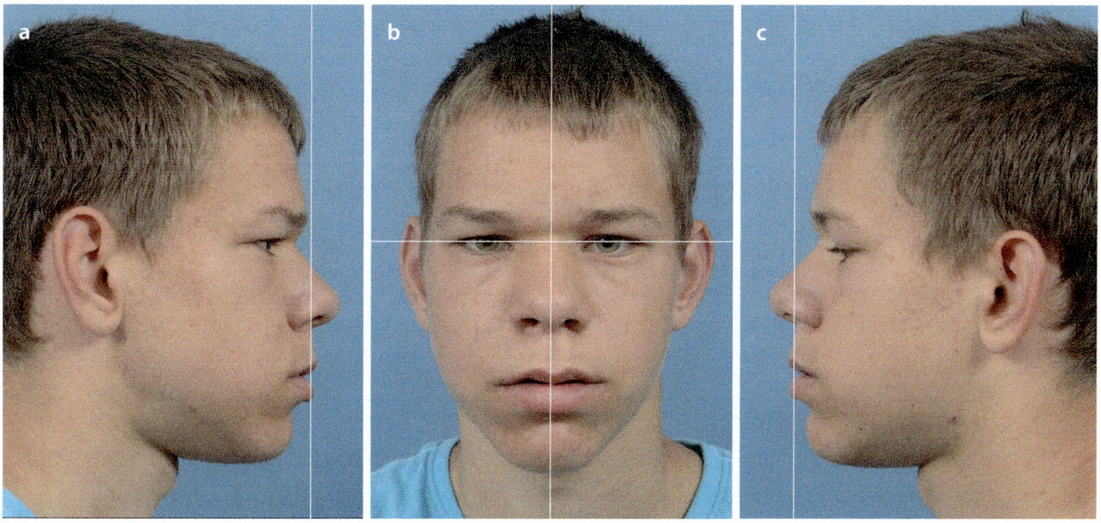

Fig. 6.196 Pre-surgical clinical right profile (**a**), frontal (**b**) and left profile (**c**) views of patient D.B. in his *c*-NHP in rest, at the time of the workup, approximately 3 weeks prior to surgery

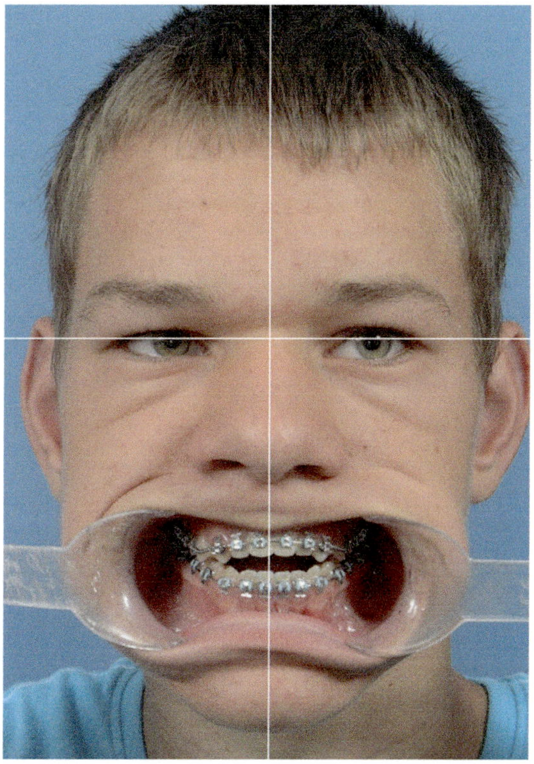

Fig. 6.197 Pre-surgical clinical frontal view with cheek retractors of patient D.B. at the time of the workup, approximately 3 weeks prior to surgery. Note the deviation of the upper and lower dental midline to the left

Case 6: Class III, Anterior Open Bite (AOB), *v*-NHP and PHP

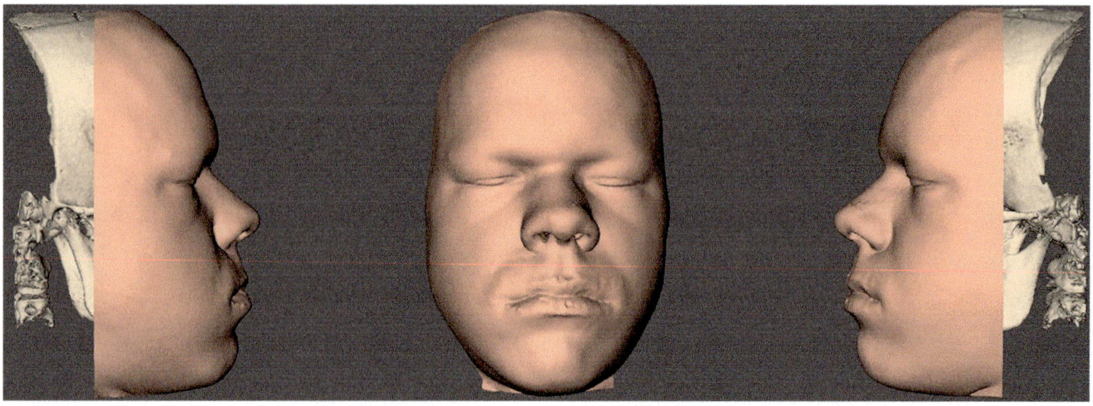

Fig. 6.198 Pre-surgical 3D "surface-rendered" right profile, frontal and left profile soft and hard tissue representations of the head of patient D.B., as generated during standardised CBCT image acquisition, at the time of the workup (Maxilim v. 2.3.0.3). Note the incorrect position and orientation of the virtual head compared to the clinical pictures of patient D.B. (Fig. 6.196), although it was attempted to scan the patient in his correct *c*-NHP in rest

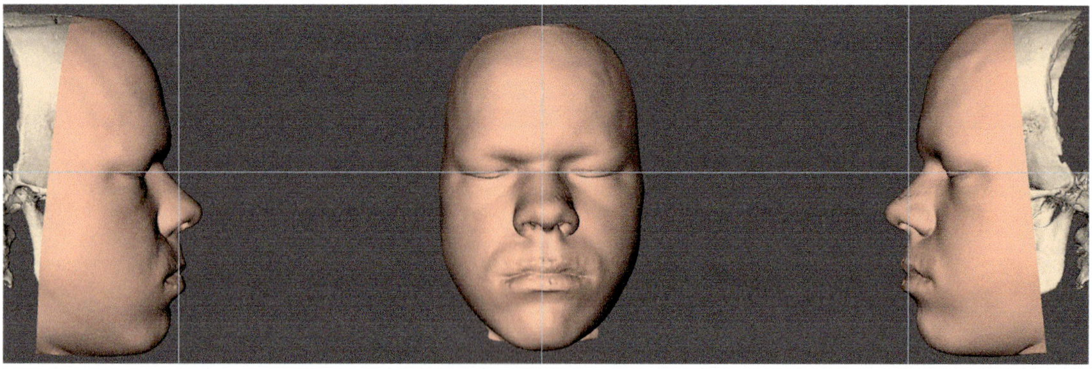

Fig. 6.199 Following a standardised "step-by-step" approach (see Sect. 3.1), the scanned head position of patient D.B. (Fig. 6.198) was virtually modified towards his *c*-NHP (Fig. 6.196), which results in his *v*-NHP and corresponds to his individual "Planning Head Position (PHP)" (3D "surface-rendered" representations, Maxilim v. 2.3.0.3). Note that since both clinical profile photographs (Fig. 6.196a, c) showed a different *c*-NHP, it was clinically decided to virtually modify to a *v*-NHP in between

Case 6: Class III, Anterior Open Bite (AOB)

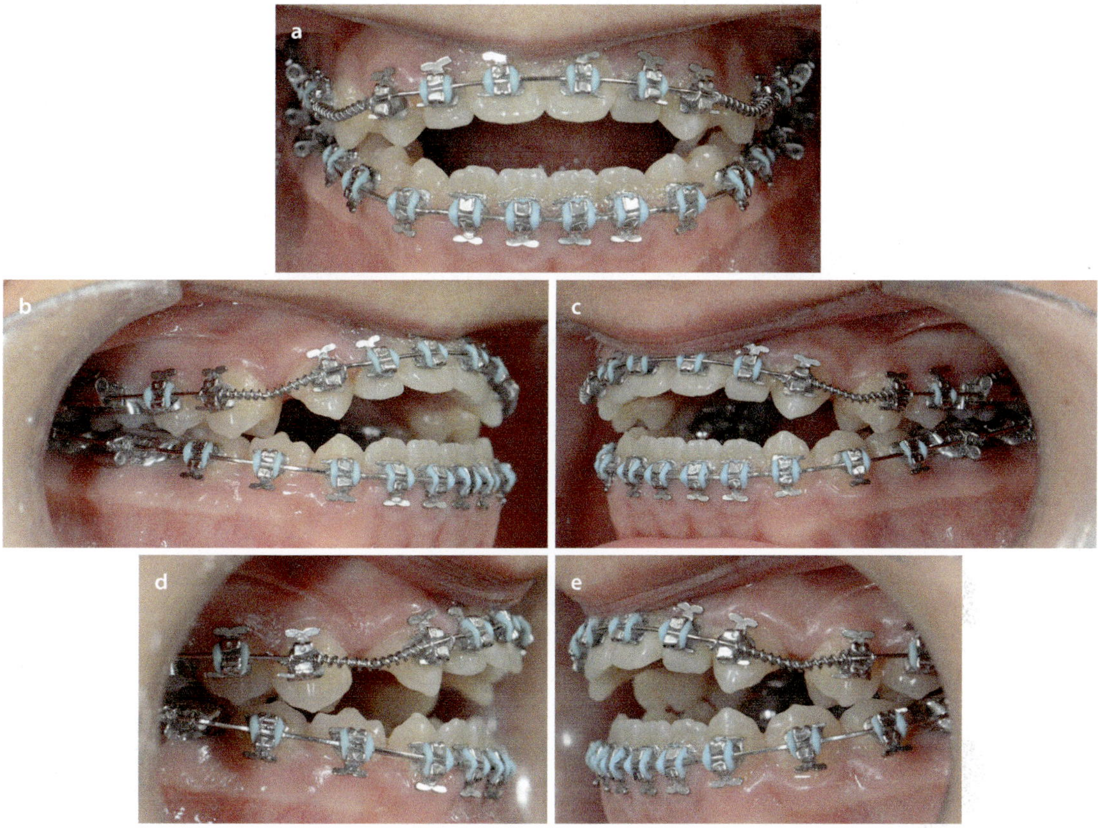

Fig. 6.200 Pre-surgical frontal (**a**), right (**b**, **d**) and left (**c**, **e**) intra-oral views of the occlusion of patient D.B. at the time of the workup, approximately 3 weeks prior to surgery. Note that prior to surgery, left and right diasteme were orthodontically prepared distally from the canines to facilitate the anterior segmental osteotomy

▪ Case 6: 3D-VPS$_5$ Step 1 Maxillary Occlusal Cant Evaluation/Correction ("Roll")

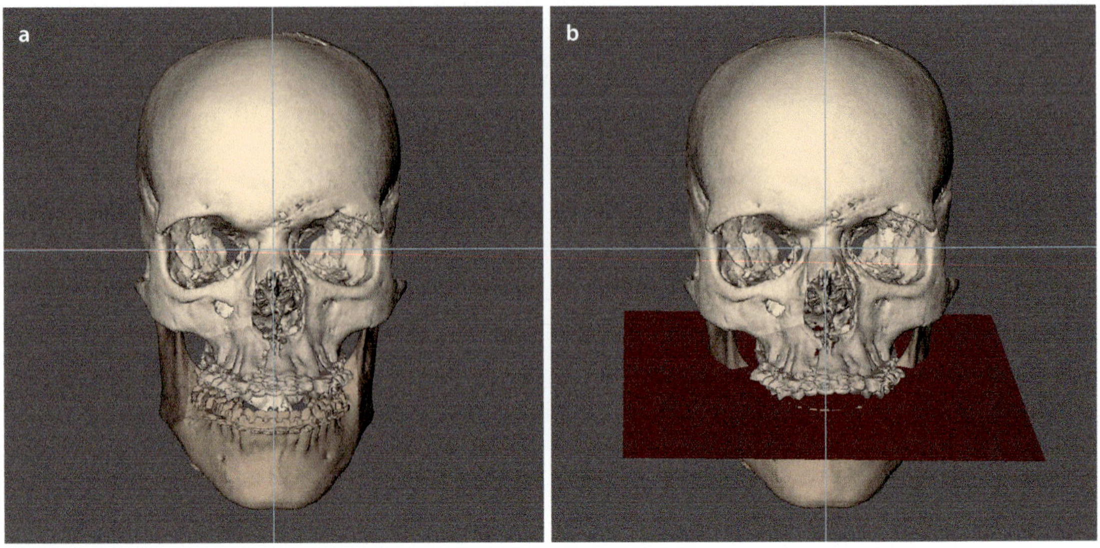

Fig. 6.201 The maxillary occlusal plane is evaluated both clinically (Fig. 6.197) and virtually (**a**) towards the horizontal 3D PHP reference plane in patient D.B. and shows virtually a slight cant (**b**) (3D "surface-rendered" representations, Maxilim v. 2.3.0.3). Note that this cant is clinically (Fig. 6.197) not so obvious

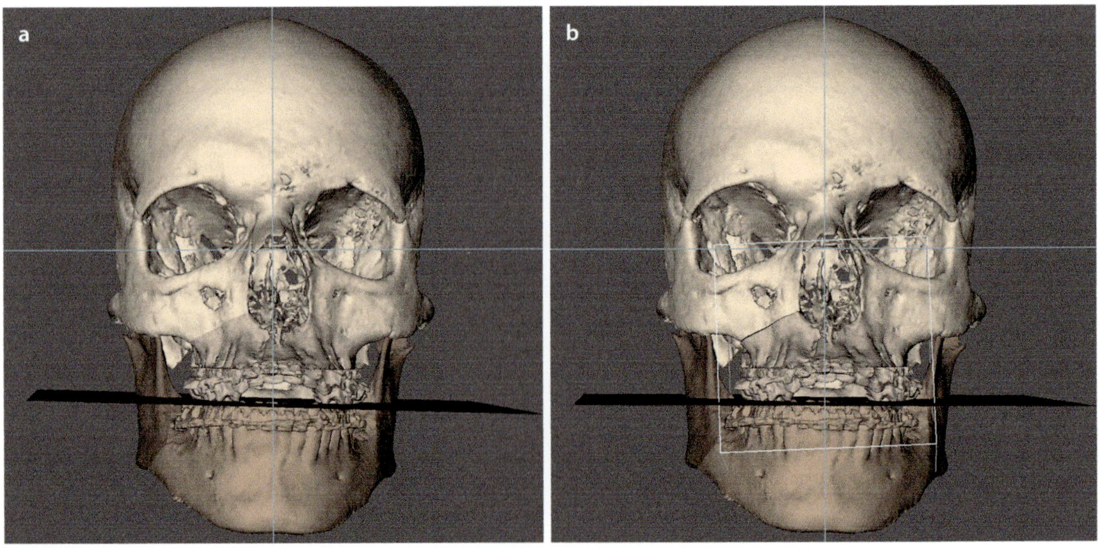

Fig. 6.202 The maxillary cant (**a**) in patient D.B. is corrected towards the horizontal 3D PHP reference plane by a CCW "Roll" rotational movement (**b**) (3D "surface-rendered" representations, Maxilim v. 2.3.0.3)

■ Case 6: 3D-VPS$_5$ Step 2 Upper Dental Midline Evaluation/Correction

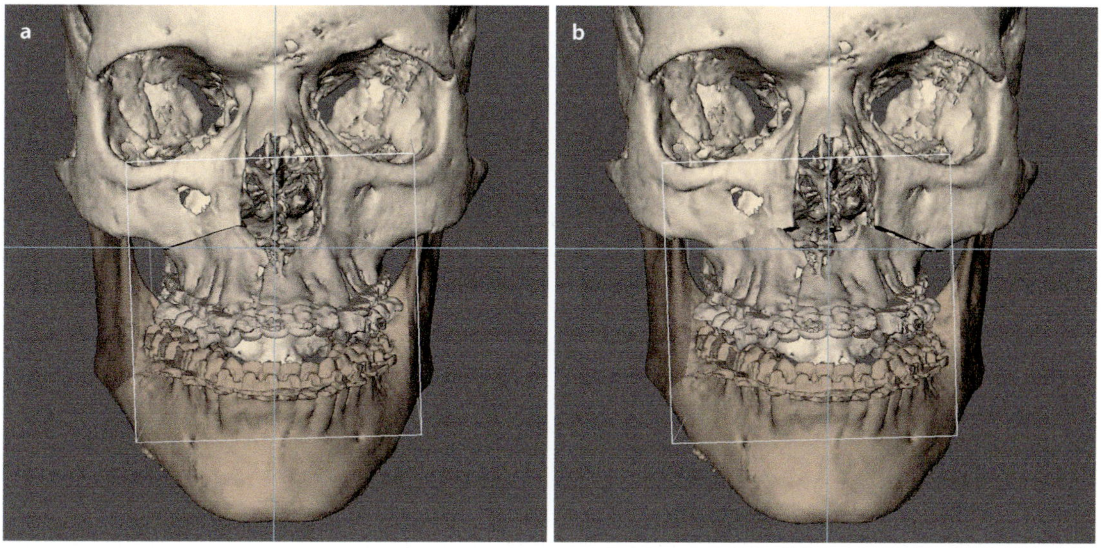

Fig. 6.203 The 3 mm deviation of the upper dental midline to the left (**a**) is corrected towards the facial midline 3D PHP reference plane, by a combination of a translation to the right and a CCW "Yaw" rotational movement to the left in patient D.B. (**b**) (3D "surface-rendered" representations, Maxilim v. 2.3.0.3)

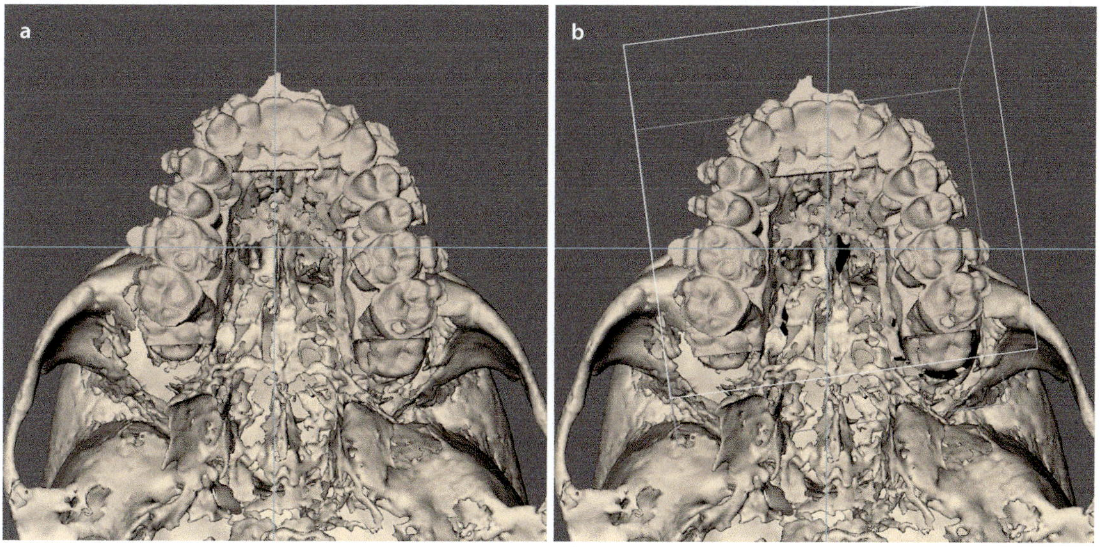

Fig. 6.204 The 3 mm deviation of the upper dental midline to the left (**a**) is corrected towards the facial midline 3D PHP reference plane, by a combination of a translation to the right and a CCW "Yaw" rotational movement to the left in patient D.B. (**b**) (3D "surface-rendered" representations, Maxilim v. 2.3.0.3)

Case 6: 3D-VPS$_5$ Step 3 Overall Evaluation of Facial Asymmetry After Virtual Occlusal Definition

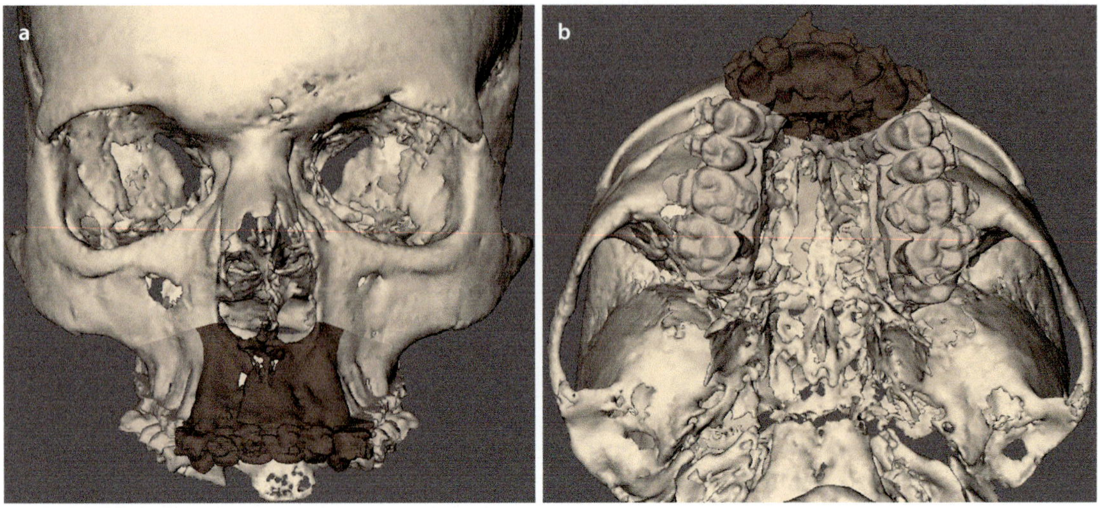

Fig. 6.205 In order to close the anterior open bite (AOB) in patient D.B., a maxillary segmental osteotomy is virtually performed (**a**) with additional bone cuts between 14–13 and 23–24 (**b**) (3D "surface-rendered" representations, Maxilim v. 2.3.0.3)

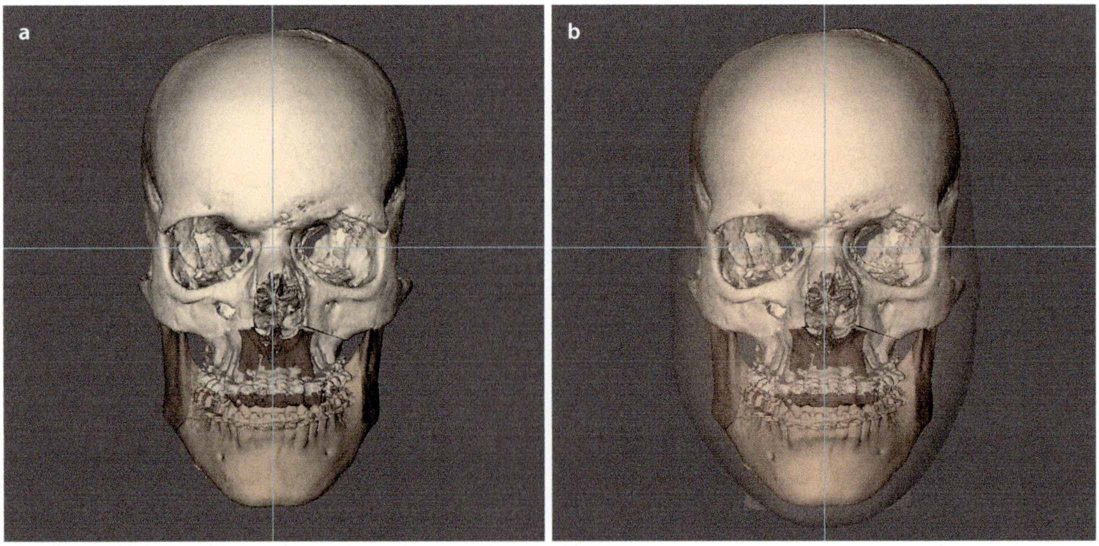

Fig. 6.206 After virtual segmental occlusal definition in patient D.B., the mandibular and midfacial contour are evaluated both virtually at the bony level (**a**) and on the soft tissues in transparency (**b**) (3D "surface-rendered" representations, Maxilim v. 2.3.0.3). Note virtually the adequate facial symmetry

Case 6: 3D-VPS$_5$ Step 4 Evaluation/Correction of Flaring ("Yaw")

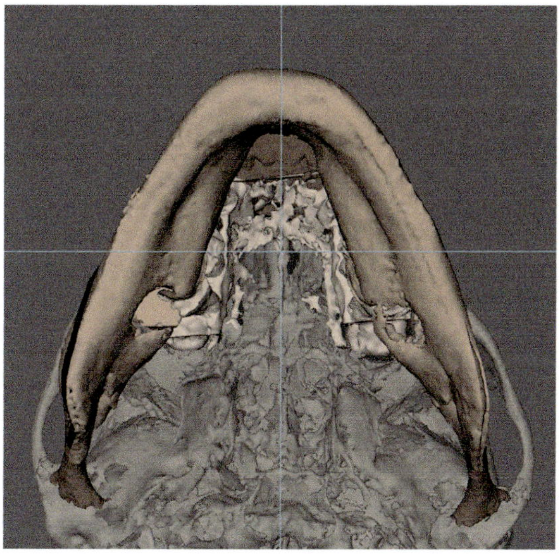

Fig. 6.207 The base view shows no flaring of the mandibular body after correction in "step 2" of the deviation of the upper dental midline by a combined translation to the right and CCW "Yaw" rotational movement of the segmented maxilla to the left in patient D.B. (3D "surface-rendered" representations, Maxilim v. 2.3.0.3)

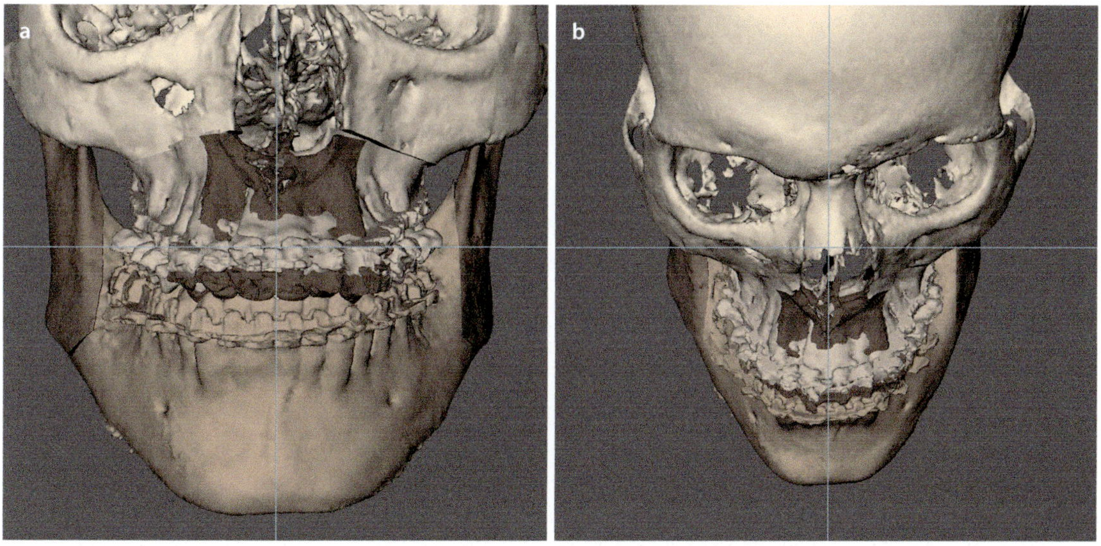

Fig. 6.208 Overall assessment of facial bony contour at this stage does not show mandibular flaring in patient D.B. (3D "surface-rendered" representations, Maxilim v. 2.3.0.3). Frontal (**a**) and frontal downward inclined (**b**) views

■ Case 6: 3D-VPS$_5$ Step 5 Upper Vertical Incisal Position Evaluation/Correction

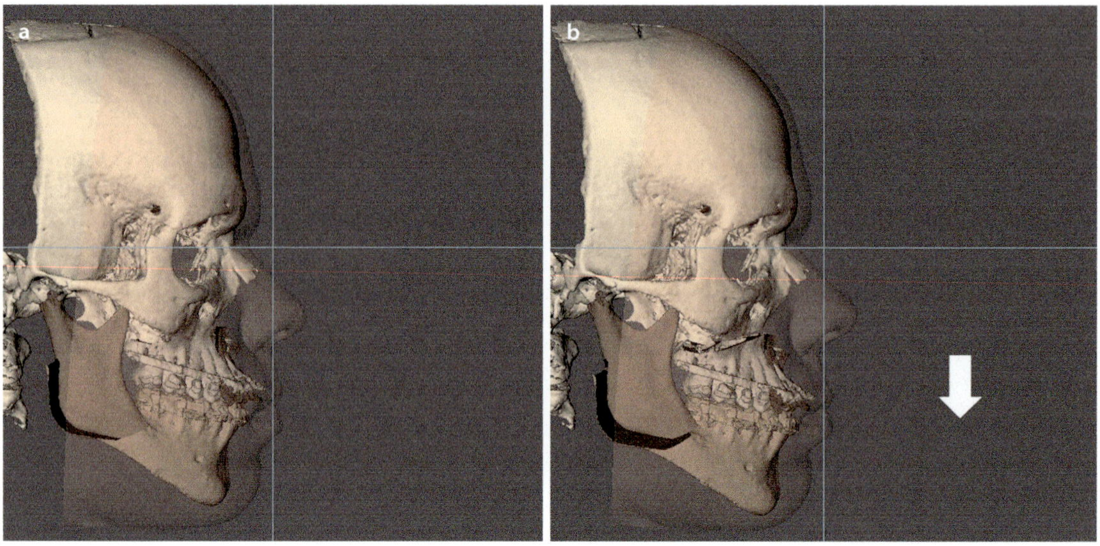

Fig. 6.209 Since patient D.B. has neither in rest nor during spontaneous smiling any incisal exposure, it was decided clinically at this stage in "step 5" to virtually extrude the segmented maxilla 4 mm which results in an extrusion of 10 mm at the upper incisal level (3D "surface-rendered" representations, Maxilim v. 2.3.0.3): before (**a**) and after (**b**) correction

■ Case 6: 3D-VPS$_5$ Step 6 Sagittal Upper Incisal Position Evaluation/Correction

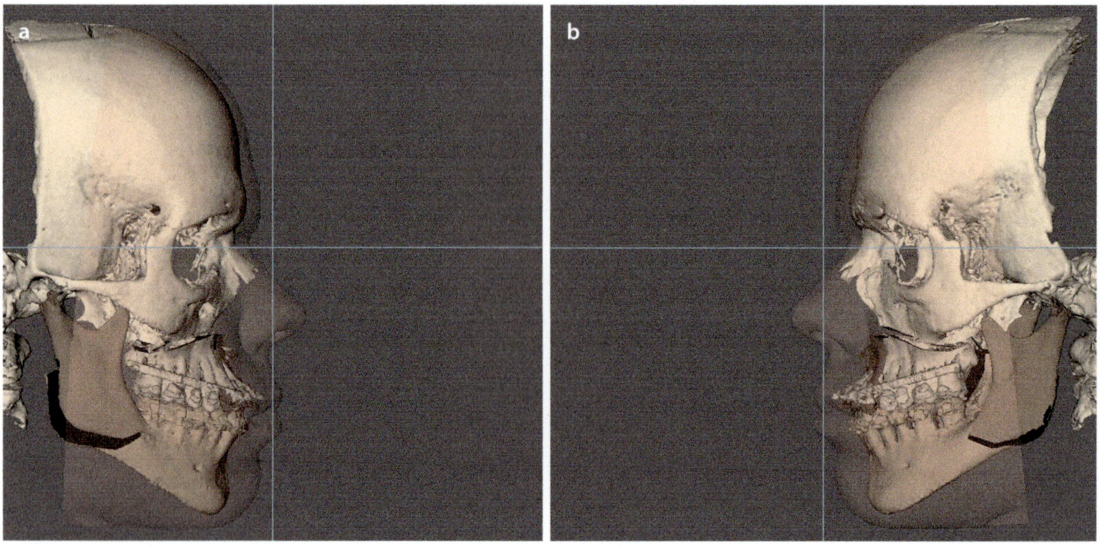

Fig. 6.210 From clinical examination but also 3D cephalometric analysis, it was decided in "step 6" not to advance the "maxillo-mandibular complex in final occlusion" in patient D.B. (3D "surface-rendered" representations, Maxilim v. 2.3.0.3). Profile left (**a**) and right (**b**) views

Case 6: 3D-VPS$_5$ Step 7 Profile Evaluation/Occlusal Plane Correction ("Pitch")

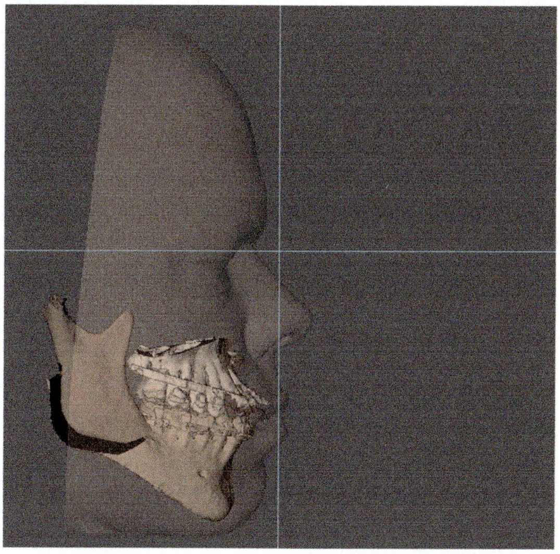

Fig. 6.211 At this stage in "step 7", the profile and dento-alveolar support of the upper lip are evaluated in patient D.B. (3D "surface-rendered" representations, Maxilim v. 2.3.0.3)

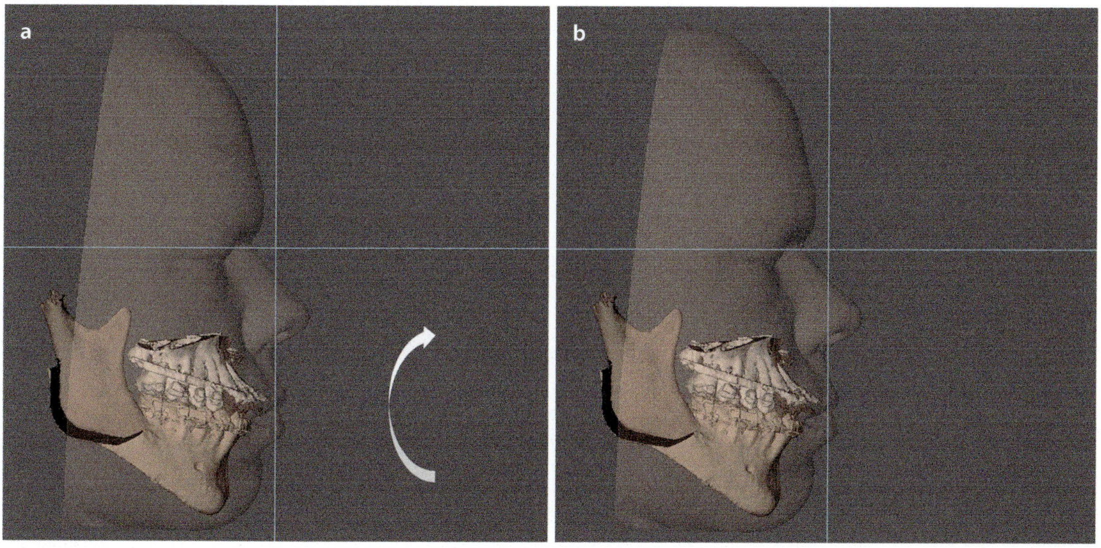

Fig. 6.212 It was decided to perform a 2° CW occlusal plane rotation with the centre of rotation at the incisal level by a "Pitch" rotational movement (3D "surface-rendered" representations, patient D.B., Maxilim v. 2.3.0.3): before (**a**) and after (**b**) correction

■ Case 6: 3D-VPS$_5$ Step 8 3D Chin Position Evaluation/Correction

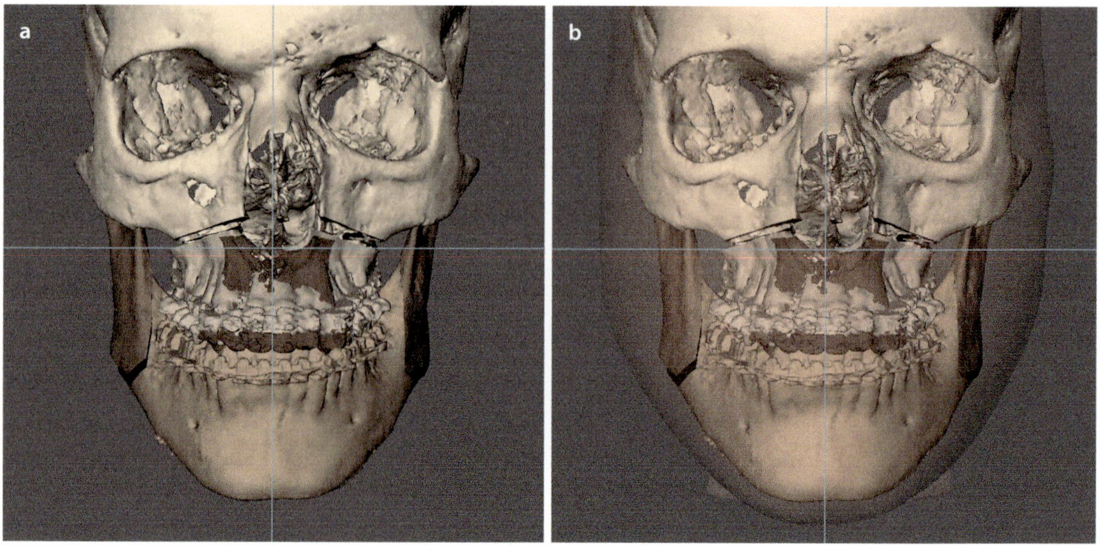

Fig. 6.213 Evaluation of the chin position in the frontal plane without (**a**) and with (**b**) the patient's 3D facial soft tissue mask in transparency (3D "surface-rendered" representations, patient D.B., Maxilim v. 2.3.0.3) does not show any obvious skeletal chin deviation neither asymmetry

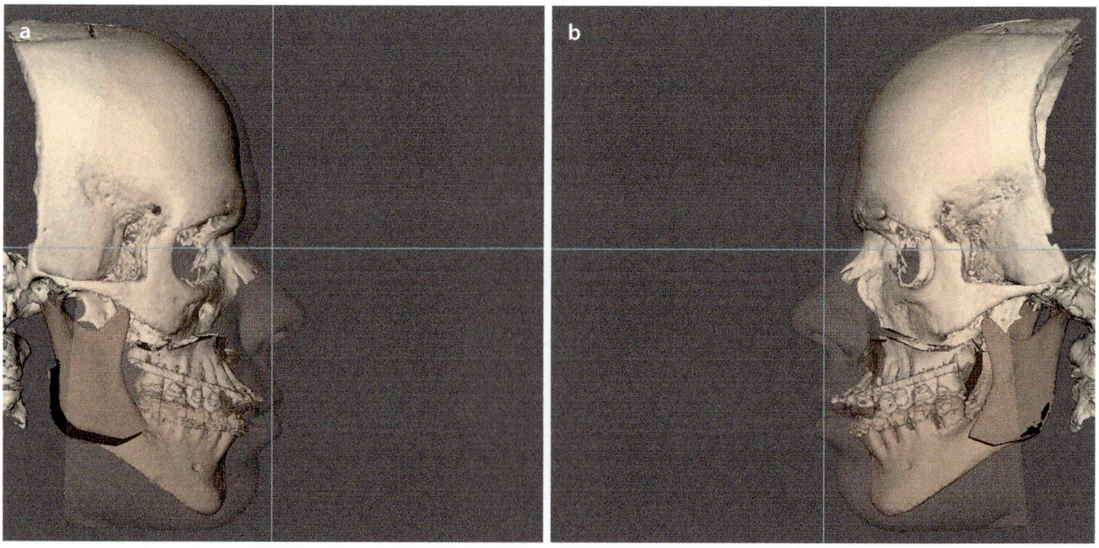

Fig. 6.214 Evaluation of the right (**a**) and left profile (**b**) views shows an adequate sagittal position of the chin towards the "true vertical (TV)" (3D "surface-rendered" representations, patient D.B., Maxilim v. 2.3.0.3)

▪ Case 6: 3D-VPS$_5$ Step 9 Patient Communication of the Individualised Treatment Plan

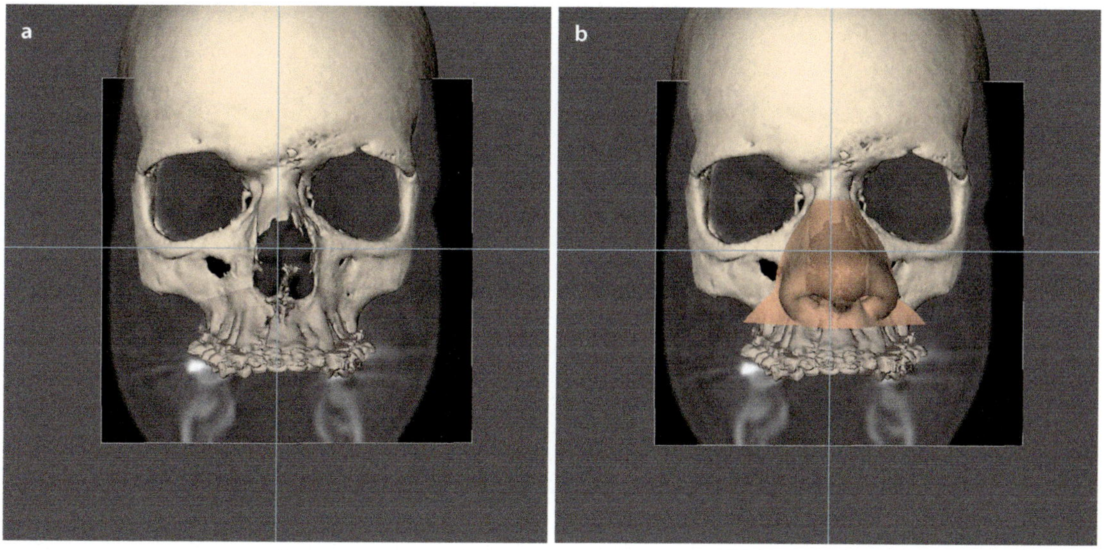

Fig. 6.215 Combination of 3D virtual evaluation of the underlying coronal slices, the virtual maxilla, the bony skull (**a**) and the virtual soft tissue of the nose (**b**) shows an important deviation of the anterior nasal spine (ANS) and nasal septum to the left, which pushes the nasal tip to the left in patient D.B. although the bony nasal pyramid is straight (3D "surface-rendered" representations, Maxilim v. 2.3.0.3)

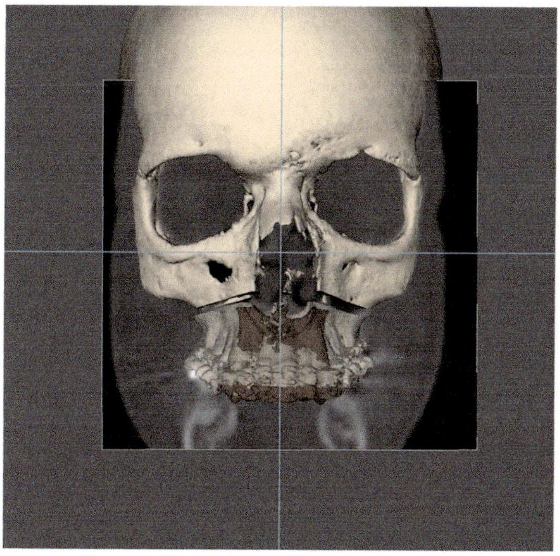

Fig. 6.216 3D virtual repositioning of the segmented maxilla shows correction of the anterior nasal spine (ANS) and nasal base (3D "surface-rendered" representations, Maxilim v. 2.3.0.3)

Case 6: 3D-VPS$_5$ Step 10 Final Adjustments of the 3D Virtual Treatment Plan

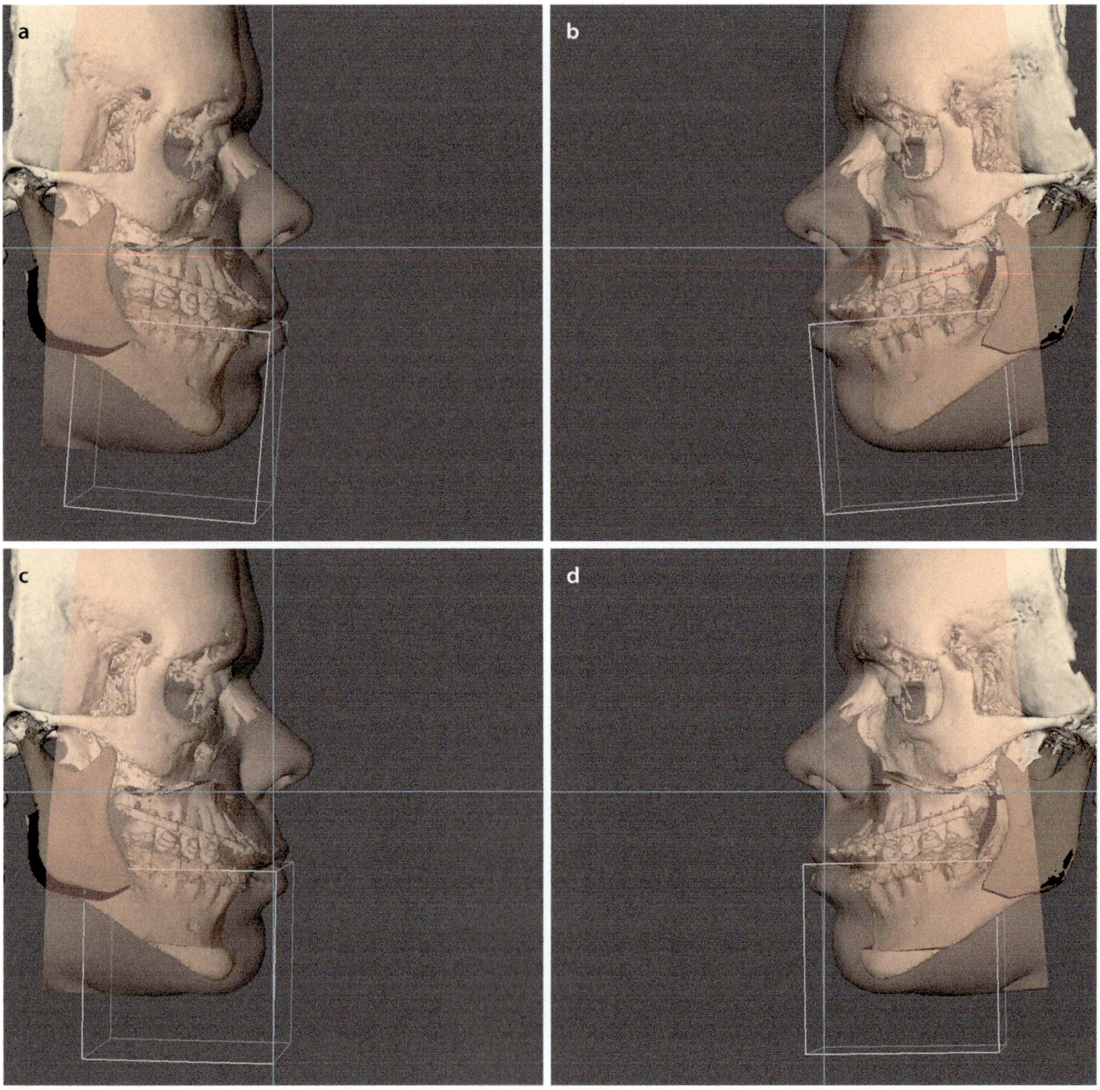

Fig. 6.217 Profile views before (**a**, **b**) and after (**c**, **d**) a virtual additional straight-line 4 mm sagittal chin advancement. In "step 10", it was decided after the final communication with patient D.B. not to perform final adjustments of the 3D virtual treatment plan anymore (3D "surface-rendered" representations, patient D.B., Maxilim v. 2.3.0.3)

Case 6: 3D-VPS$_5$- Final Integrated "Individualised 3D Virtual Treatment Plan"

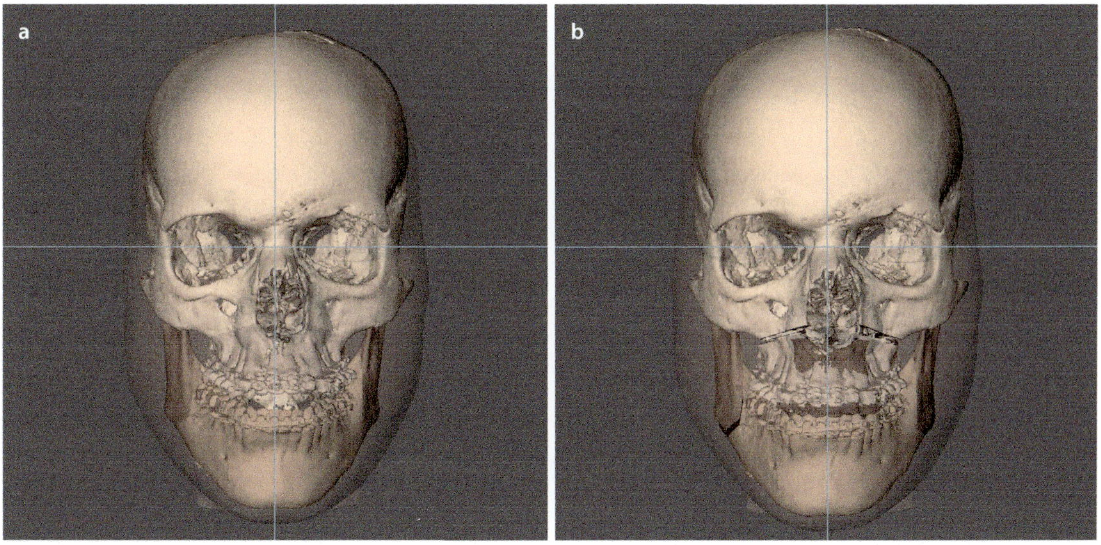

Fig. 6.218 Initial situation (**a**), and final "Individualised 3D Virtual Treatment Plan" (**b**), in the frontal plane (3D "surface-rendered" representations, patient D.B., Maxilim v. 2.3.0.3)

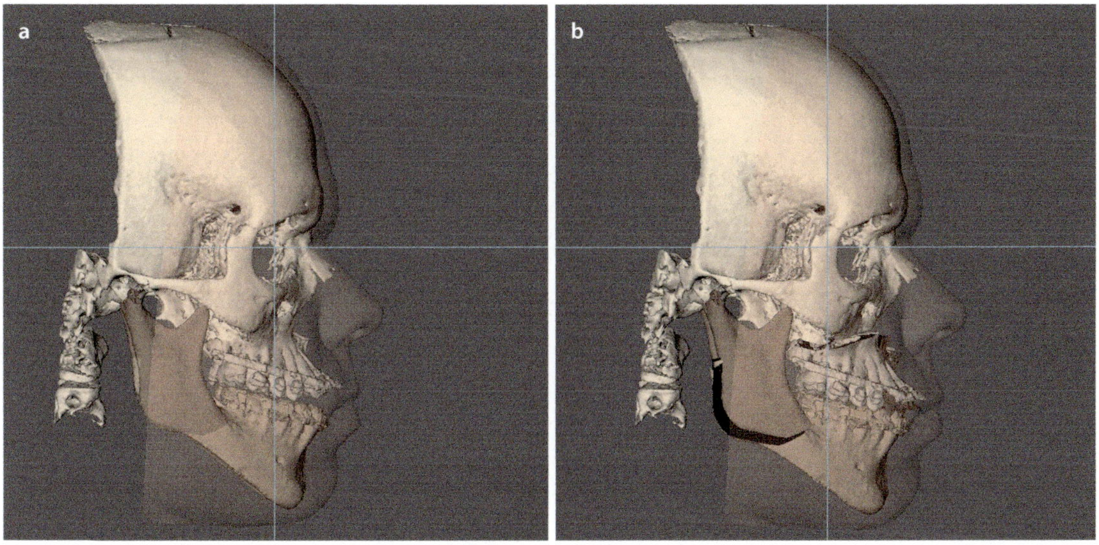

Fig. 6.219 Initial situation (**a**), and final "Individualised 3D Virtual Treatment Plan" (**b**), in the right profile plane (3D "surface-rendered" representations, patient D.B., Maxilim v. 2.3.0.3)

Case 6: 3D-VPS$_5$- Final Integrated "Individualised 3D Virtual Treatment Plan"

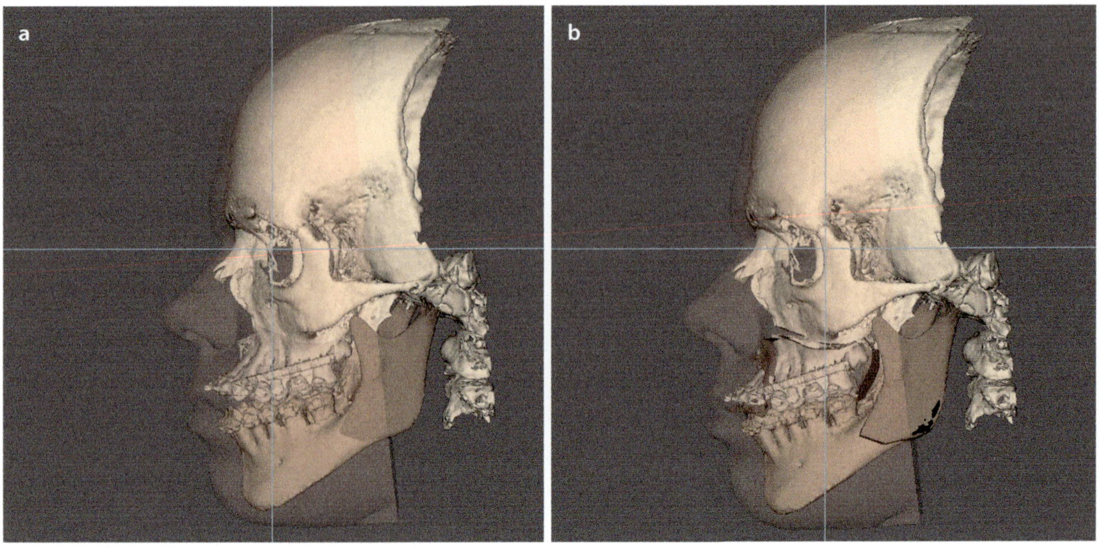

Fig. 6.220 Initial situation (**a**), and final "Individualised 3D Virtual Treatment Plan" (**b**), in the left profile plane (3D "surface-rendered" representations, patient D.B., Maxilim v. 2.3.0.3)

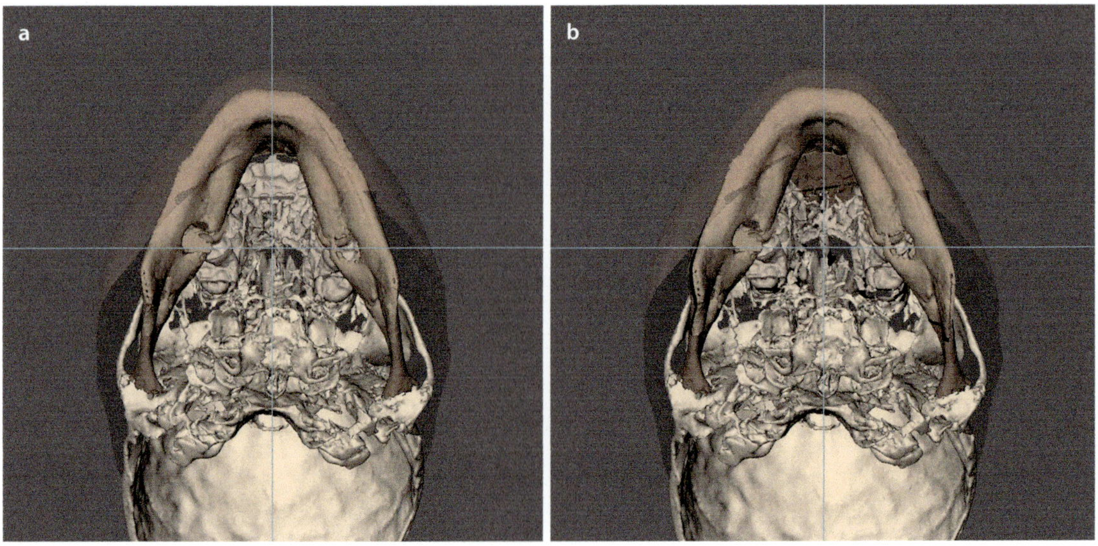

Fig. 6.221 Initial situation (**a**), and final "Individualised 3D Virtual Treatment Plan" (**b**), in the base plane (3D "surface-rendered" representations, patient D.B., Maxilim v. 2.3.0.3)

Case 6: "3D Virtual Treatment Planning, OR" Template

Maxillary osteotomy

- ■ Le Fort: ■I ☐II ☐III
- ☐ One-piece
- ■ Segmental:
  - Pieces: 2
  - Interdental: 13/14 - 23/24
- ■ Advancement: 0.0 mm
- ☐ Set-back :
- ■ Midline: 3.0 mm ■R ☐L
- ☐ Midline after Le Fort 1:
- ■ Vertical: (➔)
- ■ "Yaw" correction: CCW to the left
- ■ Other: CW "Pitch"

Mandibular osteotomy

- ■ SSO ■R ■L
- ☐ Inverted-L ☐R ☐L
- ☐ VRO ☐R ☐L
- ■ Advancement: R .... L 1 mm
- ■ Set-back: R 3 mm L ....
- ☐ CW "Pitch" rotation
- ☐ CCW "Pitch" rotation
- ☐ Midline split
- ■ IAN course: R lingual L center
- ■ Midline after BSSO: 2/3 mesial 11
- ☐ Other: lingual shortening of the distal fragment at the left side

Chin osteotomy

- ☐ Advancement:
- ☐ Set-back:
- ☐ Midline: ☐R ☐L
- ☐ Intrusion:
  - ☐ Anterior:
  - ☐ Posterior: R ...... L ......
- ☐ Extrusion:
  - ☐ Anterior:
  - ☐ Posterior: R ...... L ......
- ☐ "Shield" osteotomy
- ☐ "Chin wing" osteotomy
  - *Mental Foramen level:*
    - ☐ Symmetric
    - ☐ Asymmetric
- ☐ Other:

Planning Requirements

- ☐ Maxilla first
- ■ Mandible first
- ☐ Minimally Invasive Le Fort I
- ☐ IO-CBCT
- ☐ Kobayashi wires :
- ■ Skeletal anchorage : frontal
- ☐ Orthodontic buttons :
- ■ Occlusal grinding :
- ☐ Other :

3.5 mm	4.5 mm	10.0 mm	4.0 mm	3.0 mm
16	14	11	24	26

"Roll" correction: ☐ CW ■ CCW

Miscellaneous

- ■ Para-nasal cross sutures
- ☐ Alar cinch
- ■ Septoplasty
- ☐ Inferior turbinectomy
- ■ ANS: ☐Shortening ■ Midline
- ☐ Nasal base plasty ■R ■L
- ■ Lateral nasal wall plasty ■R ☐L
- ■ Bone graft(s): right mandibular bony gap
- ☐ Extraction(s):
- ☐ Other:

Adjuvant Cosmetic Procedures

- ☐ Bichatectomy ☐R ☐L
- ☐ Zygoma osteotomies ☐R ☐L
  - *Infraorbital Foramen level:*
    - ☐ Symmetric
    - ☐ Asymmetric
- ☐ Otoplasty: ☐R ☐L
- ☐ Rhinoplasty:
- ☐ Browlift:
- ☐ Blepharoplasty:
  - ☐Upper ☐Lower
- ☐ Facelift:
- ☐ Necklift:
- ☐ Liposuction:
- ☐ Lipofilling:
- ☐ Other:

Case 6: Class III, Anterior Open Bite (AOB)

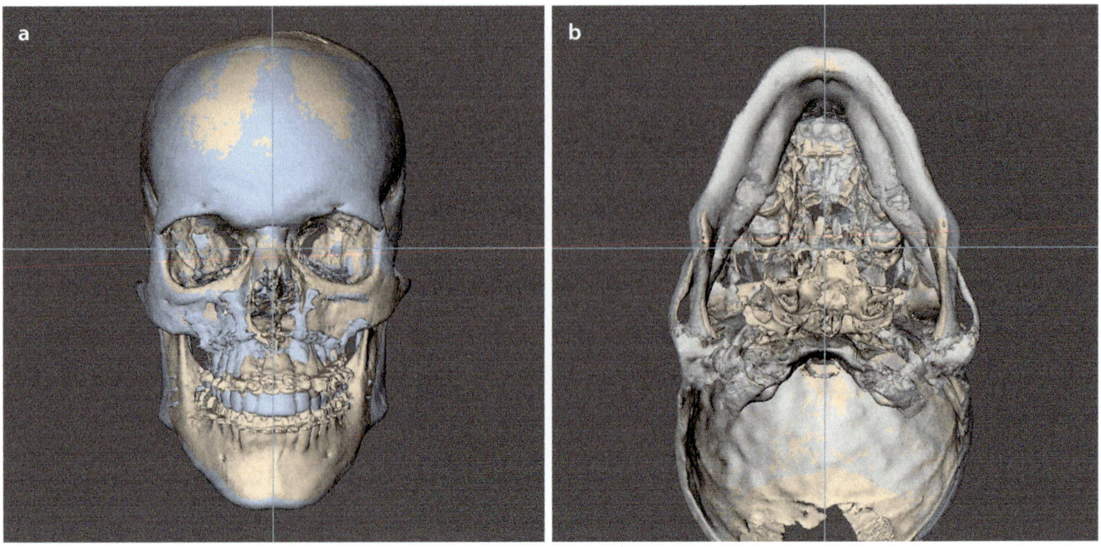

Fig. 6.222 Voxel-based superimposition on the cranial base of the pre-surgical and 10 months post-surgical (*blue*) 3D "surface-rendered" hard tissue representations. Frontal (**a**) and base (**b**) views (i-CAT, Imaging Sciences International Inc., Maxilim v. 2.3.0.3) (patient D.B.)

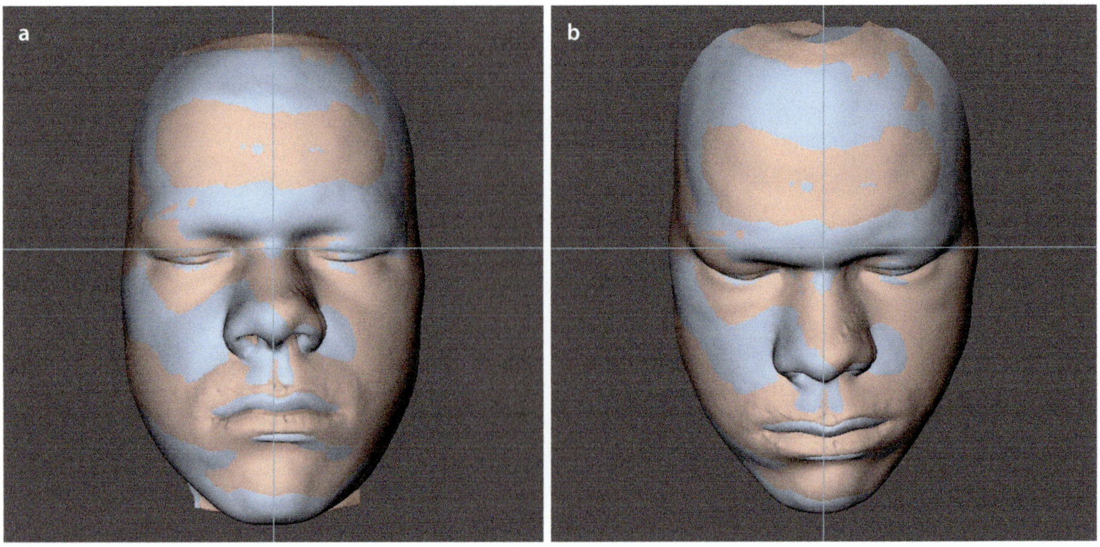

Fig. 6.223 Voxel-based superimposition on the cranial base of the pre-surgical and 10 months post-surgical (*blue*) 3D "surface-rendered" soft tissue representations. Frontal (**a**) and downward inclined (**b**) views (i-CAT, Imaging Sciences International Inc., Maxilim v. 2.3.0.3) (patient D.B.). Note the correction of the nasal tip to the right and the correction of the left nostril which came downward and was corrected to the right. Also note that although the upper dental midline was post-surgically centred (Fig. 6.222a), the philtrum is still deviated to the left which is myofunctionally related

Case 6: Class III, Anterior Open Bite (AOB)

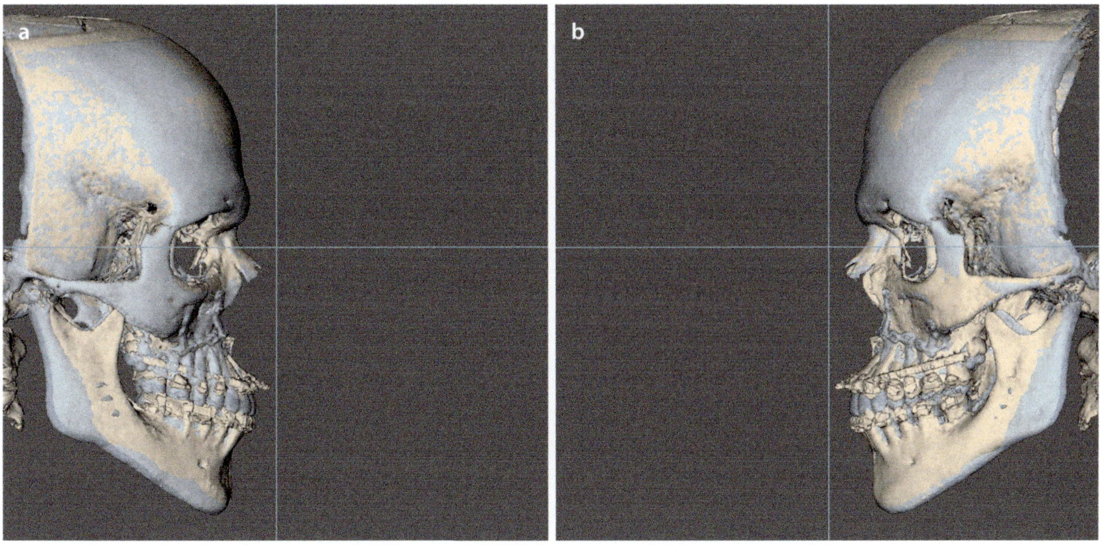

Fig. 6.224 Voxel-based superimposition on the cranial base of the pre-surgical and 10 months post-surgical (*blue*) 3D "surface-rendered" hard tissue representations. Right (**a**) and left profile (**b**) views (i-CAT, Imaging Sciences International Inc., Maxilim v. 2.3.0.3) (patient D.B.). Note the AOB closure

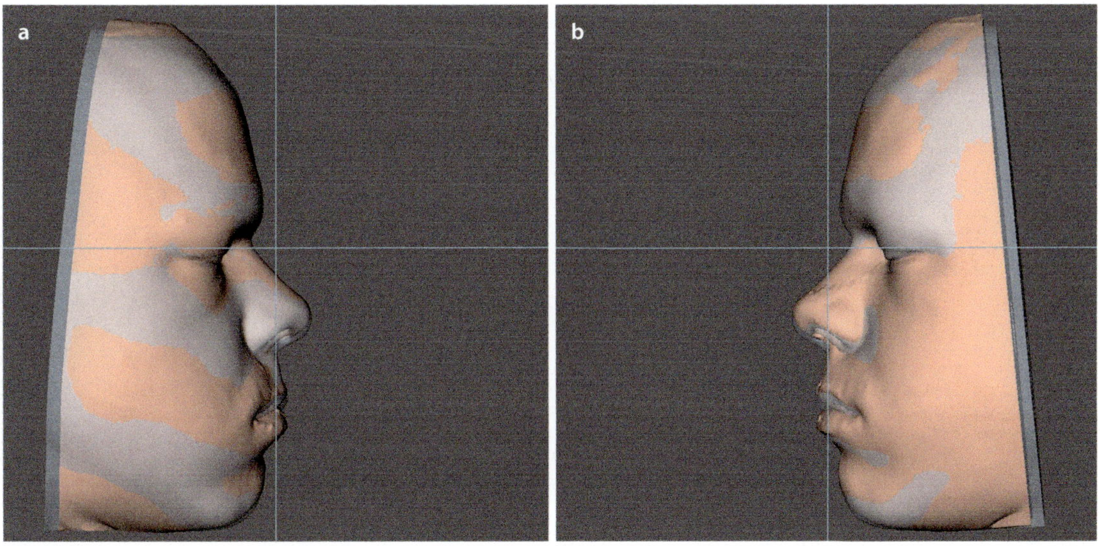

Fig. 6.225 Voxel-based superimposition on the cranial base of the pre-surgical and 10 months post-surgical (*blue*) 3D "surface-rendered" soft tissue representations. Right (**a**) and left profile (**b**) views (i-CAT, Imaging Sciences International Inc., Maxilim v. 2.3.0.3) (patient D.B.). Note that the entire nasolabial aesthetic unit came downwards during AOB closure by the anterior segmental osteotomy

■ Case 6: Class III, Anterior Open Bite (AOB), Clinical Treatment Outcome

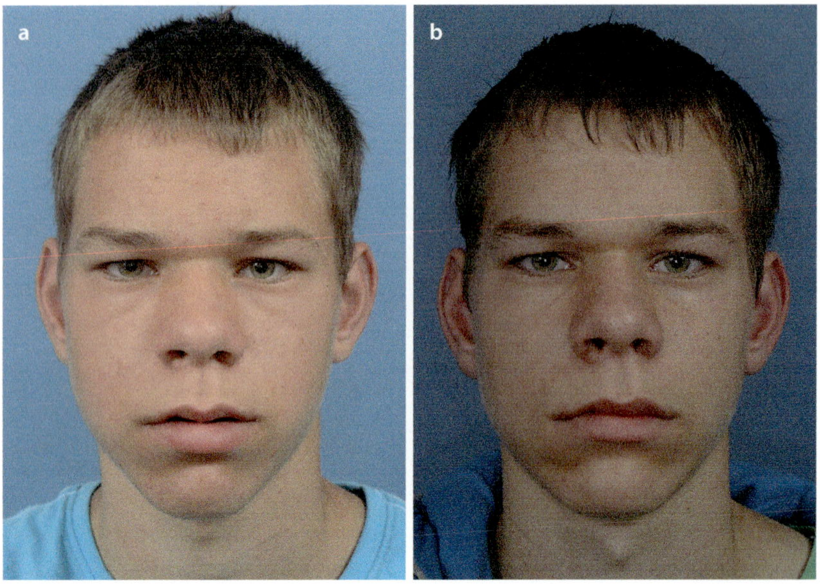

Fig. 6.226 Frontal views in rest, pre-surgical (**a**) and 6 months after (**b**) combined orthodontic-surgical treatment (patient D.B.)

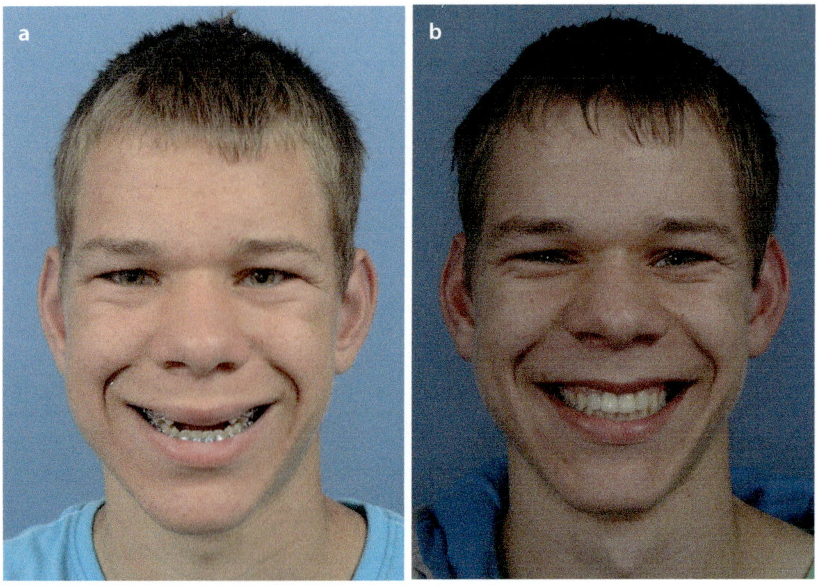

Fig. 6.227 Frontal views during smiling, pre-surgical (**a**) and 6 months after (**b**) combined orthodontic-surgical treatment (patient D.B.)

Case 6: Class III, Anterior Open Bite (AOB), Clinical Treatment Outcome

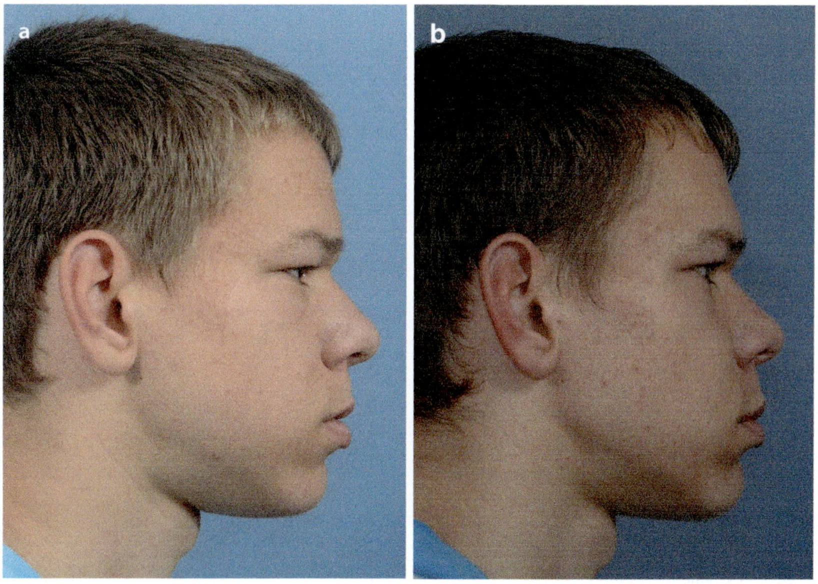

Fig. 6.228 Right profile views in rest, pre-surgical (**a**) and 6 months after (**b**) combined orthodontic-surgical treatment (patient D.B.)

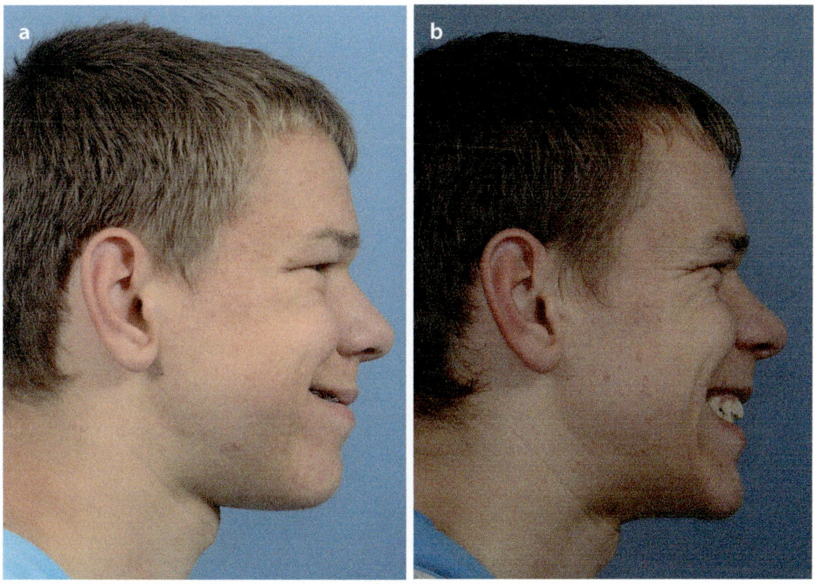

Fig. 6.229 Right profile views during smiling, pre-surgical (**a**) and 6 months after (**b**) combined orthodontic-surgical treatment (patient D.B.)

Case 6: Class III, Anterior Open Bite (AOB), Clinical Treatment Outcome

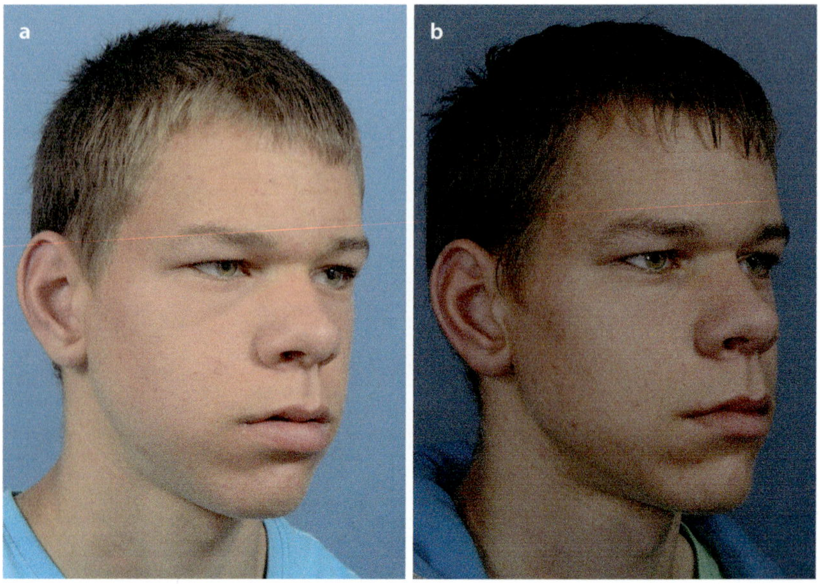

Fig. 6.230 2/3 right profile views in rest, pre-surgical (**a**) and 6 months after (**b**) combined orthodontic-surgical treatment (patient D.B.)

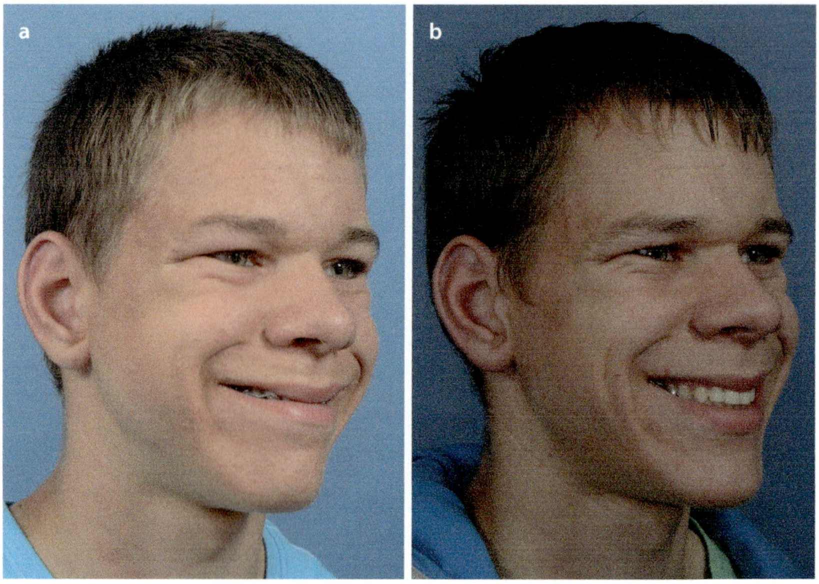

Fig. 6.231 2/3 right profile views during smiling, pre-surgical (**a**) and 6 months after (**b**) combined orthodontic-surgical treatment (patient D.B.)

Case 6: Class III, Anterior Open Bite (AOB), Clinical Treatment Outcome

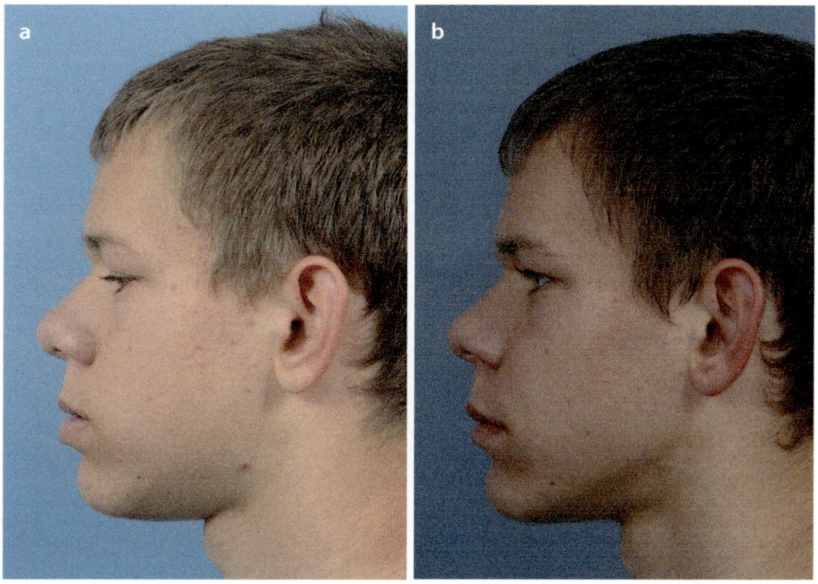

Fig. 6.232 Left profile views in rest, pre-surgical (**a**) and 6 months after (**b**) combined orthodontic-surgical treatment (patient D.B.)

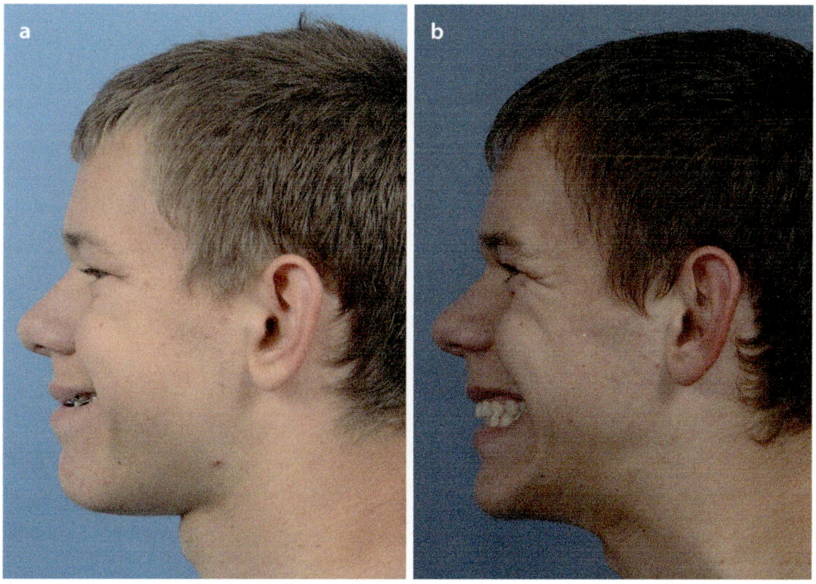

Fig. 6.233 Left profile views during smiling, pre-surgical (**a**) and 6 months after (**b**) combined orthodontic-surgical treatment (patient D.B.)

Case 6: Class III, Anterior Open Bite (AOB), Clinical Treatment Outcome

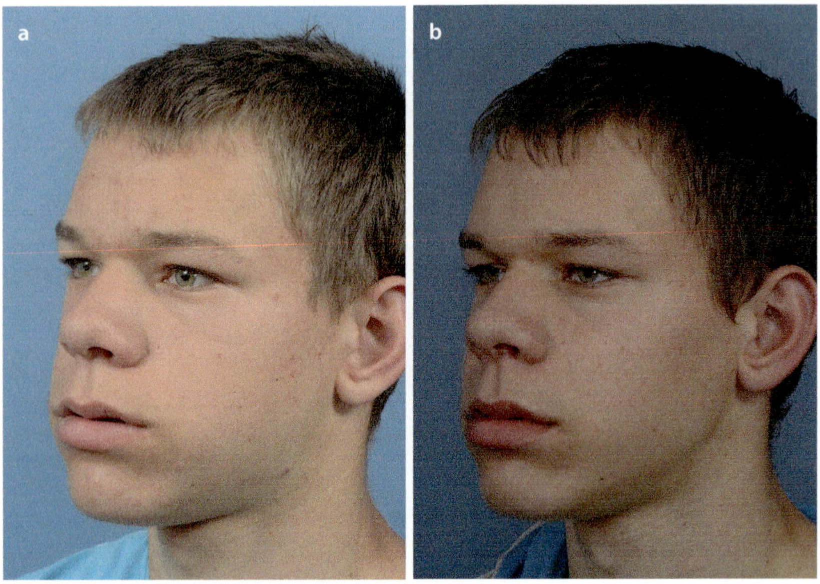

Fig. 6.234 2/3 left profile views in rest, pre-surgical (**a**) and 6 months after (**b**) combined orthodontic-surgical treatment (patient D.B.)

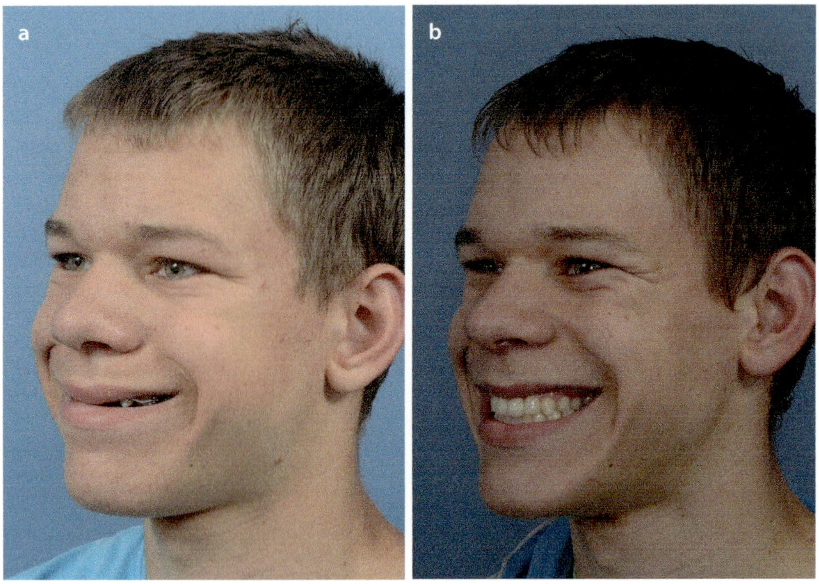

Fig. 6.235 2/3 left profile views during smiling, pre-surgical (**a**) and 6 months after (**b**) combined orthodontic-surgical treatment (patient D.B.)

Case 6: Class III, Anterior Open Bite (AOB), Clinical Treatment Outcome

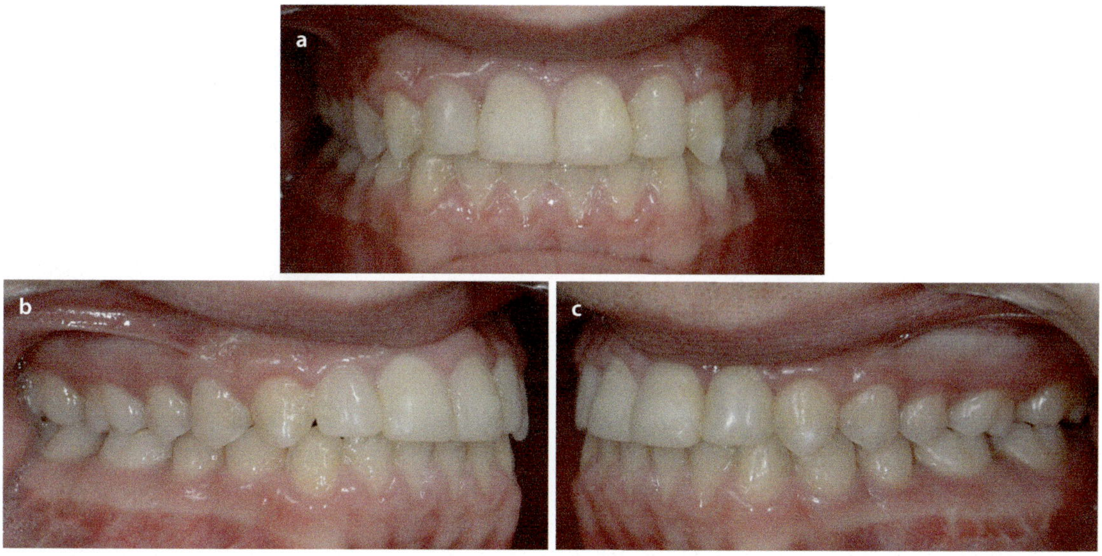

Fig. 6.236 Frontal (**a**), right (**b**) and left (**c**) intra-oral views of the patient's occlusion 6 months after combined orthodontic-surgical treatment (patient D.B.). The author acknowledges Bavo Verhoeven and Prof. Guy De Pauw for the orthodontic treatment

▪ Case 7: Hemimandibular Hyperplasia (HH)

Patient A.A. is a 24-year-old male with a short-face and mandibular asymmetry due to hemimandibular hyperplasia (HH). A bone scintigraphy was performed and did not show any active condylar growth. In the frontal view, he is clinically presenting with a mandibular asymmetry with right mandibular hyperplasia. In rest, he has no incisal display, while during spontaneous smiling, he only has 7 mm incisal exposure with an incisal crown length of 10 mm. Moreover, he presents with asymmetric ears having a prominent left ear with a poorly developed antihelical fold and right conchal cartilage hypertrophy. In the profile view, he presents with a Class II profile with a prominent chin. He has an Angle Class II malocclusion with adequate transversal relationship and a 1 mm upper dental midline deviation to the right. There is no history of TMJ dysfunction neither pain.

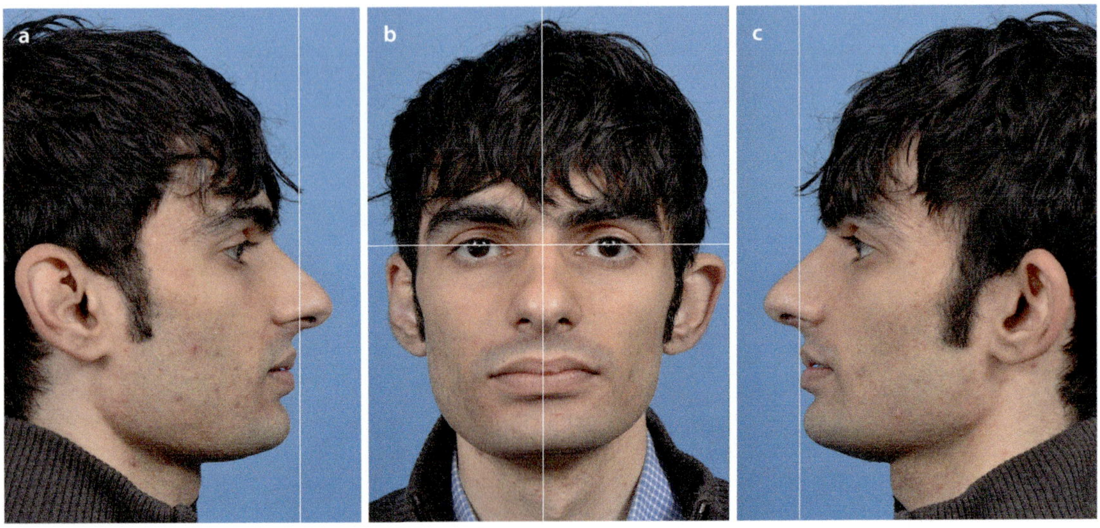

Fig. 6.237 Pre-surgical clinical right profile (**a**), frontal (**b**) and left profile (**c**) views of patient A.A. in its *c*-NHP in rest, at the time of the workup, approximately 3 weeks prior to surgery (patient A.A.). Note the right mandibular border asymmetry due to HH

Case 7: Hemimandibular Hyperplasia (HH)

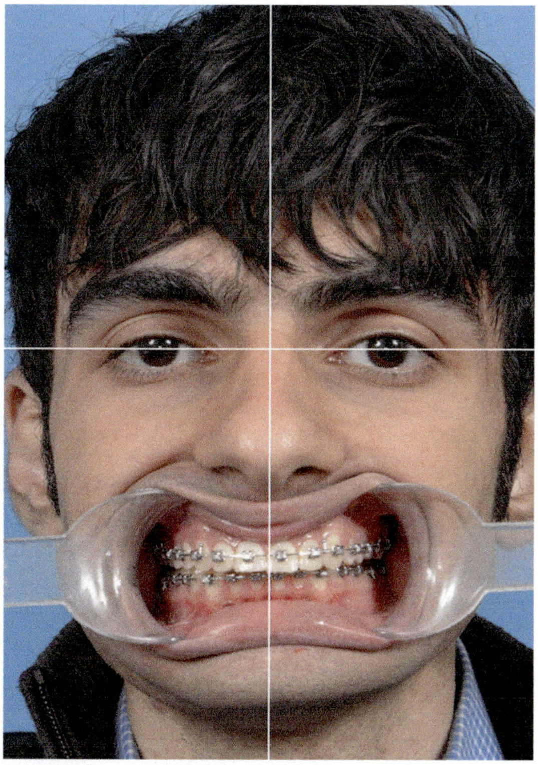

Fig. 6.238 Pre-surgical clinical frontal view of patient A.A. with cheek retractors at the time of the workup, approximately 3 weeks prior to surgery. Note that there is clinically a discrete cant of the maxilla

Case 7: Hemimandibular Hyperplasia (HH), v-NHP and PHP

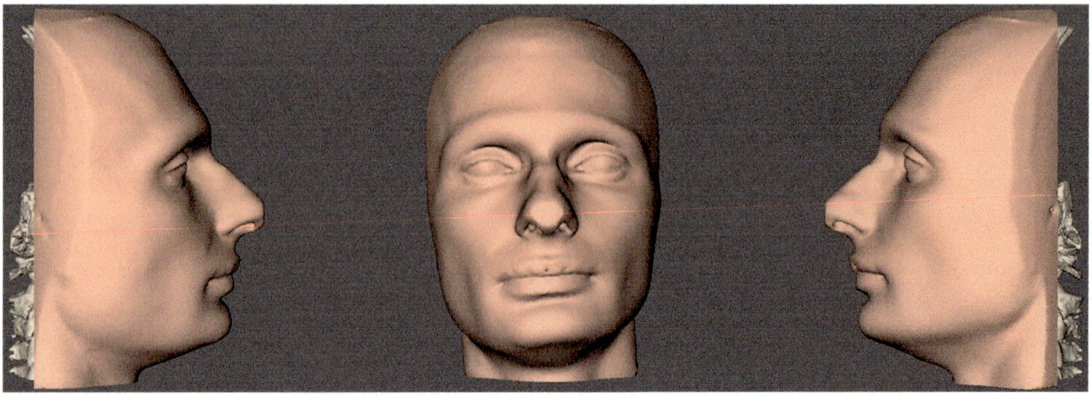

Fig. 6.239 Pre-surgical 3D "surface-rendered" right profile, frontal and left profile soft and hard tissue representations of the head of patient A.A., as generated during standardised CBCT image acquisition, at the time of the workup (Maxilim v. 2.3.0.3). Note the incorrect position and orientation of the virtual head compared to the clinical pictures of patient A.A. (Fig. 6.237), although it was attempted to scan patient A.A. in his correct *c*-NHP in rest

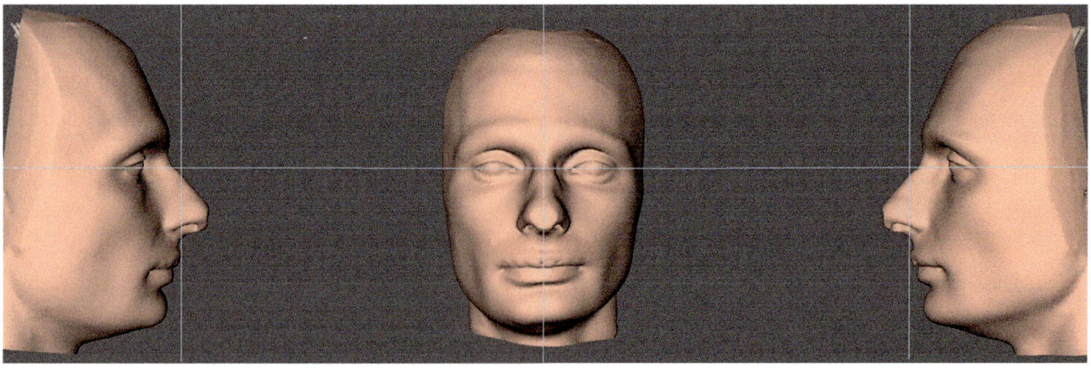

Fig. 6.240 Following a standardised "step-by-step" approach (▶ see Sect. 3.1), the scanned head position of patient A.A. (Fig. 6.239) was virtually modified towards his *c*-NHP (Fig. 6.237), which results in his *v*-NHP and corresponds to his individual "Planning Head Position (PHP)" (3D "surface-rendered" representations, Maxilim v. 2.3.0.3)

Case 7: Hemimandibular Hyperplasia (HH)

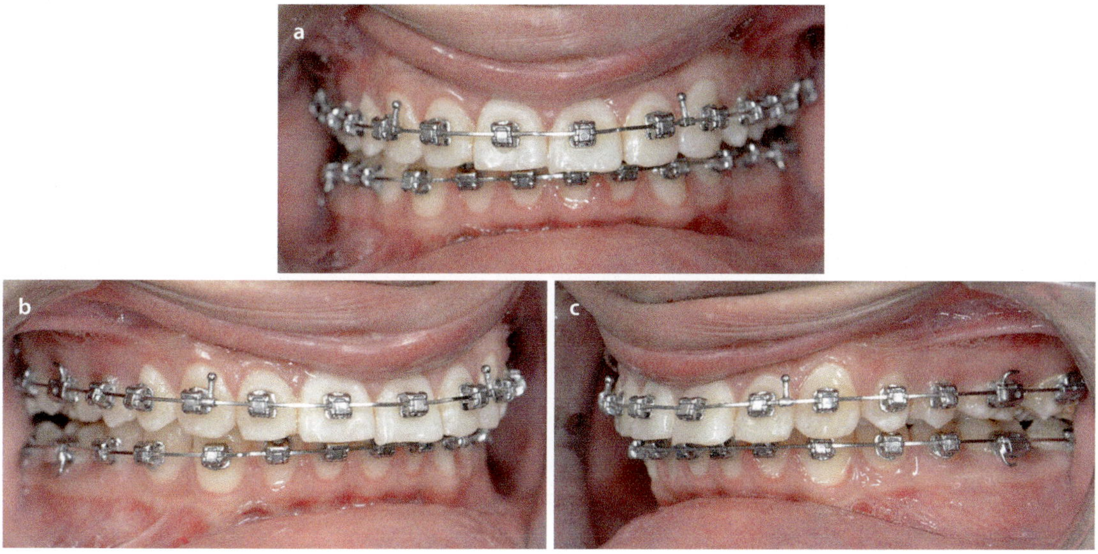

Fig. 6.241 Pre-surgical frontal (**a**), right (**b**) and left (**c**) intra-oral views of the occlusion of patient A.A. at the time of the workup, approximately 3 weeks prior to surgery

▪ Case 7: 3D-VPS$_5$ Step 1 Maxillary Occlusal Cant Evaluation/Correction ("Roll")

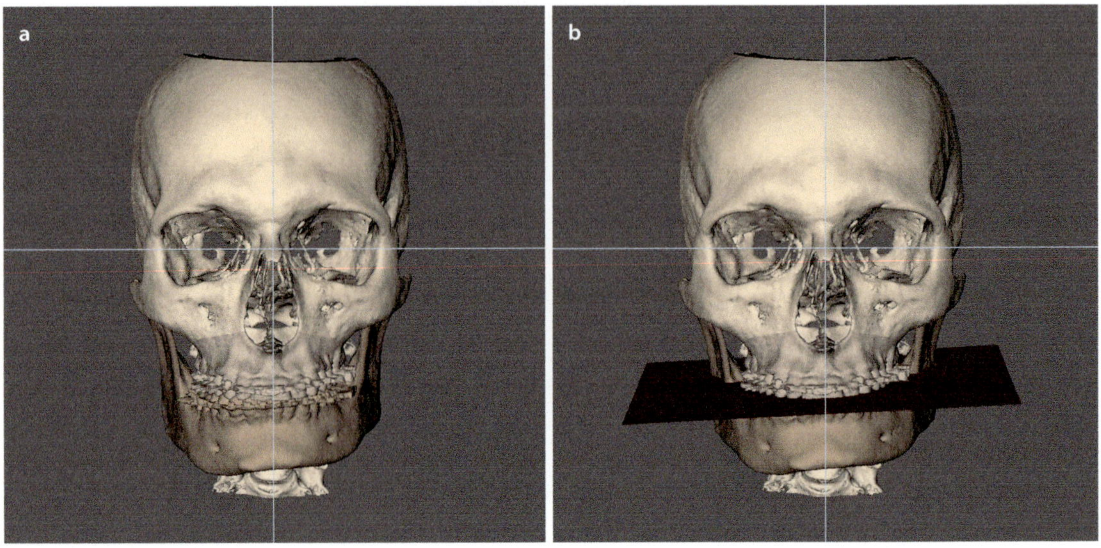

Fig. 6.242 The maxillary occlusal plane is evaluated both clinically (Fig. 6.238) and virtually (**a**) towards the horizontal 3D PHP reference plane in patient A.A. and shows virtually an important cant (**b**) (3D "surface-rendered" representations, Maxilim v. 2.3.0.3). Note that this maxillary cant is clinically (Fig. 6.238) less obvious

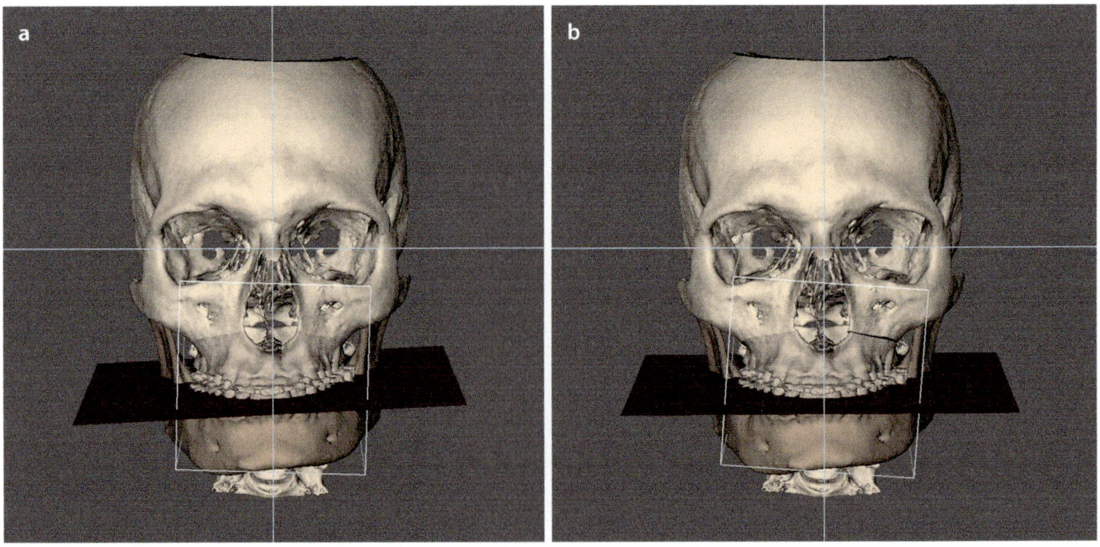

Fig. 6.243 The maxillary cant (**a**) in patient A.A. is corrected towards the horizontal 3D PHP reference plane by a CW "Roll" rotational movement (**b**) (3D "surface-rendered" representations, Maxilim v. 2.3.0.3)

▪ Case 7: 3D-VPS$_5$ Step 2 Upper Dental Midline Evaluation/Correction

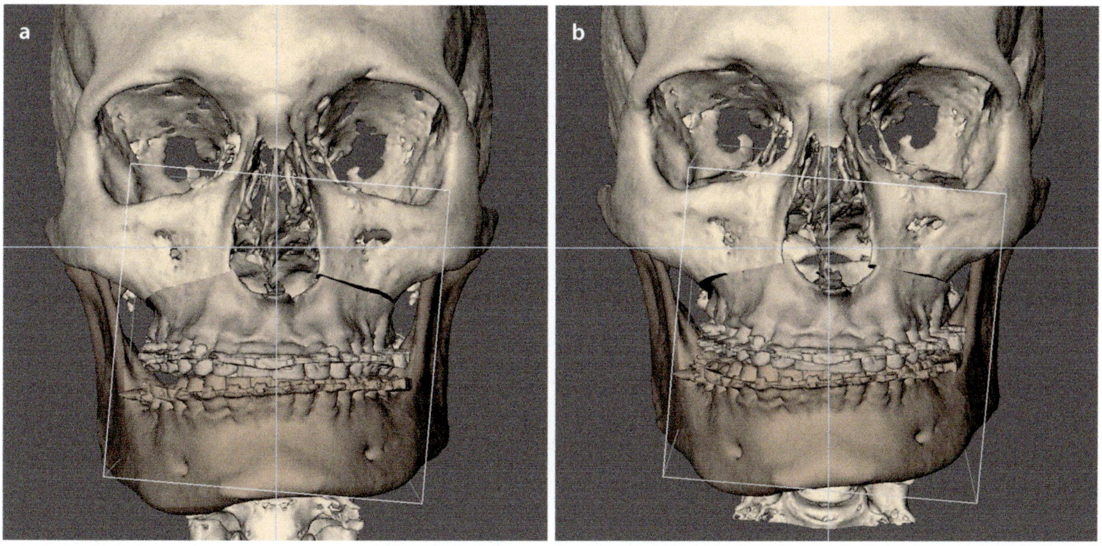

Fig. 6.244 The 1 mm deviation of the upper dental midline to the right (**a**) is corrected towards the facial midline 3D PHP reference plane, by a pure translational movement to the left in patient A.A. (**b**) (3D "surface-rendered" representations, Maxilim v. 2.3.0.3)

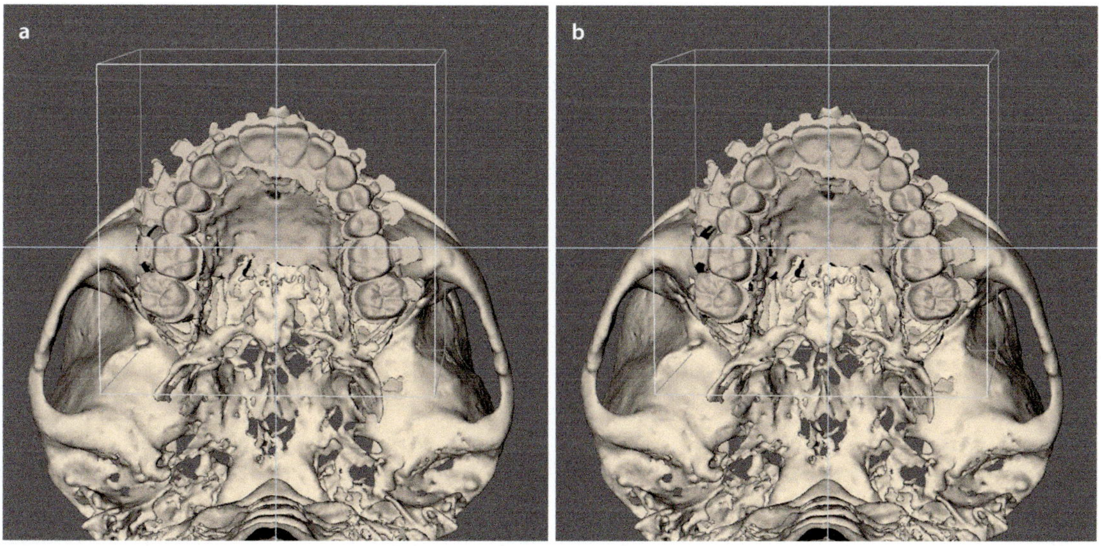

Fig. 6.245 The base views illustrate that the 1 mm deviation of the upper dental midline to the right (**a**) is corrected towards the facial midline 3D PHP reference plane, by a pure translational movement to the left (**b**) in patient A.A. (3D "surface-rendered" representations, Maxilim v. 2.3.0.3)

▪ Case 7: 3D-VPS$_5$ Step 3 Overall Evaluation of Facial Asymmetry After Virtual Occlusal Definition

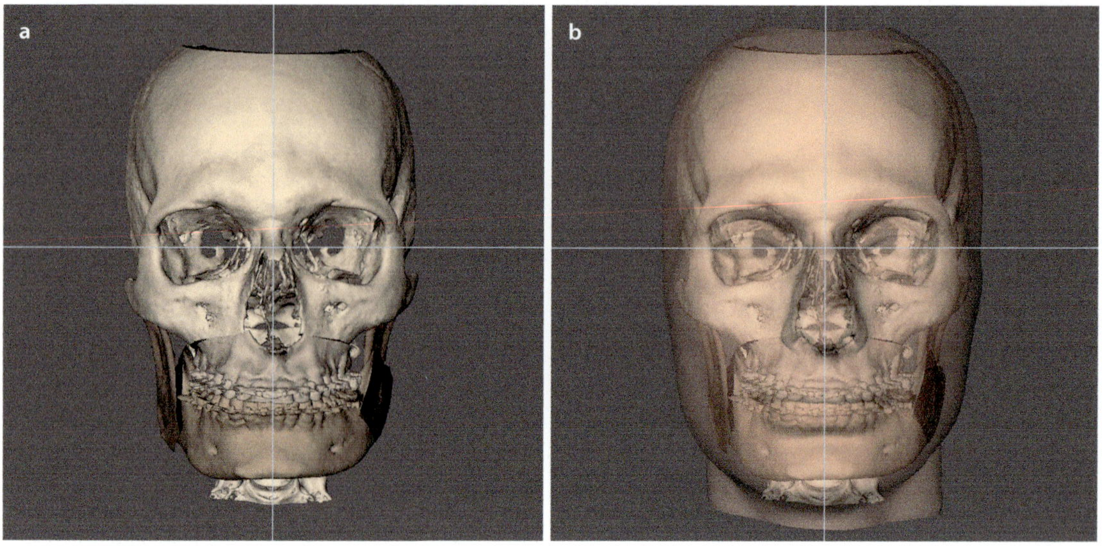

Fig. 6.246 Overall facial asymmetry of the head of patient A.A. (**a**) with transparent soft tissues (**b**) is assessed after virtual occlusal definition in the frontal view towards both the horizontal and facial midline 3D PHP reference planes (3D "surface-rendered" representations, Maxilim v. 2.3.0.3). Note the important flaring of the mandibular body to the left

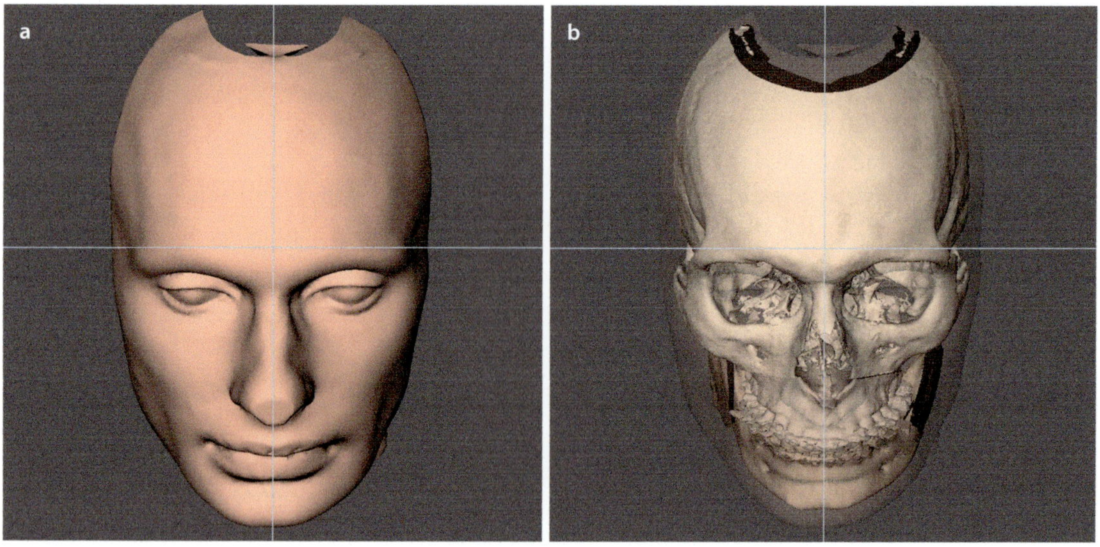

Fig. 6.247 To evaluate the overall facial asymmetry after virtual occlusal definition, the mandibular contour is evaluated both virtually on the soft tissues (**a**) and at the bony level towards the contour of the zygomatic bones and arches with soft tissues in transparency (**b**) (3D "surface-rendered" representations, patient D.C.M., Maxilim v. 2.3.0.3). Note the flaring of the mandibular body (**b**) to the left

Case 7: 3D-VPS$_5$ Step 4 Evaluation/Correction of Flaring ("Yaw")

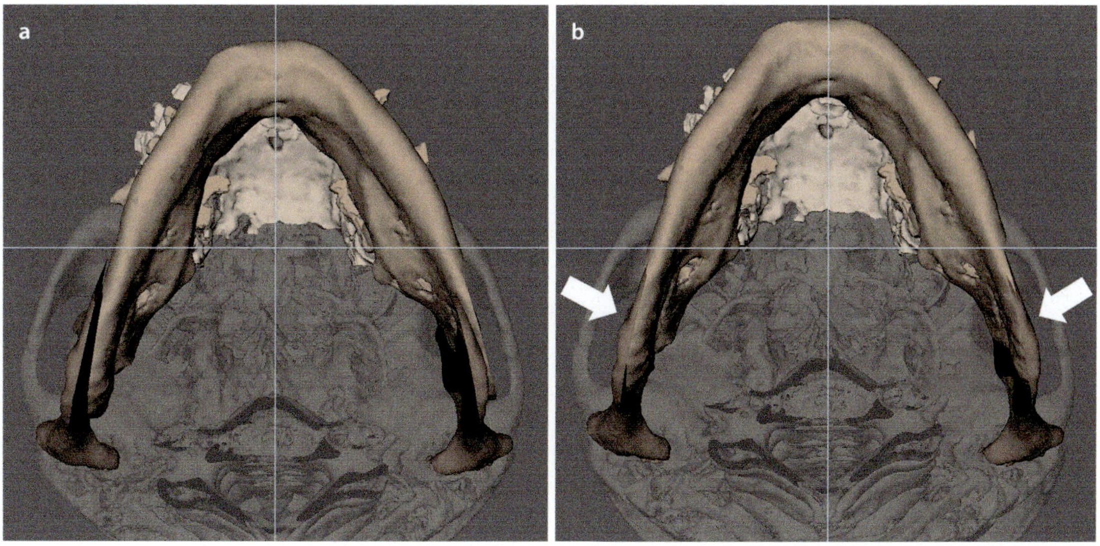

Fig. 6.248 The base views show that the flaring of the mandibular body to the left (**a**) is corrected by a CW "Yaw" rotational movement to the right (**b**) in patient A.A. (3D "surface-rendered" representations, patient A.A., Maxilim v. 2.3.0.3). Note the discrete virtual bony overlap between the distal and proximal mandibular fragments at the left side

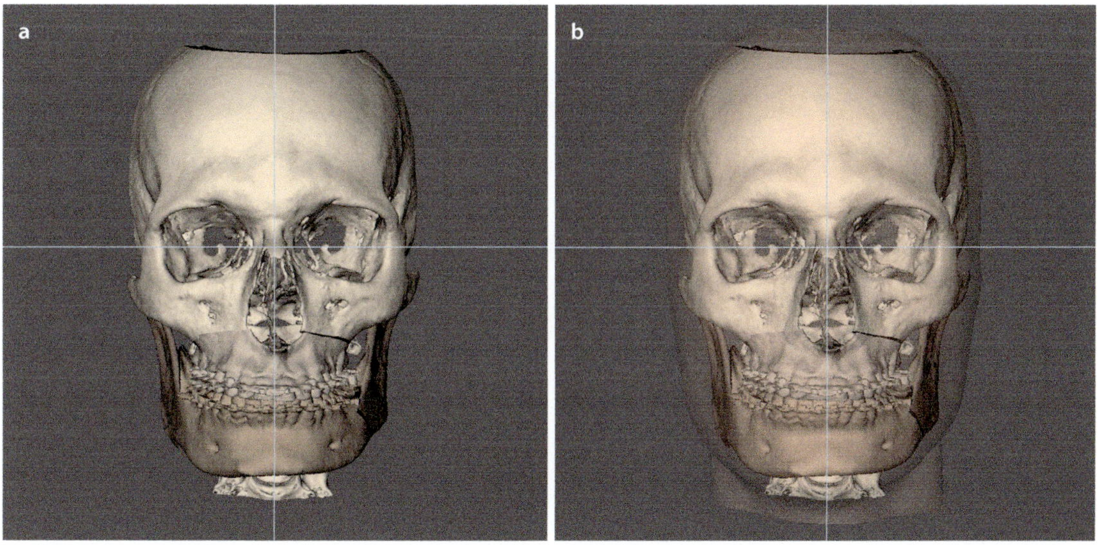

Fig. 6.249 Overall assessment of facial bony contour (**a**) with transparent soft tissues (**b**) after correction of flaring to the left by a "Yaw" rotational movement of the maxillo-mandibular complex to the right (3D "surface-rendered" representations, patient A.A., Maxilim v. 2.3.0.3)

Case 7: 3D-VPS$_5$ Step 5 Upper Vertical Incisal Position Evaluation/Correction

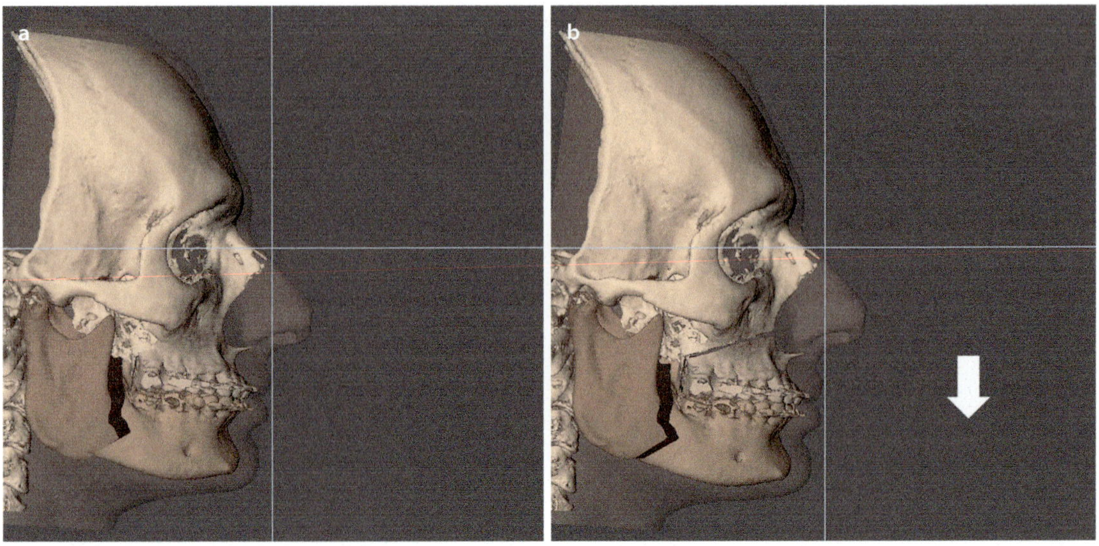

Fig. 6.250 Since patient A.A. has in rest only 1 mm and during spontaneous smiling only 7 mm incisal exposure with an incisal crown length of 10 mm, it was decided clinically at this stage to already virtually extrude the maxilla 2 mm at the upper incisal level (3D "surface-rendered" representations, Maxilim v. 2.3.0.3): before (**a**) and after (**b**) correction

Case 7: 3D-VPS$_5$ Step 6 Sagittal Upper Incisal Position Evaluation/Correction

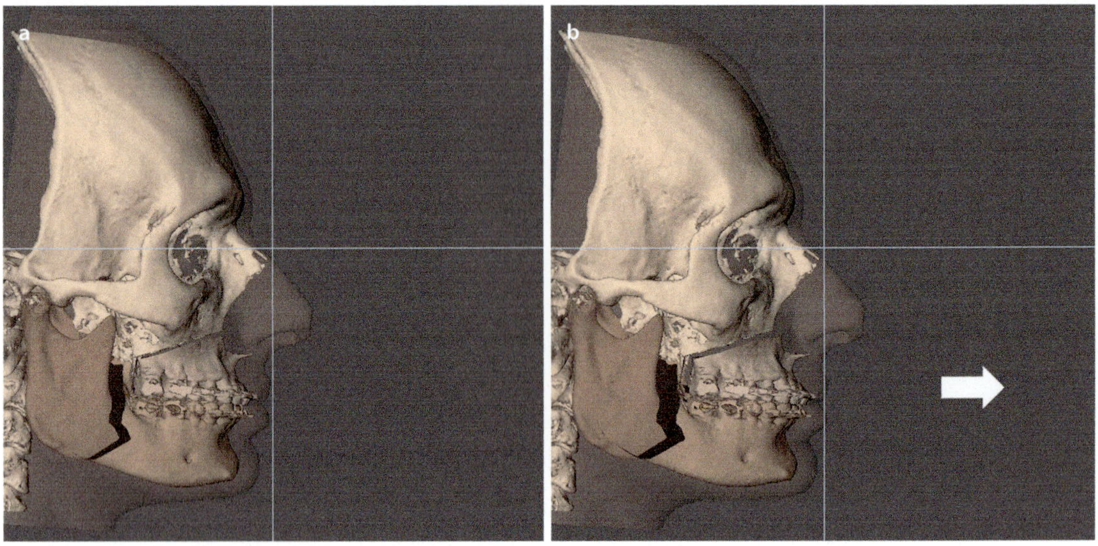

Fig. 6.251 From especially clinical examination but also 3D cephalometric analysis (**a**), it was decided to advance the "maxillo-mandibular complex in final occlusion" 3 mm at the upper incisal level (**b**) (3D "surface-rendered" representations, patient A.A., Maxilim v. 2.3.0.3). Note that it is clinically judged that this will lead to an additional 1 mm incisal exposure resulting in 4 mm incisal exposure in rest and full incisal exposure during spontaneous smiling

Case 7: 3D-VPS$_5$ Step 7 Profile Evaluation/Occlusal Plane Correction ("Pitch")

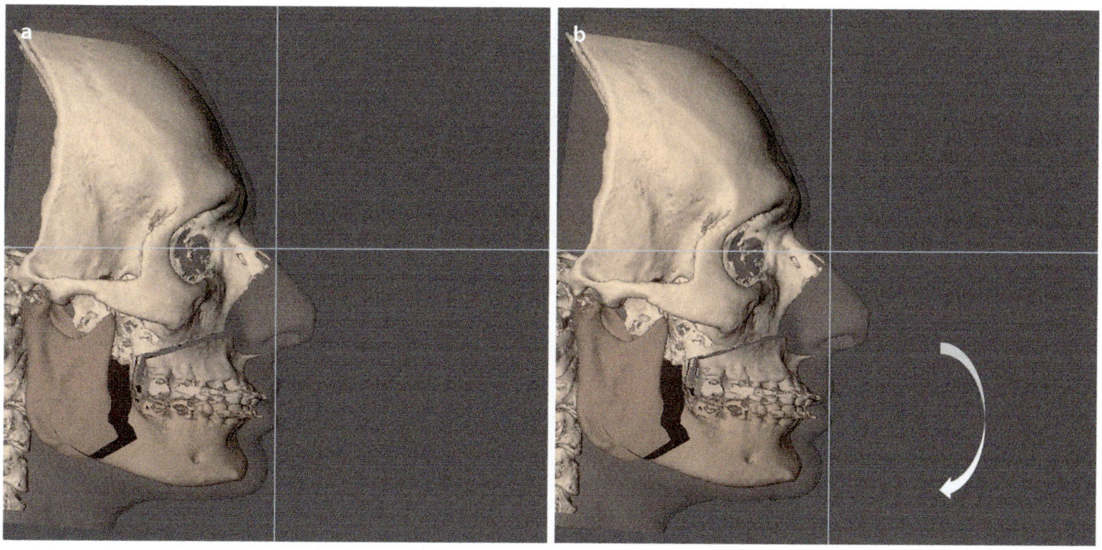

Fig. 6.252 At this stage in "step 7", the profile and dento-alveolar support of the upper lip are evaluated in patient A.A. It was decided to perform a 1.5° CW occlusal plane rotation with the centre of rotation at the incisal level by a "Pitch" rotational movement, which results in a differential extrusion of 0.5 mm and 2.0 mm at the right and left first molars, respectively (3D "surface-rendered" representations, Maxilim v. 2.3.0.3): before (**a**) and after (**b**) correction

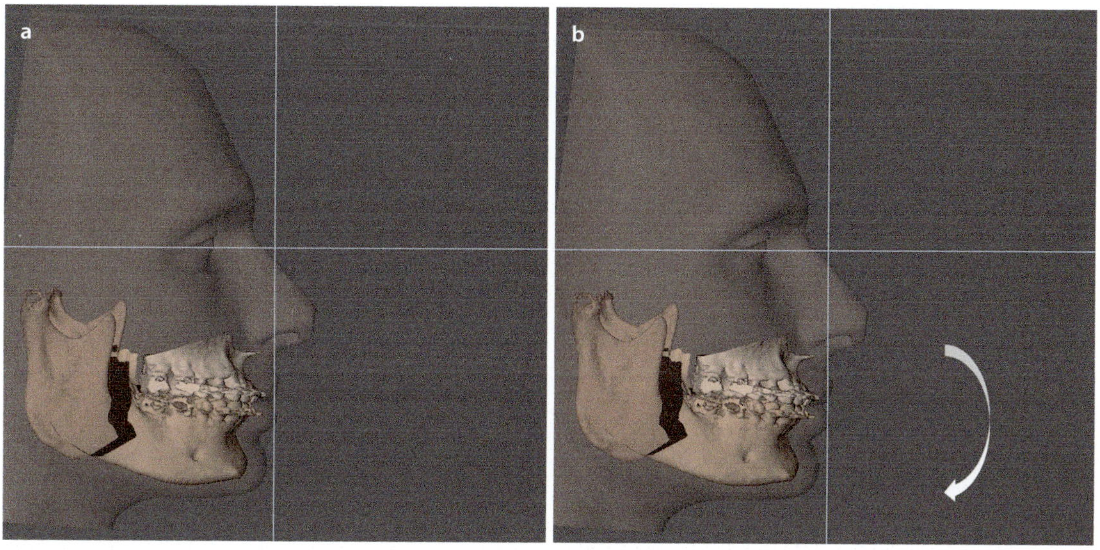

Fig. 6.253 At this stage in "step 7", the profile and dento-alveolar support of the upper lip are evaluated in patient A.A. It was decided to perform a 1.5° CW occlusal plane rotation with the centre of rotation at the incisal level by a "Pitch" rotational movement, which results in a differential extrusion of 0.5 and 2.0 mm at the right and left first molars, respectively (3D "surface-rendered" representations of the bimaxillary complex with transparent soft tissues, Maxilim v. 2.3.0.3): before (**a**) and after (**b**) correction

■ Case 7: 3D-VPS$_5$ Step 8 3D Chin Position Evaluation/Correction

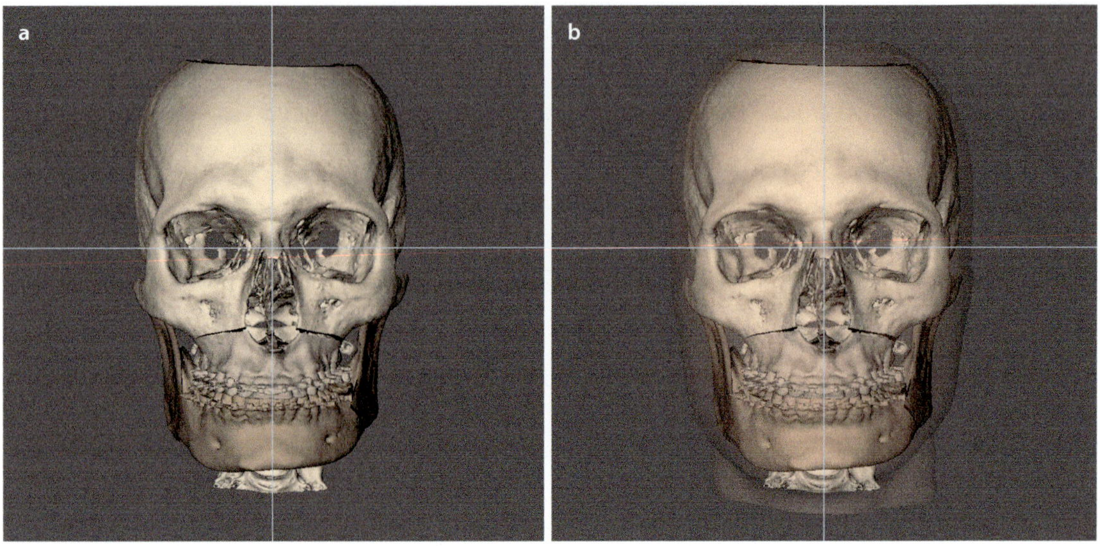

Fig. 6.254 Evaluation of the bony chin in the frontal plane without (**a**) and with (**b**) the patient's 3D facial soft tissue mask in transparency (3D "surface-rendered" representations, Maxilim v. 2.3.0.3). Note that the bony chin is centred to the median 3D PHP reference plane but is asymmetric due to the right HH in patient A.A.

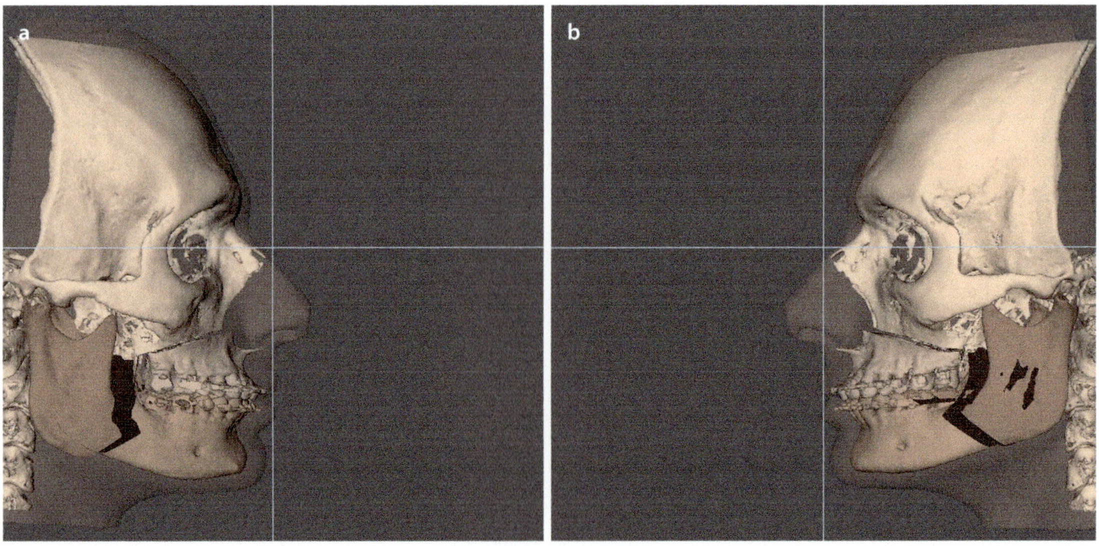

Fig. 6.255 Evaluation of the sagittal chin position in the right (**a**) and left profile (**b**) views needs to be individually assessed (3D "surface-rendered" representations, Maxilim v. 2.3.0.3). Note the adequate profile chin position with a well-defined plica labio-mentalis and mento-cervical angle in patient A.A.

Case 7: 3D-VPS$_5$ Step 9 Patient Communication of the Individualised Treatment Plan

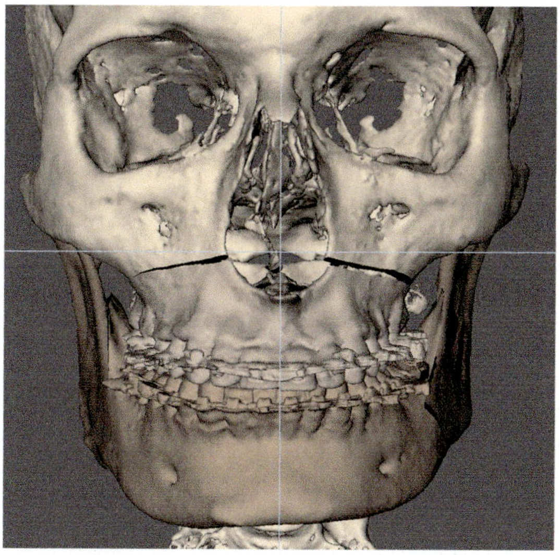

Fig. 6.256 In "step 9", the "Individualised 3D Virtual Treatment Plan" is discussed with the patient (3D "surface-rendered" representations, Maxilim v. 2.3.0.3). The persistent asymmetry of the right mandibular lower border, chin and gonial angle due to the right HH is explained to patient A.A.

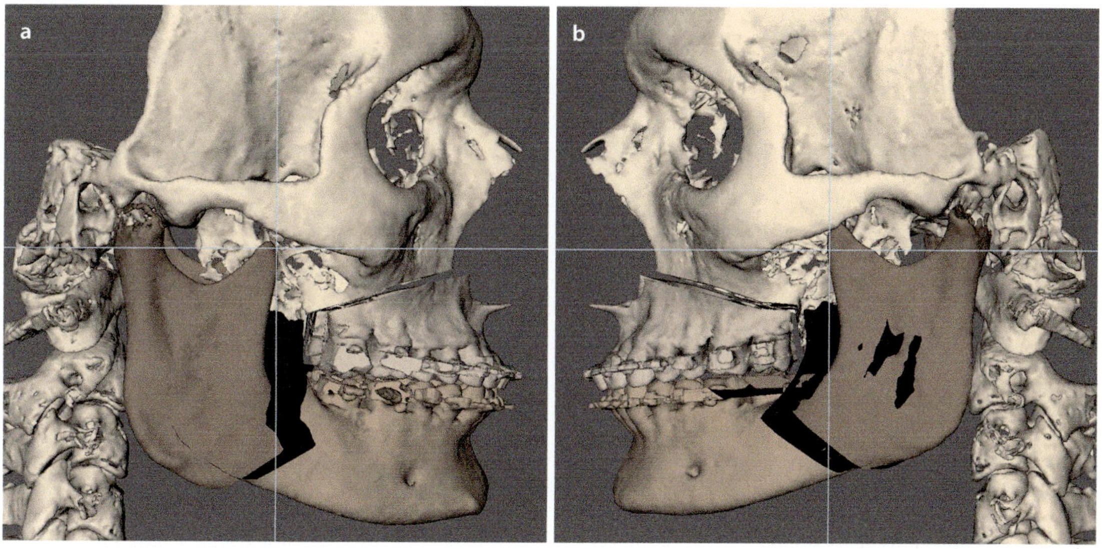

Fig. 6.257 In "step 9", the right (**a**) and left (**b**) bony profiles of the "Individualised 3D Virtual Treatment Plan" are discussed with the patient (3D "surface-rendered" representations, Maxilim v. 2.3.0.3). The persistent asymmetry of the right mandibular lower border, chin and gonial angle due to the right HH is explained to patient A.A.

▪ Case 7: 3D-VPS$_5$ Step 10 Final Adjustments of the 3D Virtual Treatment Plan

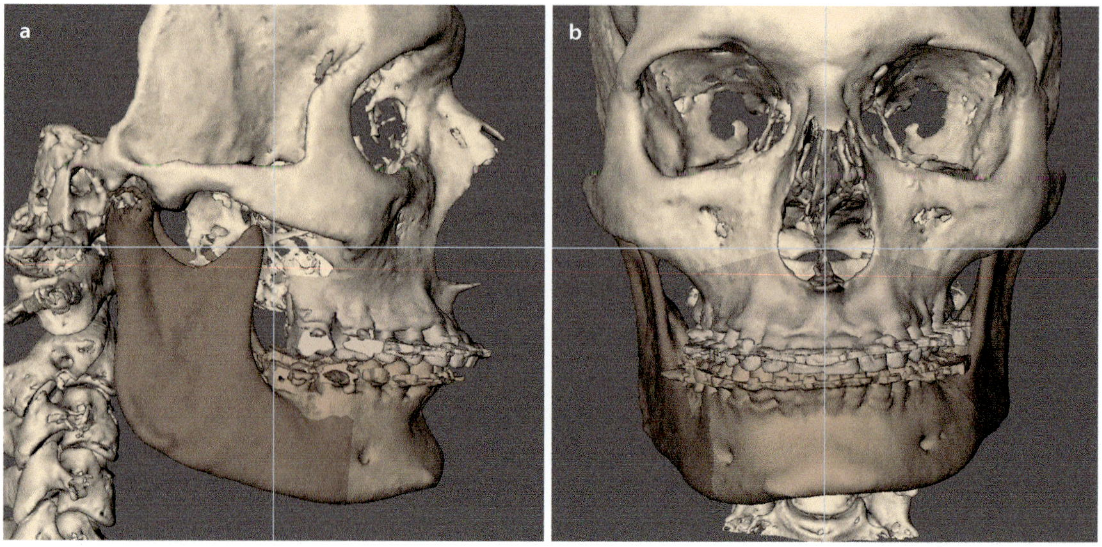

Fig. 6.258 Final adjustments of the "Individualised 3D Virtual Treatment Plan". It was decided to perform an extended right sagittal split osteotomy with the buccal corticotomy positioned just behind the right foramen mentale to facilitate a "safe" resection of the right mandibular lower border in patient A.A. (3D "surface-rendered" representations, Maxilim v. 2.3.0.3). Right profile (**a**) and frontal (**b**) views

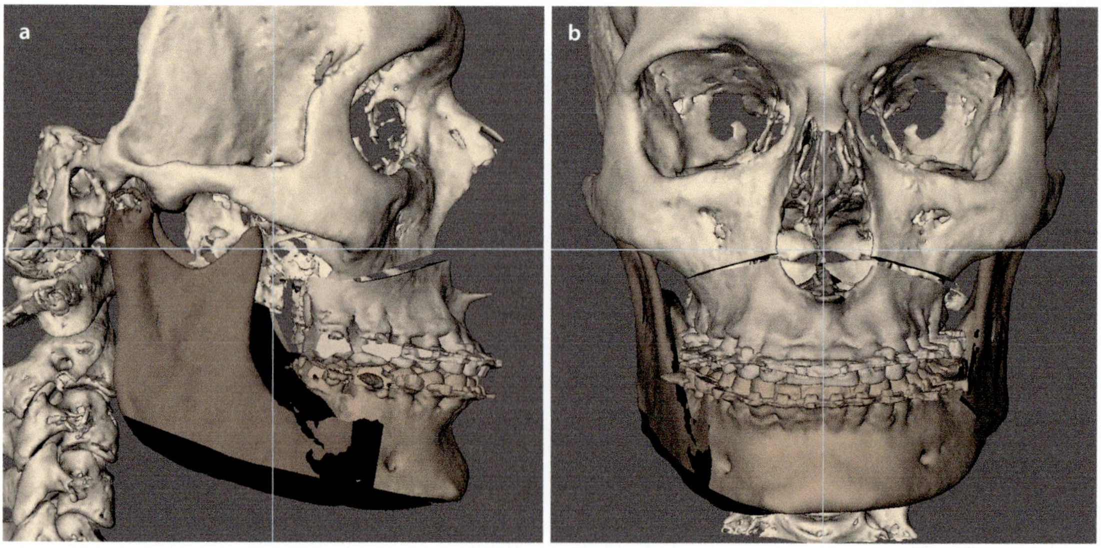

Fig. 6.259 Final adjustments of the "Individualised 3D Virtual Treatment Plan". After an extended right sagittal split osteotomy, virtual resection of the mandibular lower border was planned, from the gonial angle towards the symphysis, in patient A.A. (3D "surface-rendered" representations, Maxilim v. 2.3.0.3). Right profile (**a**) and frontal (**b**) views

Case 7: 3D-VPS$_5$- Final Integrated "Individualised 3D Virtual Treatment Plan"

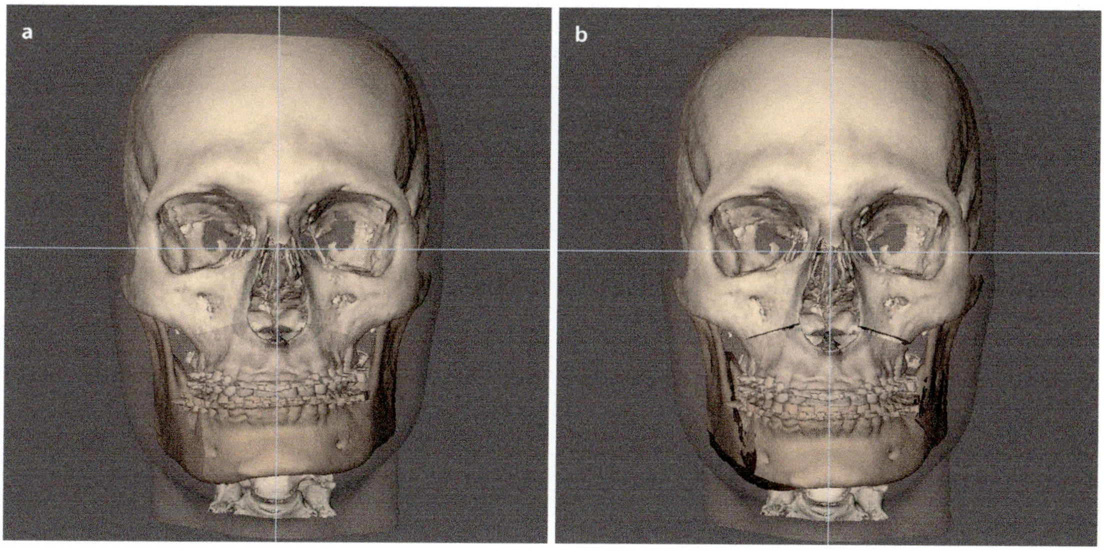

Fig. 6.260 Initial situation (**a**), and final "Individualised 3D Virtual Treatment Plan" (**b**), in the frontal plane (3D "surface-rendered" representations, patient A.A., Maxilim v. 2.3.0.3)

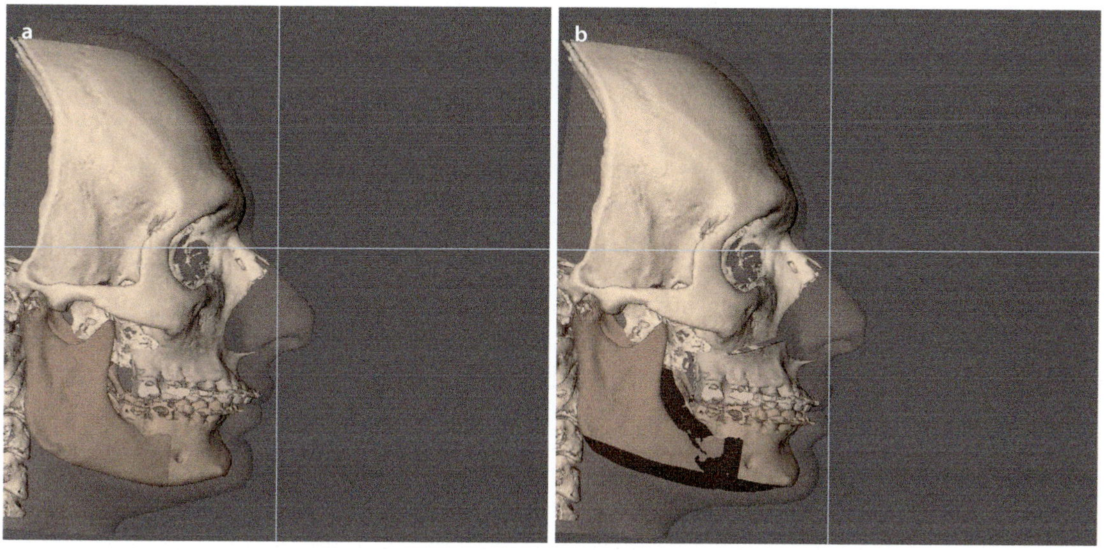

Fig. 6.261 Initial situation (**a**), and final "Individualised 3D Virtual Treatment Plan" (**b**), in the right profile plane (3D "surface-rendered" representations, patient A.A., Maxilim v. 2.3.0.3)

Case 7: 3D-VPS$_5$- Final Integrated "Individualised 3D Virtual Treatment Plan"

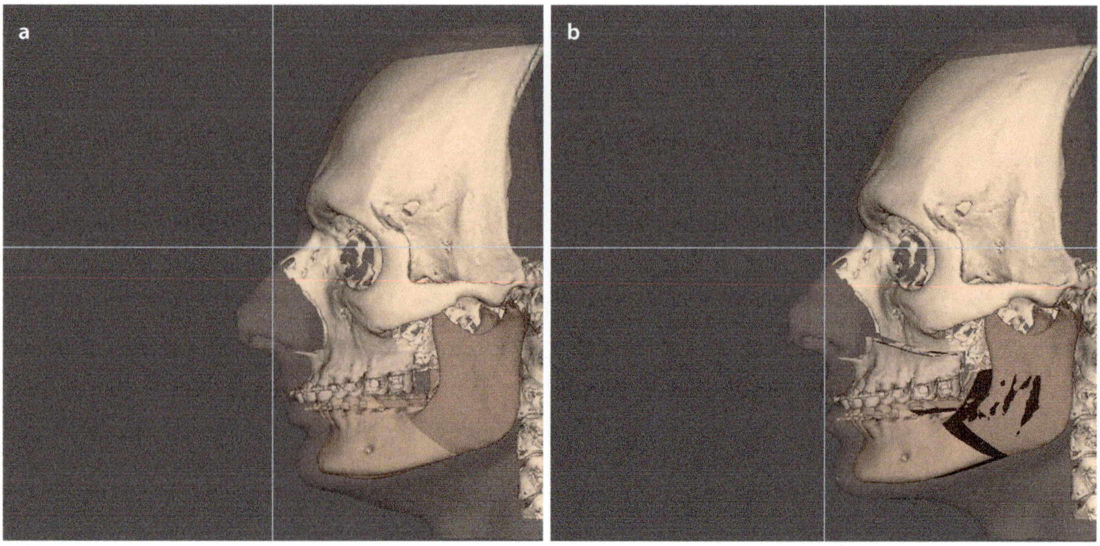

Fig. 6.262 Initial situation (**a**), and final "Individualised 3D Virtual Treatment Plan" (**b**), in the left profile plane (3D "surface-rendered" representations, patient A.A., Maxilim v. 2.3.0.3)

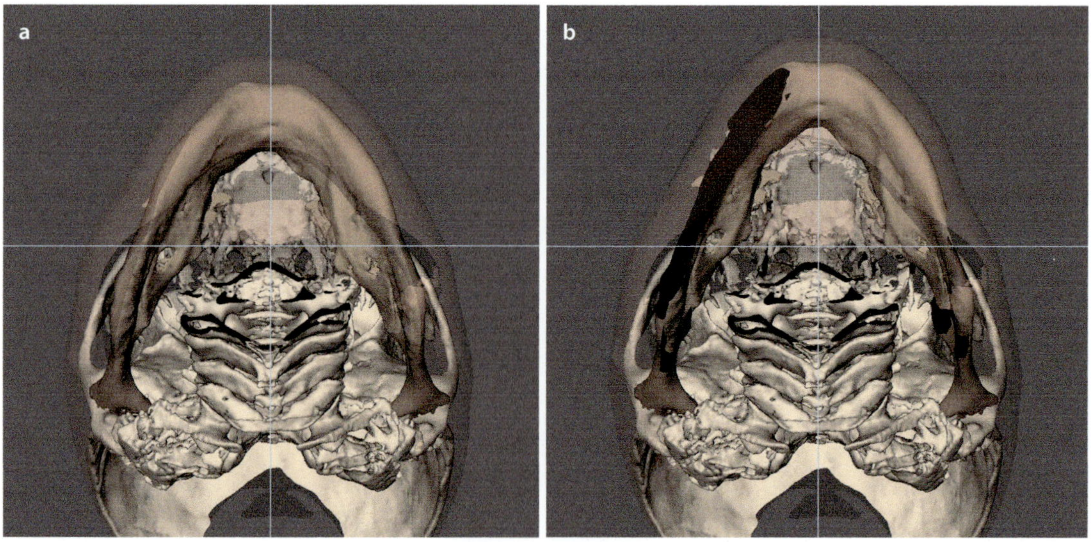

Fig. 6.263 Initial situation (**a**), and final "Individualised 3D Virtual Treatment Plan" (**b**), in the base plane (3D "surface-rendered" representations, patient A.A., Maxilim v. 2.3.0.3)

Case 7: "3D Virtual Treatment Planning, OR" Template

Maxillary osteotomy

- ■ Le Fort: ■ I ☐ II ☐ III
- ■ One-piece
- ☐ Segmental:
  - Pieces: ....
  - Interdental: ....
- ■ Advancement: 3.0 mm
- ☐ Set-back: ....
- ■ Midline: 1.0 mm ☐ R ■ L
- ■ Midline after Le Fort 1: 1/3 mesial 31
- ■ Vertical: (→)
- ■ "Yaw" correction: to the right
- ☐ Other: ....

Mandibular osteotomy

- ■ SSO ■ R ■ L
- ☐ Inverted-L ☐ R ☐ L
- ☐ VRO ☐ R ☐ L
- ■ Advancement: R 5.0 mm L 10.0 mm
- ☐ Set-back: R .... L ....
- ☐ CW rotation
- ■ CCW "Pitch" rotation
- ☐ Midline split
- ■ IAN course: R lingual L lingual
- ☐ Midline after BSSO: ....
- ■ Other: right lower border resection

Chin osteotomy

- ☐ Advancement: ....
- ☐ Set-back: ....
- ☐ Midline: .... ☐ R ☐ L
- ☐ Intrusion:
  - ☐ Anterior: ....
  - ☐ Posterior: R ...... L ......
- ☐ Extrusion:
  - ☐ Anterior: ....
  - ☐ Posterior: R ...... L ......
- ☐ "Shield" osteotomy
- ☐ "Chin wing" osteotomy
  - *Mental Foramen level:*
  - ☐ Symmetric
  - ■ Asymmetric
- ■ Other: right lower border resection

Planning Requirements

- ■ Maxilla first
- ☐ Mandible first
- ■ Minimally Invasive Le Fort I
- ■ IO-CBCT
- ☐ Kobayashi wires: ....
- ☐ Skeletal anchorage: ....
- ☐ Orthodontic buttons: ....
- ☐ Occlusal grinding: ....
- ☐ Other: ....

↓	↓	↓	↓	↓
0.5 mm	1.5 mm	2.0 mm	2.5 mm	2.0 mm
16	13	11	23	26

"Roll" correction: ■ CW ☐ CCW

Miscellaneous

- ■ Para-nasal cross sutures
- ☐ Alar cinch
- ☐ Septoplasty
- ☐ Inferior turbinectomy
- ■ ANS: ☐ Shortening ■ Midline
- ☐ Nasal base plasty ■ R ☐ L
- ■ Lateral nasal wall plasty ☐ R ■ L
- ■ Bone graft(s): right lower border
- ☐ Extraction(s): ....
- ☐ Other: ....

Adjuvant Cosmetic Procedures

- ☐ Bichatectomy ☐ R ☐ L
- ☐ Zygoma osteotomies ☐ R ☐ L
  - *Infraorbital Foramen level:*
  - ☐ Symmetric
  - ☐ Asymmetric
- ■ Otoplasty: ☐ R ■ L
- ☐ Rhinoplasty: ....
- ☐ Browlift: ....
- ☐ Blepharoplasty: ....
  - ☐ Upper ☐ Lower
- ☐ Facelift: ....
- ☐ Necklift: ....
- ☐ Liposuction: ....
- ☐ Lipofilling: ....
- ☐ Other: ....

Addendum Template. Prof. Gwen Swennen and Dr. Martin Gaboury, Maxillofacial and Facial Plastic Surgery.

■ Case 7: Hemimandibular Hyperplasia (HH), Intra-operative Cone-Beam CT (IO-CBCT)

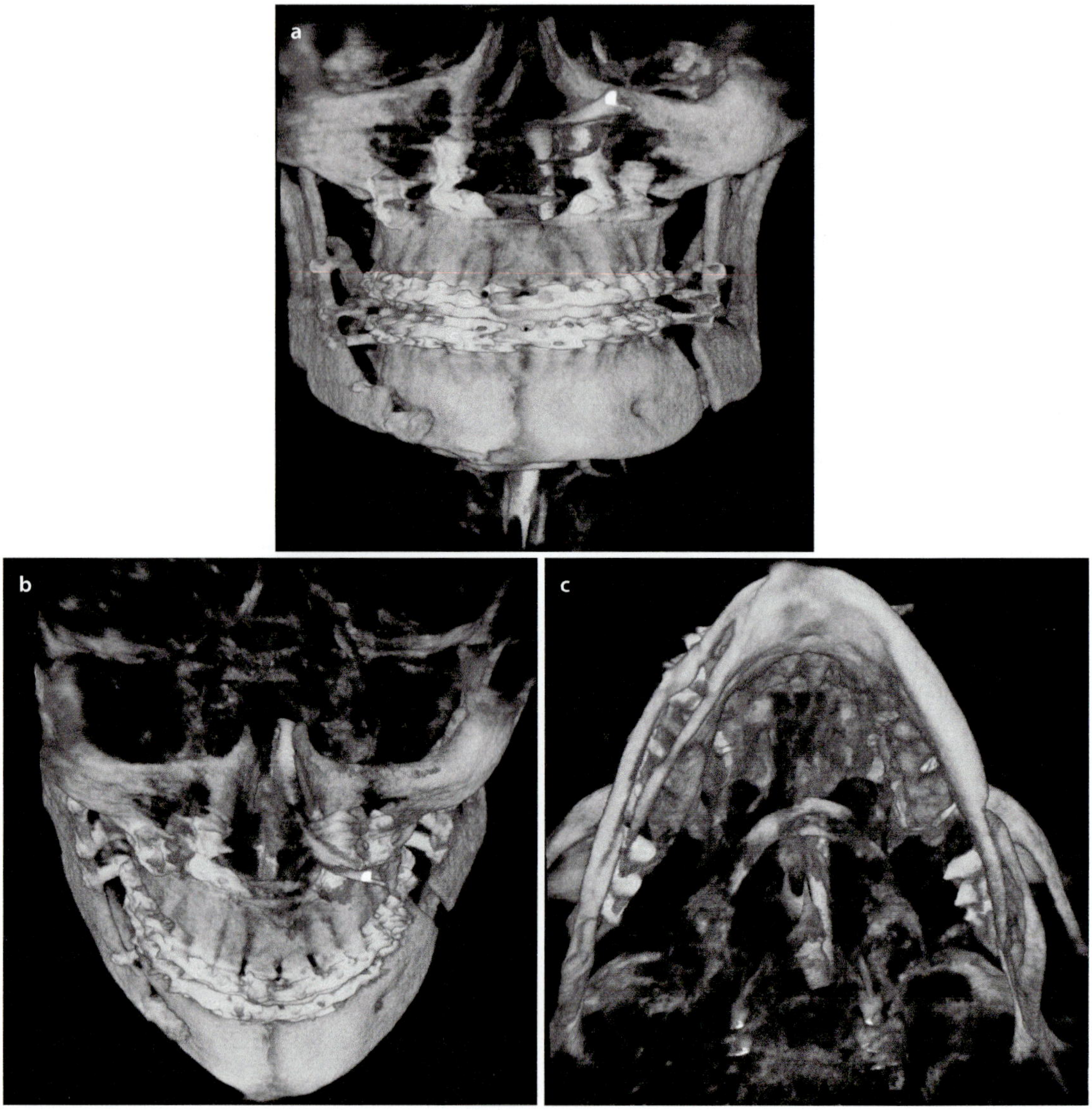

Fig. 6.264 Frontal (**a**), downward inclined (**b**) and base (**c**) views of IO-CBCT imaging after repositioning of the maxillo-mandibular complex with right mandibular lower border resection (3D "volume-rendered" representations, patient A.A., Arcadis® Orbic 3D C-arm, Siemens Healthcare GmbH)

Case 7: Hemimandibular Hyperplasia (HH), Intra-operative Cone-Beam CT (IO-CBCT)

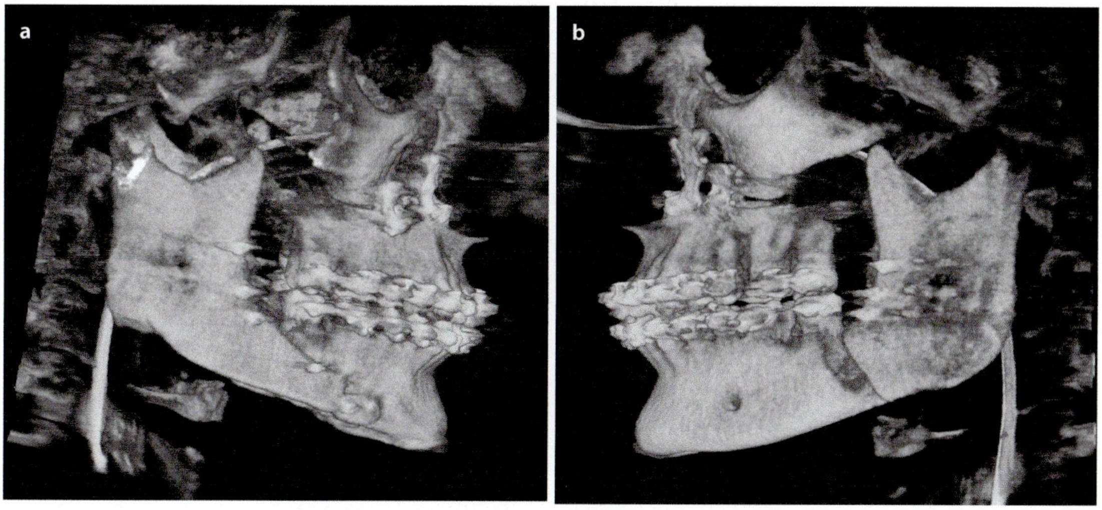

Fig. 6.265 Right (**a**) and left profile (**b**) views of IO-CBCT imaging after repositioning of the maxillo-mandibular complex with right mandibular lower border resection (3D "volume-rendered" representations, patient A.A., Arcadis® Orbic 3D C-arm, Siemens Healthcare GmbH)

Case 7: Hemimandibular Hyperplasia (HH), 3D Virtual Treatment Outcome

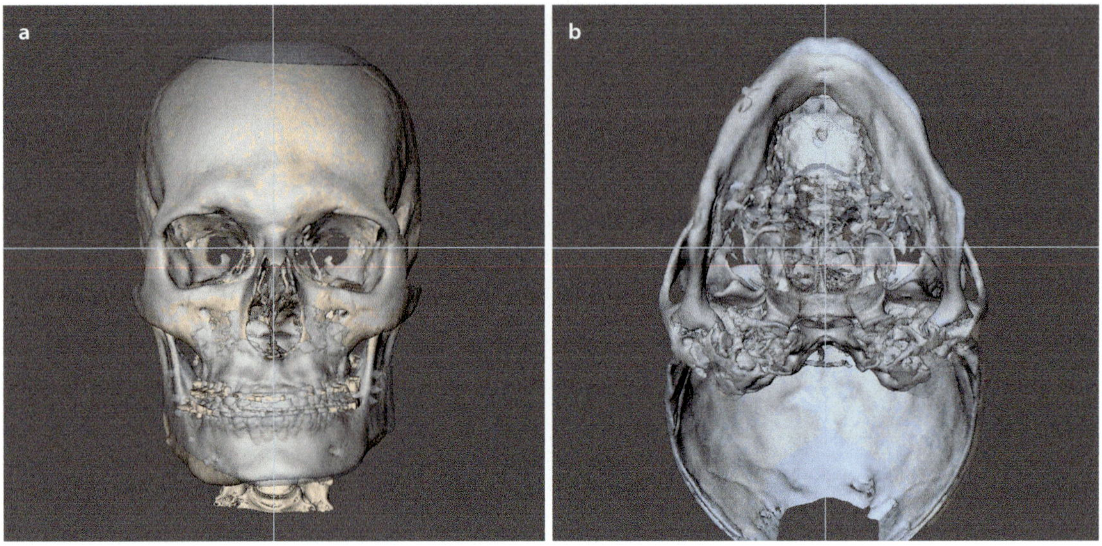

Fig. 6.266 Voxel-based superimposition on the cranial base of the pre-surgical and 9 months post-surgical (*blue*) 3D "surface-rendered" hard tissue representations. Frontal (**a**) and base (**b**) views (i-CAT, Imaging Sciences International Inc., Maxilim v. 2.3.0.3) (patient A.A.). Note the correction of the mandibular border asymmetry and adequate post-surgical mandibular bony contour

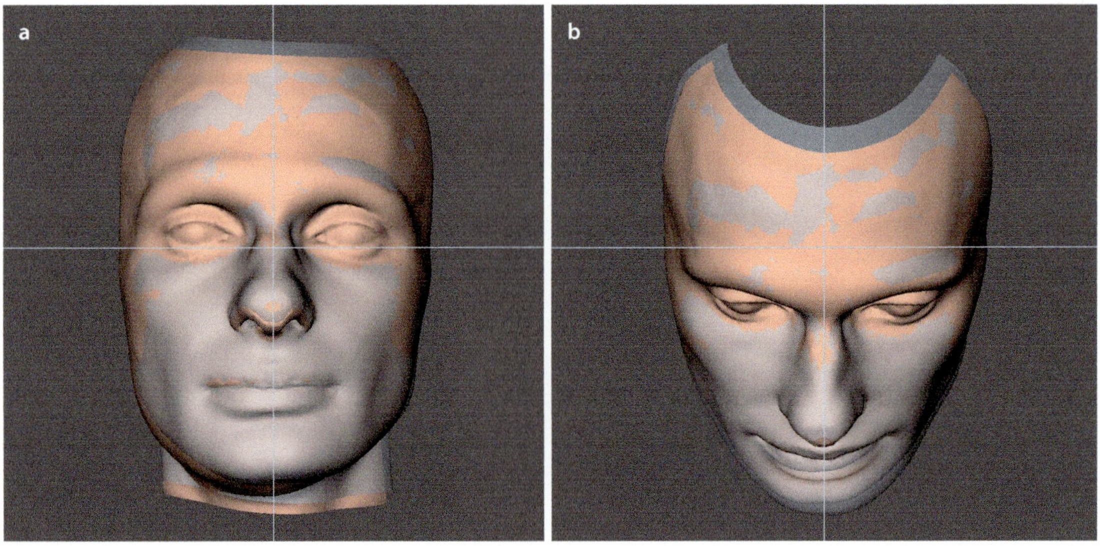

Fig. 6.267 Voxel-based superimposition on the cranial base of the pre-surgical and 9 months post-surgical (*blue*) 3D "surface-rendered" soft tissue representations. Frontal (**a**) and downward inclined (**b**) views (i-CAT, Imaging Sciences International Inc., Maxilim v. 2.3.0.3) (patient A.A.). Note the post-surgical (*blue*) facial symmetry and harmony

Case 7: Hemimandibular Hyperplasia (HH), 3D Virtual Treatment Outcome

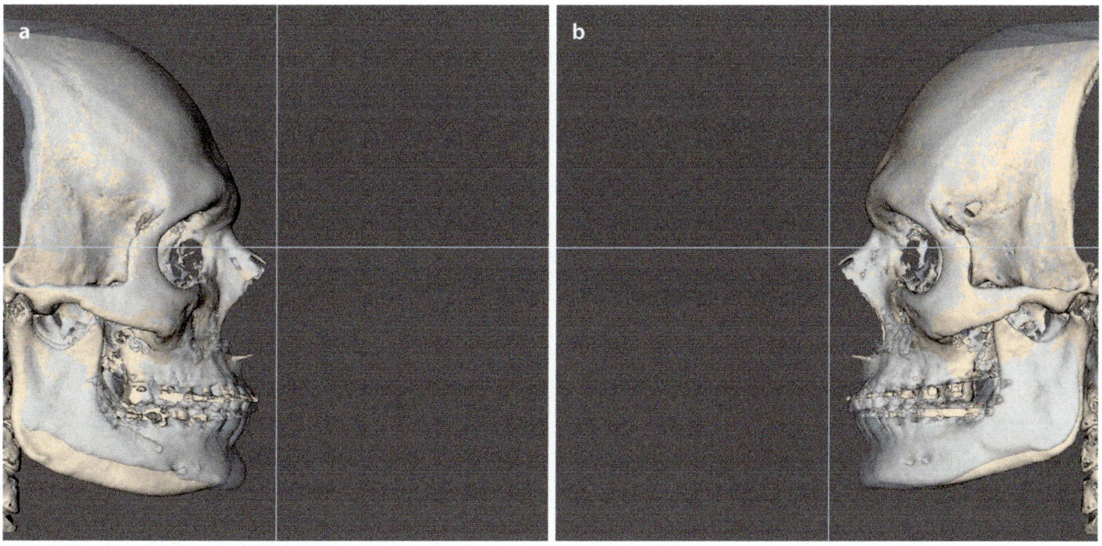

Fig. 6.268 Voxel-based superimposition on the cranial base of the pre-surgical and 9 months post-surgical 3D "surface-rendered" hard tissue representations. Right (**a**) and left profile (**b**) views (i-CAT, Imaging Sciences International Inc., Maxilim v. 2.3.0.3) (patient A.A.)

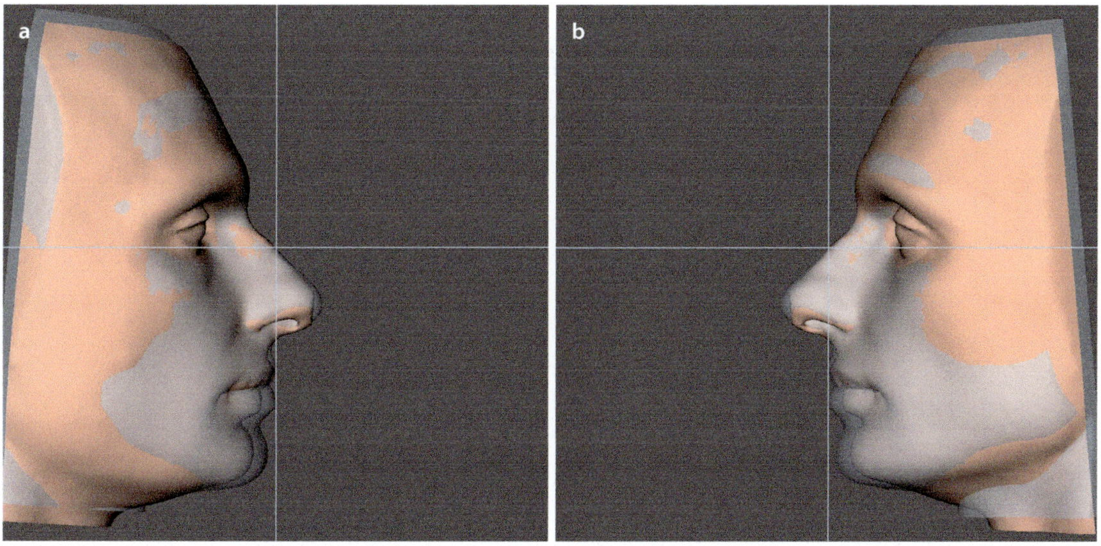

Fig. 6.269 Voxel-based superimposition on the cranial base of the pre-surgical and 9 months post-surgical (*blue*) 3D "surface-rendered" soft tissue representations. Right (**a**) and left profile (**b**) views (i-CAT, Imaging Sciences International Inc., Maxilim v. 2.3.0.3) (patient A.A.). Note the post-surgical postural changes of the upper and lower lips

Case 7: Hemimandibular Hyperplasia (HH), Clinical Treatment Outcome

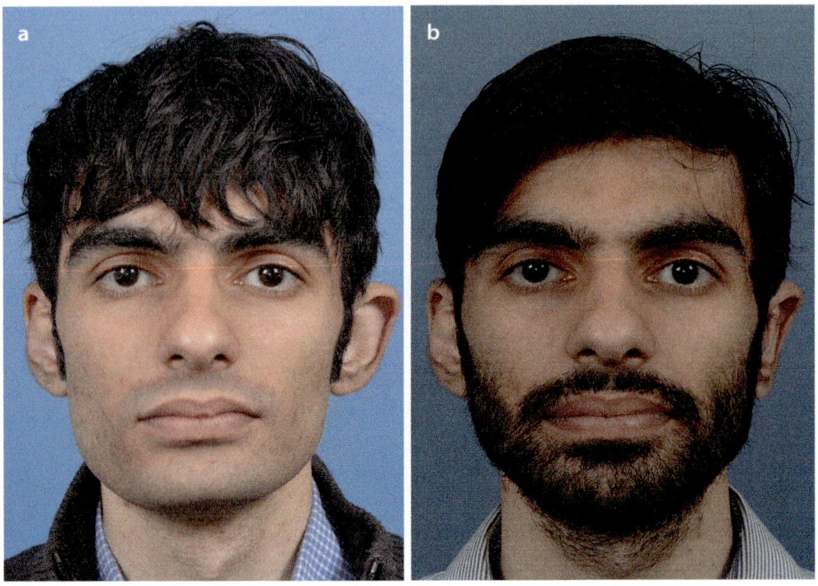

Fig. 6.270 Frontal views in rest, pre-surgical (**a**) and 5 months after (**b**) combined orthodontic-surgical treatment with right mandibular lower border resection and left otoplasty (patient A.A.)

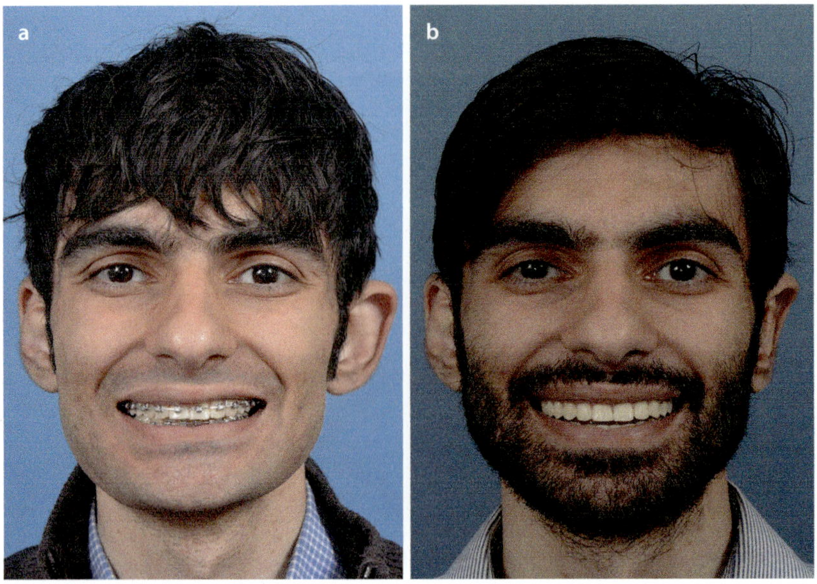

Fig. 6.271 Frontal views during smiling, pre-surgical (**a**) and 5 months after (**b**) combined orthodontic-surgical treatment with right mandibular lower border resection and left otoplasty (patient A.A.)

Case 7: Hemimandibular Hyperplasia (HH), Clinical Treatment Outcome

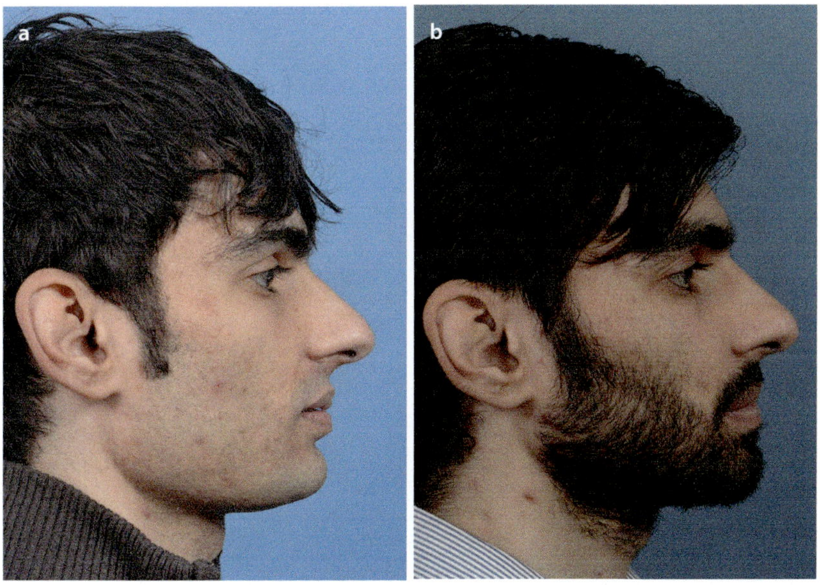

Fig. 6.272 Right profile views in rest, pre-surgical (**a**) and 5 months after (**b**) combined orthodontic-surgical treatment with right mandibular lower border resection (patient A.A.)

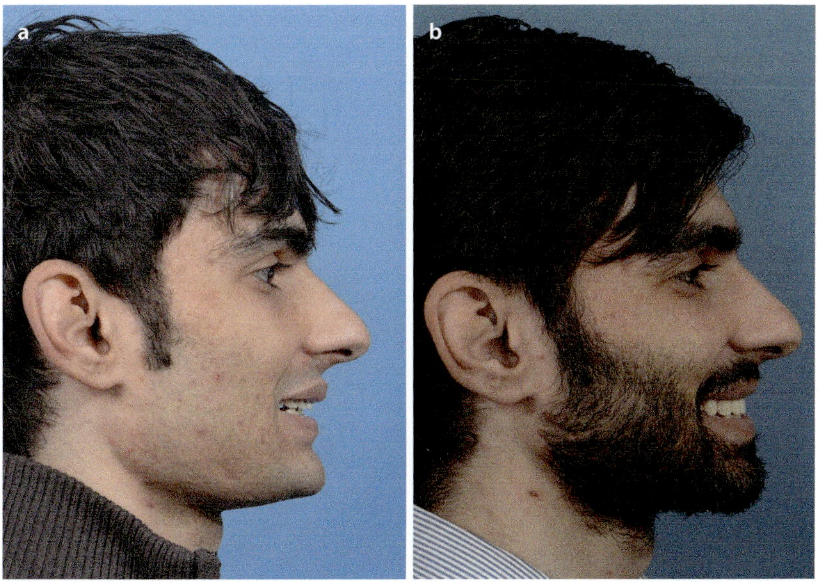

Fig. 6.273 Right profile views during smiling, pre-surgical (**a**) and 5 months after (**b**) combined orthodontic-surgical treatment with right mandibular lower border resection (patient A.A.)

Case 7: Hemimandibular Hyperplasia (HH), Clinical Treatment Outcome

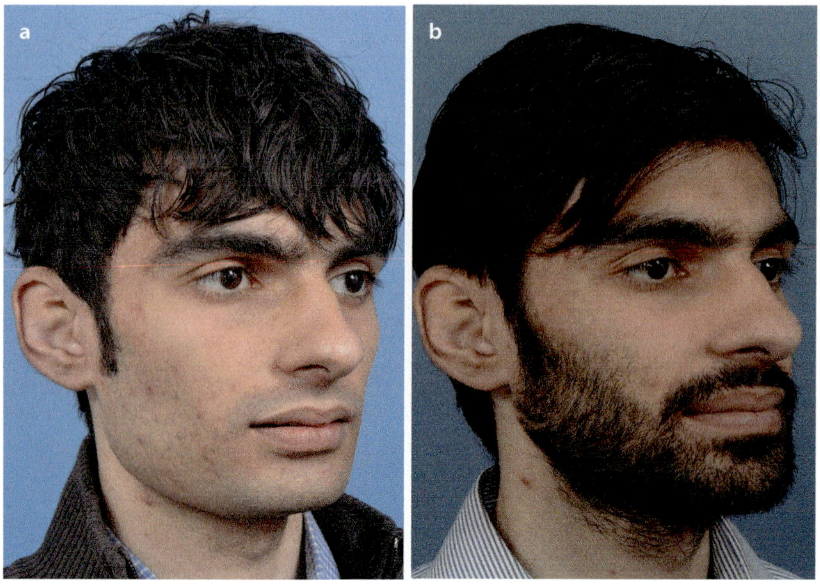

Fig. 6.274 2/3 right profile views in rest, pre-surgical (**a**) and 5 months after (**b**) combined orthodontic-surgical treatment with right mandibular lower border resection (patient A.A.)

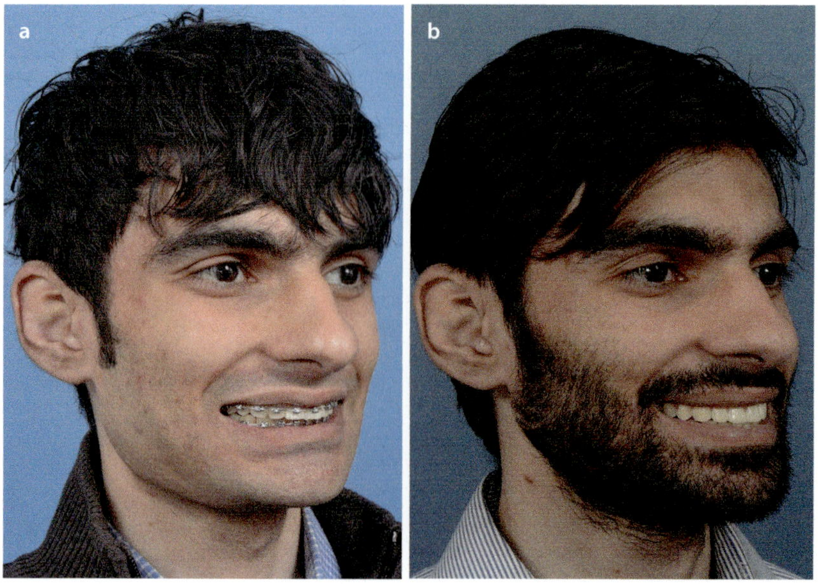

Fig. 6.275 2/3 right profile views during smiling, pre-surgical (**a**) and 5 months after (**b**) combined orthodontic-surgical treatment with right mandibular lower border resection (patient A.A.)

Case 7: Hemimandibular Hyperplasia (HH), Clinical Treatment Outcome

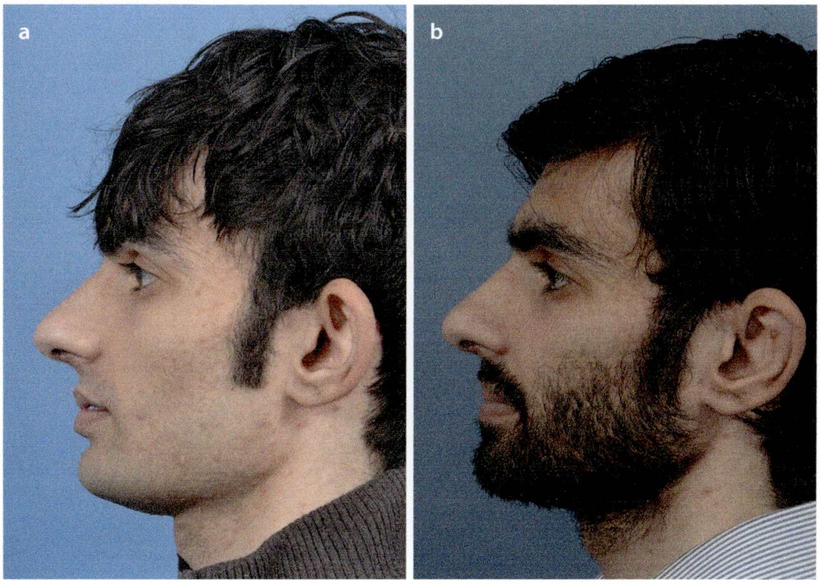

Fig. 6.276 Left profile views in rest, pre-surgical (**a**) and 5 months after (**b**) combined orthodontic-surgical treatment with right mandibular lower border resection and left otoplasty (patient A.A.)

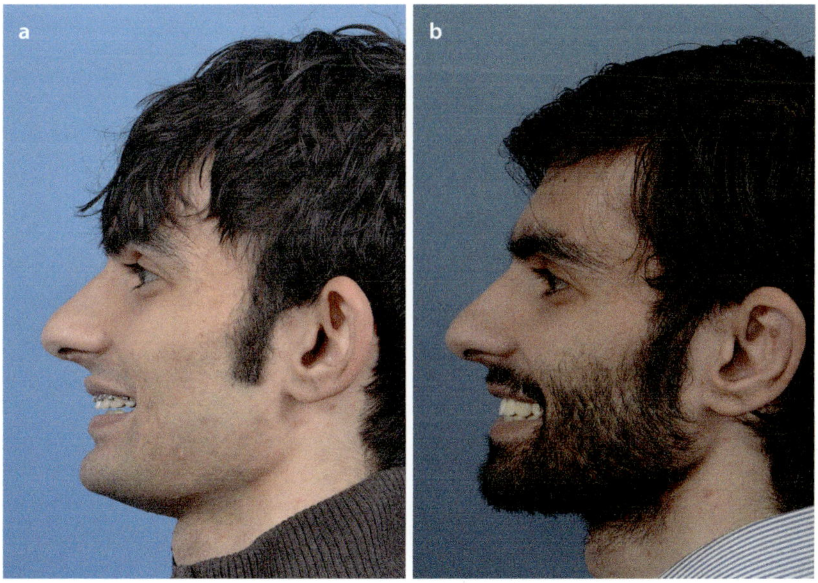

Fig. 6.277 Left profile views during smiling, pre-surgical (**a**) and 5 months after (**b**) combined orthodontic-surgical treatment with right mandibular lower border resection and left otoplasty (patient A.A.)

Case 7: Hemimandibular Hyperplasia (HH), Clinical Treatment Outcome

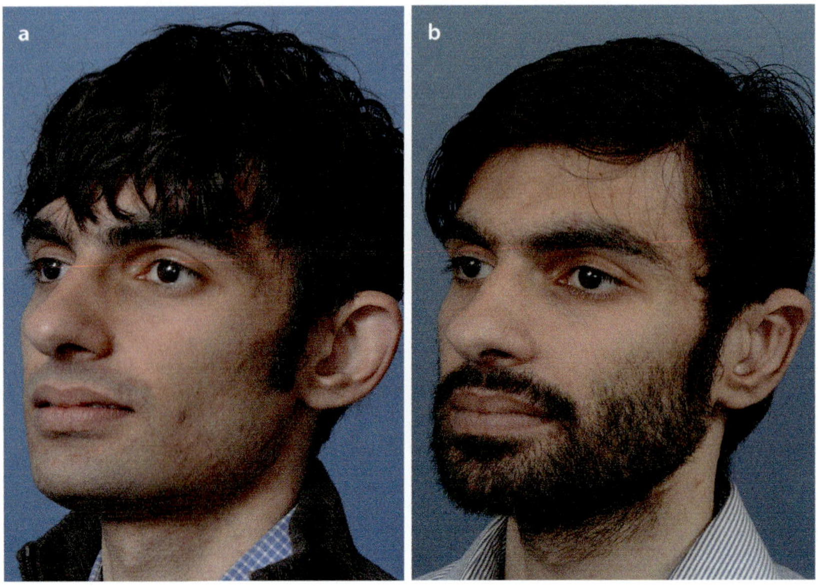

Fig. 6.278 2/3 left profile views in rest, pre-surgical (**a**) and 5 months after (**b**) combined orthodontic-surgical treatment with right mandibular lower border resection and left otoplasty (patient A.A.)

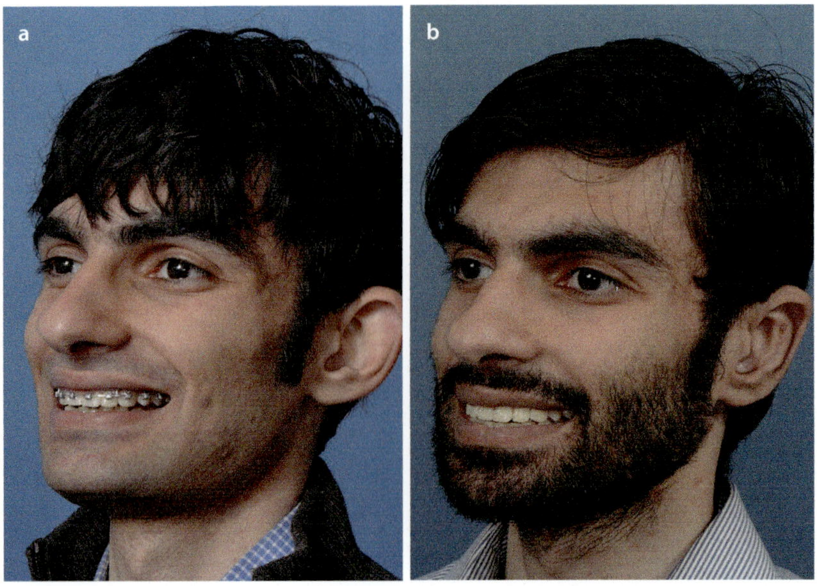

Fig. 6.279 2/3 left profile views during smiling, pre-surgical (**a**) and 5 months after (**b**) combined orthodontic-surgical treatment with right mandibular lower border resection and left otoplasty (patient A.A.)

Case 7: Hemimandibular Hyperplasia (HH), Clinical Treatment Outcome

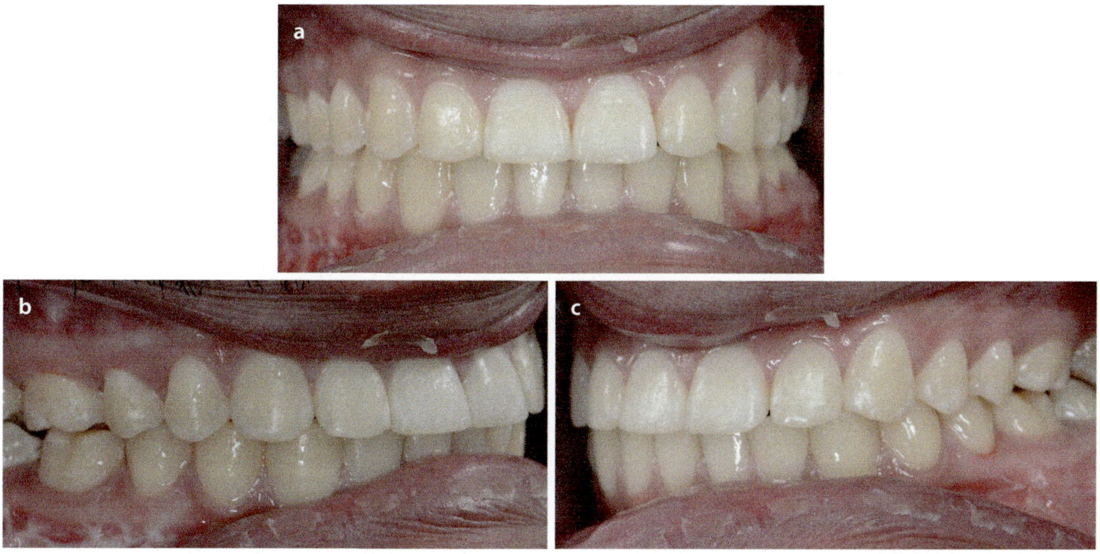

Fig. 6.280 Frontal (**a**), right (**b**) and left (**c**) intra-oral views of the patient's occlusion 5 months after combined orthodontic-surgical treatment (patient A.A.). The author acknowledges Bénédicte Rèchler for the orthodontic treatment

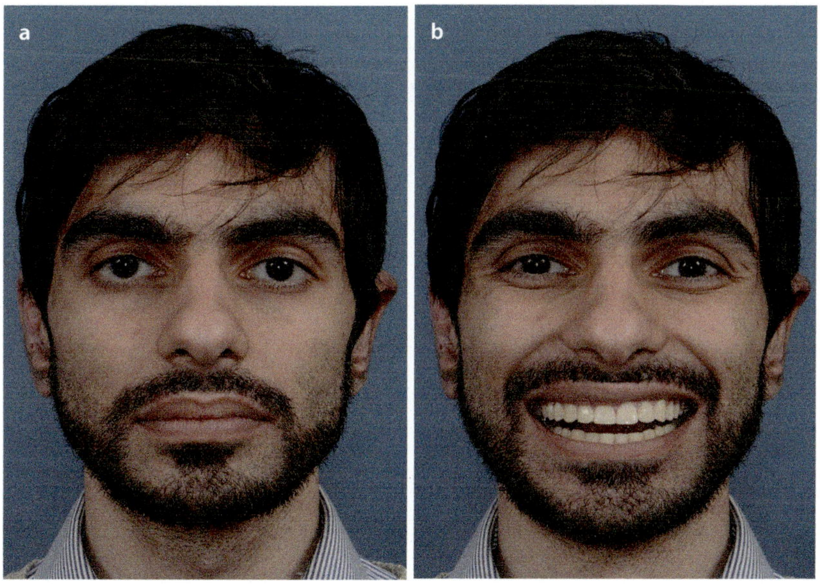

Fig. 6.281 Long-term frontal in rest (**a**) and smiling (**b**) views after an additional right otoplasty performed under local anaesthesia by the author (patient A.A.). Note that the ears are still slightly asymmetric

Case 8: IPS CaseDesigner

Finally, IPS CaseDesigner is illustrated on patient V.E.W. (▶ see also Case 1, Chap. 6), which is used throughout the book (▶ Chaps. 1, 2, 3, 4 and 5) to introduce the potential of a more enhanced, intuitive and user-friendly 3D software platform towards "3D virtual treatment planning of orthognathic surgery".

After an appropriate CBCT image acquisition, "step-by-step" Quality Control of the patient's AUM and virtual modification of the patient's virtual head towards its clinical NHP (c-NHP) is essential PRIOR to start a "3D virtual treatment planning of orthognathic surgery".

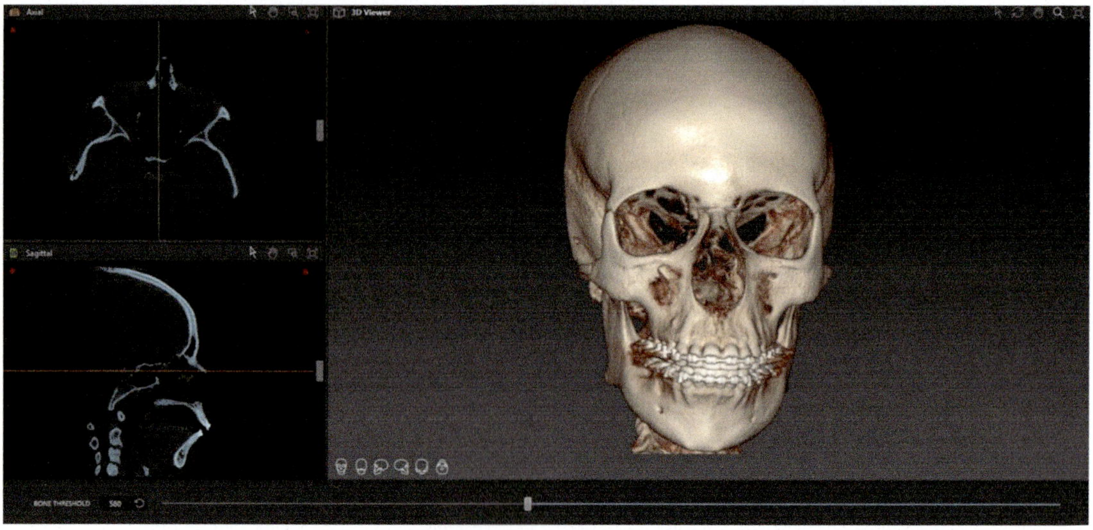

Fig. 6.282 "Volume rendering" of the hard tissues of the head of patient V.E.W. after proper CBCT image acquisition. The threshold is adjusted to optimise the visualisation of the hard tissues (i-CAT^{TM}, Imaging Sciences International, Inc., Hatfield, USA, "extended field" modus; FOV, 17 cm diameter, 22 cm height; scan time 2 × 20s; voxel size 0.4 mm at 120 kV according to DICOM field, 0018,0060 KVP, and 48 mA according to DICOM field, 0018,1151 XRayTubeCurrent) (IPS CaseDesigner v 1.1.3.1)

Case 8: IPS CaseDesigner, Step-by-Step Quality Control, Accuracy of the AUM

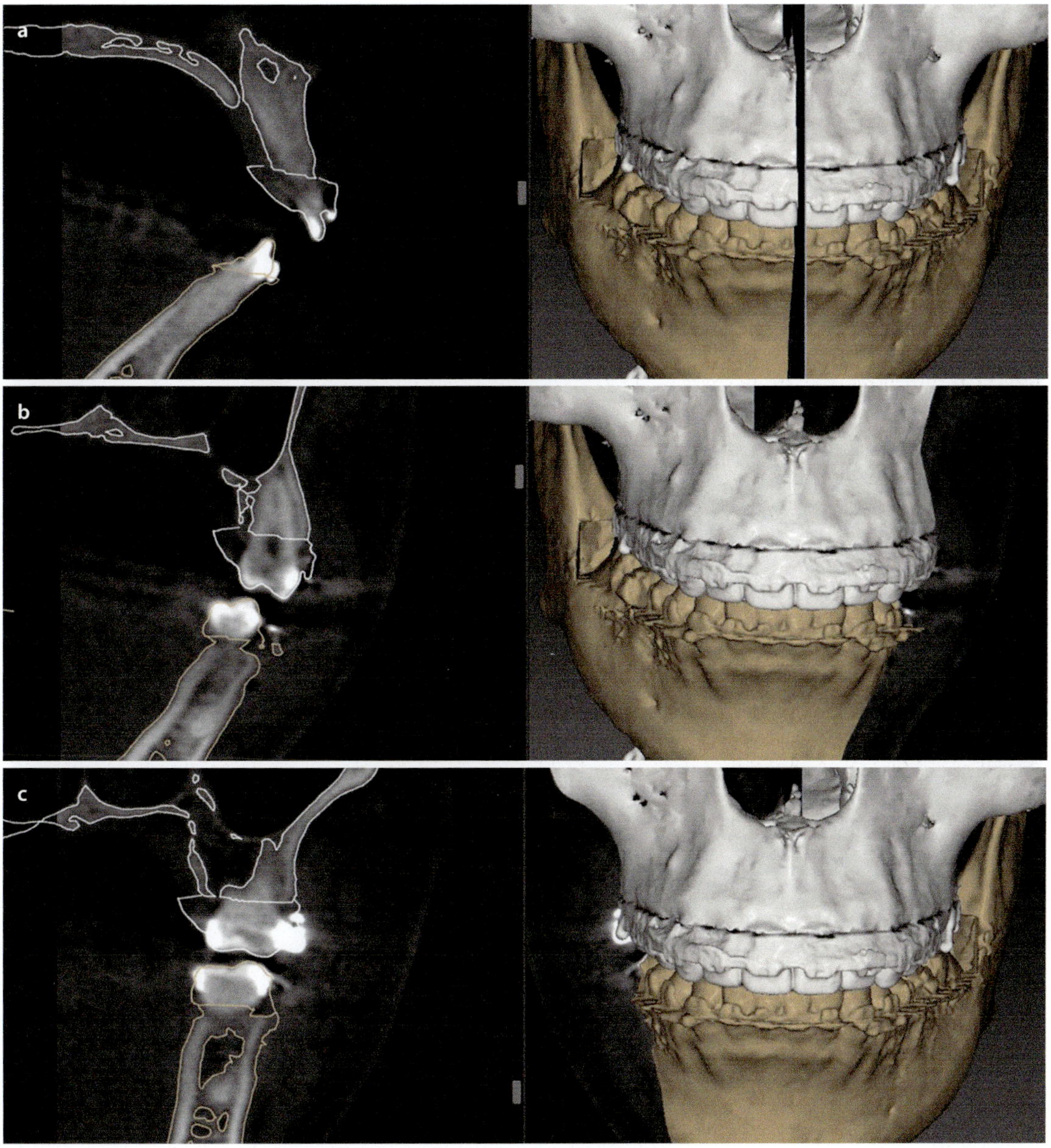

Fig. 6.283 In "step 1" of the "Step-by-Step Quality Control Checklist" (see also Sect. 1.2), the accuracy of registration of the upper and lower dental arches in the AUM of the patient is semiautomatically and dynamically verified along the dental arches (i-CAT, Imaging Sciences International Inc., IPS CaseDesigner v 1.1.3.1, patient V.E.W.): e.g. at the dental midlines (**a**), left (**b**) and right (**c**) molar regions

▪ Case 8: IPS CaseDesigner, "Step-by-Step" Quality Control, Condyle (CR) Position

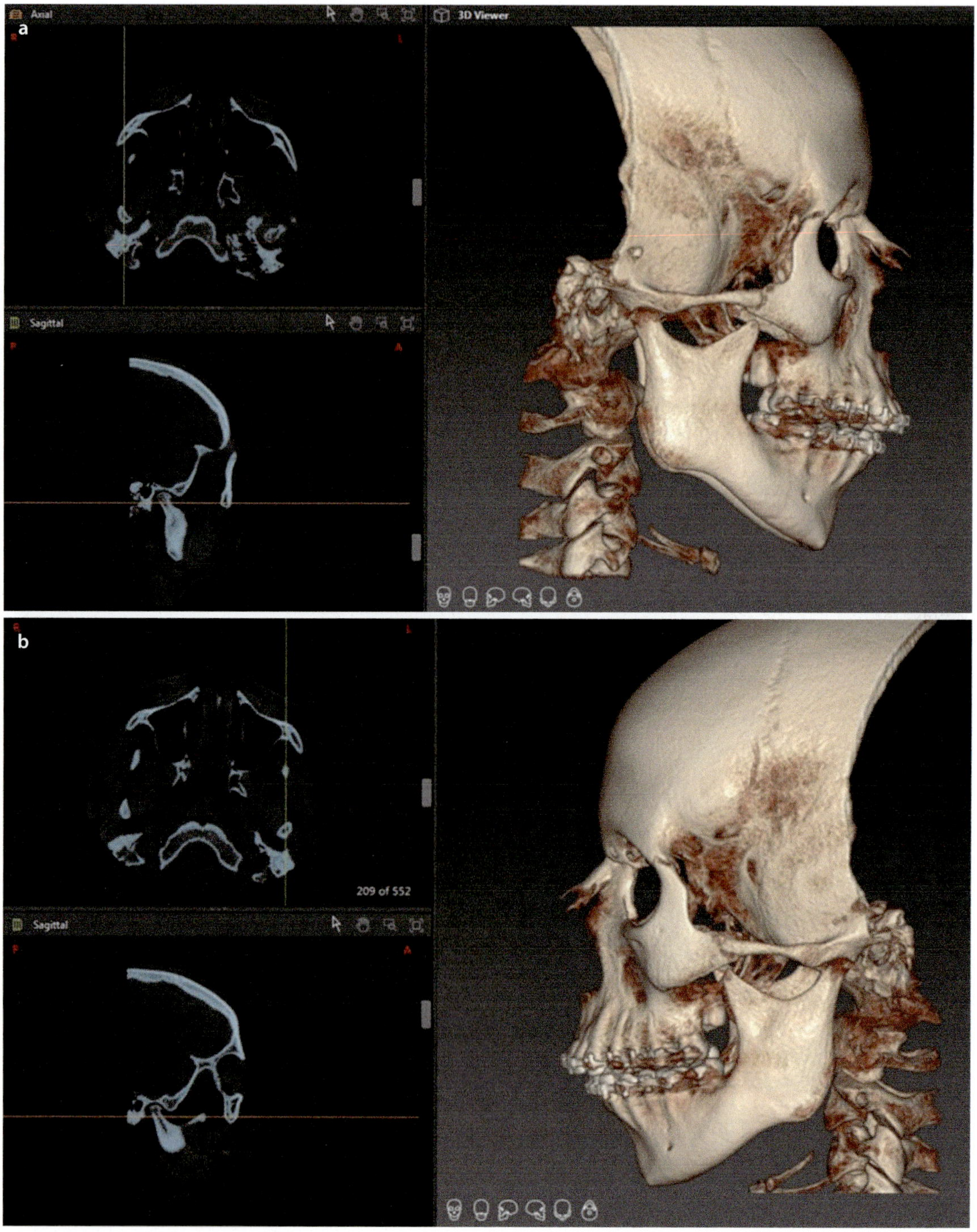

Fig. 6.284 In "step 2" of the "Step-by-Step Quality Control Checklist" (see also Sect. 1.2), proper seating of the condyles in CR is verified by semiautomatic evaluation of a combination of axial and sagittal slices and the 3D "volume-rendered" hard tissue representation of patient V.E.W. (i-CAT, Imaging Sciences International Inc., IPS CaseDesigner v 1.1.3.1). Note the appropriate seating of the right (**a**) and left (**b**) condyles

■ Case 8: IPS CaseDesigner, "Step-by-Step" Quality Control, Soft Tissue Quality

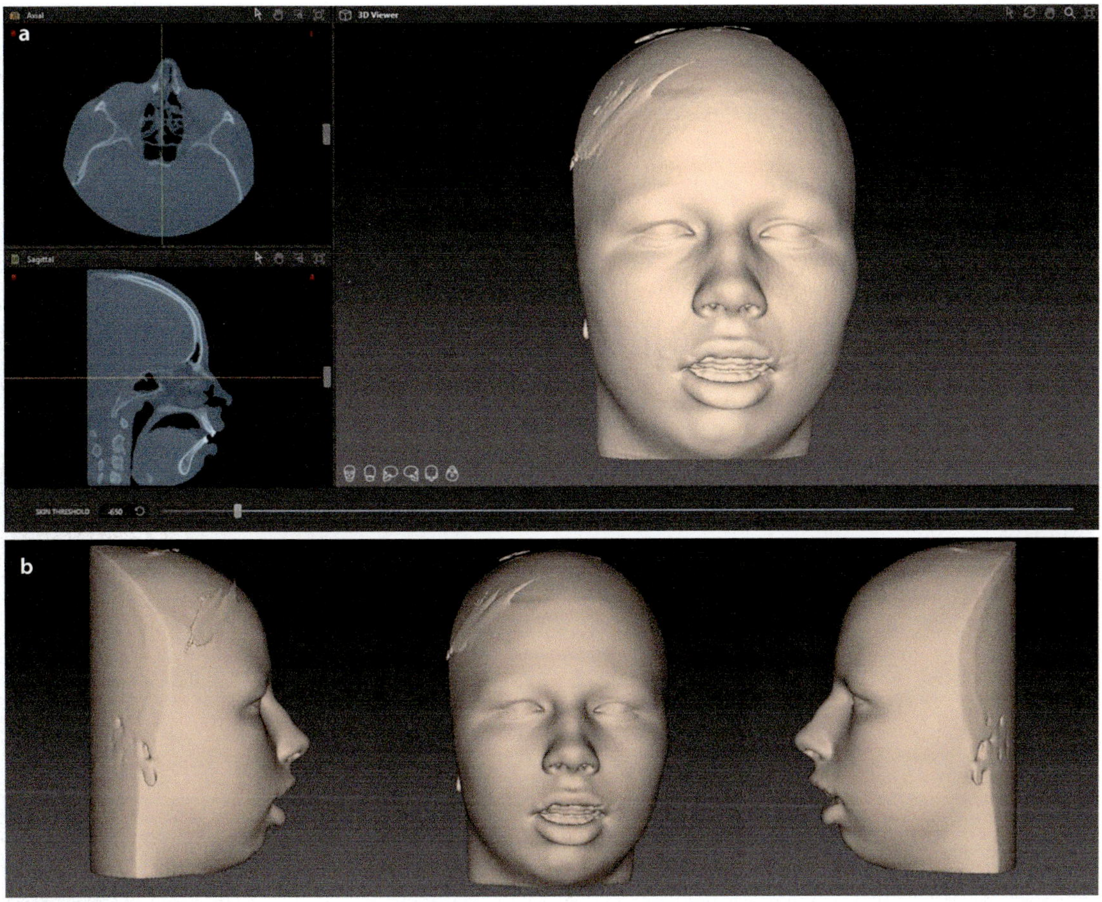

Fig. 6.285 In "step 3" of the "Step-by-Step Quality Control Checklist" (see also Sect. 1.2), the overall soft tissue quality after appropriate rendering (**a**) is evaluated on the AUM of patient V.E.W. (**b**) (i-CAT, Imaging Sciences International Inc., "volume-rendered" surface representations, IPS CaseDesigner v 1.1.3.1). Note that there is no distortion of the fronto-temporal soft tissues due to proper position of the head fixation band during CBCT scanning. Also note the absence of lip and chin distortion, as well as the absence of lip and mentalis muscle contraction

▪ Case 8: IPS CaseDesigner, *v*-NHP and PHP

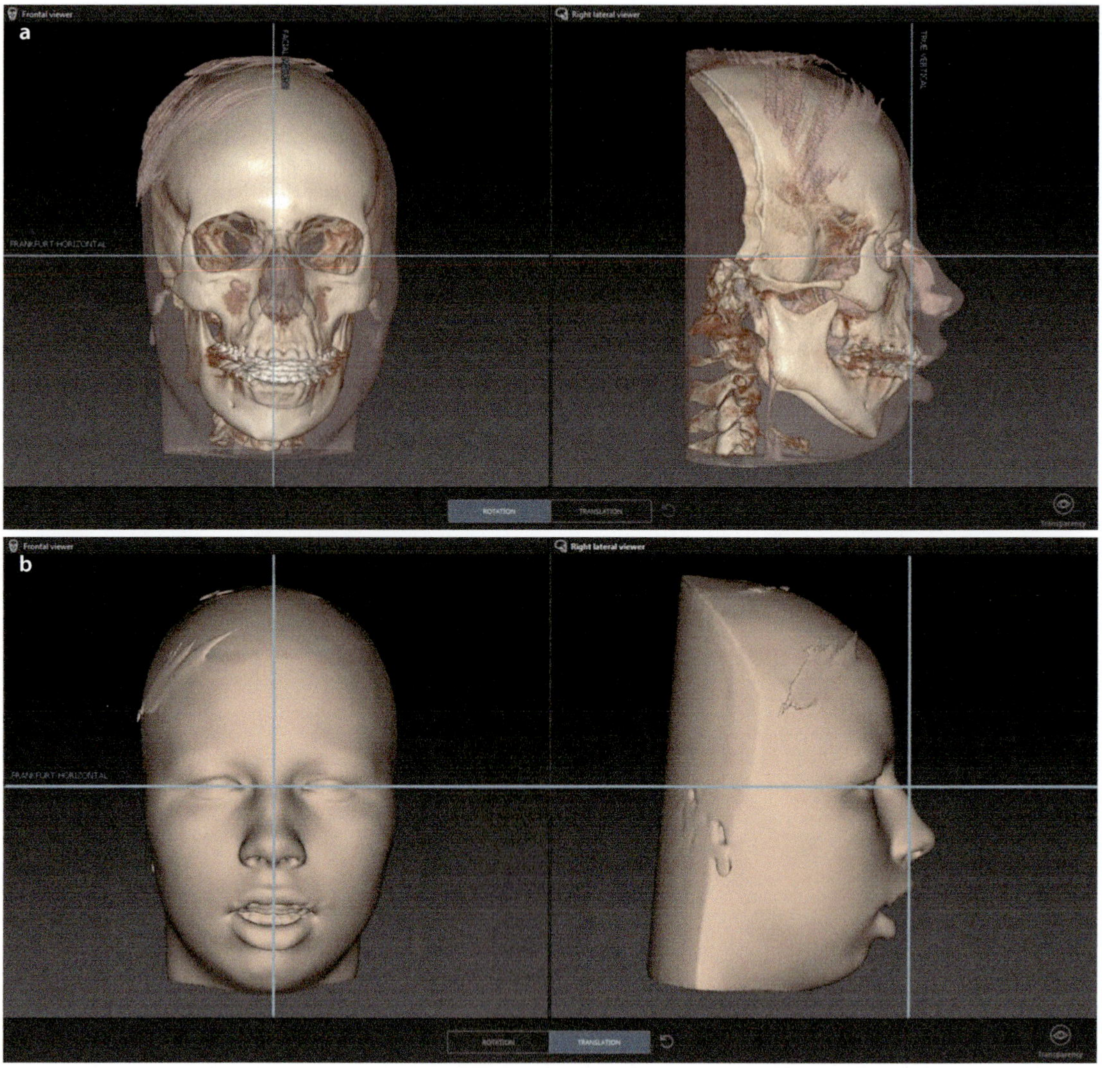

Fig. 6.286 Following a standardised "step-by-step" approach (▶ see Sect. 3.1), the scanned head position of patient V.E.W. (**a**) is virtually semiautomatically modified towards her *c*-NHP, which results in her *v*-NHP and corresponds to her individual "Planning Head Position (PHP)" (**b**) (3D "surface-rendered" representations, IPS CaseDesigner v 1.1.3.1)

■ Case 8: 3D-VPS$_5$ Step 1 Maxillary Occlusal Cant Evaluation/Correction (*"Roll"*)

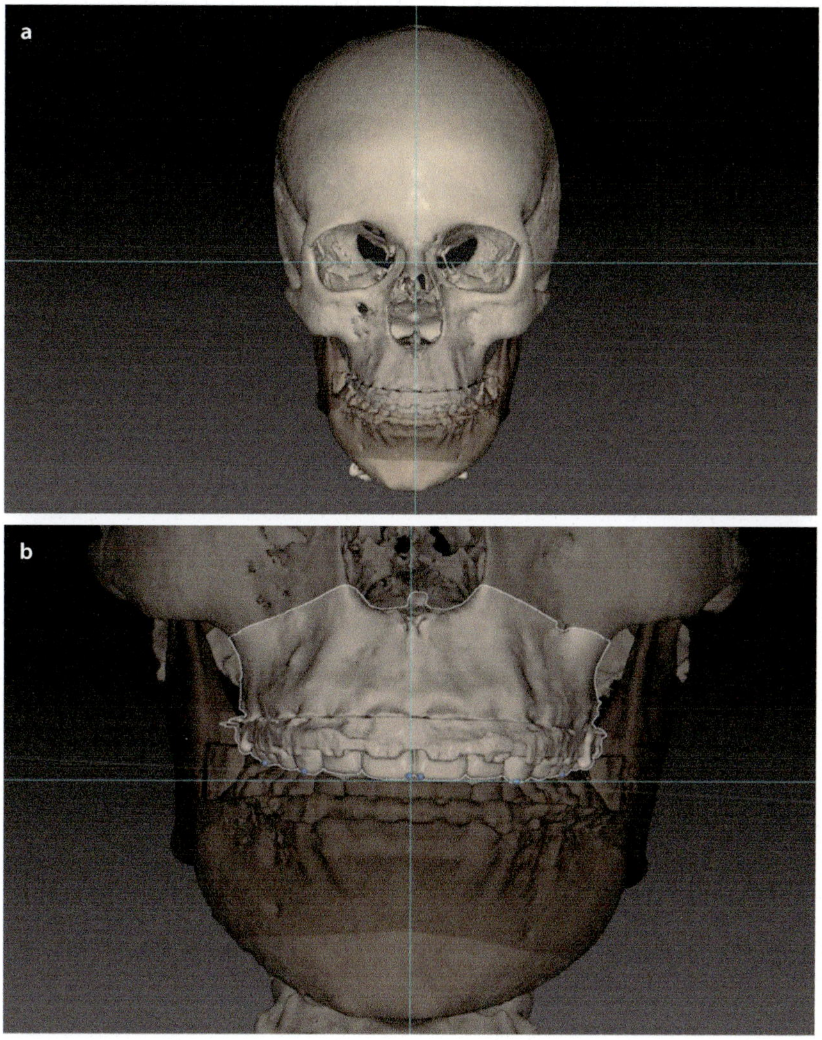

Fig. 6.287 The maxillary occlusal plane is evaluated both clinically (Fig. 3.52) and virtually towards the horizontal 3D PHP reference plane in patient V.E.W. (3D "surface-rendered" representations, IPS CaseDesigner v 1.1.3.1). Frontal (**a**) and detailed (**b**) views

■ Case 8: 3D-VPS$_5$ Step 1 Maxillary Occlusal Cant Evaluation/Correction ("Roll")

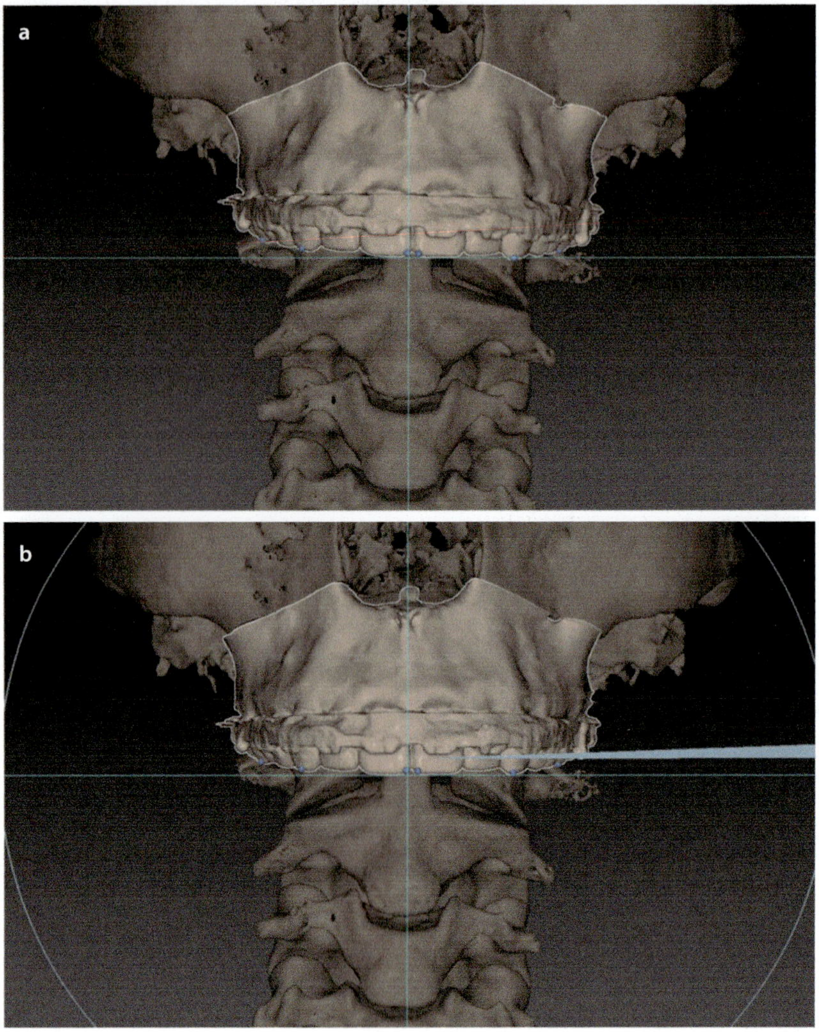

Fig. 6.288 The maxillary occlusal plane (**a**) is corrected towards the horizontal 3D PHP reference plane by a CCW "Roll" rotational movement (**b**) in patient V.E.W. (3D "surface-rendered" representations, IPS CaseDesigner v 1.1.3.1)

Case 8: 3D-VPS$_5$ Step 2 Upper Dental Midline Evaluation/Correction

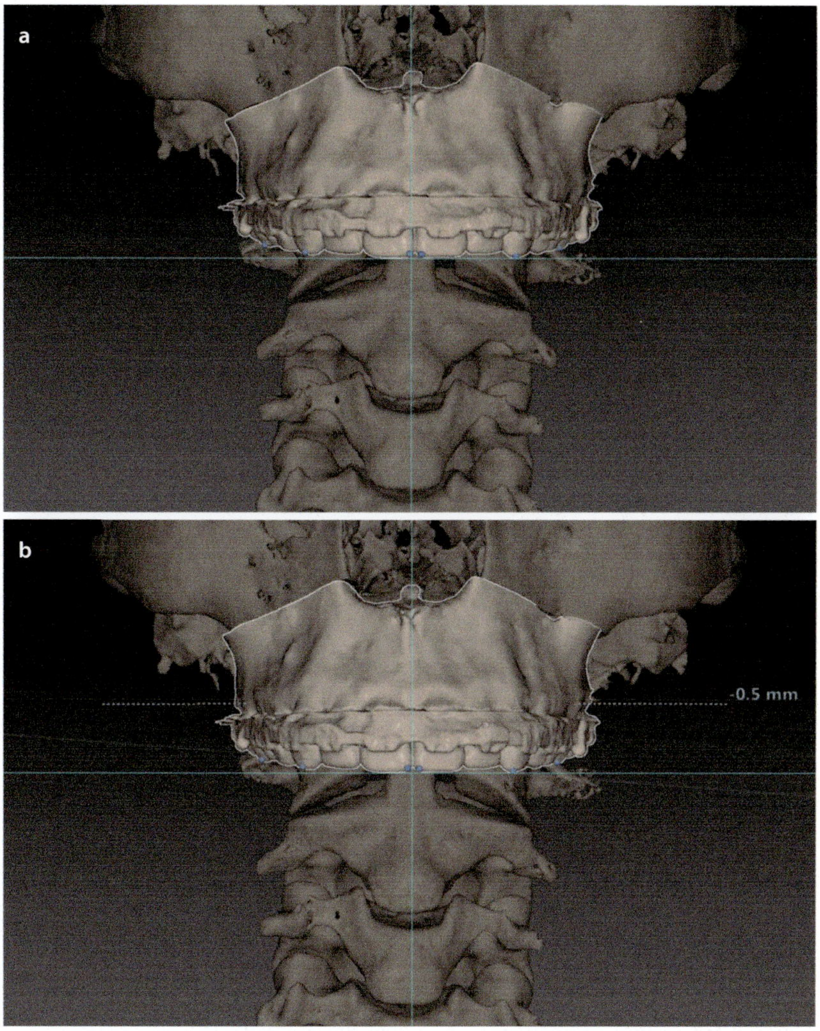

Fig. 6.289 The deviation of the upper dental midline to the left (**a**) is corrected towards the facial midline 3D PHP reference plane, by a pure translational movement to the right (**b**) in patient V.E.W. (3D "surface-rendered" representations, IPS CaseDesigner v 1.1.3.1)

Case 8: 3D-VPS$_5$ Step 2 Upper Dental Midline Evaluation/Correction

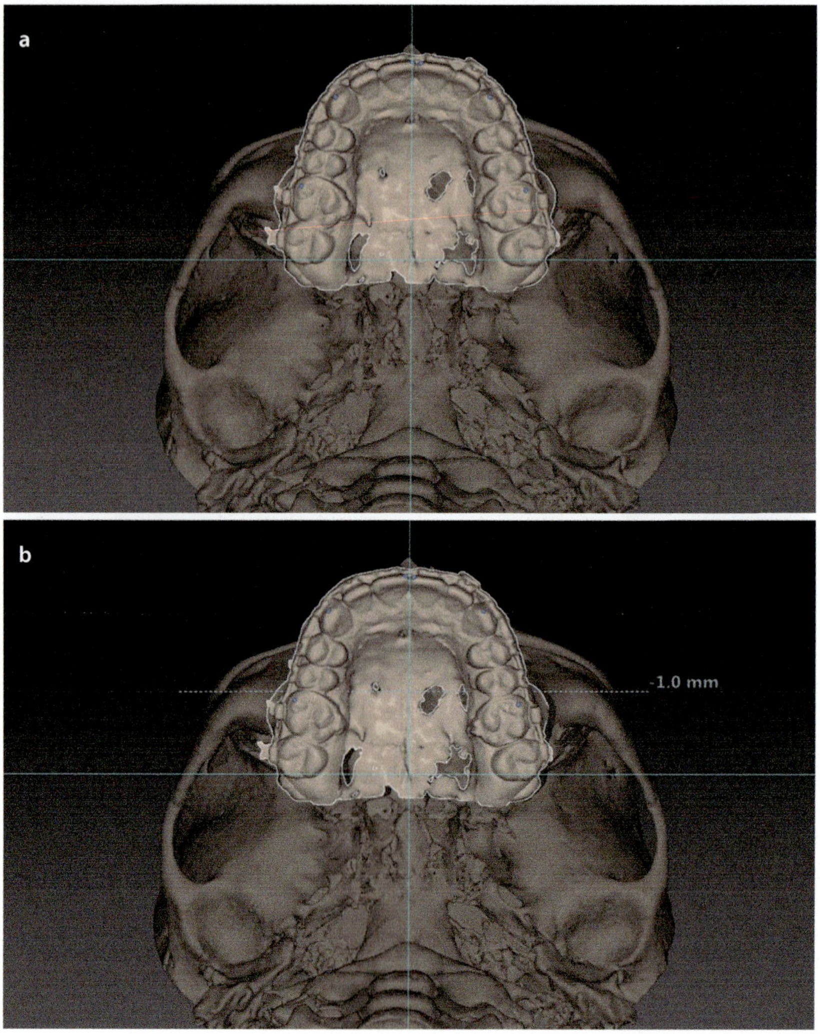

Fig. 6.290 The base views illustrate that the deviation of the upper dental midline to the left (**a**) is corrected towards the facial midline 3D PHP reference plane, by a pure translational movement to the right (**b**) (3D "surface-rendered" representations, patient V.E.W., IPS CaseDesigner v 1.1.3.1)

Case 8: 3D-VPS$_5$ Step 3 Overall Evaluation of Facial Asymmetry After Virtual Occlusal Definition

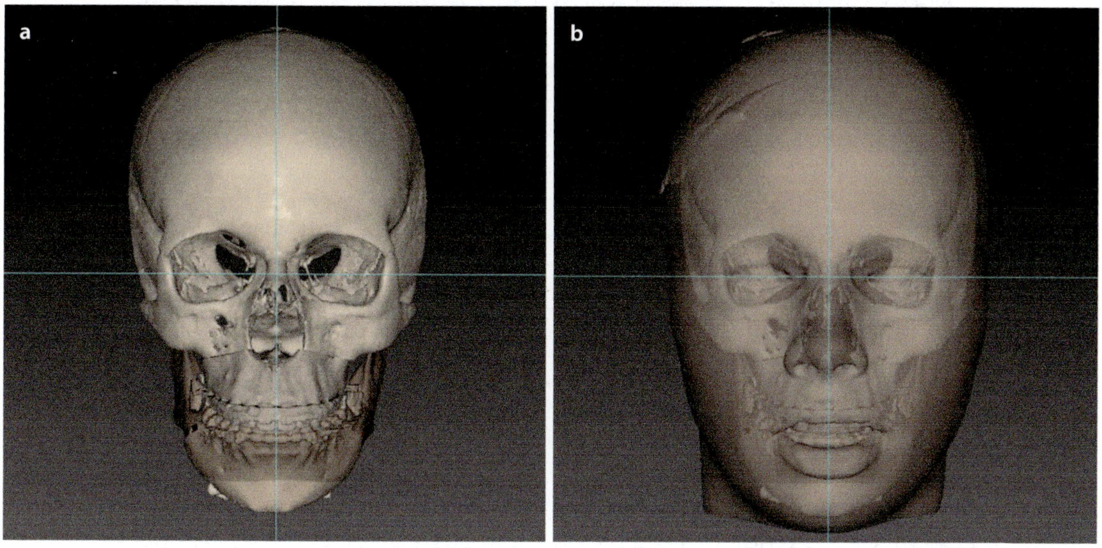

Fig. 6.291 Overall facial asymmetry of the skull of patient V.E.W. (**a**) with transparent soft tissues (**b**) is assessed after virtual occlusal definition in the frontal view towards both the horizontal and facial midline 3D PHP reference planes. (3D "surface-rendered" representations, IPS CaseDesigner v 1.1.3.1). Note the persistent chin deviation to the right

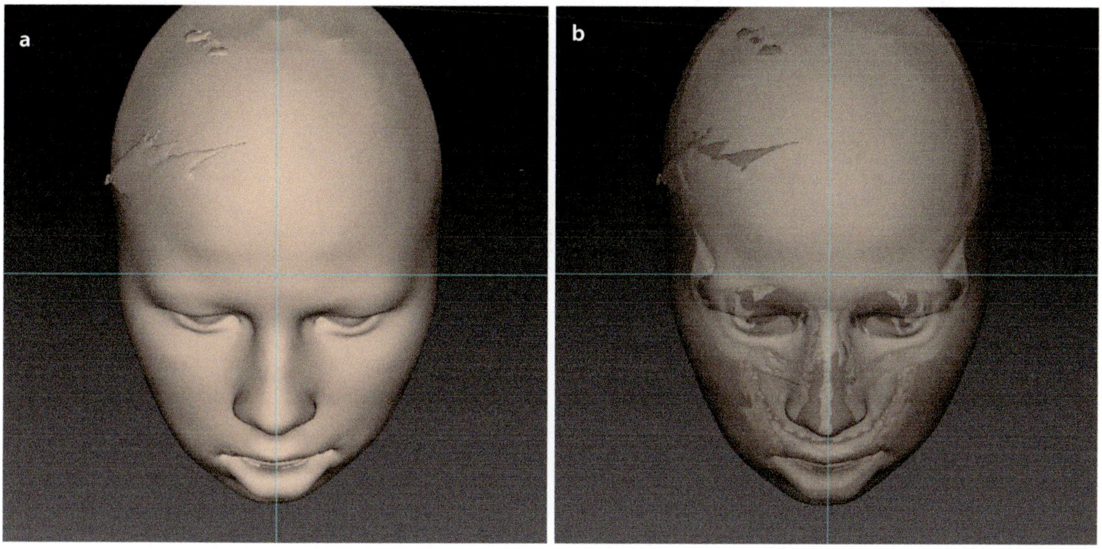

Fig. 6.292 To evaluate the overall facial asymmetry after virtual occlusal definition, the mandibular contour is evaluated both virtually on the soft tissues (**a**) and at the bony level towards the contour of the zygomatic bones and arches with soft tissues in transparency (**b**) (3D "surface-rendered" representations, patient V.E.W., IPS CaseDesigner v 1.1.3.1)

▪ Case 8: 3D-VPS$_5$ Step 4 Evaluation/Correction of Flaring ("Yaw")

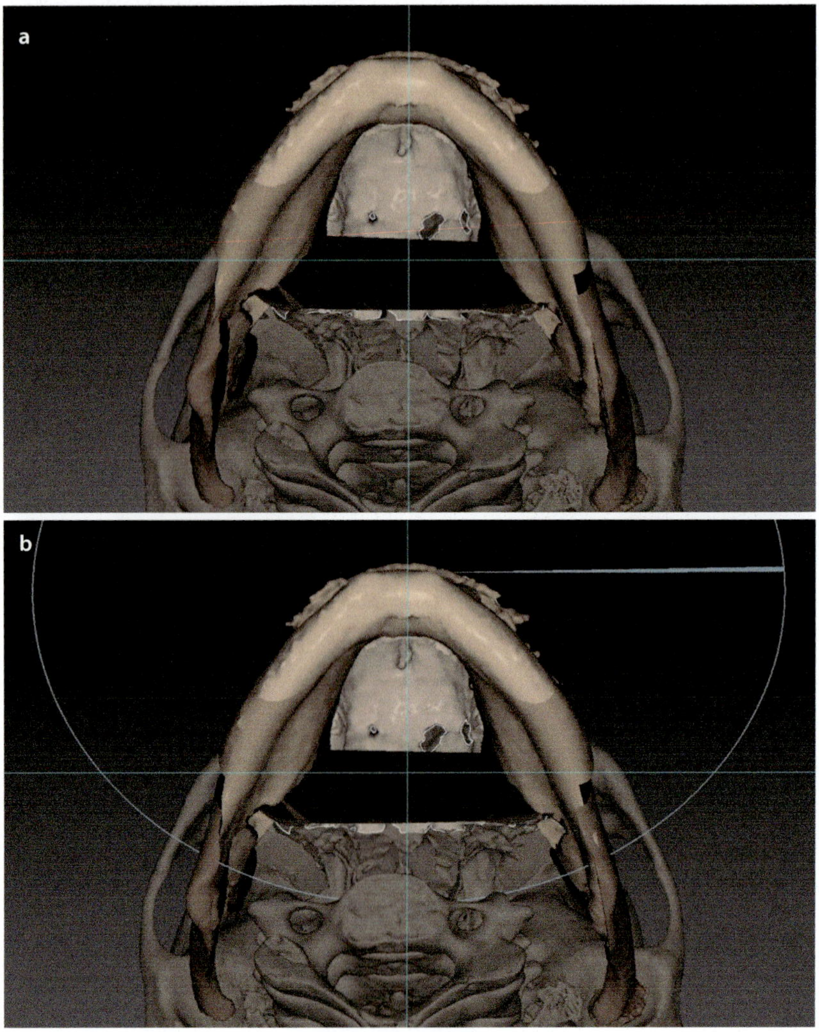

Fig. 6.293 The base views show that the flaring of the mandibular body to the right (**a**) is corrected by a CCW "Yaw" rotational movement to the left (**b**) (3D "surface-rendered" representations, patient V.E.W., IPS CaseDesigner v 1.1.3.1). Note the asymmetric bony overlaps between the distal and both proximal mandibular fragments

Case 8: 3D-VPS$_5$ Step 4 Evaluation/Correction of Flaring ("Yaw")

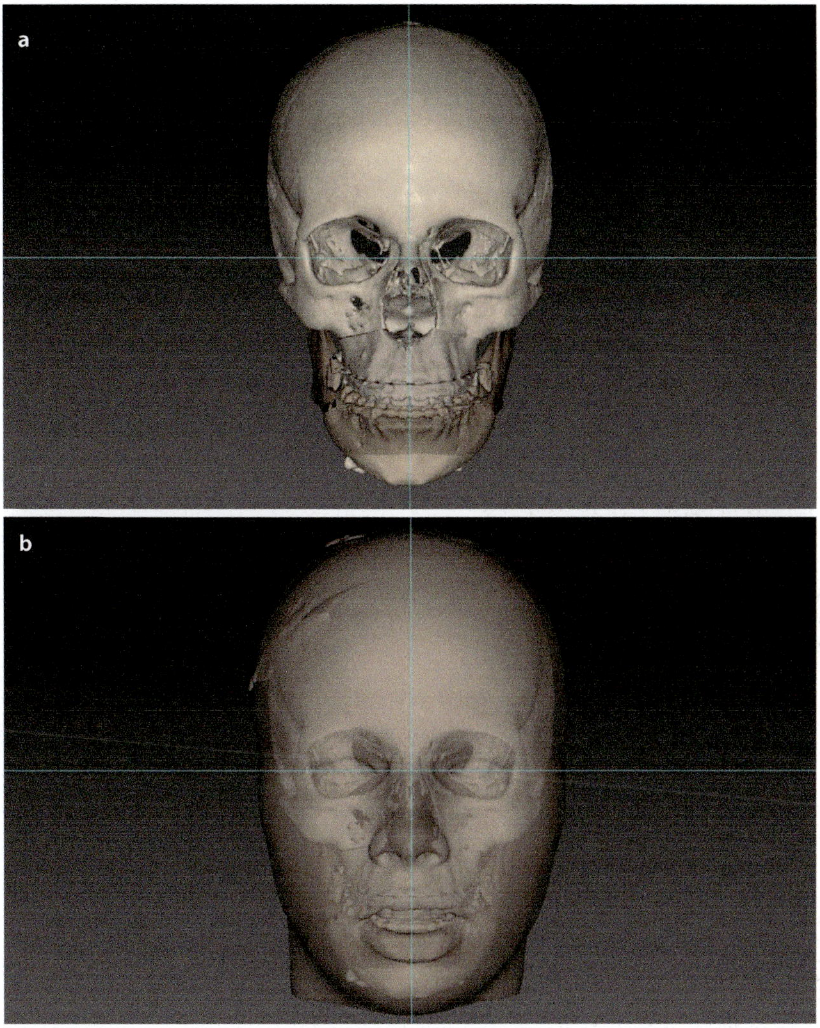

Fig. 6.294 Overall assessment of the facial bony contour of patient V.E.W. (**a**) with transparent soft tissues (**b**) after correction of flaring to the right by a "Yaw" rotational movement of the maxillo-mandibular complex to the left (3D "surface-rendered" representations, IPS CaseDesigner v 1.1.3.1)

Case 8: 3D-VPS$_5$ Step 5 Upper Vertical Incisal Position Evaluation/Correction

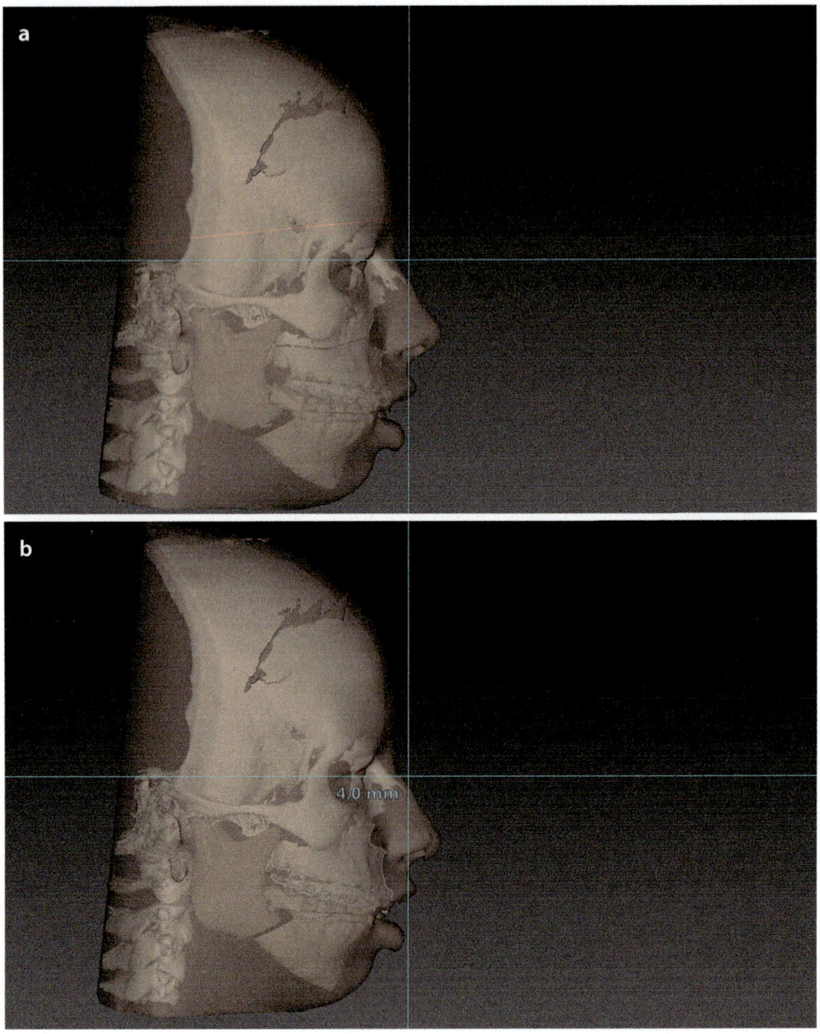

Fig. 6.295 Since patient V.E.W. has an upper incisal exposure in rest of 8 mm and a gingival exposure of 4 mm, it was decided clinically at this stage to virtually intrude the maxilla 4 mm at the upper incisal level. Note the current limit of 3D soft tissue simulation: despite a vertical incisal intrusion of 4 mm, there is no change in lip morphology and interlabial distance (3D "surface-rendered" representations, patient V.E.W., Maxilim v. 2.3.0.3): before (**a**) and after (**b**) correction

■ Case 8: 3D-VPS$_5$ Step 6 Sagittal Upper Incisal Position Evaluation/Correction

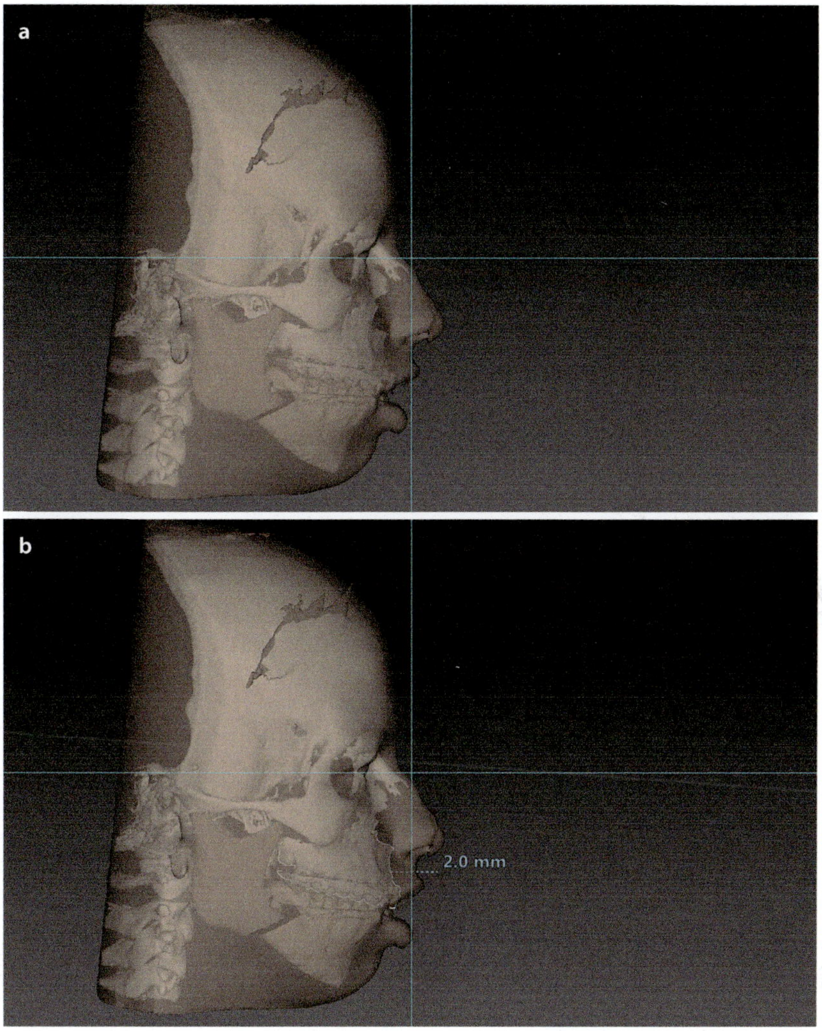

Fig. 6.296 From especially clinical examination but also 3D cephalometric analysis, it was decided to advance the "maxillo-mandibular complex in final occlusion" 2 mm at the upper incisal level in patient V.E.W. (3D "surface-rendered" representations, patient V.E.W., Maxilim v. 2.3.0.3): before (**a**) and after (**b**) correction

Case 8: 3D-VPS$_5$ Step 7 Profile Evaluation/Occlusal Plane Correction ("Pitch")

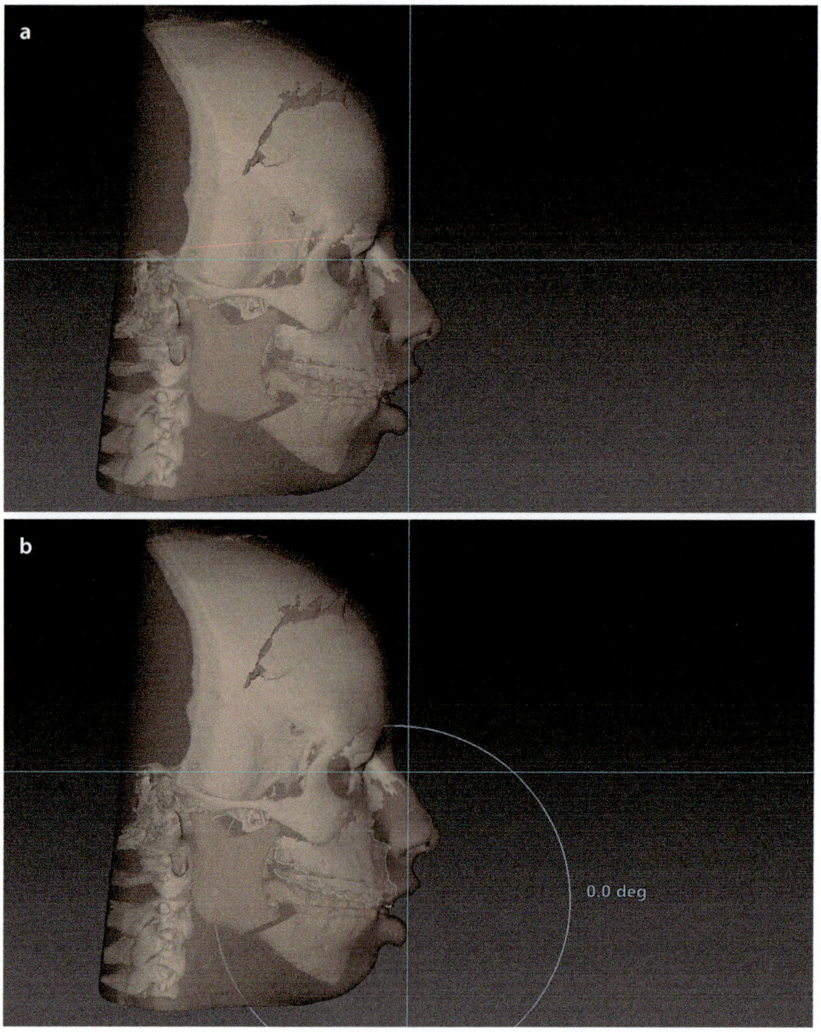

Fig. 6.297 At this stage in "step 7", the profile and dento-alveolar support of the upper lip are evaluated (**a**) (3D "surface-rendered" representations, IPS CaseDesigner v 1.1.3.1). At this stage, it was clinically decided not to alter the occlusal plane and therefore no "Pitch" movement was performed in patient V.E.W. (**b**)

▪ Case 8: 3D-VPS$_5$ Step 8 3D Chin Position Evaluation/Correction

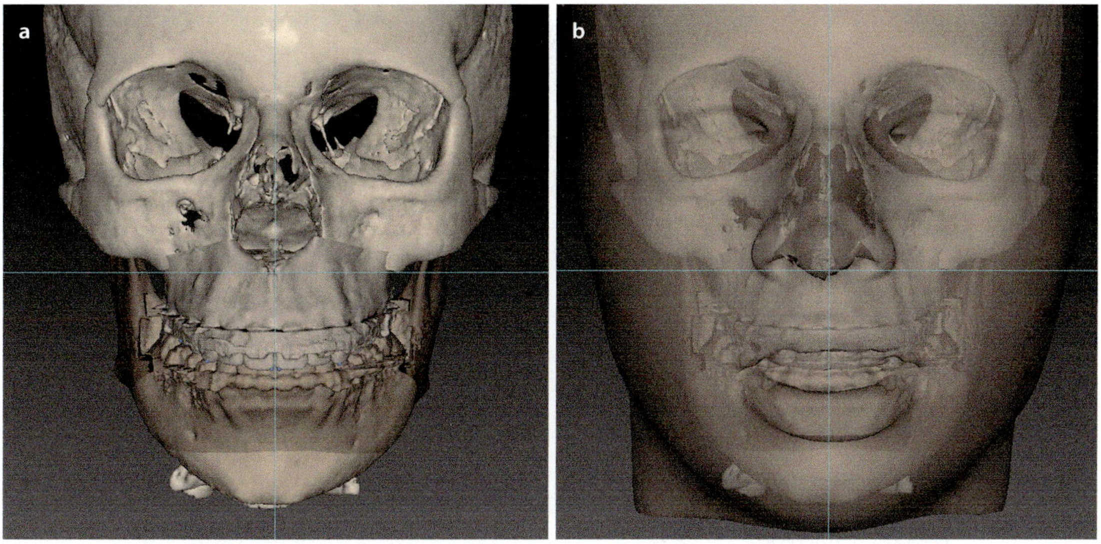

Fig. 6.298 Evaluation of the chin position in the frontal plane without (**a**) and with (**b**) the patient's 3D facial soft tissue mask in transparency (3D "surface-rendered" representations, IPS CaseDesigner v 1.1.3.1). Note the persistent cant of the mandibular symphysis and chin point deviation to the right

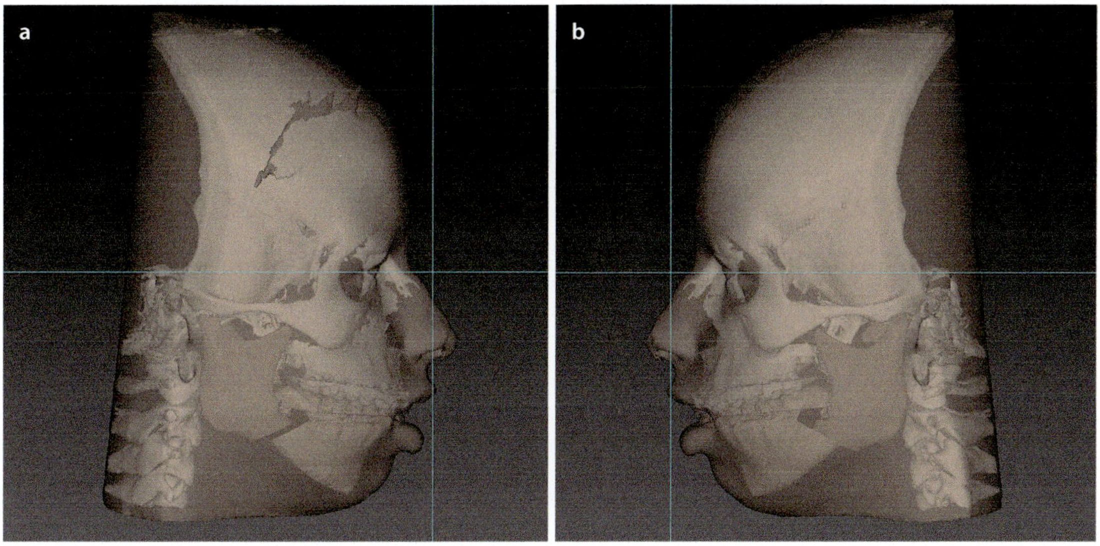

Fig. 6.299 Evaluation of the sagittal chin position in the right (**a**) and left profile (**b**) views needs to be individually assessed (3D "surface-rendered" representations, IPS CaseDesigner v 1.1.3.1). Note the retruded chin with the absence of a well-defined plica labio-mentalis

▪ Case 8: 3D-VPS$_5$ Step 8 3D Chin Position Evaluation/Correction

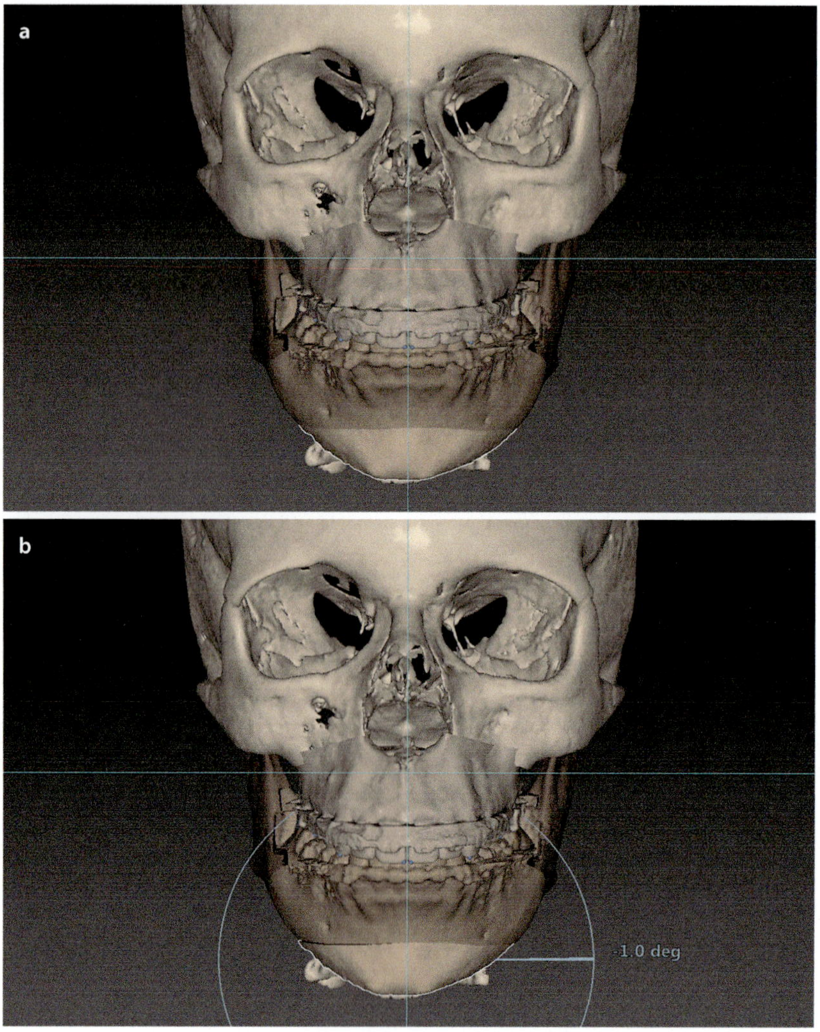

Fig. 6.300 After assessment in the frontal plane (**a**), a 1° CCW "Roll" movement (**b**) of the chin was virtually planned in patient V.E.W. to correct the slight cant (3D "surface-rendered" representations, IPS CaseDesigner v 1.1.3.1)

Case 8: 3D-VPS$_5$ Step 8 3D Chin Position Evaluation/Correction

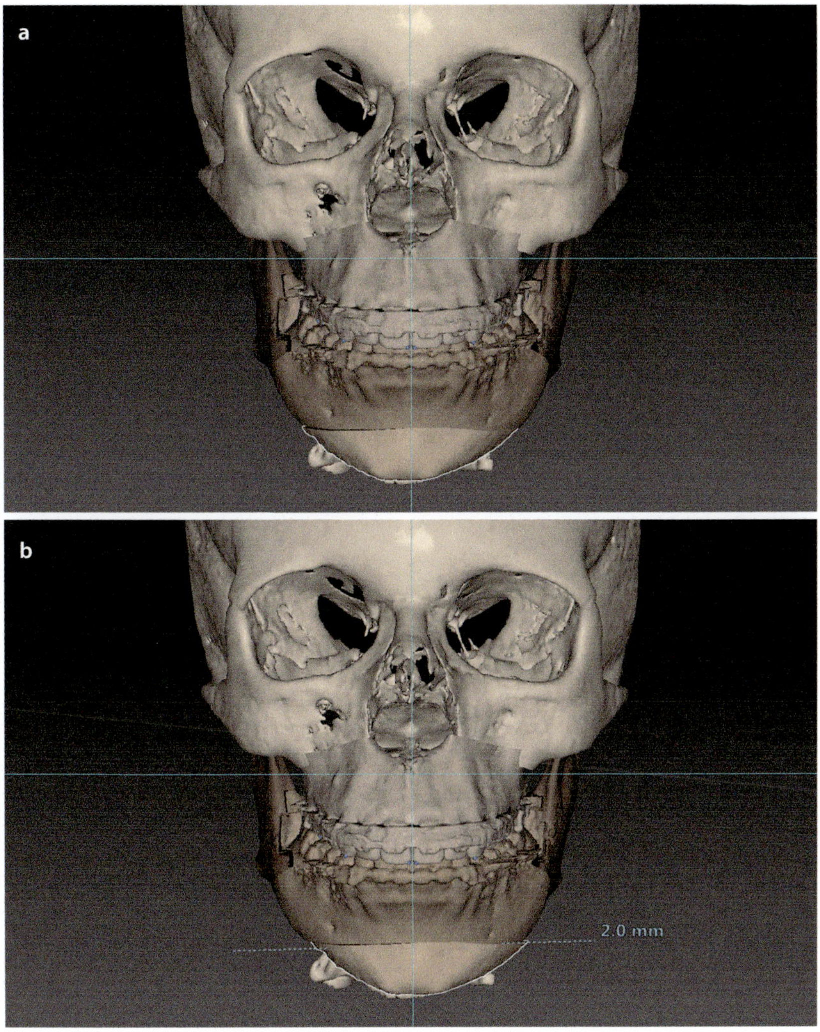

Fig. 6.301 Additionally, in the frontal plane (**a**), a midline correction of 2 mm to the left (**b**) was virtually planned to correct the mandibular symphysis deviation in patient V.E.W. (3D "surface-rendered" representations, IPS CaseDesigner v 1.1.3.1)

Case 8: 3D-VPS$_5$ Step 8 3D Chin Position Evaluation/Correction

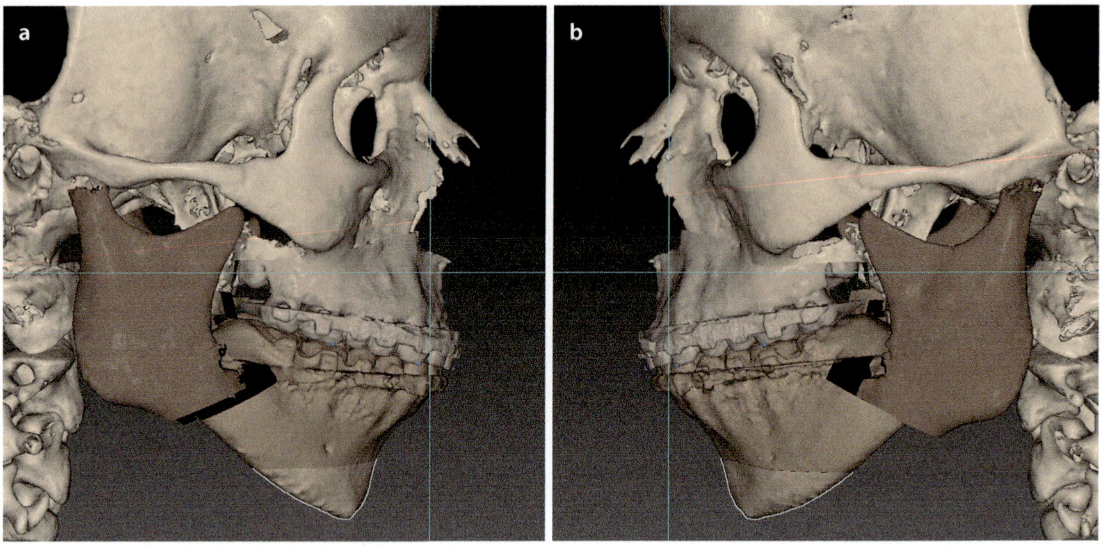

Fig. 6.302 The sagittal position of the bony chin is evaluated in the right (**a**) and left profile (**b**) views in patient V.E.W. (3D "surface-rendered" representations, IPS CaseDesigner v 1.1.3.1)

Case 8: 3D-VPS$_5$ Step 8 3D Chin Position Evaluation/Correction

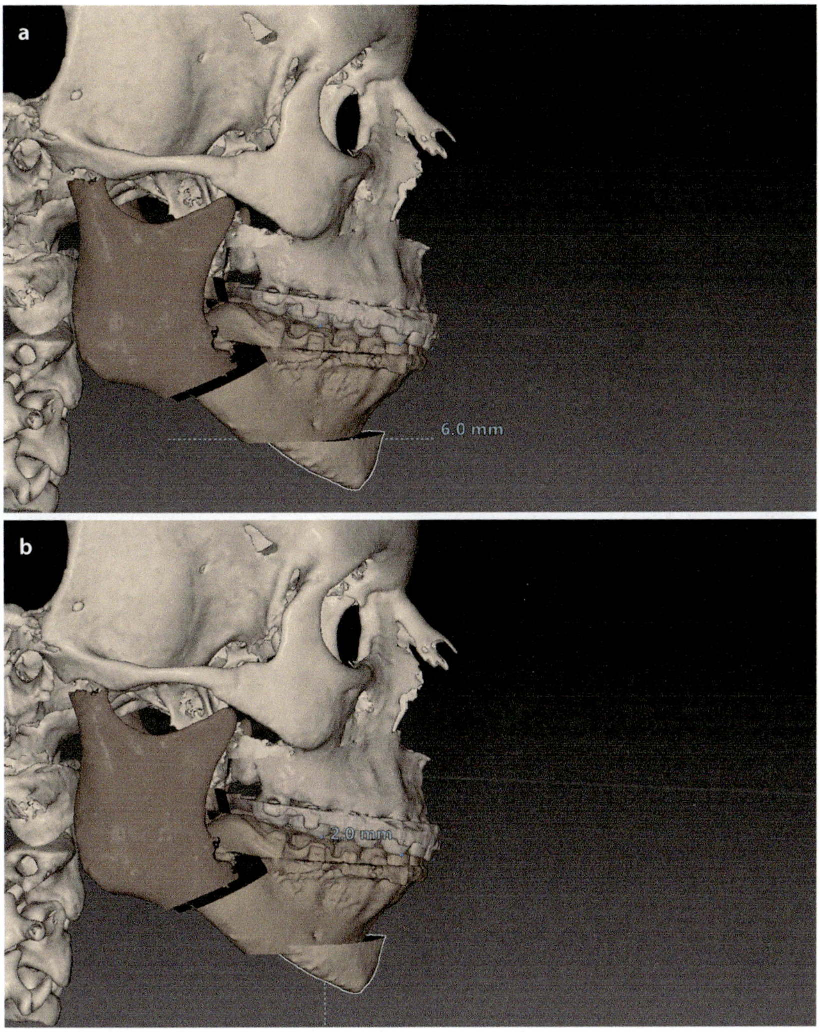

Fig. 6.303 The right profile views show that a chin advancement of 6 mm (**a**) with 2 mm anterior and 1 mm posterior intrusion at the right (**b**) was virtually planned in patient V.E.W. (3D "surface-rendered" representations, IPS CaseDesigner v 1.1.3.1)

Case 8: 3D-VPS$_5$ Step 8 3D Chin Position Evaluation/Correction

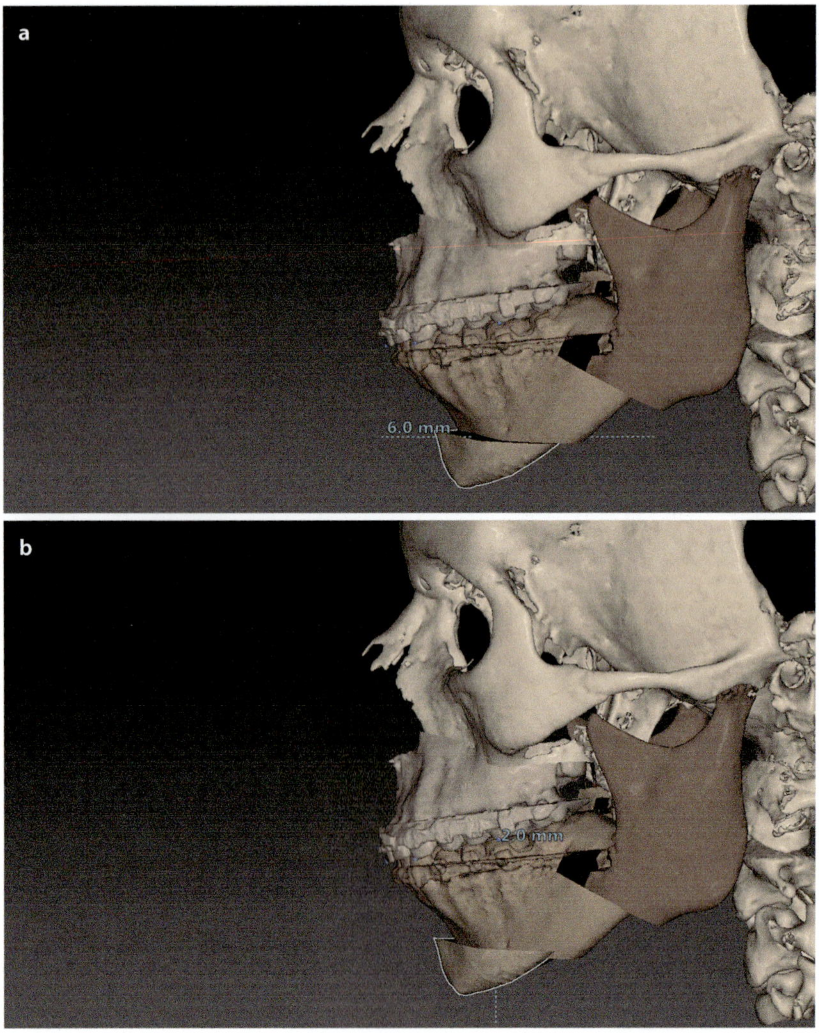

Fig. 6.304 The left profile views show that a chin advancement of 6 mm (**a**) with 2 mm anterior and 2.5 mm posterior intrusion (**b**) at the left was virtually planned in patient V.E.W. (3D "surface-rendered" representations, IPS CaseDesigner v 1.1.3.1)

Case 8: 3D-VPS$_5$ Step 8 3D Chin Position Evaluation/Correction

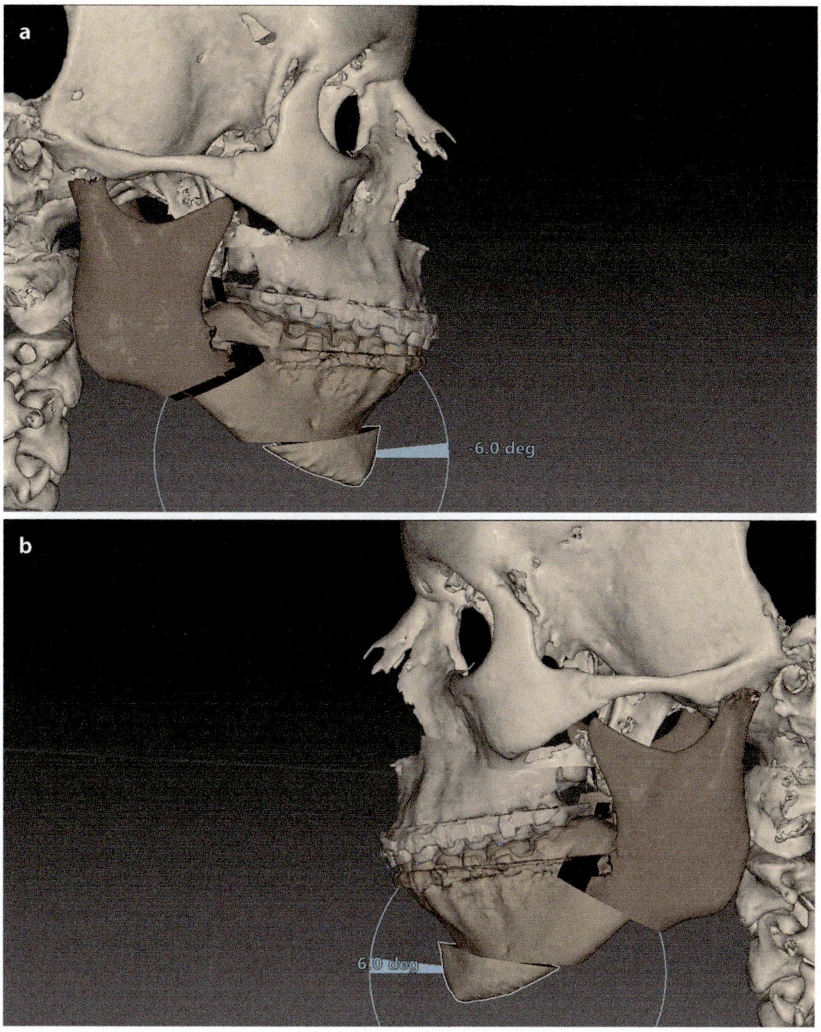

Fig. 6.305 The right (**a**) and left (**b**) profile views show that a 6° CCW "Pitch" rotational movement of the chin was virtually planned in patient V.E.W. to better align the bony segments at the inferior mandibular border level (3D "surface-rendered" representations, IPS CaseDesigner v 1.1.3.1)

Case 8: 3D-VPS$_5$ Step 8 3D Chin Position Evaluation/Correction

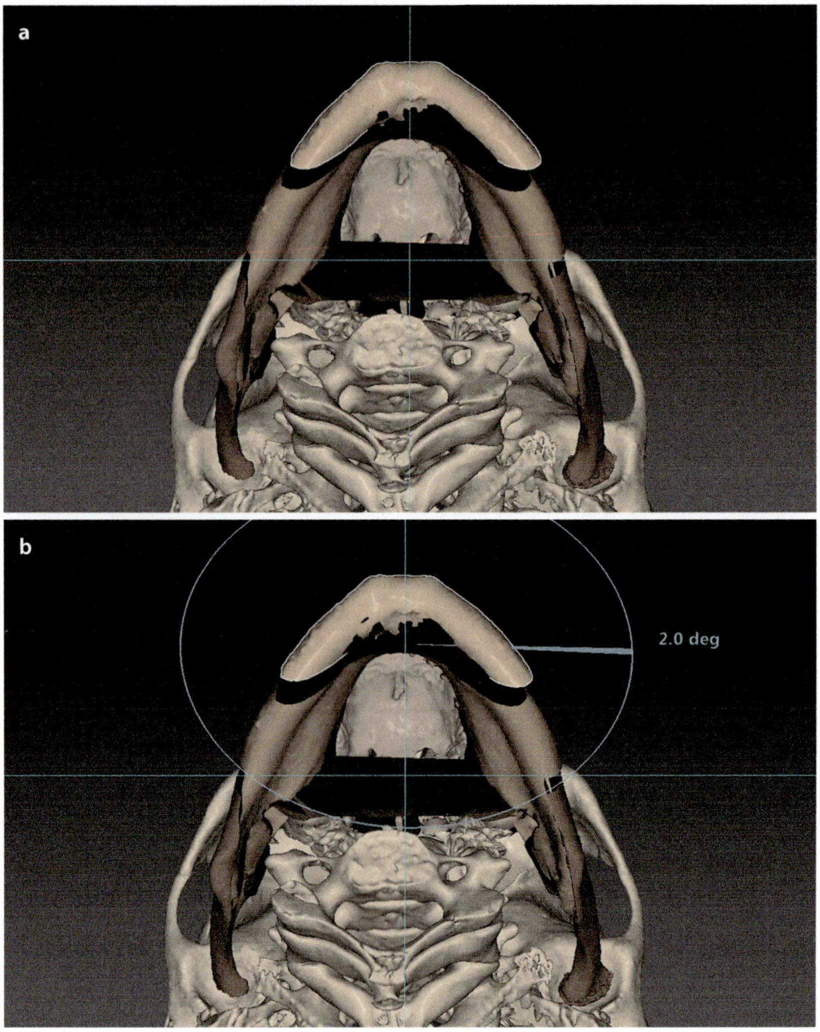

Fig. 6.306 The base views (**a**) show that additionally a 2° CW "Yaw" rotational movement (**b**) of the chin was virtually planned in patient V.E.W. (3D "surface-rendered" representations, IPS CaseDesigner v 1.1.3.1)

Case 8: 3D-VPS$_5$ Step 9 Patient Communication of the Individualised Treatment Plan

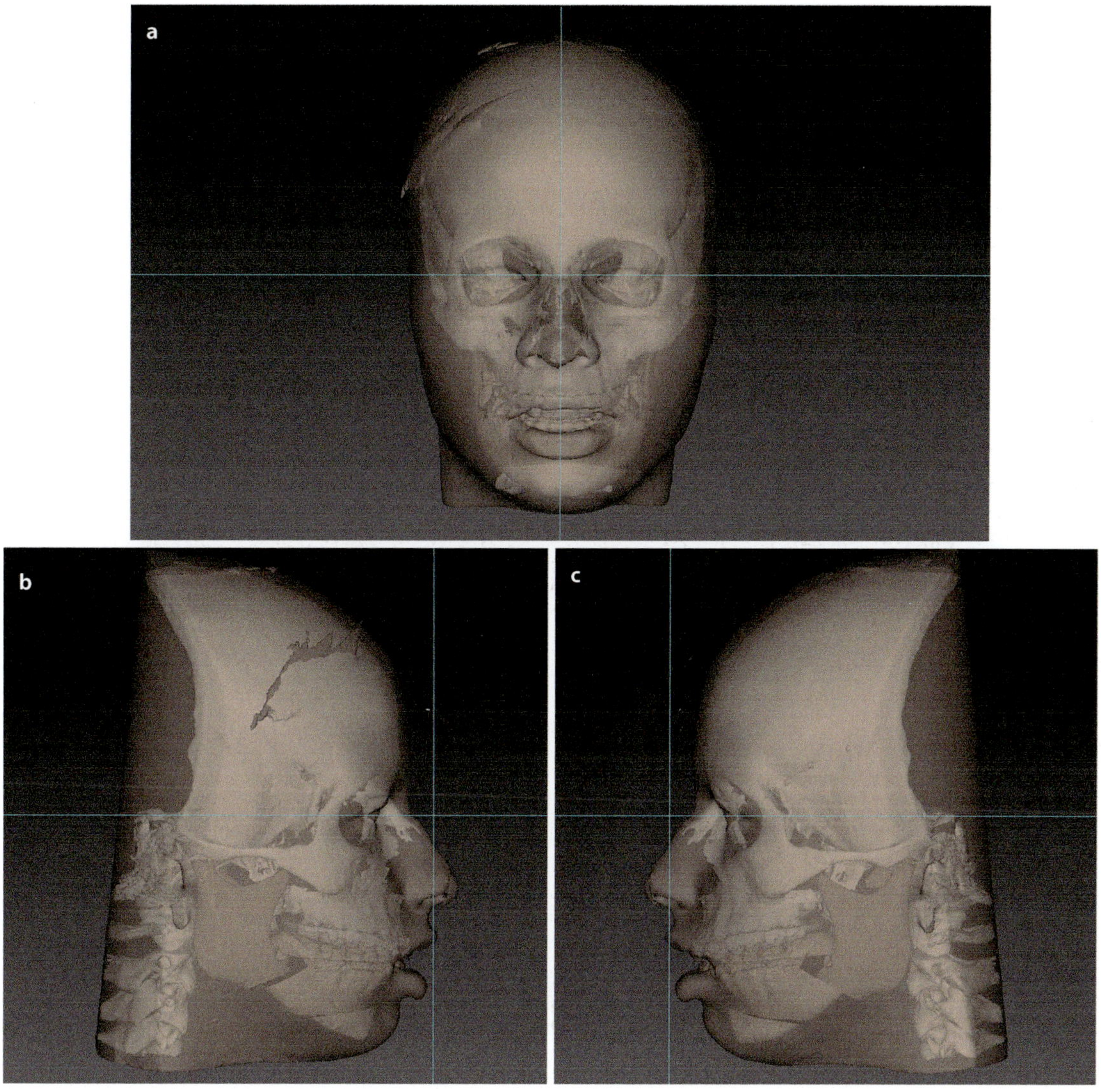

Fig. 6.307 Frontal (**a**), profile right (**b**) and left (**c**) views of the "Individualised 3D Virtual Treatment Plan", as presented to patient V.E.W., before the actual surgery (3D "surface-rendered" representations, IPS CaseDesigner v 1.1.3.1). Note the current limit of 3D soft tissue simulation at the level of the lips

▪ Case 8: 3D-VPS$_5$ Step 10 Final Adjustments of the 3D Virtual Treatment Plan

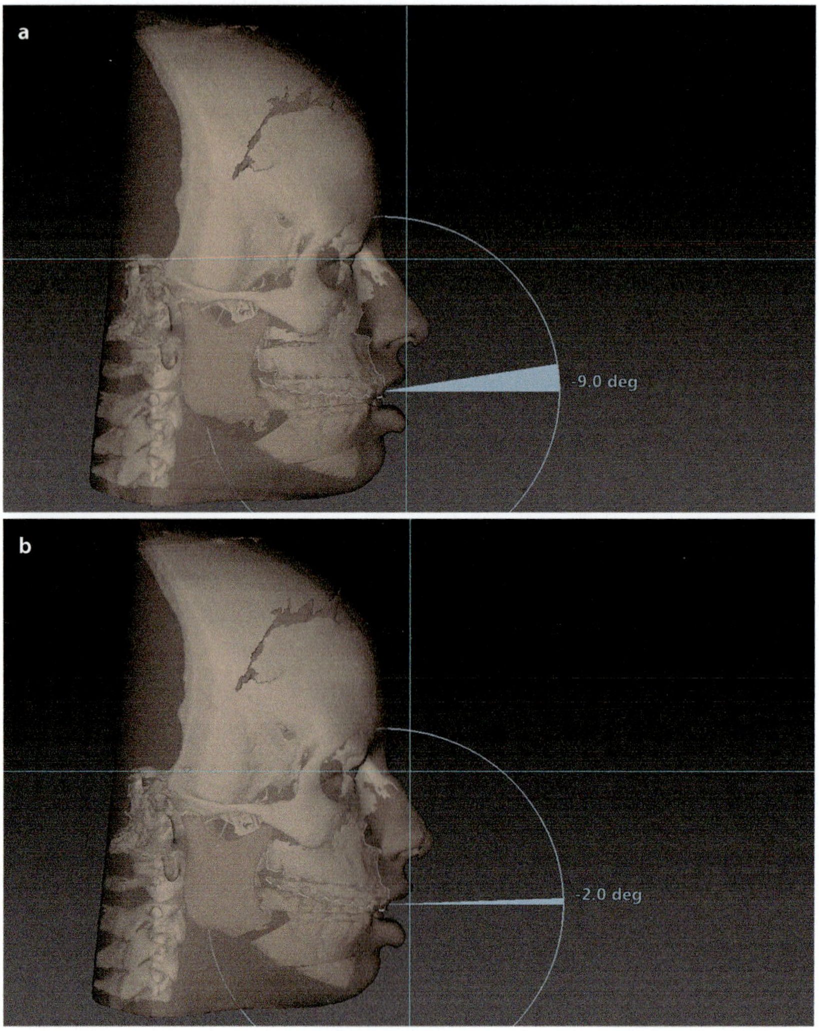

Fig. 6.308 Right profile views show potential adjustments of the "Individualised 3D Virtual Treatment Plan" consisting of more CCW "Pitch" movement of the "maxillo-mandibular complex", to provide more chin advancement: 9° (**a**) (3D "surface-rendered" representations, IPS CaseDesigner v 1.1.3.1). Finally it was decided after patient communication to perform an additional 2° CCW "Pitch" rotation of the "maxillo-mandibular complex" (**b**)

Case 8: 3D-VPS$_5$ Step 10 Final Adjustments of the 3D Virtual Treatment Plan

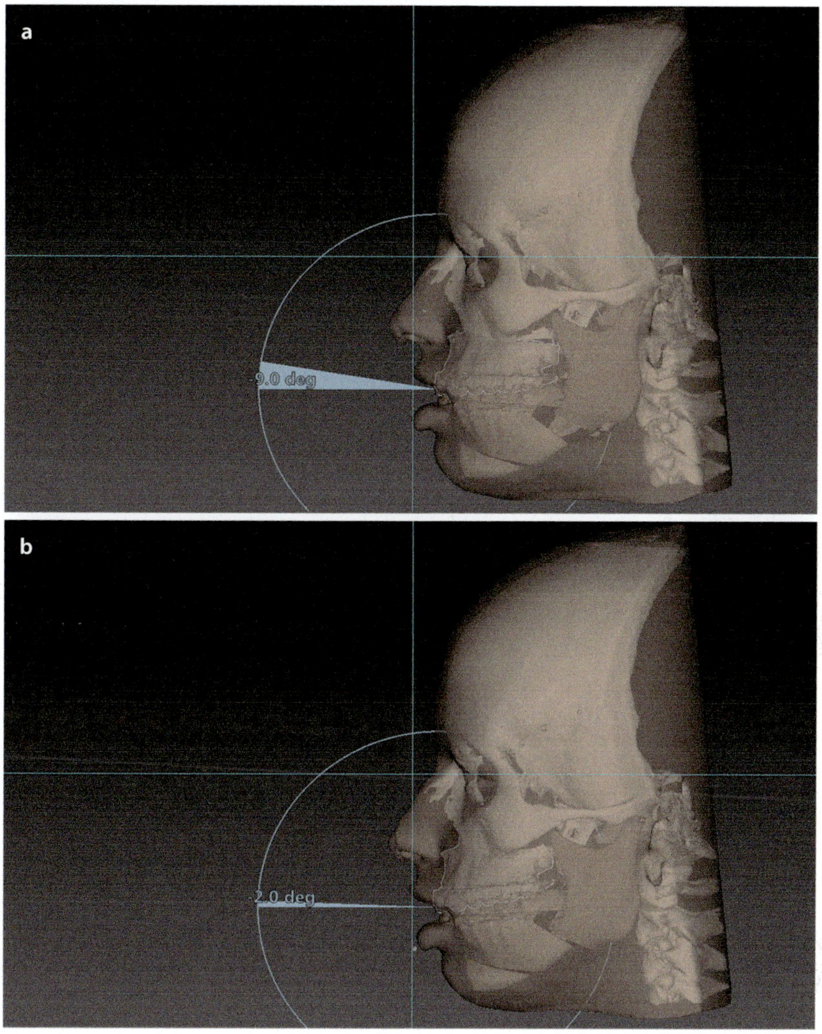

Fig. 6.309 Left profile views show potential adjustments of the "Individualised 3D Virtual Treatment Plan" consisting of more CCW "Pitch" movement of the "maxillo-mandibular complex", to provide more chin advancement: 9° (**a**) (3D "surface-rendered" representations, IPS CaseDesigner v 1.1.3.1). Finally it was decided after patient communication to perform an additional 2° CCW "Pitch" rotation of the "maxillo-mandibular complex" (**b**)

▪ Case 8: 3D-VPS$_5$- Final integrated "Individualised 3D Virtual Treatment Plan"

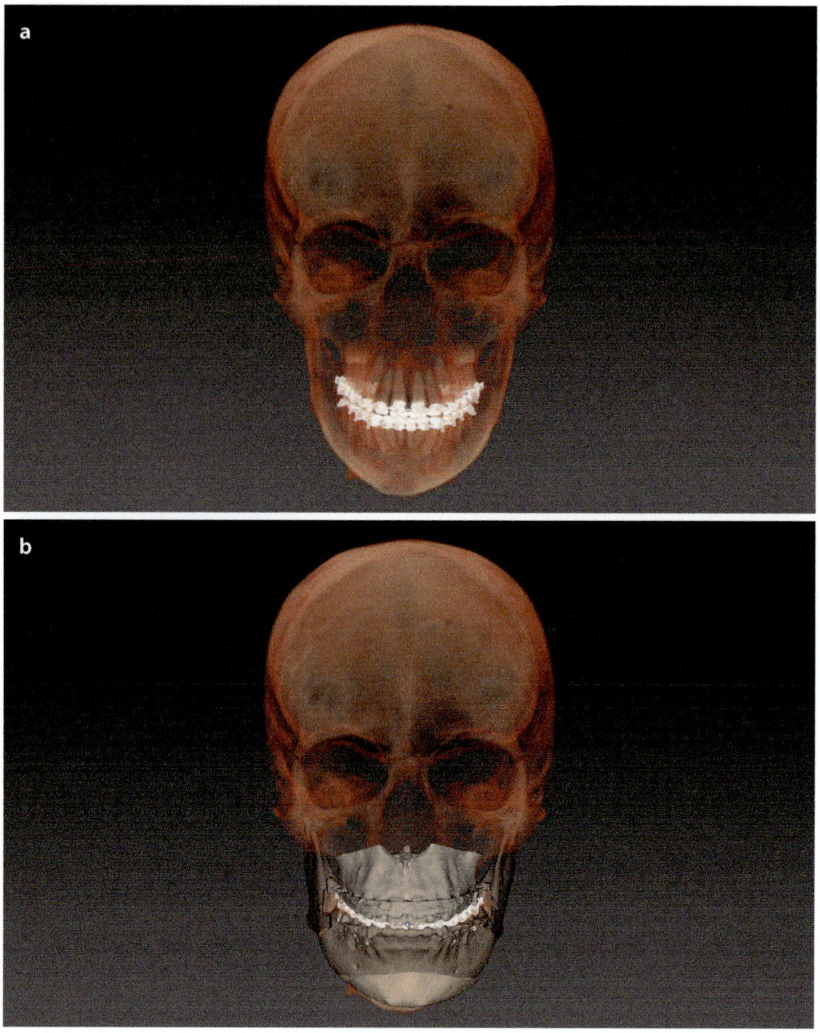

Fig. 6.310 Initial situation (**a**), and final "Individualised 3D Virtual Treatment Plan" (**b**), of patient V.E.W. in the frontal plane (3D combined "volume- and surface-rendered" hard tissue representations, IPS CaseDesigner v 1.1.3.1)

Case 8: 3D-VPS$_5$- Final Integrated "Individualised 3D Virtual Treatment Plan"

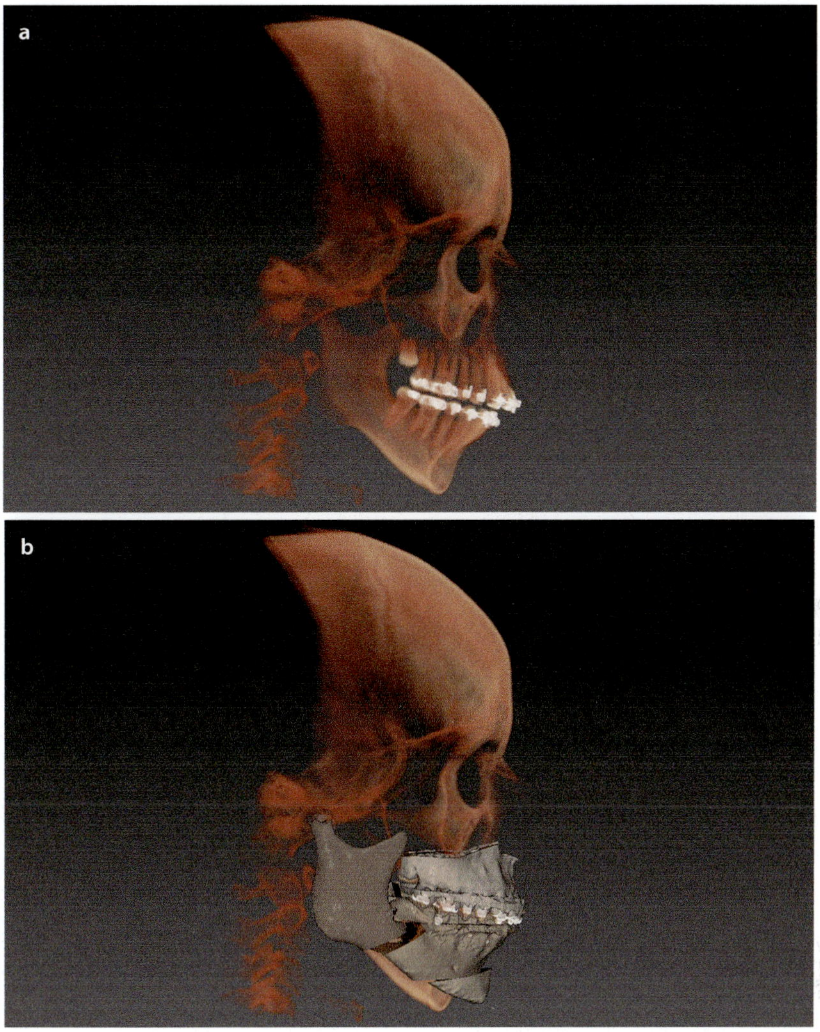

Fig. 6.311 Initial situation (**a**), and final "Individualised 3D Virtual Treatment Plan" (**b**), of patient V.E.W. in the right profile plane (3D combined "volume- and surface-rendered" hard tissue representations, IPS CaseDesigner v 1.1.3.1)

Case 8: 3D-VPS$_5$- Final Integrated "Individualised 3D Virtual Treatment Plan"

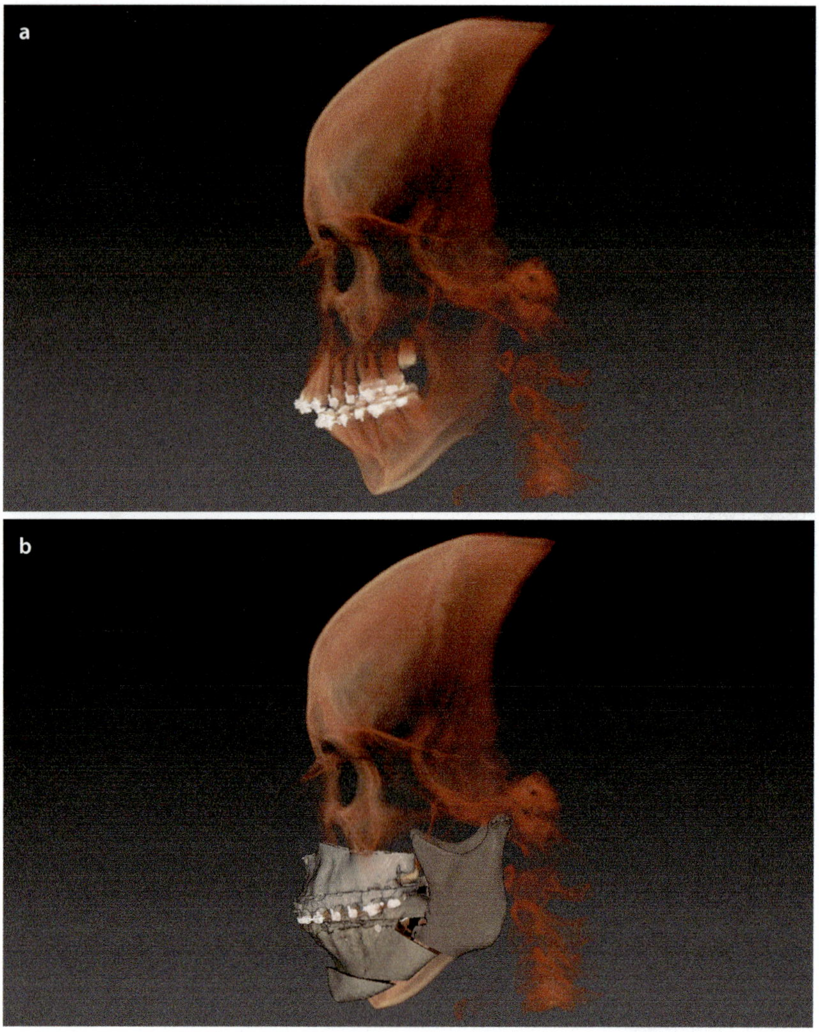

Fig. 6.312 Initial situation (**a**), and final "Individualised 3D Virtual Treatment Plan" (**b**), of patient V.E.W. in the left profile plane (3D combined "volume- and surface-rendered" hard tissue representations, IPS CaseDesigner v 1.1.3.1)

Case 8: 3D-VPS$_5$- Final Integrated "Individualised 3D Virtual Treatment Plan"

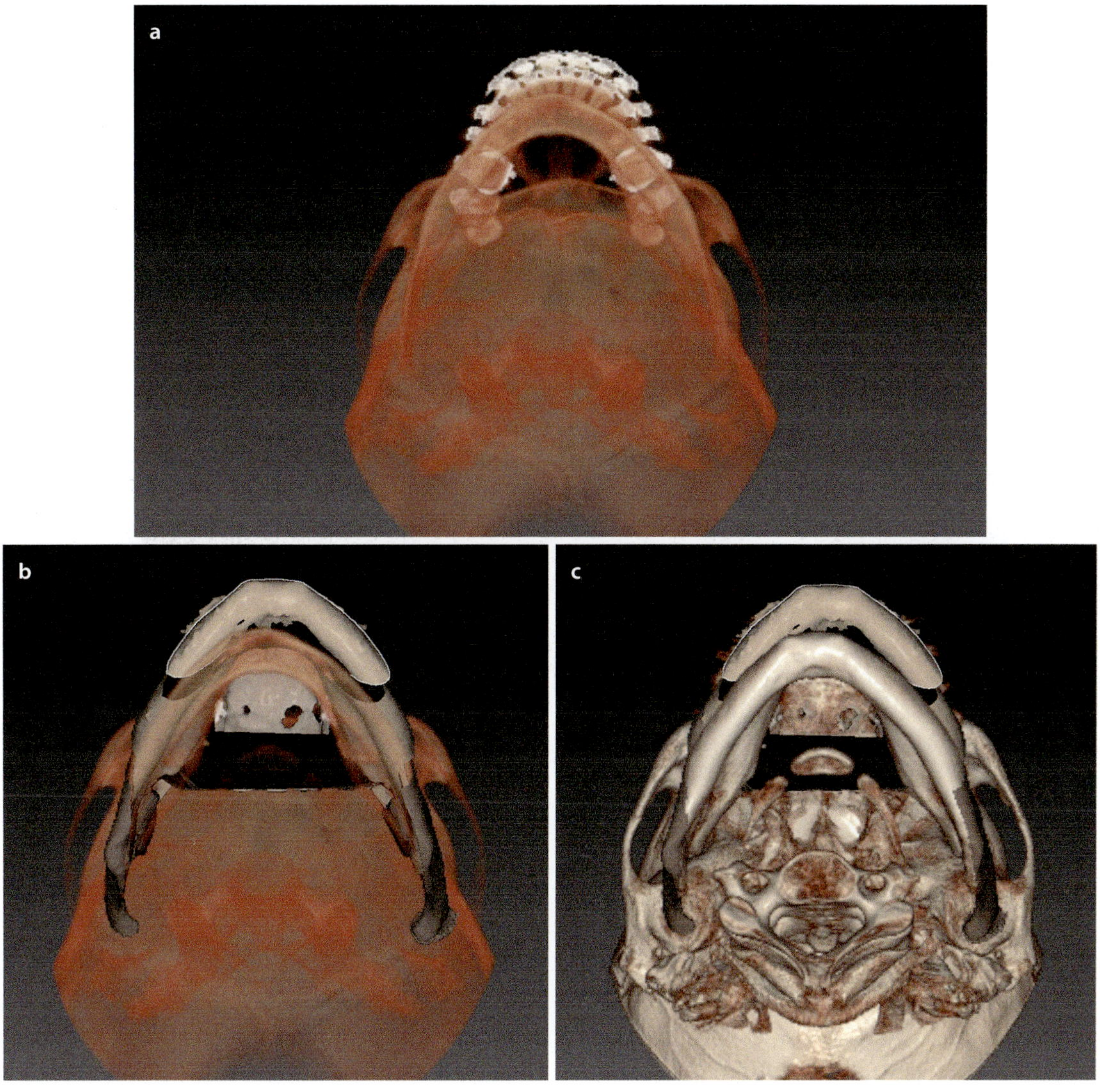

Fig. 6.313 Initial situation (**a**), and final "Individualised 3D Virtual Treatment Plan" (**b**, **c**), of patient V.E.W. in the base plane (3D combined "volume- and surface-rendered" hard tissue representations, IPS CaseDesigner v 1.1.3.1)

■ Case 8: IPS CaseDesigner "3D Virtual Treatment Planning, OR" Template

Maxillary osteotomy

- ■ Le Fort: ■I ☐II ☐III
- ■ One-piece
- ☐ Segmental:
  - Pieces: ....
  - Interdental: ....
- ■ Advancement: 2.0 mm
- ☐ Set-back : ....
- ■ Midline: 1.5 mm ■R ☐L
- ■ Midline after Le Fort 1: inbetween 31/41
- ■ Vertical: ( )
- ■ "Yaw" correction: CCW to the left
- ☐ Other: ....

Mandibular osteotomy

- ■ SSO ■R ■L
- ☐ Inverted-L ☐R ☐L
- ☐ VRO ☐R ☐L
- ■ Advancement: R 6.0 mm L 5.0 mm
- ☐ Set-back: R .... L ....
- ☐ CW "Pitch" rotation
- ■ CCW "Pitch" rotation
- ☐ Midline split
- ■ IAN course: R lingual L lingual
- ☐ Midline after BSSO: ....
- ☐ Other: ....

Chin osteotomy

- ■ Advancement: 6.0 mm
- ☐ Set-back: ....
- ■ Midline: 2.0 mm ☐R ■L
- ■ Intrusion:
  - ■ Anterior: 2.0 mm
  - ■ Posterior: R 1.0 L 2.5 mm
- ☐ Extrusion:
  - ☐ Anterior: ....
  - ☐ Posterior: R ...... L ......
- ☐ "Shield" osteotomy
- ☐ "Chin wing" osteotomy
  - *Mental Foramen level:*
    - ☐ Symmetric
    - ■ Asymmetric
- ■ Other: CCW "Roll" / CW "Yaw" rotation

Planning Requirements

- ■ Maxilla first
- ☐ Mandible first
- ☐ Minimally Invasive Le Fort I
- ☐ IO-CBCT
- ☐ Kobayashi wires : ....
- ☐ Skeletal anchorage : ....
- ☐ Orthodontic buttons : ....
- ☐ Occlusal grinding : ....
- ☐ Other : ....

16	13	11	23	26
↑ 2.5mm	↑ 3.5mm	↑ 4.5mm	↑ 4.5mm	↑ 3.5mm

"Roll" correction: ☐CW ■CCW

Miscellaneous

- ■ Para-nasal cross sutures
- ☐ Alar cinch
- ■ Septoplasty
- ■ Inferior turbinectomy
- ■ ANS: ■Shortening ■ Midline
- ■ Nasal base plasty ■R ■L
- ■ Lateral nasal wall plasty ■R ☐L
- ☐ Bone graft(s): ....
- ☐ Extraction(s): ....
- ☐ Other: ....

Adjuvant Cosmetic Procedures

- ☐ Bichatectomy ☐R ☐L
- ☐ Zygoma osteotomies ☐R ☐L
  - *Infraorbital Foramen level:*
    - ☐ Symmetric
    - ☐ Asymmetric
- ☐ Otoplasty: ☐R ☐L
- ■ Rhinoplasty: Closed
- ☐ Browlift: ....
- ☐ Blepharoplasty: ....
  - ☐Upper ☐Lower
- ☐ Facelift: ....
- ☐ Necklift: ....
- ☐ Liposuction: ....
- ☐ Lipofilling: ....
- ☐ Other: ....

Addendum Templates

G.R.J. Swennen (ed.), *3D Virtual Treatment Planning of Orthognathic Surgery*,
DOI 10.1007/978-3-662-47389-4

"3D Virtual Step-by-Step Quality Control Checklist" Template

(1) Verification of the overall Augmented Model (AUM) of the patient by the clinician

- ☐ Accuracy of Registration of the upper dental arch
- ☐ Accuracy of Registration of the lower dental arch

This is verified by evaluation of multiplanar orthogonal slices at molar, canine and incisal level and correlation with clinical photographs.

- ☐ Quality of the 3D rendering of the bone
- ☐ Quality of the 3D rendering of the soft tissues

....

(2) Verification of the condyle (CR) position in the AUM of the patient by the clinician

- ☐ Right condyle well seated in CR
- ☐ Left condyle well seated in CR

This is verified by evaluation of sagittal and coronal slices.

....

(3) Verification of the overall soft tissue quality of the AUM of the patient by the clinician

- ☐ Absence of eyebrow distortion (> fixation band during CBCT scanning)
- ☐ Absence of lip distortion (> wax bite)
- ☐ Lips in repose
- ☐ Mentalis muscle relaxed
- ☐ Absence of chin distortion (> chin support during CBCT scanning)

This is verified by correlation with clinical photographs and the clinical examination.

....

(4) Verification of the PHP of the patient by the clinician

- ☐ In the frontal plane towards the NHP*
- ☐ In the profile planes towards the TVP

This is verified by correlation with clinical photographs and the clinical examination.
* be always aware of the potential of a modified habitual NHP

....

(5) Verification of the final virtual occlusion by the clinician

- ☐ Dental midline
- ☐ Angle class I canine relationship
- ☐ Angle class I molar relationship
- ☐ Absence of "yaw" at molar level

....

"3D Virtual Treatment Planning: OR" Template

Maxillary osteotomy

- ☐ Le Fort: ☐ I ☐ II ☐ III
- ☐ One-piece
- ☐ Segmental:
  - Pieces:.........................
  - Interdental:....................
- ☐ Advancement: ....
- ☐ Set-back : ....
- ☐ Midline: .... ☐ R ☐ L
- ☐ Midline after Le Fort I: ....
- ☐ Vertical: (→)
- ☐ "Yaw" correction: ....
- ☐ Other: ....

Mandibular osteotomy

- ☐ SSO ☐ R ☐ L
- ☐ Inverted-L ☐ R ☐ L
- ☐ VRO ☐ R ☐ L
- ☐ Advancement: R .... L ....
- ☐ Set-back: R .... L ....
- ☐ CW "Pitch" rotation
- ☐ CCW "Pitch" rotation
- ☐ Midline split
- ☐ IAN course: R .... L ....
- ☐ Midline after BSSO: ....
- ☐ Other: ....

Chin osteotomy

- ☐ Advancement: ....
- ☐ Set-back: ....
- ☐ Midline: .... ☐ R ☐ L
- ☐ Intrusion:
  - ☐ Anterior: ....
  - ☐ Posterior: R ..... L .....
- ☐ Extrusion:
  - ☐ Anterior:...................
  - ☐ Posterior: R ..... L......
- ☐ "Shield" osteotomy
- ☐ "Chin wing" osteotomy
  - *Mental Foramen level:*
    - ☐ Symmetric
    - ☐ Asymmetric
- ☐ Other: ....

Planning Requirements

- ☐ Maxilla first
- ☐ Mandible first
- ☐ Minimally Invasive Le Fort I
- ☐ IO-CBCT
- ☐ Kobayashi wires: ....
- ☐ Skeletal anchorage: ....
- ☐ Orthodontic buttons: ....
- ☐ Occlusal grinding:......................
- ☐ Other: ....

____16____13____**11**____23____26____

"Roll" correction: ☐ CW ☐ CCW

Miscellaneous

- ☐ Para-nasal cross sutures
- ☐ Alar cinch
- ☐ Septoplasty
- ☐ Inferior turbinectomy
- ☐ ANS: ☐ Shortening ☐ Midline
- ☐ Nasal base plasty ☐ R ☐ L
- ☐ Lateral nasal wall plasty ☐ R ☐ L
- ☐ Bone graft(s): ....
- ☐ Extraction(s): ....
- ☐ Other: ....

Adjuvant Cosmetic Procedures

- ☐ Bichatectomy ☐ R ☐ L
- ☐ Zygoma osteotomies ☐ R ☐ L
  - *Infraorbital Foramen level:*
    - ☐ Symmetric
    - ☐ Asymmetric
- ☐ Otoplasty: ☐ R ☐ L
- ☐ Rhinoplasty: ....
- ☐ Browlift: ....
- ☐ Blepharoplasty: ....
  - ☐ Upper ☐ Lower
- ☐ Facelift: ....
- ☐ Necklift: ....
- ☐ Liposuction: ....
- ☐ Lipofilling: ....
- ☐ Other: ....

Definitions

Additive Manufacturing A group of production technologies to manufacture a 3D object by adding material (in contrast with milling, where material is being removed gradually). The process typically adds material layer by layer by a chemical reaction or sintering (also called rapid prototyping technology in the past).

Augmented Model (AUM) The patient's "surface-rendered" hard and/or soft tissue representations of the head, respectively, enhanced with detailed dental surfaces and/or texture and colour from other 3D image datasets.

Augmented Virtual Reality An innovative technology allowing co-registration of data from the real environment with virtual information, creating a hybrid world which is simultaneously visualised on a stereoscopic video display.

Euclidian Distance The straight-line distance between two points, defined as the square root of the sum of the squares of the differences between the corresponding coordinates of the points.

$$d(p,q) = \sqrt{(p_1 - q_1)^2 + (p_2 - q_2)^2 + (p_3 - q_3)^2}$$

Field of View (FOV) The scanned volume of the image dataset. In CT imaging the FOV is typically adjustable according to the area of interest; however for some CBCT apparatus, the FOV is fixed.

Iterative Closest Point (ICP) Algorithm The iterative closest point algorithm aligns two surfaces by minimising the root mean square (RMS) of the distances between the point clouds of the two surfaces.

Image Fusion The process of fusing data from two or more image datasets that were aligned using "Image Registration".

Image Registration The process of geometrically aligning image data from two or more image acquisitions.

Image Segmentation The process of partitioning a digital image into multiple data segments, for example, by thresholding.

Natural Head Position (NHP) The head orientation of the patient in a standing position with relaxed body and head posture looking at a distant point at eye level, perceived by the clinician based on general experience.

Clinical Natural Head Position (*c*-NHP) Natural head position of the subject, as recorded during the clinical examination.

Virtual Natural Head Position (*v*-NHP) Virtual modification of the scanned head position of the patient towards its *c*-NHP, which is defined by the clinician.

Pitch Rotational movement around the "x-axis" in the profile plane that can be performed CW or CCW.

Planning Head Position (PHP) At the onset of 3D virtual treatment planning, the *v*-NHP is set as the PHP of the patient, which defines the 3D PHP coordinate (Cartesian) reference frame.

Rendering The process of generating an image from a 2D or 3D dataset by visualisation algorithms.

Rigid Registration An algorithm that searches a rotation and translation which geometrically aligns the datasets. Different types of rigid registration exist: point-based, surface-based, voxel-based and surface to image (STI) registration.

Roll Rotational movement around the "z-axis" in the frontal plane that can be performed CW or CCW.

Stereolithography The process of making a 3D object, in which a computer-controlled moving laser beam is used to build up the required structure, layer by layer, from a liquid monomer that polymerises with laser light.

Surface Rendering The process of generating a view of a surface from a specific direction with specific lighting conditions. In medical visualisation of anatomical objects, this surface is typically generated by segmentation out of 3D image data (grey values).

Thresholding The process of defining a boundary between pixels or voxels with a value higher and lower than the threshold. When a 3D grey value image is segmented with thresholding, an isovalue surface is obtained, while with a 2D image, a contour is obtained.

Volume of Interest (VOI) An area or volume of particular interest to be imaged during the acquisition procedure or to be further analysed.

Volume Rendering A method to visualise a 3D image volume consisting of voxels by assigning to each voxel a colour and opacity and to further enhance the visualisation based on the variations in the image volume.

Yaw Rotational movement around the "y-axis" in the base or frontal plane that can be performed CW or CCW, but sometimes more simply described to the right or to the left.

Index

G.R.J. Swennen (ed.), *3D Virtual Treatment Planning of Orthognathic Surgery*,
DOI 10.1007/978-3-662-47389-4

U

V

Printed by Printforce, the Netherlands